ANTIOXIDANTS AND CARDIOVASCULAR DISEASE

SECOND EDITION

Developments in Cardiovascular Medicine

232. A. Bayés de Luna, F. Furlanello, B.J. Maron and D.P. Zipes (eds.):
     Arrhythmias and Sudden Death in Athletes. 2000   ISBN: 0-7923-6337-X
233. J-C. Tardif and M.G. Bourassa (eds): *Antioxidants and Cardiovascular Disease.*
     2000.   ISBN: 0-7923-7829-6
234. J. Candell-Riera, J. Castell-Conesa, S. Aguadé Bruiz (eds): *Myocardium at*
     Risk and Viable Myocardium Evaluation by SPET. 2000.ISBN: 0-7923-6724-3
235. M.H. Ellestad and E. Amsterdam (eds): Exercise Testing: New Concepts for the
     New Century. 2001.   ISBN: 0-7923-7378-2
236. Douglas L. Mann (ed.): The Role of Inflammatory Mediators in the Failing
     Heart. 2001   ISBN: 0-7923-7381-2
237. Donald M. Bers (ed.): Excitation-Contraction Coupling and Cardiac
     Contractile Force, Second Edition. 2001   ISBN: 0-7923-7157-7
238. Brian D. Hoit, Richard A. Walsh (eds.): Cardiovascular Physiology in the
     Genetically Engineered Mouse, Second Edition. 2001   ISBN 0-7923-7536-X
239. Pieter A. Doevendans, A.A.M. Wilde (eds.): Cardiovascular Genetics for Clinicians
     2001   ISBN 1-4020-0097-9
240. Stephen M. Factor, Maria A.Lamberti-Abadi, Jacobo Abadi (eds.): Handbook of
     Pathology and Pathophysiology of Cardiovascular Disease. 2001
                                                 ISBN 0-7923-7542-4
241. Liong Bing Liem, Eugene Downar (eds): Progress in Catheter Ablation. 2001
                                                 ISBN 1-4020-0147-9
242. Pieter A. Doevendans, Stefan Kääb (eds): Cardiovascular Genomics: New
     Pathophysiological Concepts. 2002   ISBN 1-4020-7022-5
243. Daan Kromhout, Alessandro Menotti, Henry Blackburn (eds.): Prevention
     of Coronary Heart Disease: Diet, Lifestyle and Risk Factors in the Seven
     Countries Study. 2002   ISBN 1-4020-7123-X
244. Antonio Pacifico (ed.), Philip D. Henry, Gust H. Bardy, Martin Borggrefe,
     Francis E. Marchlinski, Andrea Natale, Bruce L. Wilkoff (assoc. eds):
     Implantable Defibrillator Therapy: A Clinical Guide. 2002   ISBN 1-4020-7143-4
245. Hein J.J. Wellens, Anton P.M. Gorgels, Pieter A. Doevendans (eds.):
     The ECG in Acute Myocardial Infarction and Unstable Angina: Diagnosis and Risk
     Stratification. 2002   ISBN 1-4020-7214-7
246. Jack Rychik, Gil Wernovsky (eds.): Hypoplastic Left Heart Syndrome. 2003
                                                 ISBN 1-4020-7319-4
247. Thomas H. Marwick: Stress Echocardiography. Its Role in the Diagnosis and Evaluation
     of Coronary Artery Disease 2nd Edition.   ISBN 1-4020-7369-0
248. Akira Matsumori: Cardiomyopathies and Heart Failure: Biomolecular, Infectious
     and Immune Mechanisms. 2003   ISBN 1-4020-7438-7
249. Ralph Shabetai: The Pericardium. 2003   ISBN 1-4020-7639-8
250. Irene D. Turpie; George A. Heckman (eds.): Aging Issues in Cardiology. 2004
                                                 ISBN 1-40207674-6
251. C.H. Peels; L.H.B. Baur (eds.): Valve Surgery at the Turn of the Millennium. 2004
                                                 ISBN 1-4020-7834-X
252. Jason X.-J. Yuan (ed.): Hypoxic Pulmonary Vasoconstriction: Cellular and Molecular
     Mechanisms. 2004   ISBN 1-4020-7857-9
253. Francisco J. Villarreal (ed.): Interstitial Fibrosis In Heart Failure 2004
                                                 ISBN 0-387-22824-1
254. Xander H.T. Wehrens; Andrew R. Marks (eds.): Ryanodine Receptors: Structure, function
     and dysfunction in clinical disease. 2005   ISBN 0-387-23187-0
255. Guillem Pons-Lladó; Francesc Carreras (eds.): Atlas of Practical Applications of
     Cardiovascular Magnetic Resonance. 2005   ISBN 0-387-23632-5
256. José Marín-García : Mitochondria and the Heart. 2005   ISBN 0-387-25574-5
257. Macdonald Dick II: Clinical Cardiac Electrophysiology in the Young 2006
                                                 ISBN 0-387-29164-4
258. Martial G. Bourassa, Jean-Claude Tardif (eds.): Antioxidants and Cardiovascular
     Disease, 2nd Edition. 2006   ISBN 0-387-29552-6
Previous volumes are still available

ANTIOXIDANTS AND CARDIOVASCULAR DISEASE

SECOND EDITION

Edited by

Martial G. Bourassa

Montreal Heart Institute,
Research Center and Department of Medicine, Faculty of Medicine,
University of Montreal
Montreal, Quebec, Canada

And

Jean-Claude Tardif

Montreal Heart Institute,
Research Center and Department of Medicine, Faculty of Medicine,
University of Montreal
Montreal, Quebec, Canada

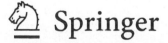 Springer

Martial G. Bourassa
Montreal Heart Institute
Research Center and Department of Medicine, Faculty of Medicine
Montreal, Quebec, Canada

Jean-Claude Tardif
Montreal Heart Institute
Research Center and Department of Medicine, Faculty of Medicine
University of Montreal
Montreal, Quebec, Canada

Library of Congress Control Number: 2005933858

ISBN-13: 978-0387-29552-7
ISBN-10: 0-387-29552-6

e-ISBN-13: 978-0387-29553-4
e-ISBN-10: 0-387-29553-4

Printed on acid-free paper.

Printed in the United States of America.

9 8 7 6 5 4 3 2 1   SPIN 11054375

springeronline.com

Contents

Contributing authors

Ayman Al Haj Zen
> Service de Cardiologie, Hôpital Européen Georges Pompidou (HEGP), 20 rue Leblanc, 75908 Paris 15, France

Juan J. Badimon
> Cardiovascular Biology Research Laboratory, Cardiovascular Institute, Mount Sinai Medical Center, One Gustave Levy Pl. Box 1030, New York, N.Y. 10029-6574 USA

Charlene Bierl
> Whitaker Cardiovascular Institute, and Evans Department of Medicine, Boston University School of Medicine, 88 East Newton Street, Boston, MA 02118-2308 USA

Christian Binggeli
> Cardiology, University Hospital, Ramistrasse 100, CH-8091 Zurich, Switzerland

Ian A. Blair
> The Institute for Translational Medicine and Therapeutics, Departments of Pharmacology, Pediatrics and Chemistry, and The Center for Cancer Pharmacology, 153 Johnson Pavilion, University of Pennsylvania, Philadelphia PA 19104-6084 USA

Martial G. Bourassa*
> Research Center, Montreal Heart Institute, 5000 Belanger Street East, Montreal, Quebec, Canada H1T 1C8. E-mail: martial.bourassa@icm-mhi.org.
> *Corresponding author.

Camille Brasselet
> Service de Cardiologie, Hôpital Européen Georges Pompidou (HEGP), 20 rue Leblanc, 75908 Paris 15, France.

Xilin Chen
> Discovery Research, AtheroGenics, Inc., 8995 Westside Parkway, Alpharetta, GA 30004 USA.

Jean-Louis Chiasson*
> Research Centre, CHUM-Hôtel-Dieu, 3850 St. Urbain Street, Montreal, Québec, Canada H2W 1T8. E-mail: jean.louis.chiasson@umontreal.ca.
> *Corresponding author.

Wilson S. Colucci*
> Cardiovascular Section, Boston University Medical Center, 88 East Newton Street, Boston, MA 02118 USA. E-mail: wilson.colucci@bmc.org.
> *Corresponding author.

Francesco Cosentino
> Cardiology, University Hospital, Ramistrasse 100, CH-8091 Zurich, Switzerland.

Tillman Cyrus
> University of Pennsylvania, Department of Pharmacology, 124 John Morgan Building, 3620 Hamilton Walk, Philadelphia PA 19104-6084 USA.

Michel de Lorgeril*
> Laboratoire Nutrition, Vieillissement et Maladies Cardiovasculaires (NVMCV), UFR de Médecine et Pharmacie, Domaine de la Merci, 38706 La Tronche, France. E-mail: michel.delorgeril@ujf-grenoble.fr.
> *Corresponding author.

Sergey Dikalov
> Division of Cardiology, Emory University School of Medicine, 1639 Pierce Drive, 319 WMB, Atlanta, GA 30322 USA.

Helmut Drexler*
> Abteilung Kardiologie und Angiologie, Medizinische Hochschule Hannover (MHH), Carl-Neuberg Str. 1, 30625 Hannover, Germany. E-mail : drexler.helmut@mh-hannover.de.
> *Corresponding author.

Anique Ducharme
 Research Center, Montreal Heart Institute, 5000 Belanger Street East, Montreal, Quebec, Canada H1T 1C8

Eric Durand
 Service de Cardiologie, Hôpital Européen Georges Pompidou (HEGP), 20 rue Leblanc, 75908 Paris 15, France.

Garrett A. FitzGerald*
 The Institute for Translational Medicine and Therapeutics, and Department of Pharmacology, 153 Johnson Pavilion, University of Pennsylvania, Philadelphia PA 19104-6084 USA. E-mail: garret@spirit.gcrc.upenn.edu.
 *Corresponding author.

Marc Forgione
 Whitaker Cardiovascular Institute, and Evans Department of Medicine, Boston University School of Medicine, 88 East Newton Street, Boston, MA 02118-2308 USA.

Valentin Fuster*
 Cardiovascular Institute, Mount Sinai Medical Center, One Gustave Levy Pl., Box 1030, New York, N.Y. 10029-6574 USA. E-mail: valentin.fuster@mssm.edu.
 *Corresponding author.

David G. Harrison*
 Division of Cardiology, Emory University School of Medicine, 1639 Pierce Drive, 319 WMB, Atlanta, GA 30322 USA. E-mail: dharr02@emory.edu.
 *Corresponding author.

Charles H. Hennekens*
 Agatston Research Institute (ARI), Miami Beach, FL; Departments of Medicine & Epidemiology and Public Health, University of Miami School of Medicine, Boca Raton, FL 33432 USA. E-mail: profchhmd@prodigy.net.
 *Corresponding author.

Danielle Hollar
 Agatston Research Institute (ARI), 4302 Alton Road, Suite 710, Miami Beach, FL 33140 USA.

Harry Ischiropoulos
    Department of Pharmacology and Pediatrics, 153 Johnson
    Pavilion, University of Pennsylvania, Philadelphia PA 19104-6084
    USA.

Charles Kunsch*
    Department of Discovery Research, AtheroGenics, Inc., 8995
    Westside Parkway, Alpharetta, GA 30004 USA. E-mail:
    ckunsch@atherogenics.com
    *Corresponding author.

Antoine Lafont*
    Service de Cardiologie, Hôpital Européen Georges Pompidou
    (HEGP), 20 rue Leblanc, 75908 Paris 15, France. E-mail:
    lafont@necker.fr.
    *Corresponding author.

Ulf Landmesser
    Abteilung Kardiologie und Angiologie, Medizinische Hochschule
    Hannover (MHH), Carl Neuberg Str. 1, 30625 Hannover, Germany

John A. Lawson
    The Institute for Translational Medicine and Therapeutics, and
    Department of Pharmacology, 153 Johnson Pavilion, University of
    Pennsylvania, Philadelphia PA 19104-6084 USA.

Joseph Loscalzo*
    Whitaker Cardiovascular Institute, and Evans Department of
    Medicine, Boston University School of Medicine, 88 East Newton
    Street, Boston, MA 02118-2308 USA. E-mail:
    joseph.loscalzo@bmc.org.
    *Corresponding author.

Thomas F. Luscher*
    Cardiology, University Hospital, Ramistrasse 100, CH-8091 Zurich,
    Switzerland. E-mail: karlue@usz.unizh.ch.
    *Corresponding author.

Ryan E. Moore
    University of Pennsylvania Medical Center, 654 Biochemical
    Research Building II/III, 421, Curie Blvd, Philadelphia PA 19104
    USA.

Georg Noll
    Cardiology, University Hospital, Ramistrasse 100, CH-8091 Zurich,
    Switzerland.

Domenico Pratico*
University of Pennsylvania, Department of Pharmacology, 124 John Morgan Building, 3620 Hamilton Walk, Philadelphia PA 19104-6084 USA. E-mail: domenico.pratico@spirit.gcrc.upenn.edu.
*Corresponding author.

Rémi Rabasa-Lhoret
Research Centre, CHUM-Hôtel-Dieu, 3850 St. Urbain Street, Montreal, Quebec, Canada H2W 1T8.

Daniel J. Rader*
University of Pennsylvania Medical Center, 654 Biomedical Research Building II/III, 421 Curie Blvd, Philadelphia, PA 19104 USA. E-mail: rader@mail.med.upenn.edu.
*Corresponding author.

Jean L. Rouleau*
Dean's Office, Faculty of Medicine, University of Montreal, Pavillon Principal, 2900 Edouard-Montpetit, Local P407, Montreal, Quebec, Canada H3T 1J4.E-mail: jean.rouleau@umontreal.ca.
*Corresponding author.

Patricia Salen
Laboratoire Nutrition, Vieillissement et Maladies Cardiovasculaires (NVMCV), UFR de Médecine et Pharmacie, Domaine de la Merci, 38706 La Tronche, France.

Douglas B. Sawyer
Cardiovascular Section, Boston University Medical Center, 88 East Newton Street, Boston, MA 02118 USA.

Ernesto L. Schiffrin*
Clinical Research Institute of Montreal, University of Montreal, 110 Pine Avenue West, Montreal, Quebec, Canada H2W 1R7. E-mail: ernesto.schiffrin@ircm.qc.ca.
*Corresponding author.

Ashok Srivastava
Research Centre, CHUM-Hôtel-Dieu, 3850 St. Urbain Street, Montreal, Quebec, Canada H2W 1T8.

Isabella Sudano
Cardiology, University Hospital, Ramistrasse 100, CH-8091 Zurich, Switzerland.

Jean-Claude Tardif
        Research Center, Montreal Heart Institute, 5000 Belanger Street
        East, Montreal, Quebec, Canada H1T 1C8

Rhian M. Touyz
        Clinical Research Institute of Montreal, University of Montreal, 110
        Pine Avenue West, Montreal, Quebec, Canada H2W 1R7.

Sotirios Tsimikas*
        Department of Medicine, Cardiology, University of California, San
        Diego (UCSD), 9350 Campus Point Dr., La Jolla, CA 92037-0682
        USA. E-mail: stsimikas@ucsd.edu
        *Corresponding author.

Bernd van der Loo
        Cardiology, University Hospital, Ramistrasse 100, CH-8091 Zurich,
        Switzerland.

Juan Viles-Gonzalez
        Cardiovascular Biology Research Laboratory, Cardiovascular
        Institute, Mount Sinai Medical Center, One Gustave Levy Pl., Box
        1030, New York, N.Y., 10029-6574 USA.

Michel White
        Research Center, Montreal Heart Institute, 5000 Belanger Street
        East. Montreal, Quebec, Canada H1T 1C8

Preface

The role and mechanisms of oxidative stress and of antioxidant molecules in patients with cardiovascular disease have been the subject of intense experimental and clinical research recently. Rapid accumulation of new knowledge in this field since the beginning of the 21st century amply justifies this second edition of the book *Antioxidants & Cardiovascular Disease.*

The generation of reactive oxygen species (ROS) is an unavoidable consequence of life in an aerobic environment. Cells produce ROS as part of their general metabolic activity. ROS are a family of molecules derived from oxygen, and characterized by their high chemical reactivity and ability to act as oxidants. ROS encompass free radicals (species containing highly reactive unpaired electrons) such as superoxide (O2-) and hydroxyl radicals (OH), as well as other molecules such as hydrogen peroxide (H2O2) and peroxynitrite (ONOO), which are not free radicals, but can also act as oxidizing agents in biological systems. Under physiological conditions, there is a balance between ROS generation and the activity of enzymatic (superoxide dismutase, catalase, glutathione peroxidase) and non-enzymatic (glutathione, alpha-tocopherol, ascorbate, thioredoxin) antioxidant defences that decrease ROS concentrations. ROS are normally produced in low concentrations and exert important physiological functions in the vessel wall. However, increased production of ROS or decreased antioxidant defences result in excess production of ROS, a condition referred to as oxidative stress. Oxidative stress can lead to free radical-induced oxidation and damage to bio-molecules such as lipids, DNA and proteins. ROS-mediated cellular damage has been associated with the pathogenesis of many diseases including Alzheimer's disease, rheumatoid arthritis, asthma, diabetes and especially cardiovascular disease.

Major cardiovascular risk factors, such as hypertension, dyslipidemia, diabetes and smoking, are associated with a marked increase in vascular ROS production. Increased ROS induce significant tissue damage and modification of lipids and proteins in the vessel wall. Over two decades ago, the antioxidant hypothesis focused mainly on the oxidative modification of LDL rendering it more atherogenic to promote foam cell formation in the intima. Although the exact mechanisms leading to LDL oxidation *in vivo* are still not entirely understood, it appears to be one of the earliest atherogenic changes leading to progression of atherosclerosis. In addition, oxidized LDL is intimately involved in the transition of stable atherosclerotic lesions to vulnerable plaques and plaque disruption. A variety of lipid and protein modifications of LDL, which are generated from lipid peroxidation, make it atherogenic. However, LDL oxidation alone may not explain the complex relation of oxidative stress and atherosclerosis.

Atherosclerosis originates from endothelial dysfunction and inflammation. Increased ROS production is a major cause of endothelial dysfunction in experimental and clinical atherosclerosis. Endothelial dysfunction leads to a rapid decrease in nitric oxide (NO) production or availability, due in part to inactivation of NO by superoxide. In addition to its vasodilator effect, NO protects against vascular injury, inflammation and thrombosis. Endothelial dysfunction is a strong independent predictor of future cardiovascular events in patients with cardiovascular risk factors, coronary artery disease and acute coronary syndromes. ROS are involved in endothelial and vascular smooth muscle cell pro-inflammatory signaling, particularly in the regulation of endothelial adhesion molecules (VCAM-1) and chemokine (MCP-1) expression. Moreover, ROS are involved in signaling cascades (redox signaling) leading to vascular pro-inflammatory and pro-thrombotic gene expression involving the transcription factor NF-kappa B. Finally, ROS activate matrix metallo-proteinases (MMPs), contributing to plaque instability and rupture.

One of the most convincing arguments for a major role of oxidative stress in the pathogenesis of atherosclerosis and cardiovascular disease has been the documentation, in numerous experimental and clinical studies, that antioxidant molecules can revert the atherosclerotic process and can reduce subsequent cardiovascular events. There is a consensus, based on several recent negative clinical trials, that supplementation with natural antioxidants such as vitamins (vitamin A, C, and E) and minerals (zinc and selenium) should not be recommended routinely. The reasons underlying the lack of efficacy of these natural antioxidants in patients with cardiovascular disease or cardiovascular risk factors are still poorly understood. On the other hand, a diet rich in antioxidant-macro-nutrients, particularly fruits and vegetables, is recommended for all individuals, and some types of diets such as the Mediterranean diet, have been shown to be highly beneficial in the prevention of cardiovascular events in patients with coronary heart disease. Some of the beneficial effects of aspirin, beta-blockers, calcium channel blockers, statins and ACE inhibitors (or angiotensin receptor blockers) in patients with cardiovascular disease are potentially related to their known antioxidant properties. These relationships must be more clearly delineated, however. Other potentially beneficial candidates also deserve to be investigated further. For example, acarbose has been shown to be beneficial in patients with diabetes mellitus. Probucol, a potent antioxidant, has been shown in numerous experimental and clinical studies to prevent atherosclerosis and restenosis after percutaneous coronary interventions. This agent is no longer in clinical use because of unacceptable side effects. An analog of probucol, AGI-1067, has recently been shown by our group to possess antioxidant properties which are comparable to those of probucol, but without the undesirable side effects of the latter. AGI-1067 has been shown to have similar beneficial effects on prevention of coronary atherosclerosis and coronary restenosis in humans and it is currently being investigated for its ability to reduce long-term clinical events in patients with coronary heart disease. Finally, this still represents a very novel approach, which may ultimately lead to major prevention of atherosclerosis and its vascular complications.

In summary, this book addresses a complex but very timely and fascinating problem in cardiovascular medicine. It is written by recognized experts in the fields of atherosclerosis and antioxidants. It should be of interest not only to academicians but also to practicing physicians. The first five chapters review the general concepts of oxidative stress and their relationship to lipid metabolism, endothelial dysfunction, genetics and transcriptional factors. The next seven chapters describe recently defined markers of oxidative stress, pharmacological compounds with antioxidant activity, natural antioxidants found in micronutrients and in nutrient-rich diets, and reviews the recent evidence for their efficacy or lack of efficacy in patients with cardiovascular disease or cardiovascular risk factors. The last seven chapters discuss the potential therapeutic benefits of antioxidants in a number of cardiovascular conditions which include atherosclerosis, restenosis after percutaneous coronary intervention, major cardiovascular risk factors such as hypertension, diabetes mellitus and dyslipidemia, and left ventricular dysfunction and congestive heart failure.

The editors are grateful to the authors and co-authors of the different chapters of the book, and wish to thank them for their excellent contributions.

Martial G. Bourassa   Jean-Claude Tardif

Chapter 1

GENERAL CONCEPTS ABOUT OXIDATIVE STRESS

Ulf Landmesser and Helmut Drexler
Abteilung Kardiologie und Angiologie, Medizinische Hochschule Hannover, Hannover, Germany

Introduction

This chapter focuses on general concepts about the role and mechanisms of oxidative stress in atherosclerosis and its resultant cardiovascular events. There is convincing evidence, from both experimental and clinical studies, that the major cardiovascular risk factors are associated with a marked increase of vascular production of reactive oxygen species (ROS) and lipid oxidation. To what extent, however, ROS contribute causally to the pathophysiology of human cardiovascular disease is an area of intense ongoing research.

Whereas initially the oxidative modification hypothesis of atherosclerosis was focused on the oxidative modification of low-density lipoprotein (LDL), rendering it more atherogenic to promote foam cell formation in the intimal space, a large body of evidence has now underscored numerous additional, likely important, oxidative events in cardiovascular disease.

Increased ROS production has been identified as a major cause of endothelial dysfunction in experimental and clinical atherosclerosis, that is associated with a rapid loss of anti-atherogenic and anti-inflammatory properties of endothelium-derived nitric oxide (NO$^{\bullet}$), in part due to increased inactivation of NO$^{\bullet}$ by superoxide. Moreover, ROS have been shown to be critically involved in signaling cascades leading to vascular pro-inflammatory and pro-thrombotic gene expression, in part involving the transcription factor nuclear factor(NF)-kappaB. Redox signaling may represent a highly localized and specific role of ROS.

In addition, ROS are potent activators of matrix metallo-proteinases (MMPs) that may represent a mechanism thereby ROS could contribute to plaque destabilization and rupture.

The refined understanding of the complexity of oxidative events, that have different cellular localization and involve different ROS as well as potential physiological functions of ROS need to be taken into account when antioxidative treatment strategies are considered.

Reactive oxygen species (ROS)

ROS encompass a variety of diverse chemical species, including both free radicals (containing highly reactive unpaired electrons), such as superoxide ($O_2^{\bullet-}$) and hydroxyl radicals ($OH^{\bullet}$), and other molecular species, such as hydrogen peroxide (H_2O_2) and peroxynitrite ($ONOO^-$). Accordingly, some of these species, such as superoxide and hydroxyl radicals, are extremely unstable, whereas others, like hydrogen peroxide, are freely diffusible and relatively long-lived [1].

Of note, besides the suggested pathological role of increased ROS production in cardiovascular diseases as discussed below and in other diseases, such as neurodegenerative disease[2], there are likely also physiologically important functions of ROS. For example, ROS play a role in cellular proliferation and host defense. Increased vascular production of ROS, however, may contribute to important processes in the pathophysiology of cardiovascular disease.

Evidence for increased oxidative stress in cardiovascular disease

Over the past decade, accumulating data from both experimental studies and studies in patients with coronary disease or cardiovascular risk factors, such as hypercholesterolemia, hypertension, diabetes and smoking, have convincingly demonstrated that there is an association of cardiovascular risk factors with an increased vascular production of ROS. In animal studies, an increased vascular production of ROS, in particular of superoxide, has been shown directly by chemiluminescence and electron spin resonance spectroscopy measurements[3-7]. In humans, increased oxidative stress has been demonstrated in patients with cardiovascular risk factors or coronary disease by increased levels of F_2 isoprostanes, stable, free radical-catalyzed products of arachidonic acid reflecting lipid peroxidation in vivo[8-11]. In addition, the urinary excretion of the F_2-isoprostane 8-iso-prostaglandin $F_{2\alpha}$ (8-iso-PGF$_{2\alpha}$) was correlated with the number of cardiovascular risk factors[12].

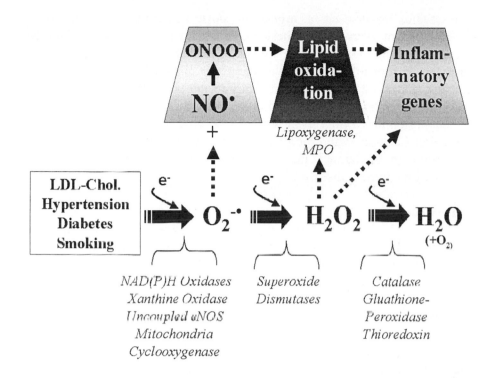

Figure 1. **Reactive oxygen species (ROS) and oxidant and antioxidant enzyme systems involved in the production and detoxification of ROS are shown.** Cardiovascular risk factors, such as hypercholesterolemia, hypertension, diabetes and smoking, increase the vascular production of ROS, in particular superoxide. This may be mediated by some of the oxidant enzyme systems shown. Superoxide reacts then rapidly with nitric oxide (NO·) resulting in reduced NO· bioactivity with loss of its vasculoprotective functions and formation of peroxynitrite (ONOO-), that may contribute to lipid oxidation. Superoxide dismutase converts superoxide to hydrogen peroxide. Myeloperoxidase and lipoxygenase are enzyme systems that are likely involved in lipid oxidation. Myeloperoxidase produces hypochlorous acid by using hydrogen peroxide. ROS, in particular hydrogen peroxide, have been suggested to play a critical role in pro-inflammatory signaling.

Moreover, in human atherosclerotic coronary arteries, an intense staining of superoxide has been shown in the plaque shoulder[13], that is rich in macrophages and prone to rupture, that is thought to underly a majority of clinical cardiovascular events.

Furthermore, increased oxidant stress in human cardiovascular disease has been suggested by several studies analyzing the effect of antioxidants on endothelial dysfunction in patients with coronary disease or cardiovascular risk factors. In these studies structurally different antioxidants, in particular a high local dose of the antioxidant vitamin C, could improve endothelium-dependent vasodilation[14-21]. It is important to note, however, that most of these studies have used a *high-local dose* of vitamin C. The local concentration of vitamin C in these studies may exceed up to 100-fold the plasma concentrations achieved by oral treatment with vitamin C. It is therefore questionable whether vitamin C as administered in large scale clinical trials (i.e. 250 mg vitamin C/day in the Heart Protection Study[22]; can achieve similar effects on endothelial function. In fact, recent studies have suggested that a high local dose of vitamin C is required to impact on endothelial function[23] and long-term oral treatment with 800 IE of vitamin E and 1000 mg of vitamin C per day had no effect on endothelial function in patients with coronary disease[24]

Lipid oxidation

Brown and Goldstein have originally put forward the concept that circulating low-density lipoprotein (LDL) must undergo some kind of structural modification before it becomes fully proatherogenic[25]. Several different modifications of LDL have been described, including oxidation, aggregation, enzymatic modification, and possibly others, that convert LDL to a form that is recognized by one or more of the macrophage scavenger receptors. The best studied of these and the one for which there is good in vivo evidence is oxidative modification[26]. Oxidation of LDL modifies its bioactivity extensively in vitro, conferring properties associated with disease pathogenesis. The oxidative modification hypothesis will be discussed in more detail in chapter 4.

This concept alone, however, may not explain the complexity of oxidative stress and atherosclerosis. For example, Witting et al.[27] observed that the antioxidant probucol and its metabolite bisphenol had a similar effect on vascular lipid oxidation, but the effect of the antioxidant probucol on atherosclerotic lesion formation was more pronounced. Although this study has several limitations[28], it may point to the notion that other oxidant mechanisms are also important in atherosclerosis.

Endothelial dysfunction

Originally, oxidative stress was primarily implicated in atherosclerosis by damaging lipids. Whereas oxidized LDL may contribute to endothelial dysfunction, it has now been recognized that oxygen radicals may directly cause endothelial dysfunction, i.e. by reducing endothelial $NO^\bullet$ bioavailability[29,30]. In particular, superoxide ($O_2^{\bullet-}$) reacts rapidly with $NO^\bullet$, resulting in formation of peroxynitrite and loss of $NO^\bullet$'s bioactivity. Endothelial dysfunction in experimental atherosclerosis could be reversed by administration of superoxide scavengers, suggesting that increased vascular superoxide production represents a major cause of endothelial dysfunction[3,4]. Recently it has been recognized that ROS, and especially peroxynitrite, can oxidize tetrahydrobiopterin, a critical co-factor for endothelial NO• synthase[4,31], that leads to dysfunction ("uncoupling") of the enzyme.

Proposed pathophysiological mechanisms of oxidative stress and cardiovascular disease

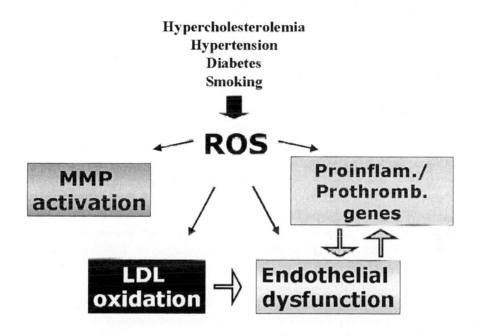

Figure 2. **Proposed mechanisms of how increased vascular ROS production, as stimulated by cardiovascular risk factors, may contribute to cardiovascular disease.** Initially, the oxidative modification hypothesis of atherosclerosis was focused on the oxidative modification of LDL cholesterol rendering it fully pro-atherogenic to promote foam cell formation and vascular inflammation. Increased ROS production has now also been identified as a major cause of endothelial dysfunction, in part resulting from increased inactivation of endothelial NO· by superoxide. In addition, accumulating data indicate ROS as critical signaling molecules involved in vascular pro-inflammatory and pro-thrombotic gene expression, i.e. endothelial leukocyte adhesion molecule and chemokine expression. ROS are potent activators of matrix metallo-proteinases that are expressed in the shoulder region of atherosclerotic plaques, that could importantly contribute to plaque destabilisation and rupture, thought to underlie a large number of clinical cardiovascular events

NO• not only produces vasodilation, but also has anti-atherogenic properties[32-34]. These include inhibition of leukocyte adhesion molecule expression, inhibition of platelet aggregation and prevention of smooth muscle cell proliferation. Thus, the loss of NO• not only alters vascular tone, but also likely contributes importantly to the development, progression and clinical complications of atherosclerosis. This concept is supported by a growing number of clinical studies indicating that the degree of endothelial dysfunction, measured as impaired endothelium-dependent vasomotion, represents a strong and independent predictor of future cardiovascular events in patients with cardiovascular risk factors, coronary disease, acute coronary syndromes and peripheral artery disease[35-40]. In fact, the effect of a *high local dose* of the antioxidant vitamin C on endothelium-dependent vasodilation has been shown to predict future cardiovascular events in a study following 179 patients with coronary disease[41], suggesting that oxidative stress-induced endothelial dysfunction has prognostic implications.

ROS and vascular inflammation

There is accumulating evidence supporting the concept that, both development of atherosclerotic lesions and clinical cardiovascular complications of atherosclerotic disease, are related to vascular inflammation[42,43]. In experimental studies, it has been shown that inhibition of leukocyte adhesion and infiltration, regulated by leukocyte adhesion molecules, such as vascular cell adhesion molecule-1 (VCAM-1), and chemokines, such as monocyte chemoattractant protein (MCP-1), prevents atherosclerotic lesion development[44-46]. Notably, it has been suggested that ROS are importantly involved in endothelial and vascular smooth muscle cell (VSMC) pro-inflammatory signaling, i.e. the regulation of endothelial adhesion molecules and chemokine expression, that may represent an important link of oxygen radicals and vascular disease[47]. The stimulating effect of cytokines, such as TNF-alpha and interleukin 1, or angiotensin II on endothelial expression of the adhesion molecule VCAM-1[48,49] or the chemokine MCP-1[50,51] was suppressed by different ROS scavengers, suggesting that ROS are critical mediators of pro-inflammatory signaling in the endothelium. Some of these redox-sensitive pro-inflammatory signaling pathways may involve the transcription factor NF-kappaB-[52].

In contrast, endothelial NO• production has been shown to exert important anti-inflammatory effects. NO• has been shown to reduce endothelial adhesion molecule and chemokine expression in vitro[53,54]. Moreover, NO• synthase gene therapy rapidly reduces hypercholesterolemia-induced leukocyte adhesion molecule expression, i.e. VCAM-1, and ameliorates monocyte infiltration into the arterial wall of cholesterol-fed rabbits[55]. The loss of endothelial NO• as a result of increased ROS production may therefore represent an important mechanism whereby oxidative stress promotes a pro-inflammatory phenotype of the endothelium.

Of note, recent evidence suggests that "redox signaling", i.e. via kinase signaling pathways may be distinct from "oxidative stress," and could be mediated by discrete, localized redox circuitry[56]. Taken together, there are several important links between increased endothelial oxidative stress and ROS production with vascular inflammation. Furthermore, inflammation per se may augment vascular oxidative stress[57]. Therefore, the observed association of vascular oxidative stress and inflammatory markers in patients with coronary disease[58] may indicate that oxidative stress promotes vascular inflammation, but also that inflammation augments oxidant stress, a potential vicious cycle.

ROS and thrombosis

Increased ROS production has been shown to be critically involved in the up regulation of tissue factor in VSMCs in response to activated platelets[59]. Tissue factor (TF) initiates the extrinsic coagulation cascade leading to thrombin formation. Thrombin induces tissue factor mRNA in human VSMCs by a redox-sensitive, NAD(P)H oxidase dependent mechanism, that may contribute to prolonged procoagulant activity and enhanced thrombogenicity at sites of vascular injury[60]. These findings suggest that vascular pro-thrombotic gene expression is redox-sensitive that may link increased oxidant stress to vascular thrombotic events.

In addition, endothelial NO$^{•}$ has several important anti-thrombotic effects and inhibits platelet adhesion to the endothelium, an effect that is lost after oxidative inactivation of NO$^{•}$. Taken together, ROS have been identified as important mediators of vascular pro-inflammatory and pro-thrombotic gene expression that together with oxidative inactivation of endothelial NO$^{•}$ may promote a pro-inflammatory and pro-thrombotic phenotype of the endothelium.

ROS activate matrix metallo-proteinases: relevance to plaque instability?

Plaque rupture is the most common type of plaque complication, and is thought to account for ≈70% of fatal acute myocardial infarctions and/or sudden coronary deaths[61,62]. The expression of MMPs, i.e. MMP-2 (gelatinase A, which degrades collagen IV) and MMP-9 (gelatinase B, which acts on collagen I fibers) that are secreted by macrophages and vascular myocytes, is increased in the rupture-prone shoulders of atherosclerotic plaques[63]. Notably, ROS have been shown to importantly modulate MMPs, that could contribute to lesion instability[64]. It has been demonstrated that pro-MMP-9 and pro-MMP-2 from VSMCs are activated in vitro by ROS[64]. Furthermore, cyclic strain-induced MMP-2 expression in VSMCs was dependent on activation of the oxidant enzyme NAD(P)H-oxidase[65]. Sorescu et al. have recently demonstrated particularly high levels of superoxide in the shoulder region of human coronary atherosclerotic plaques[13]. Thus, MMP activation by ROS could contribute to plaque rupture.

Other mechanisms linking ROS and cardiovascular disease

There are additional mechanisms that may link increased oxidant stress and cardiovascular disease. ROS have been suggested to play a major role in mediating VSMC and cardiomyocyte hypertrophy in response to stimuli such as angiotensin II or mechanical stretch, that may contribute to vascular and cardiac remodeling processes.

Another interesting novel concept that needs to be further explored suggests a link between increased oxidative stress and insulin resistance[66]. In rats over-expressing angiotensin II, superoxide scavenging could improve skeletal muscle insulin-dependent glucose uptake and whole body insulin resistance[67], indicating that oxidative stress plays an important role in angiotensin II mediated insulin resistance.

Sources of ROS in cardiovascular disease

There are numerous potential sources of ROS that have been studied intensely over the past years (*figure 1*), and may play a different role for several cardiovascular risk factors. With respect to lipid oxidation, it is still not entirely understood what are the exact mechanisms leading to LDL oxidation in vivo. There is, however, evidence to suggest that *12/15-lipoxygenase* may initiate lipid peroxidation[68,69]. Notably, when 12/15-lipoxygenase deficient mice are crossed with animals deficient in ApoE, atherosclerotic lesion formation is dramatically inhibited[68,69]. *Myeloperoxidase* (MPO)-generated ROS, i.e. HOCl, may represent a plausible pathway for converting LDL into an atherogenic form[70,71]. Notably, increased MPO serum levels could identify patients at risk for cardiac events who presented with chest pain in the absence of myocardial necrosis[72] or an acute coronary syndrome[73].

With respect to ROS-induced impairment of endothelial function, that may have important prognostic implications, the following three superoxide producing oxidant enzyme systems have received most attention, the vascular *NAD(P)H oxidase*, *xanthine oxidase* and *uncoupled endothelial nitric oxide synthase* (*figure 3*)[29,74]. Increased vascular activity of the NADPH oxidase and xanthine oxidase have been demonstrated in experimental and clinical atherosclerosis[6,13,75,76]. Of note, a deficiency of the cytosolic NAD(P)H oxidase component p47phox was associated with a markedly reduced atherosclerotic lesion formation in the apoE-deficiency mouse model of atherosclerosis[77].

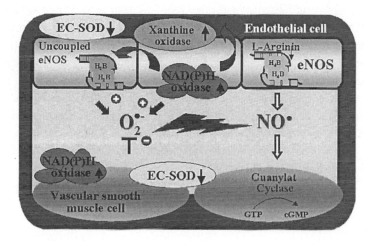

Figure 3. **Oxidant and antioxidant enzyme systems are shown that have been implicated as important sources of increased vascular superoxide production in atherosclerosis leading to rapid inactivation of NO causing endothelial dysfunction.** Experimental and clinical evidence suggests an activation of the vascular NAD(P)H oxidase system. This may further promote endothelial oxidant stress by increasing endothelial xanthine oxidase levels[81] and by causing uncoupling of the endothelial nitric oxide synthase (eNOS) due to oxidative inactivation of the eNOS cofactor tetrahydrobiopterin (H4B)(31). In advanced atherosclerosis the vascular activity of the superoxide scavenging enzyme extracellular superoxide dismutase (ecSOD) has been shown to be reduced[20].

More recent studies suggest, that intracellular ROS production may also be derived from the *mitochondria*. The production of mitochondrial superoxide radicals occurs primarily at two discrete points in the electron transport chain, namely at complex I (NADH dehydrogenase) and at complex III (ubiquinone–cytochrome *c* reductase)[1]. This could play a role in atherosclerosis and hyperglycemia[78,79].

Besides increased activation of oxidant enzyme systems in atherosclerosis, a reduced activity of several antioxidant scavenging enzyme systems has been observed in advanced human atherosclerotic disease. In particular, *extracellular superoxide dismutase*[20] and *glutathione peroxidase* activities[80] have been shown to display reduced activities in human atherosclerotic arteries.

Summary and conclusion

In summary, there is convincing evidence of an association of increased oxidant stress and cardiovascular risk factors or atherosclerosis in experimental studies and in humans. There is an increasing understanding of the complexity of oxidant mechanisms that may importantly contribute to key pathophysiological processes such as vascular inflammation, thrombosis and plaque rupture, far beyond oxidative modification of lipids. To what extent these mechanisms play a causal role for the development, progression and the complications of human atherosclerosis is an exciting and important area of ongoing intense research.

References

1. Finkel T, Holbrook NJ. Oxidants, oxidative stress and the biology of ageing. Nature 2000;408:239-47.
2. Andersen JK. Oxidative stress in neurodegeneration: cause or consequence? Nat Med 2004;10 Suppl:S18-25.
3. Ohara Y, Peterson TE, Harrison DG. Hypercholesterolemia increases endothelial superoxide anion production. J Clin Invest 1993;91:2546-51.
4. Laursen JB, Somers M, Kurz S, et al. Endothelial regulation of vasomotion in apoE-deficient mice: implications for interactions between peroxynitrite and tetrahydrobiopterin. Circulation 2001;103:1282-8.
5. Hink U, Li H, Mollnau H, et al. Mechanisms underlying endothelial dysfunction in diabetes mellitus. Circ Res 2001;88:E14-22.
6. Warnholtz A, Nickenig G, Schulz E, et al. Increased NADH-oxidase-mediated superoxide production in the early stages of atherosclerosis: evidence for involvement of the renin- angiotensin system. Circulation 1999;99:2027-33.
7. White CR, Darley-Usmar V, Berrington WR, et al. Circulating plasma xanthine oxidase contributes to vascular dysfunction in hypercholesterolemic rabbits. Proc Natl Acad Sci U S A 1996;93:8745-9.
8. Davi G, Alessandrini P, Mezzetti A, et al. In vivo formation of 8-Epi-prostaglandin F2 alpha is increased in hypercholesterolemia. Arterioscler Thromb Vasc Biol 1997;17:3230-5.
9. Reilly MP, Pratico D, Delanty N, et al. Increased formation of distinct F2 isoprostanes in hypercholesterolemia. Circulation 1998;98:2822-8.
10. Minuz P, Patrignani P, Gaino S, et al. Increased oxidative stress and platelet activation in patients with hypertension and renovascular disease. Circulation 2002;106:2800-5.
11. Morrow JD, Frei B, Longmire AW, et al. Increase in circulating products of lipid peroxidation (F2-isoprostanes) in smokers. Smoking as a cause of oxidative damage. N Engl J Med 1995;332:1198-203.
12. Schwedhelm E, Bartling A, Lenzen H, et al. Urinary 8-iso-prostaglandin F2alpha as a risk marker in patients with coronary heart disease: a matched case-control study. Circulation 2004;109:843-8.
13. Sorescu D, Weiss D, Lassegue B, et al. Superoxide production and expression of nox family proteins in human atherosclerosis. Circulation 2002;105:1429-35.
14. Ting HH, Timimi FK, Boles KS, et al. Vitamin C improves endothelium-dependent vasodilation in patients with non-insulin-dependent diabetes mellitus. J Clin Invest 1996;97:22-8.
15. Levine GN, Frei B, Koulouris SN, et al. Ascorbic acid reverses endothelial vasomotor dysfunction in patients with coronary artery disease. Circulation 1996;93:1107-13.
16. Heitzer T, Just H, Munzel T. Antioxidant vitamin C improves endothelial dysfunction in chronic smokers. Circulation 1996;94:6-9.

17. Ting HH, Timimi FK, Haley EA, et al. Vitamin C improves endothelium-dependent vasodilation in forearm resistance vessels of humans with hypercholesterolemia. Circulation 1997;95:2617-22.

18. Taddei S, Virdis A, Ghiadoni L, et al. Vitamin C improves endothelium-dependent vasodilation by restoring nitric oxide activity in essential hypertension. Circulation 1998;97:2222-9.

19. Hornig B, Arakawa N, Kohler C, et al. Vitamin C improves endothelial function of conduit arteries in patients with chronic heart failure. Circulation 1998;97:363-8.

20. Landmesser U, Merten R, Spiekermann S, et al. Vascular extracellular superoxide dismutase activity in patients with coronary artery disease: relation to endothelium-dependent vasodilation. Circulation 2000;101:2264-70.

21. Higashi Y, Sasaki S, Nakagawa K, et al. Endothelial function and oxidative stress in renovascular hypertension. N Engl J Med 2002;346:1954-62.

22. MRC/BHF Heart Protection Study of antioxidant vitamin supplementation in 20,536 high-risk individuals: a randomised placebo-controlled trial. Lancet 2002;360:23-33.

23. Sherman DL, Keaney JF, Biegelsen ES, et al. Pharmacological concentrations of ascorbic acid are required for the beneficial effect on endothelial vasomotor function in hypertension. Hypertension 2000;35:936-41.

24. Kinlay S, Behrendt D, Fang JC, et al. Long-term effect of combined vitamins E and C on coronary and peripheral endothelial function. J Am Coll Cardiol 2004;4:629-34.

25. Brown MS, Goldstein JL. Lipoprotein metabolism in the macrophage: implications for cholesterol deposition in atherosclerosis. Annu Rev Biochem 1983;52:223-61.

26. Steinberg D, Witztum JL. Is the oxidative modification hypothesis relevant to human atherosclerosis? Do the antioxidant trials conducted to date refute the hypothesis? Circulation 2002;105:2107-11.

27. Witting P, Pettersson K, Ostlund-Lindqvist AM, et al. Dissociation of atherogenesis from aortic accumulation of lipid hydro(pero)xides in Watanabe heritable hyperlipidemic rabbits. J Clin Invest 1999;104:213-20.

28. Heinecke JW. Is lipid peroxidation relevant to atherogenesis? J Clin Invest 1999;104:135-6.

29. Cai H, Harrison DG. Endothelial dysfunction in cardiovascular diseases: the role of oxidant stress. Circ Res 2000;87:840-4.

30. Landmesser U, Harrison DG. Oxidant stress as a marker for cardiovascular events: Ox marks the spot. Circulation 2001;104:2638-40.

31. Landmesser U, Dikalov S, Price SR, et al. Oxidation of tetrahydrobiopterin leads to uncoupling of endothelial cell nitric oxide synthase in hypertension. J Clin Invest 2003;111:1201-9.

32. Cooke JP, Dzau VJ. Derangements of the nitric oxide synthase pathway, L-arginine, and cardiovascular diseases. Circulation 1997;96:379-82.

33. Kuhlencordt PJ, Gyurko R, Han F, et al. Accelerated atherosclerosis, aortic aneurysm formation, and ischemic heart disease in apolipoprotein E/endothelial nitric oxide synthase double-knockout mice. Circulation 2001;104:448-54.

34. Landmesser U, Hornig B, Drexler H. Endothelial function: a critical determinant in atherosclerosis? Circulation 2004;109(Suppl 1):II27-33.
35. Suwaidi JA, Hamasaki S, Higano ST, et al. Long-term follow-up of patients with mild coronary artery disease and endothelial dysfunction. Circulation 2000;101:948-54.
36. Schachinger V, Britten MB, Zeiher AM. Prognostic impact of coronary vasodilator dysfunction on adverse long- term outcome of coronary heart disease. Circulation 2000;101:1899-906.
37. Halcox JPJ, Schenke WH, Zalos G, et al. Prognostic value of coronary vascular endothelial dysfunction. Circulation 2002;106:653-8.
38. Perticone F, Ceravolo R, Pujia A, et al. Prognostic significance of endothelial dysfunction in hypertensive patients. Circulation 2001;104:191-6.
39. Gokce N, Keaney JF, Hunter LM, et al. Predictive value of noninvasively determined endothelial dysfunction for long-term cardiovascular events in patients with peripheral vascular disease. J Am Coll Cardiol 2003;41:1769-75.
40. Fichtlscherer S, Breuer S, Zeiher AM. Prognostic value of systemic endothelial dysfunction in patients with acute coronary syndromes. Further evidence for the existence of the "vulnerable" patient. Circulation 2004;110:1926-32.
41. Heitzer T, Schlinzig T, Krohn K, et al. Endothelial dysfunction, oxidative stress, and risk of cardiovascular events in patients with coronary artery disease. Circulation 2001;104:2673-8.
42. Ross R. Atherosclerosis--an inflammatory disease. N Engl J Med 1999;340:115-26.
43. Libby P, Ridker PM, Maseri A. Inflammation and atherosclerosis. Circulation 2002;105:1135-43.
44. Boring L, Gosling J, Cleary M, et al. Decreased lesion formation in CCR2-/- mice reveals a role for chemokines in the initiation of atherosclerosis. Nature 1998;394:894-7.
45. Cybulsky MI, Iiyama K, Li H, et al. A major role for VCAM-1, but not ICAM-1, in early atherosclerosis. J Clin Invest 2001;107:1255-62.
46. Rosenfeld ME. Leukocyte recruitment into developing atherosclerotic lesions: the complex interaction between multiple molecules keeps getting more complex. Arterioscler Thromb Vasc Biol 2002;22:361-3.
47. Kunsch C, Medford RM. Oxidative stress as a regulator of gene expression in the vasculature. Circ Res 1999;85:753-66.
48. Marui N, Offermann MK, Swerlick R, et al. Vascular cell adhesion molecule-1 (VCAM-1) gene transcription and expression are regulated through an antioxidant-sensitive mechanism in human vascular endothelial cells. J Clin Invest 1993;92:1866-74.
49. Chen XL, Zhang Q, Zhao R, et al. Rac1 and superoxide are required for the expression of cell adhesion molecules induced by tumor necrosis factor-alpha in endothelial cells. J Pharmacol Exp Ther 2003;305:573-80.

50. Chen XL, Tummala PE, Olbrych MT, et al. Angiotensin II induces monocyte chemoattractant protein-1 gene expression in rat vascular smooth muscle cells. Circ Res 1998;83:952-9.

51. Chen XL, Zhang Q, Zhao R, et al. Superoxide, H2O2, and iron are required for TNF-alpha-induced MCP-1 gene expression in endothelial cells: role of Rac1 and NADPH oxidase. Am J Physiol Heart Circ Physiol 2004;286:H1001-7.

52. Collins T, Cybulsky MI. NF-kappaB: pivotal mediator or innocent bystander in atherogenesis? J Clin Invest 2001;107:255-64.

53. Zeiher AM, Fisslthaler B, Schray-Utz B, et al. Nitric oxide modulates the expression of monocyte chemoattractant protein 1 in cultured human endothelial cells. Circ Res 1995;76:980-6.

54. Tomita H, Egashira K, Kubo-Inoue M, et al. Inhibition of NO synthesis induces inflammatory changes and monocyte chemoattractant protein-1 expression in rat hearts and vessels. Arterioscler Thromb Vasc Biol 1998;18:1456-64.

55. Qian H, Neplioueva V, Shetty GA, et al. Nitric oxide synthase gene therapy rapidly reduces adhesion molecule expression and inflammatory cell infiltration in carotid arteries of cholesterol-fed rabbits. Circulation 1999;99:2979-82.

56. Go YM, Gipp JJ, Mulcahy RT, et al. H2O2-dependent activation of GCLC-ARE4 reporter occurs by mitogen-activated protein kinase pathways without oxidation of cellular glutathione or thioredoxin-1. J Biol Chem 2004;279:5837-45.

57. Pleiner J, Mittermayer F, Schaller G, et al. High doses of vitamin C reverse Escherichia coli endotoxin-induced hyporeactivity to acetylcholine in the human forearm. Circulation 2002;106:1460-4.

58. Fichtlscherer S, Breuer S, Schachinger V, et al. C-reactive protein levels determine systemic nitric oxide bioavailability in patients with coronary artery disease. Eur Heart J 2004;25:1412-8.

59. Gorlach A, Brandes RP, Bassus S, et al. Oxidative stress and expression of p22phox are involved in the up-regulation of tissue factor in vascular smooth muscle cells in response to activated platelets. Faseb J 2000;14:1518-28.

60. Herkert O, Diebold I, Brandes RP, et al. NADPH oxidase mediates tissue factor-dependent surface procoagulant activity by thrombin in human vascular smooth muscle cells. Circulation 2002;105:2030-6.

61. Falk E, Shah PK, Fuster V. Coronary plaque disruption. Circulation 1995;92:657-71.

62. Naghavi M, Libby P, Falk E, et al. From vulnerable plaque to vulnerable patient: a call for new definitions and risk assessment strategies: Part I. Circulation 2004;108:1664-72.

63. Galis ZS, Sukhova GK, Lark MW, et al. Increased expression of matrix metalloproteinases and matrix degrading activity in vulnerable regions of human atherosclerotic plaques. J Clin Invest 1994;94:2493-503.

64. Rajagopalan S, Meng XP, Ramasamy S, et al. Reactive oxygen species produced by macrophage-derived foam cells regulate the activity of vascular matrix metalloproteinases in vitro. J Clin Invest 1996;98:2572-9.

65. Grote K, Flach I, Luchtefeld M, et al. Mechanical stretch enhances mRNA expression and proenzyme release of matrix metalloproteinase-2 (MMP-2) via NAD(P)H oxidase-derived reactive oxygen species. Circ Res 2003;92:e80-6.

66. Ceriello A, Motz E. Is Oxidative stress the pathogenic mechanism underlying insulin resistance, diabetes, and cardiovascular disease? The common soil hypothesis revisited. Arterioscler Thromb Vasc Biol 2004;24:816-23.

67. Blendea MC, Jacobs D, Stump CS, et al. Abrogation of oxidative stress improves insulin sensitivity in the ren2 rat model of tissue angiotensin II overexpression. Am J Physiol Endocrinol Metab 2004;Oct 19;[Epub ahead of print].

68. Cyrus T, Witztum JL, Rader DJ, et al. Disruption of the 12/15-lipoxygenase gene diminishes atherosclerosis in apo E-deficient mice. J Clin Invest 1999;103:1597-604.

69. Cyrus T, Pratico D, Zhao L, et al. Absence of 12/15-lipoxygenase expression decreases lipid peroxidation and atherogenesis in apolipoprotein e-deficient mice. Circulation 2001;103:2277-82.

70. Podrez EA, Schmitt D, Hoff III, et al. Myeloperoxidase-generated reactive nitrogen species convert LDL into an atherogenic form in vitro. J Clin Invest 1999;103:1547-60.

71. Zhang R, Brennan ML, Shen Z, et al. Myeloperoxidase functions as a major enzymatic catalyst for initiation of lipid peroxidation at sites of inflammation. J Biol Chem 2002;277:46116-22.

72. Brennan ML, Penn MS, Van Lente F, et al. Prognostic value of myeloperoxidase in patients with chest pain. N Engl J Med 2003;349:1595-604.

73. Baldus S, Heeschen C, Meinertz T, et al. Myeloperoxidase serum levels predict risk in patients with acute coronary syndromes. Circulation 2003;108:1440-5.

74. Mueller CF, Laude K, McNally JS, et al. Redox mechanisms in blood vessels. Arterioscler Thromb Vasc Biol 2004;[Epub ahead of print].

75. Azumi H, Inoue N, Takeshita S, et al. Expression of NADH/NADPH oxidase p22phox in human coronary arteries. Circulation 1999;100:1494-8.

76. Spiekermann S, Landmesser U, Dikalov S, et al. Xanthine- and NAD(P)H oxidase-activity in patients with coronary artery disease- relation to endothelium-dependent vasodilation. Circulation 2003;107:1383-9.

77. Barry-Lane PA, Patterson C, van der Merwe M, et al. p47phox is required for atherosclerotic lesion progression in ApoE(-/-) mice. J Clin Invest 2001;108:1513-22.

78. Ballinger SW, Patterson C, Knight-Lozano CA, et al. Mitochondrial integrity and function in atherogenesis. Circulation 2002;106:544-9.

79. Nishikawa T, Edelstein D, Du XL, et al. Normalizing mitochondrial superoxide production blocks three pathways of hyperglycemic damage. Nature 2000;404:787-90.

80. Lapenna D, de Gioia S, Ciofani G, et al. Glutathione-related antioxidant defenses in human atherosclerotic plaques. Circulation 1998;97:1930-4.

81. McNally JS, Davis ME, Giddens DP, et al. Role of xanthine oxidoreductase and NAD(P)H oxidase in endothelial superoxide production in response to oscillatory shear stress. Am J Physiol Heart Circ Physiol 2003;285:H2290-7.

Chapter 2

LIPOPROTEINS AND OXIDATION

Sotirios Tsimikas
University of California, San Diego, CA

Introduction

Oxidation of lipoproteins, and in particular low density lipoprotein (LDL), has been implicated as a major factor in the initiation and progression of atherosclerosis[1].Over the last 25 years, research from many laboratories has elucidated multiple mechanisms through which oxidized LDL (OxLDL) is atherogenic. Oxidation of LDL in the vessel wall leads to an inflammatory cascade that activates many atherogenic pathways, including the unregulated uptake of OxLDL by scavenger receptors of monocyte-derived macrophages leading to foam cell formation. Accumulation of foam cells leads to fatty streak formation, the earliest visible atherosclerotic lesion. It consists primarily of cholesterol ester-laden cells, mostly derived from circulating monocytes that have penetrated through the endothelial layer, but also from modified smooth muscle cells. Foam cell necrosis and/or apoptosis and continued accumulation of oxidized lipids in the extracellular space eventually lead to atheroma formation. The complex interplay of oxidized lipids, inflammatory processes, endothelial dysfunction and platelet activation and thrombus ultimately lead to plaque progression and/or disruption leading to clinical events. Inflammatory cells play a central role throughout all these events, which results in atherosclerotic lesions having many features of a chronic inflammatory disease[2].

Palinski, Napoli and colleagues have established that fatty streaks may appear as early during the development of atherosclerosis as during human fetal life. In fact, they documented that OxLDL was present in aortas of fetuses whose mothers were hypercholesterolemic even prior to monocyte entry into the vessel wall, suggesting that LDL oxidation is involved *a priori* in the recruitment of monocytes into the vessel wall[3,4]. They also showed that maternal hypercholesterolemia is an important factor in the progression of atherosclerosis of children, that, in the setting of maternal hyper-cholesterolemia in utero, there is altered gene expression that mediates subsequent atherosclerosis and that treatment of hypercholesterolemia with antioxidants or lipid lowering agents in pregnant animal models reduces progression of atherosclerosis in progeny[5,6]. These observations suggest that oxidation of LDL is one of the earliest atherogenic changes that mediate progression of atherosclerosis. More recent studies also suggest that OxLDL is intimately involved in the transition of stable atherosclerotic lesions to vulnerable plaques and plaque disruption, as will be discussed later.

Mechanisms of LDL oxidation

Each LDL particle contains approximately 700 molecules of phospholipids, 600 of free cholesterol, 1600 of cholesterol esters, 185 of triglycerides and 1 copy of apoprotein B-100, which in turn is made of 4536 amino acid residues. The protein and the lipid moieties of the LDL particle are both exquisitely sensitive to oxidation and may undergo oxidative damage. LDL in plasma is relatively stable but once it has been purified and isolated it begins to oxidize rapidly, unless a chelating agent such as EDTA, is present throughout the stages of preparation[7]. In particular, copper (5 μM) and other divalent cations are able to catalyze oxidative modification of LDL during overnight incubation, resulting in the modified LDL which becomes a ligand for the acetyl LDL receptor, leading to foam cell formation[8]. Copper-catalyzed oxidative modification of LDL results in degradation of as much as 40% of the phosphatidylcholine, present on the polyunsaturated fatty acids (PUFA) in the *sn*-2 position, which is then converted to lysophosphatidylcholine. In addition, 50-75% of the PUFA are destroyed by attacks at the double bonds[9,10]. Apoprotein B-100 is also altered by direct oxidative attack and conjugation of lipid aldehyde fragments generated from the polyunsaturated fatty acids with epsilon amino groups of lysine residues of apoprotein B-100 leads to generation of immunogenic and atherogenic oxidation-specific neoepitopes. The LDL particle becomes smaller, denser, in some cases as dense as HDL, and more negatively charged.

The term "OxLDL" does not imply one specific structure or homogenous molecular form, but a variety of lipid and protein modifications of LDL that are generated from lipid peroxidation that make it atherogenic[11]. Therefore, it is imperative that the conditions under which OxLDL is generated be well defined to allow comparison among studies. This is particularly relevant for clinical studies where measures of circulating OxLDL are increasingly being performed. For this reason, in studies measuring circulating OxLDL we have previously suggested that the antibody used to quantitate OxLDL be used in the designation of OxLDL, to reduce confusion about what is being measured and allow comparisons between published studies. For example, a plasma measure of OxLDL that has been generated by our group, OxLDL-E06, denotes the measurement of oxidized phospholipid (OxPL) epitopes on LDL that is detected by the natural murine IgM autoantibody E06[12-15].

Nonenzymatic

Nonenzymatic oxidation catalyzed by Cu^{2+} is believed to depend upon the presence of lipid hydroperoxides in the LDL[16]. These hydroperoxides are degraded to peroxy and alkoxy radicals by Cu^{2+} and in turn, those radicals can initiate a cyclic chain reaction that can generate many more hydroperoxides. The fatty acid side chains of cholesterol esters and cholesterol's polycyclic sterol ring structure are susceptible to oxidative attack[16]. Generation of minimally modified LDL (mmLDL) can be initiated by incubation of LDL with Cu^{2+} for even a few hours, resulting in inflammatory and proatherogenic biological properties[17], prior to recognition by scavenger receptors[18,19].

Cell-mediated and enzymatic

Due to the presence of abundant antioxidant defenses present in plasma, it is believed that most of the oxidation of LDL occurs in the vessel wall rather than in plasma. In fact, although oxidation-specific epitopes can be present on circulating LDL (i.e. OxLDL-E06), fully oxidized LDL, i.e. the type that is generated in vitro by prolonged exposure to copper, is not present in any significant amounts in plasma. In fact, injection of fully oxidized LDL in animal models results in the rapid elimination from plasma within minutes[20-22]. Incubation of LDL with all cells that are found in atherosclerotic lesions, such as endothelial cells, smooth muscle cells and monocyte/macrophages, and also neutrophils and fibroblasts, accelerates *in vitro* oxidative modification. LDL can also be oxidized at sites of inflammation[23].

In addition to cell mediated oxidation, a number of different enzyme systems such as lipoxygenases[24-28], and phagocyte (i.e. macrophage)-derived myeloperoxidase (MPO)[29], NADPH oxidase[30], inducible nitric oxide synthase and other peroxidases[31], potentially contribute to the oxidation of LDL. Macrophages and/or other phagocytes, which express these enzymes as mechanisms for generating antimicrobial reactive oxygen species essential for native immunity[32], likely amplify oxidative reactions in macrophage-rich areas of atherosclerotic lesions.

Convincing data for a role of the enzyme 12/15-lipoxygenase (LO) in enhancing in vivo oxidation and accelerating murine atherogenesis has recently been demonstrated[33-35]. 12-15 LO "seeds" LDL in tissue fluid, resulting in initiation of lipid peroxidation by hydroperoxides, generation of proinflammatory OxLDL and subsequent enhanced uptake by macrophages[36]. Atherosclerotic lesions of rabbits and humans, but not normal arteries, contain mRNA and protein of 15-LO (the homologous enzyme in rabbits and humans)[37], and stereospecific products of the LO reaction can be found in atherosclerotic lesions, consistent with enzymatic oxidation[38,39]. Additional evidence to support this hypothesis includes the observations that incubation of LDL with isolated soybean LO leads to oxidation of LDL[24]; that inhibitors of macrophage 12/15-LO decrease the ability of macrophages to initiate oxidation of LDL[28], and that LDL incubated with fibroblasts transfected with LO become "seeded" with fatty acid hydroperoxides, which can then propagate lipid peroxidation under the proper conditions[25,40]. Also, treatment of hypercholesterolemic rabbits with specific inhibitors of 15-LO reduces the progression of atherosclerosis[41,42].

However, the most convincing evidence for the in vivo role of 12/15 LO, at least in murine atherogenesis, has been provided by showing that crossing 12/15-LO deficient mice into apoE-deficient mice caused an ~50% reduction in the extent of atherosclerotic lesions, despite similar blood lipid profiles in both groups[33-35]. Urinary and plasma levels of F_2-isoprostanes, non-enzymatic breakdown products resulting from lipid peroxidation of arachidonic acid, and OxLDL autoantibodies were also reduced and both highly correlated with plaque burden and with each other. In another study, 12/15-LO deficient mice crossed into LDLR$^{-/-}$ mice also had reduction in the extent of atherosclerosis[43]. Conversely, overexpression of 15-LO in endothelial cells led to an enhancement of atherosclerosis in LDLR-negative mice[44] and 12/15-LO overexpression in C57BL/6J mice was shown to mediate monocyte/endothelial cell interactions in the vessel wall at least in part through molecular regulation of expression of endothelial adhesion molecules[45]. Additional studies have shown that combined paraoxonase/apoE-deficient knockout mice have enhanced LDL oxidation, detected by enhanced clearance of intravenously injected LDL and faster generation of plasma levels of circulating OxLDL and immune complexes, and attendant enhanced atherosclerosis[46]. Although it is possible that 12/15-LO affected atherogenesis by other mechanisms, these studies lend strong support to the concept that a major mechanism by which 12/15-LO deficiency decreased atherosclerosis was by decreasing the extent of lipid peroxidation, and specifically, the generation of OxLDL. However, not all data are consistent in this regard and it is possible that species differences may exist as exemplified by a study showing that macrophage-specific overexpression of 15-LO led to protection against atherosclerosis in cholesterol fed-rabbits[47,48]. The reasons for these differences are unclear but the 12/15-LO deletion in the mouse studies was global, while the studies with 15-LO overexpression in rabbits were tissue-specific. Similarly, conflicting results have been observed for the contributions of endothelial and inducible nitric oxide synthases to the development of atherosclerosis in mouse models[49-52]. It is possible that mechanisms responsible for LDL oxidation differ between humans and animal models.

It is also likely that in vivo there are many mechanisms beside LO by which LDL is oxidized within the artery wall[53,54]. For example, MPO is a heme enzyme secreted by neutrophils and monocytes that generates a number of oxidants, including hypochlorous acid (HOCl), which can initiate lipid oxidation and peroxidation. MPO has been identified in human atherosclerotic lesions and is of particular interest because lipid modifications found in human atherosclerosis bear similarities to hypochlorous acid-mediated derivation of lipoprotein constituents in vitro[55]. Interestingly, a recent study showed that a single initial measurement of plasma myeloperoxidase levels in patients presenting to the emergency room with chest pain and negative troponin T levels independently predicted in-hospital risk of myocardial infarction (MI), as well as the risk of major adverse cardiac events at 30-day and 6-month periods[56]. However, in bone marrow transplantation experiments in which LDLR$^{-/-}$ mice received MPO-deficient bone marrow progenitor cells, larger lesions were observed than in LDLR$^{-/-}$ mice transplanted with wild type progenitor cells. Similar results were seen when MPO-deficient mice were crossed into LDLR$^{-/-}$ mice. However, there was no evidence for the presence of MPO in murine lesions and the types of MPO-dependent oxidation products found in human lesions were not present in murine lesions[57], suggesting that MPO could not be directly related to lesion formation in mice.

The leukocyte 5-LO has recently been identified as a significant modifier of susceptibility to atherosclerosis in inbred strains of mice[58,59]. This observation may be linked to LDL modification, but a direct association has not yet been established.

Macrophage foam cell formation

Oxidative modification of LDL

The most compelling evidence of the primacy of LDL in contributing to the pathogenesis of atherosclerosis is demonstrated by the premature atherosclerosis seen in homozygous familial hypercholesterolemia (HFH)[60]. Patients with HFH, with a prevalence of 1:1,000,000, develop plasma LDL cholesterol levels of 500-1000 mg/dl and have been documented to have MIs as early as 18 months of age and usually succumb to various manifestations of ischemic cardiovascular disease by the third decade of life. HFH, estimated to be present in 1:500 individuals, results in LDL cholesterol levels of 200-350 mg/dl, and greatly accelerated, clinically relevant, atherosclerosis as well. Before the statin era, ~5% of males had an MI by age 30 years; 25% had died of MI by age 50 years; and 50% had died by age 60 years compared to only 10% of non affected male siblings. Even 30% of FH females will have coronary artery disease by age 60[61]. This monogenic disorder manifests its phenotypic expression through one of >600 reported mutations within the LDL receptor (LDLR) gene, a membrane protein to which LDL binds with high affinity and which leads to its internalization and degradation within the cell, that reduces LDLR number and/or activity[62].

Paradoxically, patients with HFH, despite the absence of LDLR, develop excessive numbers of foam cells, manifested by the accumulation of cholesterol in subcutaneous and tendon xanthomas and in arterial lesions. Their circulating LDL, while it does show some relatively minor differences in structure from that of normal LDL, behaves metabolically like LDL from normal subjects[63]. In addition, incubation of monocyte/macrophages with very high concentrations of native LDL *in vitro* does not lead to accumulation of cholesterol[64]. The underlying mechanisms mediating macrophage foam cell formation in the absence of LDLR were clarified in 1979 by the landmark studies of Brown and Goldstein when they discovered the "acetyl LDL receptor"[64]. They demonstrated that treatment of LDL *in vitro* with acetic anhydride leading to modification of a significant fraction of the lysine residues of apoB, generated a modified form of LDL, acetyl-LDL, that was taken up much more rapidly than native LDL by a specific, saturable receptor by cultured macrophages (*Figure 1*).

Unlike the LDL receptor which downregulates as the cell cholesterol content increases, the acetyl LDL receptor, which is expressed at normal levels in patients with LDLR deficiency, is not downregulated and is fully active even as the cell cholesterol content increases markedly. Kodama et al[65] subsequently cloned and sequenced the acetyl LDL receptor which was redesignated the scavenger receptor, type A, or SR-A. In vitro, chemical acetoacetylation or conjugation of LDL with malondialdehyde (MDA) or via aggregated platelets releasing MDA generates MDA-LDL, which is recognized by SR-A[66,67]. However, the concentrations of MDA needed to generate MDA-LDL in vitro seem to be significantly higher than could be achieved in vivo, although MDA-LDL epitopes are abundant in atherosclerotic lesions[68-70].

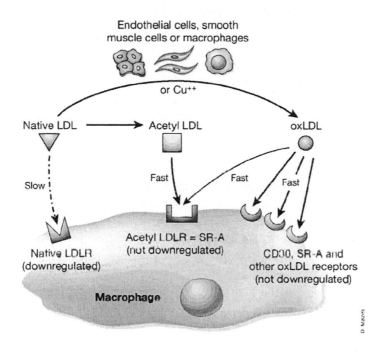

Figure 1. **Mechanisms of OxLDL uptake by monocytes.** Native LDL cannot induce foam-cell formation because uptake is slow and because the LDL receptor downregulates. Either acetyl LDL or OxLDL can induce cholesterol accumulation in macrophages resulting in foam-cell formation because uptake is rapid and the scavenger receptors do not downregulate in response to an increase in cellular cholesterol. Reproduced with permission from Steinberg.[1]

Further evidence for a potential clinically relevant mechanism of foam cell formation was provided by Steinberg and colleagues in 1981 when they showed that overnight incubation of LDL with a cultured monolayer of endothelial cells[71], vascular smooth muscle cells[72] or with peritoneal macrophages[73,74] in a medium rich in metal ions generated modified LDL with a marked increase in the rate of uptake and degradation by mouse peritoneal macrophages. The binding and uptake of the modified LDL was competitively inhibited by unlabeled acetyl LDL (~60%) indicating that a large part of the uptake was by way of SR-A and implying at the same time that additional receptors must be involved. Subsequent studies showed that these changes could be reproduced by simply incubating the LDL with copper to catalyze nonenzymatic oxidation and that all of these cell-induced changes can be blocked by adding vitamin E to the medium[8]. Morel et al[75] also observed that oxidatively modified LDL was cytotoxic for cultured endothelial cells and that antioxidants prevented generation of that cytotoxicity.

Alternative ways to account for foam cell formation

There are a number of potential alternative or complementary mechanisms by which foam cells might be generated, but these have not been as extensively studied nor as well documented as oxidative modification.

βVLDL and other lipoproteins rich in apoprotein E

βVLDL is a minor component of normal plasma and has a density like that of VLDL but beta electrophoretic mobility similar to LDL. βVLDL is enriched in apoprotein E, binds with high affinity to the LDL receptor on macrophages in vitro[76] and is taken up at a sufficiently rapid rate to increase the macrophage cholesterol content[77]. Uptake of βVLDL may occur via other receptors as well, such as LRP, perhaps assisted by binding of lipoprotein lipase (LPL)[78].

Aggregated LDL

Aggregates of LDL, generated by vigorous mixing resulting in denaturation of LDL, results in avid uptake of aggregated LDL via the native LDLR through phagocytosis, rather than endocytosis, which may result in accumulation of intracellular cholesterol in macrophages[79]. Large aggregates of LDL in the matrix of the rabbit arterial intima soon after an intravenous injection of a large single bolus of LDL can be noted[80], but whether this occurs spontaneously in vivo is unclear.

LDL-autoantibody immune complexes

Complexes of LDL or of aggregated LDL with IgG antibodies are taken up by macrophages at a markedly increased rate[81,82]. This is partly because the complex can now be taken up both by way of the LDL receptor and by way of the Fc receptor and perhaps partly because the LDL is further aggregated in the presence of a sufficient concentration of antibody. Increased levels of apoB-immune complexes have been recently documented in patients with acute coronary syndromes (ACS)[14] and following percutaneous coronary intervention (PCI)[15] and decreased levels following treatment of ACS patients with atorvastatin[83].

Complex formation between LDL and proteoglycans

LDL binds tightly to certain forms of proteoglycans, such as dextran sulfate[84,85], and after binding appears to be more susceptible to subsequent oxidative modification[86].

Enzymatically-modified LDL

Several enzyme mediated modifications of LDL (E-LDL), such as sphingomyelinase[87] and trypsin/cholesterol esterase[88,89] and cathepsin H,[90] have documented enhanced uptake by macrophages as well as C-reactive protein binding of E-LDL leading to complement activation[91].

Macrophage scavenger receptors

Macrophages express a variety of scavenger receptors, such as SR-A, CD36, SR-BI, CD68 and scavenger receptor for phosphatidylserine and oxidized lipoprotein (SR-PSOX), that mediate binding and uptake of OxLDL[92-94] (*Figure 1*). As a class, scavenger receptors tend to recognize polyanionic macromolecules and have been proposed to play physiologic roles in the recognition and clearance of pathogens, such as gram positive and negative bacteria[95-97], and apoptotic cells[98-101]. For example, mice generated with SR-A deletion were found to be more susceptible to infections[102]. Since atherosclerosis does not exert any evolutionary pressure, it is unlikely that scavenger receptors evolved as a mechanism for clearing OxLDL. In fact these receptors are found in lower mammals and, at least functionally, as far back as Drosophila[103]. CD36 has also been demonstrated to function as a fatty acid transport protein in adipose tissue and muscle[93], while SR-BI mediates selective uptake of HDL cholesterol esters in liver and steroidogenic tissues[104-106].

Studies in SR-A knockout mice comparing OxLDL binding and internalization by macrophages show that 20-30% of OxLDL uptake is attributable to SR-A[102]. In patients with total deficiency of CD36, monocyte/macrophage uptake of OxLDL is approximately 50% of total compared to patients with normal monocyte/macrophages[107]. Gene deletion and bone marrow transplantation experiments suggest that SR-A and CD36 knockouts result in a significant reduction in the progression of atherosclerosis[102,108,109], implying important quantitative roles of scavenger receptors in mediating atherogenesis. In contrast, studies of the SR-BI gene indicate that it plays an anti-atherogenic role[110,111], as it may facilitate reverse cholesterol transport by HDL by ABCA1-mediated cholesterol efflux in macrophages[112]. Macrophages from mice with combined SR-A and CD36 deficiency show a 75% decrease in uptake of OxLDL in vitro[113]. Interestingly, SR-BI/apo E double knockout mice exhibit severe atherosclerosis with evidence of plaque rupture and acute MI as early as six weeks of life, complications that are rare in other murine models of atherosclerosis this early in life[110].

Manipulation of scavenger receptor number and activity may have theoretical clinical applications. However, this is tempered by the realization that these receptors are involved in multiple beneficial functions unrelated to atherogenesis, such as clearing microorganisms and apoptotic cells. For example, mice generated with SR-A deletion were found to be more susceptible to infections[102]. Therefore, although atherosclerosis may be ameliorated, additional infectious and proliferative lesions may develop.

Cholesterol homeostasis and foam cell formation

Macrophages possess mechanisms for preserving intracellular cholesterol homeostasis via either ABCA1-mediated transport of unesterified cholesterol and phospholipids to nascent HDL and/or conversion of cholesterol to cholesteryl esters[114]. These pathways appear to be overwhelmed in the setting of atherosclerosis through scavenger receptor-mediated uptake of modified lipoproteins resulting in foam cell formation (*Figure 2*). Cholesterol esterification is carried out by acyl coenzyme A: acylcholesterol transferase (ACAT)[115]. Under conditions in which cholesterol efflux pathways become saturated, cholesterol esterification seems to be a protective response to excess free cholesterol, which can be toxic[116]. Disposal of excess cholesterol can be achieved either by delivery to extracellular acceptors, such as lipid-poor apo AI, or by conversion to more soluble forms. Recent studies indicate that members of the ABC family of transport proteins, including ABCA1, also play an important role in the mechanism by which cells transfer excess cholesterol to HDL acceptors. Loss of ABCA1 results in Tangier disease, a condition in which patients have extremely low levels of circulating HDL and massive accumulation of cholesterol in macrophage-rich organs[117-120], and an apparent increased risk of atherosclerosis[114].

Roles of PPARs and LXRs in regulating scavenger receptor activity and cholesterol homeostasis

Peroxisome proliferators activated receptors (PPARs), PPARα, PPARγ and PPARδ, are members of the nuclear receptor superfamily of ligand activated transcription factors[121].The endogenous ligands that regulate PPAR activity remain poorly characterized but are presumed to include fatty acids and their metabolites[122,123]. The prostaglandin 15-deoxy $\Delta^{12,14}$ prostaglandin J_2 and lipoxygenase products including 12 HETE and 13 HODE present in OxLDL, have been suggested to be endogenous ligands for PPARγ in macrophages[124-127]. Fibrates and thiazolidinediones are synthetic ligands for PPARα[128-130] and PPARγ[131], respectively. PPARγ is highly expressed in macrophages and foam cells of atherosclerotic lesions and several lines of evidence suggest that PPARγ agonists can exert both atherogenic and antiatherogenic effects on patterns of gene expression[127,132-134]

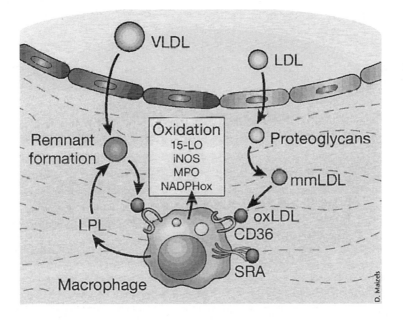

Figure 2. **Mechanisms contributing to foam cell formation.** LDL penetrates into the artery wall where it is trapped after adhering to proteoglycans. It is then highly susceptible to oxidation by enzymes such as lipoxygenases, MPO and iNOS. VLDL particles are subject to modification by lipoprotein lipase. The resulting remnant particles are also subject to trapping by proteoglycans, oxidative modification and uptake by macrophages. mmLDL, minimally modified LDL; SR-A, scavenger receptor class A. Reproduced with permission from Li et al.[206]

PPARγ stimulates expression of the scavenger receptor CD36[134]. PPARγ agonists also inhibit the program of macrophage activation in response to inflammatory mediators such as interferon γ and lipopolysaccharide[133,135,136]. In addition, PPARα and PPARγ have been reported to induce the expression of Liver X receptor α (LXRα), suggesting that PPARs may exert anti-atherogenic effects through secondary activation of LXR target genes[137,138]. LXRs induce the expression of ABC transporters that have been linked to cholesterol efflux[139], serve as an acceptor of cholesterol transported by ABCA1-dependent processes[140], and induce synthesis of fatty acids that are preferential substrates of ACAT in cholesterol esterification reactions[141]. Thus, these genes act in concert to reduce free cholesterol levels and protect macrophages from its cytotoxic effects. The use of LXR agonists indicate that LXRs exert anti-atherogenic effects in mouse models of atherosclerosis[142,143]. The net effects of TZDs in mouse models of atherosclerosis seem to be protective[142,144-146]. In addition, LDLR^-/- mice transplanted with PPARγ^-/- bone marrow progenitor cells develop more extensive atherosclerosis than animals transplanted with wild-type bone marrow, demonstrating a protective role of PPARγ in monocyte-derived macrophages[137].

Properties of oxidized LDL that make it potentially more atherogenic than native LDL

A partial list of biological properties of OxLDL that may make it more atherogenic than native LDL is shown in *Table I*. The four most important properties are described below in detail.

Table 1. **Potential mechanisms by which oxidized LDL may influence atherogenesis**

- OxLDL has enhanced uptake by macrophages leading to foam cell formation
- Products of OxLDL are chemotactic for monocytes and T-cells and inhibit the motility of tissue macrophages
- Products of OxLDL are cytotoxic, in part due to oxidized sterols, and can induce apoptosis
- OxLDL, or products, are mitogenic for smooth muscle cells and macrophages
- OxLDL, or products, can alter gene expression of vascular cells, e.g. induction of MCP-1, colony-stimulating factors, IL-1 and expression of adhesion molecules
- OxLDL, or products, can increase expression of macrophage scavenger receptors, thereby enhancing its own uptake
- OxLDL, or products, can induce proinflammatory genes, e.g. hemoxygenase, SAA and ceruloplasmin
- OxLDL can induce expression and activate PPARγ, thereby influencing many gene functions
- OxLDL is immunogenic and elicits autoantibody formation and activated T-cells
- Oxidation renders LDL more susceptible to aggregation, which independently leads to enhanced uptake. Similarly, OxLDL is a better substrate for sphyingomyelinase, which also aggregates LDL
- OxLDL may enhance procoagulant pathways, e.g. by induction of tissue factor and platelet aggregation
- Products of OxLDL can aversely impact arterial vasomotor properties
- OxLDL is involved in acute coronary syndromes and may potentially lead to plaque disruption

Modified from Tsimikas et al[207]

The ability to induce foam cell formation from monocyte/macrophages and smooth muscle cells

As discussed above, the unregulated uptake of OxLDL by macrophage scavenger receptors causing cholesterol accumulation and foam cell formation was the first observation that suggested this mechanism of the potential importance of OxLDL in atherogenesis.

Recruitment of monocytes from the circulation into the artery wall

In fetal atherosclerosis, OxLDL is present in the vessel wall prior to monocyte recruitment[3]. OxLDL is a chemoattractant for monocytes[147] and T-lymphocytes[148], which are the major cell types that are found in atherosclerotic lesions[149]. OxLDL also inhibits the motility of tissue macrophages[150] which may prevent macrophages from exiting atherosclerotic lesions. MmLDL, which is still recognized by the LDL receptor, stimulates release of monocyte chemoattractant protein-1 (MCP-1) and macrophage colony stimulating factor (M-CSF) from human aortic endothelial cells which can induce recruitment of monocytes into the vessel wall. Many of these biological effects of mmLDL are attributable to oxidized phospholipids, which exist at concentrations that would be biologically active in vivo[151,152]. Lysophosphatidylcholine, a major component of more extensively OxLDL[8], can induce the expression of adhesion molecules and thus contribute to monocyte recruitment[153].

Cytotoxicity

Several laboratories independently showed that endothelial cells or smooth muscle cells incubated in the presence of LDL showed signs of toxicity going on to cell death in 24 to 48 hours[154-156]. This was attributed primarily to conversion of LDL in the medium to OxLDL and the addition of antioxidants or whole serum completely prevented the cytotoxicity. It is not clear if such concentrations may occur in vivo, but the potential for endothelia dysfunction due to endothelial cell toxicity is obviously present.

Inhibition of vasodilatation in response to nitric oxide

Arteries exposed to OxLDL in vitro show an endothelium-dependent vasodilator impairment[157]. Clinical studies show that treatment of patients with coronary artery disease with statins and/or antioxidant compounds can improve endothelial-dependent coronary vasomotion[158,159]. Several studies have shown that circulating OxLDL levels have been associated with endothelial dysfunction[160]. For example, Tamai et al showed that a single session of LDL apheresis significantly increased brachial artery acetylcholine-induced flow mediated dilatation (FMD) within four hours. Interestingly, the best predictors of improvement in FMD were reduction in plasma levels of OxLDL and increased production in nitrate/nitrites[161]. Similarly, the extent of susceptibility of plasma LDL to oxidation[162] and the presence of elevated plasma OxLDL-E06, have been strongly correlated with coronary endothelial dysfunction in a statin regression study[160]. In addition, plasma levels of OxLDL-E06[163] and OxLDL measured by another independent assay[164] have been shown to correlate with coronary endothelial dysfunction in heart transplant recipients.

Evidence that oxidation of LDL takes place in vivo

Because oxidation of LDL is relatively easily prevented if kept in the presence of 5% serum, albumin or several different antioxidants, it suggested that the normal components of extracellular fluid were adequate to provide antioxidant protection under ordinary circumstances[165]. However, there are now many lines of evidence that oxidation of lipoproteins does occur *in vivo* and that this process is quantitatively important[166].

1) When LDL undergoes oxidative modification, a variety of oxidative neoepitopes that have been termed "oxidation-specific" epitopes by Witztum's group[68,69], are generated through the generation of highly reactive small carbon fragments of PUFA that may react with both the lipid and protein portions of autologous LDL. For example, two common epitopes are malondialdehyde (MDA) and 4-hydroxynonenal (4-HNE), which may form adducts with adjacent epsilon-amino groups of lysine residues leading to the generation of MDA-lysine adducts or Schiff base adducts and Michael-type adducts with lysine residues, respectively[69]. Many other similar modifications can be generated, yielding both lipid-protein and lipid-lipid adducts. Even subtle modification of LDL such as the nonenzymatic glycation of apoB results in adduct formation that renders autologous LDL immunogenic[167]. In order to develop antibodies that would recognize these epitopes, Witztum and colleagues prepared model OxLDLs from homologous LDL, such as MDA-LDL and 4-HNE-LDL, and used these to immunize mice to generate "oxidation-specific" murine monoclonal antibodies[68,168]. All of these antibodies immunostained such epitopes in atherosclerotic lesions in rabbits, non-human primates, and humans, but not in normal arterial tissue. Other investigators have developed similar antibodies that immunostain atherosclerotic lesions in a similar manner[169,170].

2) LDL, gently extracted from atherosclerotic tissue of rabbits and humans, shows all the physical, biological, and immunologic properties observed with LDL oxidized *in vitro*[171]. Of particular importance was the demonstration that LDL particles isolated from fatty streak lesions had

enhanced uptake by macrophage scavenger receptors and that this uptake could be competed for by *in vitro* OxLDL.

3) Oxidized lipids, including oxidized sterols, are routinely demonstrable in atherosclerotic tissue, but not in normal aortic tissue[38,39,172-174].

4) Numerous reports now document that circulating LDL displays chemical indices of early stages of oxidation[175,176] and oxidation-specific epitopes can be demonstrated in LDL particles by antibody-based immunochemical techniques[14,15,177-180].

5) Minimal modifications of autologous LDL render it immunogenic. It has been demonstrated that autoantibodies to a variety of epitopes of OxLDL can be found in sera of experimental animal models and humans with atherosclerosis[168,171,178,181]. For example, titers of autoantibodies to epitopes of OxLDL correlated significantly with the extent of atherosclerosis in apoE[-/-] and LDLR[-/-] mice[181] as well as with the presence and quantity of OxLDL in the vessel wall[182]. Furthermore the titers of such autoantibodies are related to the presence and/or the rate of progression of disease in animal models[34,182,183].

6) OxLDL autoantibodies and OxLDL-immune complexes are found in atherosclerotic lesions of mice, rabbits and humans[184,185]. Autoantibody titer to MDA-LDL was highly significant predictor of the progression of carotid intimal-medial-thickness in a group of middle-aged Finnish males[186] and in a recent Swedish cohort[187].There have been now a large number of studies in humans suggesting that the titer of antibodies to epitopes of OxLDL are associated with various clinical manifestations of atherosclerosis or with traditional risk factors for atherosclerosis such as hypertension, diabetes and smoking[188].

7) Oxidized LDL is present in the earliest human fetal lesions even before the presence of monocyte/macrophages[189].

8) Non-invasive imaging with radiolabeled murine and human antibodies show the physical presence of OxLDL in the vessel wall in vivo[70,190-192].

The role of OxLDL in human cardiovascular disease

It was first documented in 1989 by Palinski et al[168] and Ylä-Hertualla et al[171] that OxLDL exists in vivo in both animal and human atherosclerotic lesions. More recently, Nishi et al[180] documented that vulnerable carotid plaques from humans are greatly enriched in OxLDL and that plaque content of OxLDL was 70 times the plasma concentration. Statins have recently been shown to reduce the vessel wall content of OxLDL as well as the plasma levels of circulating OxLDL[83]. For example, in humans pretreated with pravastatin for three months prior to carotid endarterectomy, significantly reduced OxLDL immunostaining was noted in carotid specimens stained with the monoclonal antibody NA59[68,69], which recognizes 4-hydroxynonenal epitopes of OxLDL[193].

Autoantibodies to OxLDL were first documented in animals and patients by Witztum's laboratory in 1989[168,171]. Many human studies have been published subsequently, not all of which are consistent, showing associations with various manifestations of atherosclerosis in patients. The reasons for these inconsistencies are multiple and varied[188] and measurement of autoantibodies to OxLDL, although interesting from a pathophysiological perspective, has not thus far provided additional clinical value above and beyond traditional risk factors.

The ability to measure circulating OxLDL, however, has opened a new arena in studying the role of OxLDL in human disease. Three laboratories have developed antibody-based assays for measuring circulating early forms of OxLDL[12,194,195]. Recent studies have shown that increased levels of circulating OxLDL are found in plasma of patients with coronary[196,197] and carotid artery disease[198] and in ACS[14,179,199]. For example, circulating OxLDL measured on isolated LDL by monoclonal antibody DLH3 correlated well with the presence of OxLDL in coronary atherectomy specimens and appeared to differentiate the severity of the underlying clinical presentation[179]. Increased levels of OxLDL are also associated with increased carotid intima-media thickness[198]. In addition, plasma levels of OxLDL have been shown to correlate with coronary[160] and brachial reactivity[161] following treatment with lovastatin or LDL apheresis, respectively. Recent studies have also shown an association between plasma OxLDL levels and acute cerebral infarction[200] and strong immunostaining for MDA-LDL has been reported in brain tissue of patients with Alzheimer's disease[201]. We recently documented that OxLDL-E06 strongly reflected the presence of ACS in a prospective study with a seven-month follow-up period, showing a characteristic rise and fall in levels. In addition, we documented a strong correlation between OxLDL-E06 and Lp(a) with a correlation of 0.91. Subsequently, we measured serial levels of OxLDL-E06 in patients undergoing uncomplicated PCI for stable angina and showed a 36% and 64% rise post procedure in OxLDL-E06 and Lp(a) levels, respectively (*Figure 3*)[15]. Interestingly, the oxidized phospholipids (OxPL) measured by antibody E06 were present equally on Lp(a) and other apoB lipoproteins post PCI, but subsequently were all transferred to Lp(a) by six hours, suggesting that Lp(a) may act as a sink for OxPL and may mediate their transport and clearance. These observations support the hypothesis that OxPL are present in disrupted plaques and are released into the circulation by PCI, where they are bound by apoB-containing lipoproteins, and preferentially by Lp(a). Furthermore, they define a novel relationship between OxPL and Lp(a) and suggest new insights into the role of Lp(a) in normal physiology as well as in atherogenesis. We have proposed that Lp(a) may in fact contribute to a protective immune response by binding OxPL, similar to binding of OxPL by C-reactive protein[202], as it is highly enriched in PAF-acetylhydrolase which may serve to detoxify OxPL by cleaving the oxidized sn-2 fatty acid. On the other hand, its atherogenicity may rise from the fact that when plasma levels of Lp(a) are elevated, an enhanced number of Lp(a) particles would enter the vessel wall where Lp(a) is preferentially bound to the extra-cellular matrix and with its an enhanced content of OxPL, Lp(a) would have profound pro-inflammatory properties[18].

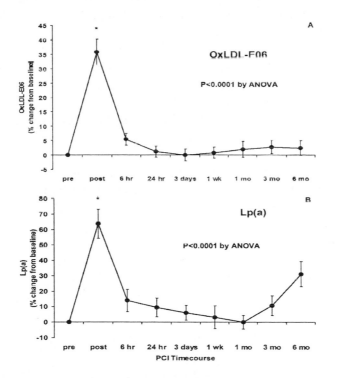

Figure 3. **Mean percent change from pre-PCI levels in OxLDL-E06 (A) and Lp(a) (B) levels following PCI.** *=P<0.001 compared to other timepoints. Reproduced with permission from Tsimikas et al.[15]

The role of OxLDL in response to treatment has not been defined. Iuliano et al[203] have shown that radiolabeled LDL injected into patients with carotid plaques undergoing endarterectomy accumulates in macrophages within these plaques and its uptake is markedly decreased by treatment with vitamin E (900 mg/day) for four weeks. Our group has also recently shown that high-dose atorvastatin (80 mg/day) significantly reduced total plasma levels of OxLDL-E06 (total apoB-OxPL, i.e. OxPL associated with all circulating apoB-100 particles) in patients with ACS in the Myocardial Ischemia Reduction with Aggressive Lipid Lowering therapy (MIRACL) study[83]. Interestingly, in that study, there was enrichment of OxPL on a smaller pool of apoB-100 particles (i.e. increased OxPL/apoB ratio), in parallel with strikingly similar increases in Lp(a), suggesting binding by Lp(a). Additional data has also shown that most of the OxPL epitopes in plasma are associated with Lp(a)[14,15,204]. Unpublished data from our laboratory and our collaborators in monkeys, rabbits, and LDLR[-/-] mice undergoing dietary regression show similar changes in OxLDL-E06 (i.e. marked reduction in total apoB-OxPL but increased in OxPL/apoB in the remaining apoB particles at steady state) in conjunction with significantly reduced OxPL epitopes in the vessel wall. These data support the hypothesis that statins or aggressive lipid lowering promote mobilization and clearance of pro-inflammatory OxPL from the vessel wall and circulation, respectively, which may contribute to a rapid reduction in ischemic events. This is also supported by a recent study showing increases in both Lp(a) and OxPL/apoB levels in patients placed on low fat diets, a condition in which one might postulate efflux of OxPL out of the vessel wall[205].

Future studies will determine if OxLDL plasma measurements provide independent diagnostic or prognostic information above and beyond any easily measured lipoprotein parameters.

References

1. Steinberg D. Atherogenesis in perspective: hypercholesterolemia and inflammation as partners in crime. Nat Med 2002;8:1211-17.
2. Libby P. Inflammation in atherosclerosis. Nature 2002;420:868-74.
3. Napoli C, D'Armiento FP, Mancini FP et al. Fatty streak formation occurs in human fetal aortas and is greatly enhanced by maternal hypercholesterolemia. Intimal accumulation of Low Density Lipoprotein and its oxidation precede monocyte recruitment into early atherosclerotic lesions. J Clin Invest 1997;100:2680-90.
4. Napoli C, Glass CK, Witztum JL et al. Influence of maternal hypercholesterolaemia during pregnancy on progression of early atherosclerotic lesions in childhood: Fate of Early Lesions in Children (FELIC) study. Lancet 1999;354:1234-41.
5. Napoli C, Witztum JL, Calara F et al. Maternal hypercholesterolemia enhances atherogenesis in normocholesterolemic rabbits, which is inhibited by antioxidant or lipid lowering intervention during pregnancy: an experimental model of atherogenic mechanisms in human fetuses. Circ Res 2000;87:946-52.
6. Napoli C, de Nigris F, Welch JS et al. Maternal hypercholesterolemia during pregnancy promotes early atherogenesis in LDL receptor-deficient mice and alters aortic gene expression determined by microarray. Circulation 2002;105:1360-7.
7. Schuh J, Fairclough GF, Jr., Haschemeyer RH. Oxygen-mediated heterogeneity of apo-low-density lipoprotein. Proc Natl Acad Sci U S A 1978;75:3173-7.
8. Steinbrecher UP, Parthasarathy S, Leake DS et al. Modification of low density lipoprotein by endothelial cells involves lipid peroxidation and degradation of low density lipoprotein phospholipids. Proc Natl Acad Sci U S A 1984;81:3883-7.
9. Esterbauer H, Jurgens G, Quehenberger O et al. Autoxidation of human low density lipoprotein: loss of polyunsaturated fatty acids and vitamin E and generation of aldehydes. J Lipid Res 1987;28:495-509.
10. Reaven P, Parthasarathy S, Grasse BJ et al. Effects of oleate-rich and linoleate-rich diets on the susceptibility of low density lipoprotein to oxidative modification in mildly hypercholesterolemic subjects. J Clin Invest 1993;91:668-76.
11. Steinberg D. Oxidized low density lipoprotein--an extreme example of lipoprotein heterogeneity. Isr J Med Sci 1996;32:469-72.
12. Hörkkö S, Bird DA, Miller E et al. Monoclonal autoantibodies specific for oxidized phospholipids or oxidized phospholipid-protein adducts inhibit macrophage uptake of oxidized low-density lipoproteins. J Clin Invest 1999;103:117-28.
13. Tsimikas S, Witztum JL. Measuring circulating oxidized low-density lipoprotein to evaluate coronary risk. Circulation 2001;103:1930-2.
14. Tsimikas S, Bergmark C, Beyer RW et al. Temporal increases in plasma markers of oxidized low-density lipoprotein strongly reflect the presence of acute coronary syndromes. J Am Coll Cardiol 2003;41:360-70.

15. Tsimikas S, Lau HK, Han KR et al. Percutaneous coronary intervention results in acute increases in oxidized phospholipids and Lp(a): Acute and long-term immunological responses to oxidized LDL. Circulation 2004;109:3164-70.

16. Esterbauer H, Gebicki J, Puhl H et al. The role of lipid peroxidation and antioxidants in oxidative modification of LDL. Free Radic Biol Med 1992;13:341-90.

17. Berliner JA, Territo MC, Sevanian A et al. Minimally modified low density lipoprotein stimulates monocyte endothelial interactions. J Clin Invest 1990;85:1260-6.

18. Berliner JA, Subbanagounder G, Leitinger N et al. Evidence for a role of phospholipid oxidation products in atherogenesis. Trends Cardiovasc Med 2001;11:142-7.

19. Navab M, Ananthramaiah GM, Reddy ST et al. Thematic review series: The pathogenesis of atherosclerosis: The oxidation hypothesis of atherogenesis: the role of oxidized phospholipids and HDL. J Lipid Res 2004;45:993-1007.

20. Van Berkel TJ, De Rijke YB, Kruijt JK. Different fate in vivo of oxidatively modified low density lipoprotein and acetylated low density lipoprotein in rats. Recognition by various scavenger receptors on Kupffer and endothelial liver cells. J Biol Chem 1991;266:2282-9.

21. Calara F, Dimayuga P, Niemann A et al. An animal model to study local oxidation of LDL and its biological effects in the arterial wall. Arterioscler Thromb Vasc Biol 1998;18:884-93.

22. Steinbrecher UP, Witztum JL, Parthasarathy S et al. Decrease in reactive amino groups during oxidation or endothelial cell modification of LDL. Correlation with changes in receptor-mediated catabolism. Arteriosclerosis 1987;7:135-43.

23. Liao F, Andalibi A, Qiao JH et al. Genetic evidence for a common pathway mediating oxidative stress, inflammatory gene induction, and aortic fatty streak formation in mice. J Clin Invest 1994;94:877-84.

24. Sparrow CP, Parthasarathy S, Steinberg D. Enzymatic modification of low density lipoprotein by purified lipoxygenase plus phospholipase A2 mimics cell-mediated oxidative modification. J Lipid Res 1988;29:745-53.

25. Benz DJ, Mol M, Ezaki M et al. Enhanced levels of lipoperoxides in low density lipoprotein incubated with murine fibroblast expressing high levels of human 15-lipoxygenase. J Biol Chem 1995;270:5191-7.

26. Parthasarathy S, Wieland E, Steinberg D. A role for endothelial cell lipoxygenase in the oxidative modification of low density lipoprotein. Proc Natl Acad Sci U S A 1989;86:1046-50.

27. Cathcart MK, McNally AK, Chisolm GM. Lipoxygenase-mediated transformation of human low density lipoprotein to an oxidized and cytotoxic complex. J Lipid Res 1991;32:63-70.

28. Rankin SM, Parthasarathy S, Steinberg D. Evidence for a dominant role of lipoxygenase(s) in the oxidation of LDL by mouse peritoneal macrophages. J Lipid Res 1991;32:449-56.

29. Savenkova ML, Mueller DM, Heinecke JW. Tyrosyl radical generated by myeloperoxidase is a physiological catalyst for the initiation of lipid peroxidation in low density lipoprotein. J Biol Chem 1994;269:20394-400.

30. McNally AK, Chisolm GM, III, Morel DW et al. Activated human monocytes oxidize low-density lipoprotein by a lipoxygenase-dependent pathway. J Immunol 1990;145:254-9.

31. Wieland E, Parthasarathy S, Steinberg D. Peroxidase-dependent metal-independent oxidation of low density lipoprotein in vitro: a model for in vivo oxidation? Proc Natl Acad Sci U S A 1993;90:5929-33.

32. Babior BM. Phagocytes and oxidative stress. Am J Med 2000;109:33-44.

33. Cyrus T, Witztum JL, Rader DJ et al. Disruption of the 12/15-lipoxygenase gene diminishes atherosclerosis in apo E deficient mice. J Clin Invest 1999;103:1597-604.

34. Cyrus T, Praticó D, Zhao L et al. Absence of 12/15-lipoxygenase expression decreases lipid peroxidation and atherogenesis in apolipoprotein E-deficient mice. Circulation 2001;103:2277-82.

35. Steinberg D. At last, direct evidence that lipoxygenases play a role in atherogenesis. J Clin Invest 1999;103:1487-8.

36. Parthasarathy S, Santanam N, Ramachandran S et al. Oxidants and antioxidants in atherogenesis. An appraisal [In Process Citation]. J Lipid Res 1999;40:2143-57.

37. Ylä-Herttuala S, Rosenfeld M, Sigal E et al. Gene expression in macrophage-rich human atherosclerotic lesions. 15-lipoxygenase and acteyl low density lipoprotein receptor messenger RNA colocalize with oxidation specific lipid- protein adducts. J Clin Invest 1991;87:1146-52.

38. Folcik VA, Nivar-Aristy RA, Krajewski LP et al. Lipoxygenase contributes to the oxidation of lipids in human atherosclerotic plaques. J Clin Invest 1995;96:504-10.

39. Kuhn H, Belkner J, Zaiss S et al. Involvement of 15-lipoxygenase in early stages of atherogenesis. J Exp Med 1994;179:1903-11.

40. Ezaki M, Witztum JL, Steinberg D. Lipoperoxides in LDL incubated with fibroblasts that overexpress 15-lipoxygenase. J Lipid Res 1995;36:1996-2004.

41. Sendobry SM, Cornicelli JA, Welch K et al. Attenuation of diet-induced atherosclerosis in rabbits with a highly selective 15-lipoxygenase inhibitor lacking significant antioxidant properties. Br J Pharmacol 1997;120:1199-206.

42. Bocan TM, Rosebury WS, Mueller SB et al. A specific 15-lipoxygenase inhibitor limits the progression and monocyte-macrophage enrichment of hypercholesterolemia-induced atherosclerosis in the rabbit. Atherosclerosis 1998;136:203-16.

43. George J, Afek A, Shaish A et al. 12/15-Lipoxygenase gene disruption attenuates atherogenesis in LDL receptor-deficient mice. Circulation 2001;104:1646-50.

44. Harats D, Shaish A, George J et al. Overexpression of 15-lipoxygenase in vascular endothelium accelerates early atherosclerosis in LDL receptor-deficient mice. Arterioscler Thromb Vasc Biol 2000;20:2100-5.

45. Reilly KB, Srinivasan S, Hatley ME et al. 12/15-Lipoxygenase activity mediates inflammatory monocyte/endothelial interactions and atherosclerosis in vivo. J Biol Chem 2004;279:9440-50.

46. Shih DM, Xia YR, Wang XP et al. Combined serum paraoxonase knockout/apolipoprotein E knockout mice exhibit increased lipoprotein oxidation and atherosclerosis. J Biol Chem 2000;275:17527-35.

47. Shen J, Herderick E, Cornhill JF et al. Macrophage-mediated 15-lipoxygenase expression protects against atherosclerosis development. J Clin Invest 1996;98:2201-8.

48. Funk CD, Cyrus T. 12/15-Lipoxygenase, oxidative modification of LDL and atherogenesis. Trends in Cardiovascular Medicine 2001;11:116-24.

49. Detmers PA, Hernandez M, Mudgett J et al. Deficiency in inducible nitric oxide synthase results in reduced atherosclerosis in apolipoprotein E-deficient mice. J Immunol 2000;165:3430-5.

50. Ihrig M, Dangler CA, Fox JG. Mice lacking inducible nitric oxide synthase develop spontaneous hypercholesterolaemia and aortic atheromas. Atherosclerosis 2001;156:103-7.

51. Niu XL, Yang X, Hoshiai K et al. Inducible nitric oxide synthase deficiency does not affect the susceptibility of mice to atherosclerosis but increases collagen content in lesions. Circulation 2001;103:1115-20.

52. Shi W, Wang X, Shih DM et al. Paradoxical reduction of fatty streak formation in mice lacking endothelial nitric oxide synthase. Circulation 2002;105:2078-82.

53. Heinecke JW. Is lipid peroxidation relevant to atherogenesis? J Clin Invest 1999;104:135-6.

54. Gaut JP, Byun J, Tran HD et al. Myeloperoxidase produces nitrating oxidants in vivo. J Clin Invest 2002;109:1311-9.

55. Daugherty A, Dunn JL, Rateri DL et al. Myeloperoxidase, a catalyst for lipoprotein oxidation, is expressed in human atherosclerotic lesions. J Clin Invest 1994;94:437-44.

56. Brennan ML, Penn MS, Van Lente F et al. Prognostic value of myeloperoxidase in patients with chest pain. N Engl J Med 2003;349:1595-604.

57. Brennan ML, Anderson MM, Shih DM et al. Increased atherosclerosis in myeloperoxidase-deficient mice. J Clin Invest 2001;107:419-30.

58. Mehrabian M, Allayee H, Wong J et al. Identification of 5-lipoxygenase as a major gene contributing to atherosclerosis susceptibility in mice. Circ Res 2002;91:120-6.

59. Mehrabian M, Allayee H. 5-lipoxygenase and atherosclerosis. Curr Opin Lipidol 2003;14:447-57.

60. Goldstein JL, Kita T, Brown MS. Defective lipoprotein receptors and atherosclerosis. Lessons from an animal counterpart of familial hypercholesterolemia. N Engl J Med 1983;309:288-96.

61. Goldstein JL, Hobbs HH, Brown MS. The metabolic and molecular bases of inherited disease. New York, NY: Mc-Graw Hill, 1995.

62. Brown MS, Goldstein JL. A receptor-mediated pathway for cholesterol homeostasis. Science 1986;232:34-47.

63. Simons LA, Reichl D, Myant NB et al. The metabolism of the apoprotein of plasma low density lipoprotein in familial hyperbetalipoproteinaemia in the homozygous form. Atherosclerosis 1975;21:283-98.
64. Goldstein JL, Ho YK, Basu SK et al. Binding site on macrophages that mediates uptake and degradation of acetylated low density lipoprotein, producing massive cholesterol deposition. Proc Natl Acad Sci U S A 1979;76:333-7.
65. Kodama T, Freeman M, Rohrer L et al. Type I macrophage scavenger receptor contains alpha-helical and collagen-like coiled coils. Nature 1990;343:531-5.
66. Fogelman AM, Shechter I, Seager J et al. Malondialdehyde alteration of low density lipoproteins leads to cholesteryl ester accumulation in human monocyte-macrophages. Proc Natl Acad Sci U S A 1980;77:2214-8.
67. Mahley RW, Innerarity TL, Weisgraber KB et al. Altered metabolism (in vivo and in vitro) of plasma lipoproteins after selective chemical modification of lysine residues of the apoproteins. J Clin Invest 1979;64:743-50.
68. Palinski W, Ylä-Herttuala S, Rosenfeld ME et al. Antisera and monoclonal antibodies specific for epitopes generated during oxidative modification of low density lipoprotein. Arteriosclerosis 1990;10:325-35.
69. Rosenfeld ME, Palinski W, Ylä-Herttuala S et al. Distribution of oxidation specific lipid-protein adducts and apolipoprotein B in atherosclerotic lesions of varying severity from WHHL rabbits. Arteriosclerosis 1990;10:336-49.
70. Tsimikas S, Shortal BP, Witztum JL et al. In vivo uptake of radiolabeled MDA2, an oxidation-specific monoclonal antibody, provides an accurate measure of atherosclerotic lesions rich in oxidized LDL and is highly sensitive to their regression. Arterioscler Thromb Vasc Biol 2000;20:689-97.
71. Henriksen T, Mahoney EM, Steinberg D. Enhanced macrophage degradation of low density lipoprotein previously incubated with cultured endothelial cells: recognition by receptors for acetylated low density lipoproteins. Proc Natl Acad Sci U S A 1981;78:6499-503.
72. Henriksen T, Mahoney EM, Steinberg D. Interactions of plasma lipoproteins with endothelial cells. Ann N Y Acad Sci 1982;401:102-16.
73. Cathcart MK, Morel DW, Chisolm GM, III. Monocytes and neutrophils oxidize low density lipoprotein making it cytotoxic. J Leukoc Biol 1985;38:341-50.
74. Parthasarathy S, Printz DJ, Boyd D et al. Macrophage oxidation of low density lipoprotein generates a modified form recognized by the scavenger receptor. Arteriosclerosis 1986;6:505-10.
75. Morel DW, Hessler JR, Chisolm GM. Low density lipoprotein cytotoxicity induced by free radical peroxidation of lipid. J Lipid Res 1983;24:1070-6.
76. Pitas RE, Innerarity TL, Mahley RW. Cell surface receptor binding of phospholipid protein complexes containing different ratios of receptor-active and -inactive E apoprotein. J Biol Chem 1980;255:5454-60.

77. Goldstein JL, Ho YK, Brown MS et al. Cholesteryl ester accumulation in macrophages resulting from receptor-mediated uptake and degradation of hypercholesterolemic canine beta-very low density lipoproteins. J Biol Chem 1980;255:1839-48.

78. Chappell DA, Inoue I, Fry GL et al. The carboxy-terminal domain of lipoprotein lipase induces cellular catabolism of normal very low density lipoproteins via the low density lipoprotein receptor-related protein/alpha 2-macroglobulin receptor. Ann N Y Acad Sci 1994;737:434-8.

79. Khoo JC, Miller E, McLoughlin P et al. Enhanced macrophage uptake of low density lipoprotein after self-aggregation. Arteriosclerosis 1988;8:348-58.

80. Nievelstein PF, Fogelman AM, Mottino G et al. Lipid accumulation in rabbit aortic intima 2 hours after bolus infusion of low density lipoprotein. A deep-etch and immunolocalization study of ultrarapidly frozen tissue. Arterioscler Thromb 1991;11:1795-805.

81. Khoo JC, Miller E, Pio F et al. Monoclonal antibodies against LDL further enhance macrophage uptake of LDL aggregates. Arterioscler Thromb 1992;12:1258-66.

82. Lopes-Virella MF, Griffith RL, Shunk KA et al. Enhanced uptake and impaired intracellular metabolism of low density lipoprotein complexed with anti-low density lipoprotein antibodies. Arterioscler Thromb 1991;11:1356-67.

83. Tsimikas S, Witztum JL, Miller ER et al. Circulating oxidized LDL markers reflect the clinical benefit noted with atorvastatin in the myocardial ischemia reduction with aggressive lipid lowering therapy (MIRACL) Trial. Circulation 2003;108:IV-479.

84. Camejo G. The interaction of lipids and lipoproteins with the intercellular matrix of arterial tissue: its possible role in atherogenesis. Adv Lipid Res 1982;19:1-53.

85. Kaplan M, Aviram M. Retention of oxidized LDL by extracellular matrix proteoglycans leads to its uptake by macrophages: an alternative approach to study lipoproteins cellular uptake. Arterioscler Thromb Vasc Biol 2001;21:386-93.

86. Hurt E, Camejo G. Effect of arterial proteoglycans on the interaction of LDL with human monocyte-derived macrophages. Atherosclerosis 1987;67:115-26.

87. Marathe S, Choi Y, Leventhal AR et al. Sphingomyelinase converts lipoproteins from apolipoprotein E knockout mice into potent inducers of macrophage foam cell formation. Arterioscler Thromb Vasc Biol 2000;20:2607-13.

88. Torzewski M, Klouche M, Hock J et al. Immunohistochemical demonstration of enzymatically modified human LDL and its colocalization with the terminal complement complex in the early atherosclerotic lesion. Arterioscler Thromb Vasc Biol 1998;18:369-78.

89. Kapinsky M, Torzewski M, Buchler C et al. Enzymatically degraded LDL preferentially binds to CD14high CD16+ monocytes and induces foam cell formation mediated only in part by the class B scavenger-receptor CD36. Arterioscler Thromb Vasc Biol 2001;21:1004-10.

90. Han SR, Momeni A, Strach K et al. Enzymatically modified LDL induces cathepsin H in human monocytes: potential relevance in early atherogenesis. Arterioscler Thromb Vasc Biol 2003;23:661-7.

91. Bhakdi S, Torzewski M, Paprotka K et al. Possible protective role for C-reactive protein in atherogenesis: complement activation by modified lipoproteins halts before detrimental terminal sequence. Circulation 2004;109:1870-6.

92. Boullier A, Gillotte KL, Hörkkö S et al. The binding of oxidized low density lipoprotein to mouse CD36 is mediated in part by oxidized phospholipids that are associated with both the lipid and protein moieties of the lipoprotein [In Process Citation]. J Biol Chem 2000;275:9163-9.

93. Febbraio M, Hajjar DP, Silverstein RL. CD36: a class B scavenger receptor involved in angiogenesis, atherosclerosis, inflammation, and lipid metabolism. J Clin Invest 2001;108:785-91.

94. Linton MF, Fazio S. Class A Scavenger receptors, macrophages, and atherosclerosis. Curr Opin Lipidol 2001;12:489-95.

95. Krieger M, Acton S, Ashkenas J et al. Molecular flypaper, host defense, and atherosclerosis. Structure, binding properties, and functions of macrophage scavenger receptors. J Biol Chem 1993;268:4569-72.

96. Binder CJ, Chang MK, Shaw PX et al. Innate and acquired immunity in atherogenesis. Nat Med 2002;8:1218-26.

97. Binder CJ, Horkko S, Dewan A et al. Pneumococcal vaccination decreases atherosclerotic lesion formation: molecular mimicry between Streptococcus pneumoniae and oxidized LDL. Nat Med 2003;9:736-43

98. Fadok VA, Savill JS, Haslett C et al. Different populations of macrophages use either the vitronectin receptor or the phosphatidylserine receptor to recognize and remove apoptotic cells. J Immunol 1992;149:4029-35.

99. Fadok VA, Voelker DR, Campbell PA et al. Exposure of phosphatidylserine on the surface of apoptotic lymphocytes triggers specific recognition and removal by macrophages. J Immunol 1992;148:2207-16.

100. Savill J, Fadok V, Henson P et al. Phagocyte recognition of cells undergoing apoptosis. Immunol Today 1993;14:131-6.

101. Chang MK, Bergmark C, Laurila A et al. Monoclonal antibodies against oxidized low-density lipoprotein bind to apoptotic cells and inhibit their phagocytosis by elicited macrophages: evidence that oxidation-specific epitopes mediate macrophage recognition. Proc Natl Acad Sci U S A 1999;96:6353-8.

102. Suzuki H, Kurihara Y, Takeya M et al. A role for macrophage scavenger receptors in atherosclerosis and susceptibility to infection. Nature 1997;386:292-6.

103. Krieger M, Herz J. Structures and functions of multiligand lipoprotein receptors: macrophage scavenger receptors and LDL receptor-related protein (LRP). Annu Rev Biochem 1994;63:601-37.

104. Acton S, Rigotti A, Landschulz KT et al. Identification of scavenger receptor SR-BI as a high density lipoprotein receptor. Science 1996;271:518-20.

105. Ji Y, Wang N, Ramakrishnan R et al. Hepatic scavenger receptor BI promotes rapid clearance of high density lipoprotein free cholesterol and its transport into bile. J Biol Chem 1999;274:33398-402.

106. Kozarsky KF, Donahee MH, Rigotti A et al. Overexpression of the HDL receptor SR-BI alters plasma HDL and bile cholesterol levels. Nature 1997;387:414-7.

107. Nozaki S, Kashiwagi H, Yamashita S et al. Reduced uptake of oxidized low density lipoproteins in monocyte-derived macrophages from CD36-deficient subjects. J Clin Invest 1995;96:1859-65.

108. Febbraio M, Podrez EA, Smith JD et al. Targeted disruption of the class B scavenger receptor CD36 protects against atherosclerotic lesion development in mice. J Clin Invest 2000;105:1049-56.

109. Sakaguchi H, Takeya M, Suzuki H et al. Role of macrophage scavenger receptors in diet-induced atherosclerosis in mice. Lab Invest 1998;78:423-34.

110. Braun A, Trigatti BL, Post MJ et al. Loss of SR-BI expression leads to the early onset of occlusive atherosclerotic coronary artery disease, spontaneous myocardial infarctions, severe cardiac dysfunction, and premature death in apolipoprotein E-deficient mice. Circ Res 2002;90:270-6.

111. Huszar D, Varban ML, Rinninger F et al. Increased LDL cholesterol and atherosclerosis in LDL receptor-deficient mice with attenuated expression of scavenger receptor B1. Arterioscler Thromb Vasc Biol 2000;20:1068-73.

112. Chen W, Silver DL, Smith JD et al. Scavenger receptor-BI inhibits ATP-binding cassette transporter 1- mediated cholesterol efflux in macrophages. J Biol Chem 2000;275:30794-800.

113. Kunjathoor VV, Febbraio M, Podrez EA et al. Scavenger receptors class A-I/II and CD36 are the principal receptors responsible for the uptake of modified low density lipoprotein leading to lipid loading in macrophages. J Biol Chem 2002;277:49982-8.

114. Tall AR, Wang N. Tangier disease as a test of the reverse cholesterol transport hypothesis. J Clin Invest 2000;106:1205-7.

115. Brewer HB, Jr. The lipid-laden foam cell: an elusive target for therapeutic intervention. J Clin Invest 2000;105:703-5.

116. Accad M, Smith SJ, Newland DL et al. Massive xanthomatosis and altered composition of atherosclerotic lesions in hyperlipidemic mice lacking acyl CoA:cholesterol acyltransferase 1. J Clin Invest 2000;105:711-9.

117. Bodzioch M, Orso E, Klucken J et al. The gene encoding ATP-binding cassette transporter 1 is mutated in Tangier disease. Nat Genet 1999;22:347-51.

118. Brooks-Wilson A, Marcil M, Clee SM et al. Mutations in ABC1 in Tangier disease and familial high-density lipoprotein deficiency. Nat Genet 1999;22:336-45.

119. Lawn RM, Wade DP, Garvin MR et al. The Tangier disease gene product ABC1 controls the cellular apolipoprotein-mediated lipid removal pathway. J Clin Invest 1999;104:R25-R31.

120. Rust S, Rosier M, Funke H. Tangier disease is caused by mutations in the gene encoding ATP-binding cassette transporter 1. Nature Genet 1999;22:352-5.

121. Willson TM, Brown PJ, Sternbach DD et al. The PPARs: from orphan receptors to drug discovery. J Med Chem 2000;43:527-50.

122. Chawla A, Lee CH, Barak Y et al. PPAR delta is a very low-density lipoprotein sensor in macrophages. Proc Natl Acad Sci U S A 2003;100:1268-73.

123. Ziouzenkova O, Perrey S, Asatryan L et al. Lipolysis of triglyceride-rich lipoproteins generates PPAR ligands: evidence for an antiinflammatory role for lipoprotein lipase. Proc Natl Acad Sci U S A 2003;100:2730-5.

124. Forman BM, Tontonoz P, Chen J et al. 15-Deoxy-delta 12, 14-prostaglandin J2 is a ligand for the adipocyte determination factor PPAR gamma. Cell 1995;83:803-12.

125. Kliewer SA, Lenhard JM, Willson TM et al. A prostaglandin J2 metabolite binds peroxisome proliferator-activated receptor gamma and promotes adipocyte differentiation. Cell 1995;83:813-9.

126. Huang JT, Welch JS, Ricote M et al. Interleukin-4-dependent production of PPAR-gamma ligands in macrophages by 12/15-lipoxygenase. Nature 1999;400:378-82.

127. Nagy L, Tontonoz P, Alvarez JG et al. Oxidized LDL regulates macrophage gene expression through ligand activation of PPAR gamma. Cell 1998;93:229-40.

128. Barak Y, Nelson MC, Ong ES et al. PPAR gamma is required for placental, cardiac, and adipose tissue development. Mol Cell 1999;4:585-95.

129. Rosen ED, Sarraf P, Troy AE et al. PPAR gamma is required for the differentiation of adipose tissue in vivo and in vitro. Mol Cell 1999;4:611-7.

130. Barbier O, Torra IP, Duguay Y et al. Pleiotropic actions of peroxisome proliferator-activated receptors in lipid metabolism and atherosclerosis. Arterioscler Thromb Vasc Biol 2002;22:717-26.

131. Lehmann JM, Moore LB, Smith-Oliver TA et al. An antidiabetic thiazolidinedione is a high affinity ligand for peroxisome proliferator-activated receptor gamma (PPAR gamma). J Biol Chem 1995;270:12953-6.

132. Ricote M, Huang J, Fajas L et al. Expression of the peroxisome proliferator-activated receptor gamma (PPAR gamma) in human atherosclerosis and regulation in macrophages by colony stimulating factors and oxidized low density lipoprotein. Proc Natl Acad Sci U S A 1998;95:7614-9.

133. Ricote M, Li AC, Willson TM et al. The peroxisome proliferator-activated receptor-gamma is a negative regulator of macrophage activation. Nature 1998;391:79-82.

134. Tontonoz P, Nagy L, Alvarez JG et al. PPAR gamma promotes monocyte/macrophage differentiation and uptake of oxidized LDL. Cell 1998;93:241-52.

135. Jiang C, Ting AT, Seed B. PPAR-gamma agonists inhibit production of monocyte inflammatory cytokines. Nature 1998;391:82-6.

136. Marx N, Schonbeck U, Lazar MA et al. Peroxisome proliferator-activated receptor gamma activators inhibit gene expression and migration in human vascular smooth muscle cells. Circ Res 1998;83:1097-103.

137. Chawla A, Boisvert WA, Lee CH et al. A PPAR gamma-LXR-ABCA1 pathway in macrophages is involved in cholesterol efflux and atherogenesis. Mol Cell 2001;7:161-71.

138. Chinetti G, Lestavel S, Bocher V et al. PPAR-alpha and PPAR-gamma activators induce cholesterol removal from human macrophage foam cells through stimulation of the ABCA1 pathway. Nat Med 2001;7:53-8.

139. Chawla A, Repa JJ, Evans RM et al. Nuclear receptors and lipid physiology: opening the X-files. Science 2001;294:1866-70.

140. Laffitte BA, Repa JJ, Joseph SB et al. LXRs control lipid-inducible expression of the apolipoprotein E gene in macrophages and adipocytes. Proc Natl Acad Sci U S A 2001;98:507-12.

141. Repa JJ, Liang G, Ou J et al. Regulation of mouse sterol regulatory element-binding protein-1c gene (SREBP-1c) by oxysterol receptors, LXRalpha and LXRbeta. Genes Dev 2000;14:2819-30.

142. Claudel T, Leibowitz MD, Fievet C et al. Reduction of atherosclerosis in apolipoprotein E knockout mice by activation of the retinoid X receptor. Proc Natl Acad Sci U S A 2001;98:2610-5.

143. Joseph SB, McKilligin E, Pei L et al. Synthetic LXR ligand inhibits the development of atherosclerosis in mice. Proc Natl Acad Sci U S A 2002;99:7604-9.

144. Chen Z, Ishibashi S, Perrey S et al. Troglitazone inhibits atherosclerosis in apolipoprotein E-knockout mice: pleiotropic effects on CD36 expression and HDL. Arterioscler Thromb Vasc Biol 2001;21:372-7.

145. Collins AR, Meehan WP, Kintscher U et al. Troglitazone inhibits formation of early atherosclerotic lesions in diabetic and nondiabetic low density lipoprotein receptor-deficient mice. Arterioscler Thromb Vasc Biol 2001;21:365-71.

146. Li AC, Brown KK, Silvestre MJ et al. Peroxisome proliferator-activated receptor gamma ligands inhibit development of atherosclerosis in LDL receptor-deficient mice. J Clin Invest 2000;106:523-31.

147. Quinn MT, Parthasarathy S, Fong LG et al. Oxidatively modified low density lipoproteins: a potential role in recruitment and retention of monocyte/macrophages during atherogenesis. Proc Natl Acad Sci U S A 1987;84:2995-8.

148. McMurray HF, Parthasarathy S, Steinberg D. Oxidatively modified low density lipoprotein is a chemoattractant for human T lymphocytes. J Clin Invest 1993;92:1004-8.

149. Jonasson L, Holm J, Skalli O et al. Regional accumulations of T cells, macrophages, and smooth muscle cells in the human atherosclerotic plaque. Arteriosclerosis 1986;6:131-8.

150. Quinn MT, Parthasarathy S, Steinberg D. Endothelial cell-derived chemotactic activity for mouse peritoneal macrophages and the effects of modified forms of low density lipoprotein. Proc Natl Acad Sci U S A 1985;82:5949-53.

151. Watson AD, Navab M, Hama SY et al. Effect of platelet activating factor-acetylhydrolase on the formation and action of minimally oxidized low density lipoprotein. J Clin Invest 1995;95:774-82.

152. Subbanagounder G, Leitinger N, Schwenke DC et al. Determinants of bioactivity of oxidized phospholipids: Specific oxidized fatty acyl groups at the sn-2 position. Arterioscler Thromb Vasc Biol 2000;20:2248-54.

153. Kume N, Cybulsky MI, Gimbrone MA, Jr. Lysophosphatidylcholine, a component of atherogenic lipoproteins, induces mononuclear leukocyte adhesion molecules in cultured human and rabbit arterial endothelial cells. J Clin Invest 1992;90:1138-44.

154. Hessler JR, Morel DW, Lewis LJ et al. Lipoprotein oxidation and lipoprotein-induced cytotoxicity. Arteriosclerosis 1983;3:215-22.

155. Henriksen T, Evensen SA, Carlander B. Injury to human endothelial cells in culture induced by low density lipoproteins. Scand J Clin Lab Invest 1979;39:361-8.

156. Morel DW, DiCorleto PE, Chisolm GM. Endothelial and smooth muscle cells alter low density lipoprotein in vitro by free radical oxidation. Arteriosclerosis 1984;4:357-64.

157. Kugiyama K, Kerns SA, Morrisett JD et al. Impairment of endothelium-dependent arterial relaxation by lysolecithin in modified low-density lipoproteins. Nature 1990;344:160-2.

158. Anderson TJ, Meredith IT, Yeung AC et al. The effect of cholesterol-lowering and antioxidant therapy on endothelium-dependent coronary vasomotion. N Engl J Med 1995;332:488-93.

159. Treasure CB, Klein JL, Weintraub WS et al. Beneficial effects of cholesterol-lowering therapy on the coronary endothelium in patients with coronary artery disease. N Engl J Med 1995;332:481-7.

160. Penny WF, Ben Yehuda O, Kuroe K et al. Improvement of coronary artery endothelial dysfunction with lipid-lowering therapy: heterogeneity of segmental response and correlation with plasma-oxidized low density lipoprotein. J Am Coll Cardiol 2001;37:766-74.

161. Tamai O, Matsuoka H, Itabe H et al. Single LDL apheresis improves endothelium-dependent vasodilatation in hypercholesterolemic humans. Circulation 1997;95:76-82.

162. Anderson TJ, Meredith IT, Charbonneau F et al. Endothelium-dependent coronary vasomotion relates to the susceptibility of LDL to oxidation in humans. Circulation 1996;93:1647-50.

163. Fang JC, Kinlay S, Behrendt D et al. Circulating autoantibodies to oxidized LDL correlate with impaired coronary endothelial function after cardiac transplantation. Arterioscler Thromb Vasc Biol 2002;22:2044-8.

164. Holvoet P, Stassen JM, Van Cleemput J et al. Oxidized low density lipoproteins in patients with transplant-associated coronary artery disease. Arterioscler Thromb Vasc Biol 1998;18:100-7.

165. Dabbagh AJ, Frei B. Human suction blister interstitial fluid prevents metal ion-dependent oxidation of low density lipoprotein by macrophages and in cell-free systems. J Clin Invest 1995;96:1958-66.

166. Witztum JL, Steinberg D. The oxidative modification hypothesis of atherosclerosis: Does it hold for humans? Trends Cardiovasc Med 2001;11:93-102.

167. Witztum JL, Steinbrecher UP, Kesaniemi YA et al. Autoantibodies to glucosylated proteins in the plasma of patients with diabetes mellitus. Proc Natl Acad Sci U S A 1984;81:3204-8.

168. Palinski W, Rosenfeld ME, Ylä-Herttuala S et al. Low density lipoprotein undergoes oxidative modification in vivo. Proc Natl Acad Sci U S A 1989;86:1372-6.

169. Haberland ME, Fong D, Cheng L. Malondialdehyde-altered protein occurs in atheroma of Watanabe heritable hyperlipidemic rabbits. Science 1988;241:215-8.

170. Boyd HC, Gown AM, Wolfbauer G et al. Direct evidence for a protein recognized by a monoclonal antibody against oxidatively modified LDL in atherosclerotic lesions from a Watanabe heritable hyperlipidemic rabbit. Am J Pathol 1989;135:815-25.

171. Ylä-Herttuala S, Palinski W, Rosenfeld ME et al. Evidence for the presence of oxidatively modified low density lipoprotein in atherosclerotic lesions of rabbit and man. J Clin Invest 1989;84:1086-95.

172. Hulten LM, Lindmark H, Diczfalusy U et al. Oxysterols present in atherosclerotic tissue decrease the expression of lipoprotein lipase messenger RNA in human monocyte-derived macrophages. J Clin Invest 1996;97:461-8.

173. Carpenter KL, Taylor SE, van der Veen C et al. Lipids and oxidised lipids in human atherosclerotic lesions at different stages of development. Biochim Biophys Acta 1995;1256:141-50.

174. Piotrowski JJ, Shah S, Alexander JJ. Mature human atherosclerotic plaque contains peroxidized phosphatidylcholine as a major lipid peroxide. Life Sci 1996;58:735-40.

175. Hodis HN, Kramsch DM, Avogaro P et al. Biochemical and cytotoxic characteristics of an in vivo circulating oxidized low density lipoprotein (LDL-). J Lipid Res 1994;35:669-77.

176. Sevanian A, Hwang J, Hodis H et al. Contribution of an in vivo oxidized LDL to LDL oxidation and its association with dense LDL subpopulations. Arterioscler Thromb Vasc Biol 1996;16:784-93.

177. Itabe H, Yamamoto H, Suzuki M et al. Oxidized phosphatidylcholines that modify proteins. Analysis by monoclonal antibody against oxidized low density lipoprotein. J Biol Chem 1996;271:33208-17.

178. Palinski W, Hörkkö S, Miller E et al. Cloning of monoclonal autoantibodies to epitopes of oxidized lipoproteins from apolipoprotein E-deficient mice. Demonstration of epitopes of oxidized low density lipoprotein in human plasma. J Clin Invest 1996;98:800-14.

179. Ehara S, Ueda M, Naruko T et al. Elevated levels of oxidized low density lipoprotein show a positive relationship with the severity of acute coronary syndromes. Circulation 2001;103:1955-60.

180. Nishi K, Itabe H, Uno M et al. Oxidized LDL in carotid plaques and plasma associates with plaque instability. Arterioscler Thromb Vasc Biol 2002;22:1649-54.

181. Palinski W, Tangirala RK, Miller E et al. Increased autoantibody titers against epitopes of oxidized LDL in LDL receptor-deficient mice with increased atherosclerosis. Arterioscler Thromb Vasc Biol 1995;15:1569-76.

182. Tsimikas S, Palinski W, Witztum JL. Circulating autoantibodies to oxidized LDL correlate with arterial accumulation and depletion of oxidized LDL in LDL receptor-deficient mice. Arterioscler Thromb Vasc Biol 2001;21:95-100.

183. Aikawa M, Sugiyama S, Hill CC et al. Lipid lowering reduces oxidative stress and endothelial cell activation in rabbit atheroma. Circulation 2002;106:1390-6.

184. Ylä-Herttuala S, Palinski W, Butler SW et al. Rabbit and human atherosclerotic lesions contain IgG that recognizes epitopes of oxidized LDL. Arterioscler Thromb 1994;14:32-40.

185. Shaw PX, Hörkkö S, Chang MK et al. Natural antibodies with the T15 idiotype may act in atherosclerosis, apoptotic clearance, and protective immunity. J Clin Invest 2000;105:1731-40.

186. Salonen JT, Ylä-Herttuala S, Yamamoto R et al. Autoantibody against oxidised LDL and progression of carotid atherosclerosis. Lancet 1992;339:883-7.

187. Hulthe J, Bokemark L, Fagerberg B. Antibodies to oxidized LDL in relation to intima-media thickness in carotid and femoral arteries in 58-year-old subjectively clinically healthy men. Arterioscler Thromb Vasc Biol 2001;21:101-7.

188. Palinski W, Witztum JL. Immune responses to oxidative neoepitopes on LDL and phospholipids modulate the development of atherosclerosis. J Intern Med 2000;247:371-80.

189. Palinski W, Napoli C. The fetal origins of atherosclerosis: maternal hypercholesterolemia, and cholesterol-lowering or antioxidant treatment during pregnancy influence in utero programming and postnatal susceptibility to atherogenesis. FASEB J 2002;16:1348-60.

190. Tsimikas S, Palinski W, Halpern SE et al. Radiolabeled MDA2, an oxidation-specific, monoclonal antibody, identifies native atherosclerotic lesions in vivo. J Nucl Cardiol 1999;6:41-53.

191. Shaw PX, Hörkkö S, Tsimikas S et al. Human-derived anti-oxidized LDL autoantibody blocks uptake of oxidized LDL by macrophages and localizes to atherosclerotic lesions in vivo. Arterioscler Thromb Vasc Biol 2001;21:1333-9.

192. Tsimikas S. Noninvasive imaging of oxidized Low-Density Lipoprotein in atherosclerotic plaques with tagged oxidation-specific antibodies. Am J Cardiol 2002;90:L22-7.

193. Crisby M, Nordin-Fredriksson G, Shah PK et al. Pravastatin treatment increases collagen content and decreases lipid content, inflammation, metalloproteinases, and cell death in human carotid plaques: Implications for plaque stabilization. Circulation 2001;103:926-33.

194. Holvoet P, Vanhaecke J, Janssens S et al. Oxidized LDL and malondialdehyde-modified LDL in patients with acute coronary syndromes and stable coronary artery disease. Circulation 1998;98:1487-94.

195. Itabe H, Yamamoto H, Imanaka T et al. Sensitive detection of oxidatively modified low density lipoprotein using a monoclonal antibody. J Lipid Res 1996;37:45-53.

196. Toshima S, Hasegawa A, Kurabayashi M et al. Circulating oxidized low density lipoprotein levels: A biochemical risk marker for coronary heart disease. Arterioscler Thromb Vasc Biol 2000;20:2243-7.

197. Holvoet P, Mertens A, Verhamme P et al. Circulating oxidized LDL is a useful marker for identifying patients with coronary artery disease. Arterioscler Thromb Vasc Biol 2001;21:844-8.

198. Hulthe J, Fagerberg B. Circulating oxidized LDL is associated with subclinical atherosclerosis development and inflammatory cytokines (AIR Study). Arterioscler Thromb Vasc Biol 2002;22:1162-7.

199. Holvoet P, Collen D, van de Werf F. Malondialdehyde-modified LDL as a marker of acute coronary syndromes. JAMA 1999;281:1718-21.

200. Uno M, Kitazato KT, Nishi K et al. Raised plasma oxidised LDL in acute cerebral infarction. J Neurol Neurosurg Psychiatry 2003;74:312-6.

201. Dei R, Takeda A, Niwa H et al. Lipid peroxidation and advanced glycation end products in the brain in normal aging and in Alzheimer's disease. Acta Neuropathol (Berl) 2002;104:113-22.

202. Chang MK, Binder CJ, Torzewski M et al. C-reactive protein binds to both oxidized LDL and apoptotic cells through recognition of a common ligand: Phosphorylcholine of oxidized phospholipids. Proc Natl Acad Sci U S A 2002;99:13043-8.

203. Iuliano L, Mauriello A, Sbarigia E et al. Radiolabeled native low-density lipoprotein injected into patients with carotid stenosis accumulates in macrophages of atherosclerotic plaque: effect of vitamin E supplementation. Circulation 2000;101:1249-54.

204. Edelstein C, Pfaffinger D, Hinman J et al. Lysine-phosphatidylcholine adducts in Kringle V impart unique immunological and potential pro-inflammatory properties to human apolipoprotein(a). J Biol Chem 2003;278:52841-7.

205. Silaste ML, Rantala M, Alfthan G et al. Changes in dietary fat intake alter plasma levels of oxidized low-density lipoprotein and lipoprotein(a). Arterioscler Thromb Vasc Biol 2004;24:498-503.

Chapter 3

PATHOGENESIS OF ATHEROSCLEROSIS

Juan Viles-Gonzalez, Juan J. Badimon, Valentin Fuster
Cardiovascular Institute, Mount Sinai Medical Center, New York, New York

Introduction

Atherosclerosis is the most prevalent disease of modern society. Coronary atherosclerosis and its thrombotic complications are responsible for over one half million deaths annually, and countless other complications, in North America alone. Coronary plaques appear early in one's life and by the end of the second decade, asymptomatic atherosclerotic lesions are present in most people. As these lesions grow, they may eventually limit blood flow to the myocardium resulting in chronic ischemic syndromes. If progression is rapid as in the case of plaque rupture accompanied by superimposed thrombosis, an acute ischemic syndrome such as unstable angina, myocardial infarction (MI), or sudden death may result from the sudden narrowing or occlusion of the artery[1].

Atherosclerosis is primarily a disease of the intima. It is global in it reach, affecting arteries as large as an aorta down to the size of tertiary branches of coronary arteries. By definition, atherosclerosis is characterized by a soft *atherosis* (lipid core) and the hard collagenous *sclerosis*. The connection, between the sclerotic and atheromatous components is uncertain, and attempts to reconstruct a dynamic sequence in the evolution of atherosclerotic plaques, based on morphology and composition, have been disappointing[2].

Fissuring or rupture of an atherosclerotic plaque in the coronary arteries is the principal event in the development of the acute coronary syndromes[3]. The concept that atherosclerotic plaques undergo disruption or rupture leading to thrombus formation was proposed many years ago. Disrupted atherosclerotic plaques are commonly associated with the formation of mural thrombi, anchored to fissures in the disruptured plaque. Angiographic, angioscopic and pathological data have established an association between plaque rupture and the development of unstable angina, acute MI and sudden ischemic death. Additionally, there is ample evidence that plaque rupture, thrombosis, and fibrous organization of the thrombus may also account for the progression of atherosclerotic disease in asymptomatic patients and in those individuals with stable coronary artery disease[4].

The response-to-injury hypothesis of atherosclerosis

During the nineteenth century, two major hypotheses were used to explain the pathogenesis of atherosclerosis. The first was the incrustation hypothesis, proposed by Rokitansky in 1852. It was suggested that intimal thickening resulted from fibrin deposition with subsequent organization by fibroblast and secondary lipid accumulation. The second theory proposed by Virchow in 1856 was the lipid hypothesis. This theory correctly described atherosclerosis as a disease involving the intima. It suggested that lipids transudate into the arterial wall, interact with the extracellular matrix and promote intimal proliferation[6,7]. In the middle half of this century, Duduid suggested that intimal thickening was an accumulation of fibrin and platelets. In the later half of this century, many investigators had demonstrated the active participation of humoral components such as inflammatory cells in the development of atherosclerotic lesions.

The most prevalent view of atherogenesis proposed by Ross integrates these theories into the more complex response-to-injury hypothesis[6]. This theory suggests that dysfunctional alterations to the endothelium result from some sort of injury. This endothelial dysfunction is the trigger for a series of successive events that will be responsible for the formation of atherosclerotic lesions[5,6]. The coexistence of one or more risk factors (hyperlipidemia, smoking, diabetes, hypertension, obesity, etc.) or local hemodynamic factors could contribute to the development of an endothelial lesion. A break in the endothelial barrier will facilitate the entrance of circulating monocytes and plasma lipids into the arterial wall, as well as platelet deposition at the sites of endothelial denudation. Damaged endothelial cells, monocytes, and aggregated platelets through the release of mitogenic factors, such as cytokines, potentiate the migration and proliferation of vascular smooth muscle cells (SMCs); together with increased receptor-mediated lipid accumulation and increased connective tissue synthesis, they eventually shape the typical atheromatous plaque. These processes may account for the slow progression of the disease. However, in some instances a much faster development is observed; thrombosis associated with a disrupted or ruptured plaque seems to be responsible for this process[7,8].

Development of atherosclerosis

The morphologic studies by Herbert C. Stary[9-12] have provided interesting answers about plaque evolution. He performed detailed studies on a cohort of patients ranging from infants to young adults, who had died from noncardiac causes. Stary observed that, in the first three decades of life, the composition of lesions is predominantly lipid and relatively predictable. From the fourth decade on, the composition of more advanced lesions becomes more unpredictable because mechanisms other than lipid accumulation, such as thrombosis, contribute to lesion progression. In 1995 the American Heart Association (AHA) Committee on Vascular Lesions characterized atherosclerotic lesions into eight types based on Stary's observations (*Figure 1*)[9].

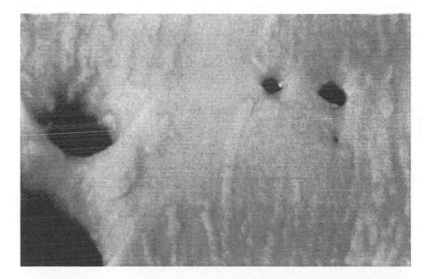

Figure 1. The evolution of atherosclerosis, according to the histological classification proposed by the American Heart Association Committee on Vascular Lesions.

The first observation was that all humans develop focal and eccentric thickening of the intima due to SMC proliferation. This lesion appears very early in life, even as early as the first year of life[13]. At certain sites in the coronary vasculature such as areas of low shear stress at bifurcation points, the endothelium is dysfunctional. There is leakage of lipoproteins into the intima where they are trapped by the extracellular matrix. Cholesterol ester rich lipoproteins undergo oxidation by oxygen free radicals, initiating the events leading to atherosclerotic plaque formation. Initially, there is SMC migration and proliferation. This initial atherosclerotic lesion (Stary type I) is only microscopically and chemically perceivable, and consists of focal intimal thickening characterized by isolated SMC proliferation. Such minimal alterations were found in the coronary arteries of 45% of infants in the first year of life. Fatty streaks (Stary type II lesion) are composed of more lipid-laden cells than initial lesions, and are macroscopically visible as fatty dots or barely raised streaks (*Figure 2*). Oxidized lipoproteins are phagocytized by macrophages resulting in the formation of foam cells. Each lesion is made up of one or more layers of lipid-filled foam cells within the intima, accompanied by occasional scattered SMCs containing lipid droplets. The constituent lipids of type II lesions consist primarily of cholesterol esters, cholesterol, and phospholipids. The main cholesterol fatty acids are cholesteryl oleate and cholesteryl linoleate. Whether a type II lesion develops further is determined in large part by the mechanical forces that act on a particular part of the vessel wall. Mechanical forces are distinct at bifurcation points and branch vessels. At these sites, the influx of lipoproteins is enhanced[10].

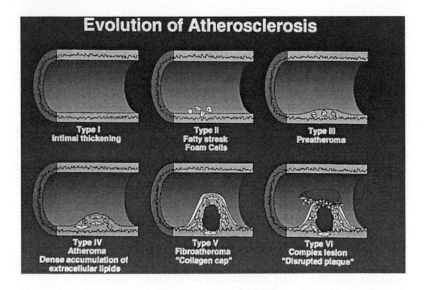

Figure 2. **A picture of a fatty streak (Stary Type II Lesion) taken from an abdominal aorta.**

Progression beyond the fatty streak stage is associated with a sequence of changes starting with the appearance of extra-cellular lipid, forming a more pronounced intimal layer (preatheroma, or Stary type III lesion). Microscopically, extracellular lipid droplets and particles accumulate to form pools deep in the intima that disrupt the structural coherence of SMCs and extracellular matrix. This lesion is, histologically, the bridge between minimal and advanced disease. The presence of a type III lesion probably signals future clinical disease at this location. The same cannot be said for type I and II lesions.

Scattered pools of extracellular lipids may progress to a large, dense and confluent accumulation of extracellular lipid, mainly as free cholesterol and its esters, forming the *lipid core* characteristic of the atheroma, or Stary type IV lesions[14]. Type IV is the first lesion type to be considered as advanced in this histological classification because of the disruption and disorganization of arterial structure caused by the large accumulation of extracellular lipid. The accumulated lipid of this lesion may not narrow the arterial lumen much; thus in many people this lesion is not angiographically visible. The disruption of the structural SMCs by the lipid allows for an increase in the outer perimeter of the arterial segment. The greater outside dimensions in atheromatous segments is necessary to accommodate the eccentric intimal thickening.

In Stary type V lesions or fibroatheroma *(Figure 3)*, SMCs migrate into and proliferate within the plaque, forming a layer over the luminal side of the lipid core. This fibrous cap initially acts as a barrier enveloping the atheromatous core attempting to prevent its extravasation into the lumen. Generally, collagen is synthesized as a reaction to the cell and tissue disruption that results from the accumulation of a lipid core. Initially, there is abundant collagen formation in the fibrous cap. Collagen often becomes the predominant feature, accounting for more of the thickness of the lesion than does the underlying lipid accumulation. As additional collagen is produced, and plaque increases in size, the lipid-rich core becomes avascular and almost totally acellular, consisting of pultaceous debris, including dead macrophages and mesenchymal cells along with abundant free cholesterol crystals (fatty gruel)[15]. Type V lesions, like type IV lesions, are susceptible to rupture and to the formation of mural thrombi. The ingrowth of SMCs and extracellular matrix into the thrombus may have erased evidence of a past plaque rupture and superimposed mural thrombus. Multiple episodes of plaque rupture, thrombus, and integration of the thrombus by SMCs may result in a multilayered appearance of type V lesion, analogous to the rings of a tree. Despite being acutely clinically silent, these repeated cycles of plaque rupture, thrombus formation and integration contribute to progression of chronic ischemic disease, by the progressive narrowing of the lumen. Thrombotic complications are thus far unpredictable. Sometimes, thrombotic episodes can be interspersed by months or years without additional episodes. On the other hand, recurrent new layers of thrombus follow in quick succession, and an occlusion can occur within hours to days. Although type IV and V lesions are usually clinically silent, their recognition by intravascular ultrasound or magnetic resonance imaging may help identify them before they develop symptom producing fissures and superimposed thrombosis[8].

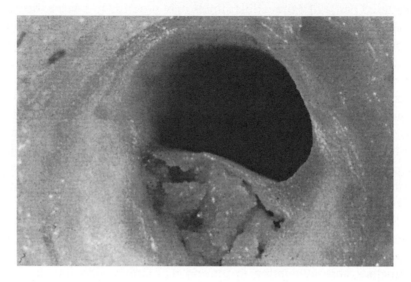

Figure 3. **A macroscopic section of a mature atherosclerotic plaque, or Fibroatheroma (Stary Type V Lesion).** Note the importance of the lipid core, and the overlying fibrous cap.

Lesions having visible thrombotic deposits and/or hemorrhage, in addition to lipid and collagen, are referred to as complicated fibroatheroma or complex lesions (Stary type VI lesions) (*Figure 4*). The clinical manifestations of acute coronary syndromes derive largely from this lesion. The superimposed thrombus accelerates progression beyond the gradual rate of growth of type IV and V lesions[16,17].

Stary type VII lesions are reserved for advanced mineralized lesions (calcific lesion). The intima of these lesions consists of layers of collagen, often hylanized, or of substantial quantities of minerals (calcium). Finally atherosclerotic lesions consisting almost entirely of fibrotic collagen, where the lipid may actually have regressed are referred to as Stary type VIII lesions. Both these lesions can represent the histological end stages of atherosclerotic lesions[18].

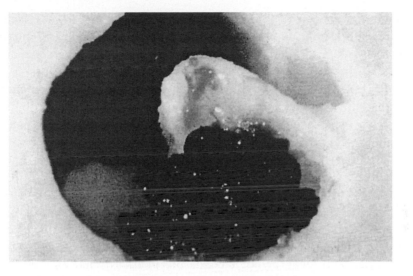

Figure 4. **A disrupted atherosclerotic plaque with superimposed thrombosis. The Complex Lesion (Stary Type VI Lesion).**

The response-to-injury hypothesis and the early atherosclerotic plaque *(Stary type I, II, III):*

Chronic injury to the endothelium is caused mainly by disturbances in blood flow in the artery. Atherosclerotic plaques tend to develop in lesion-prone areas, such as in arterial bifurcations, which are subject to repeated mechanical forces, such as oscillating shear forces[19]. It has been shown that endothelial cells undergo morphological alterations in response to change in the degree and orientation of shear stress: elongated endothelial cells are located in regions of high-shear stress: whereas polygonal endothelial cells are located in regions of low-shear stress. These alterations may be responsible for variations in endothelial permeability to lipoprotein particles[20]. In addition, stagnation in the velocity of blood flow permits increased uptake of atherogenic particles, such as lipoproteins, as a result of increased residence time or prolonged contact with the endothelium[21,22].

In addition to local shear forces and atherogenic lipoproteins, which are enhanced in arterial hypertension, other factors such as hypercholesterolemia, glycosylated products of diabetes, chemical irritants such as nicotine, circulating vasoactive amines, infection and immunocomplexes contribute to endothelial injury[23].

The endothelium

The *endothelium* is intact but dysfunctional in the early phases of atherosclerosis. Endothelial dysfunction is a systemic, reversible disorder considered the precursor that initiates the atherosclerotic process[24,25]. It is characterized by a reduction of the bioavailability of vasodilators, in particular nitric oxide (NO), whereas endothelium-derived contracting factors are increased. This imbalance leads to an impairment of endothelium-dependent vasodilation, the hallmark of endothelial dysfunction. A dysfunctional endothelium promotes lipid and cell permeability, lipoprotein oxidation, inflammation, SMC proliferation, extracellular matrix deposition or lysis, platelet activation, and thrombus formation[26]. The endothelium regulates the production of prothrombotic and antithrombotic factors, growth factors, and vasoactive substances. The clear predilection for lesion formation at arterial branching points indicates the importance of local rheologic conditions in atherosclerosis. Furthermore, endothelial cell gene expression is modulated by acute changes in flow profiles[27]. A dysfunctional endothelium generates a proatherogenic environment by creating a proinflammatory, proliferative and prothrombotic milieu that favors atherogenesis[27]. Platelets and thrombi are often found adherent to areas of *endothelial denudation*, and can become incorporated into the atherosclerotic plaque[28]. Local secretion of NO is diminished in atherosclerotic human coronary arteries[29]. In addition, platelet-derived mediators, such as serotonin, induce vasoconstriction in the presence of a dysfunctional endothelium[30]. Moreover, vasoconstrictor response to these stimuli is increased by endothelin-1[31], concentrations of which are elevated in the plasma of patients with early and advanced atherosclerosis[32], as well as in culprit lesions[33]. Endothelial dysfunction is involved in the recruitment of inflammatory cells into the vessel wall and in the initiation of atherosclerosis. Endothelial cells produce cytokines and express adhesion molecules (e.g., selectins, and vascular and intercellular cell adhesion molecules), and assist leukocytes and other blood-derived cells in "homing" and infiltration. Monocytes migrate into the subendothelium, where they transform into macrophages and modulate inflammatory reactions and the secretion of chemoattractants. Many of the cardiovascular risk factors, including hyperlipidemia, hypertension, diabetes, and smoking are associated with overproduction of reactive oxygen species or increased oxidative stress, thus reducing vascular NO bioavailability and promoting cellular damage[34]. Hence, increased oxidative stress is considered a major mechanism involved in the pathogenesis of endothelial dysfunction and may serve as a common pathogenic mechanism of the effect of risk factors on the endothelium[34,35]. In summary, endothelial dysfunction contributes to enhanced plaque vulnerability, may trigger plaque rupture, and favors thrombus formation. Thus it may be viewed as an important causal factor for several aspects of atherothrombotic disease[36], compounded by the toxic effects of oxidized low-density lipoprotein (LDL), and degradation products such as oxygen free-radicals[37,38]. An arteriographic study has shown that there is progressive impairment of endothelial vasoactive function in patients with hypercholesterolemia progressing to vasoconstriction in angiographically atherosclerotic arteries[33].

Lipid accumulation

It is now firmly established that high levels of LDL are associated with atherosclerosis. Lipids deposited in these atherosclerotic lesions are predominantly derived from plasma LDLs. Two mechanisms are involved in the internalization and intravascular accumulation of cholesterol and its esters: the first is active and depends on specific receptors located in endothelial cells, SMCs, and the extracellular matrix, the other is passive and is presumably the result of severe endothelial injury[39-41]. Modified (oxidized) LDLs (oxLDL) are a key component in endothelial injury[42]. Endothelial cells, macrophages and SMCs have all shown the ability to oxidize native LDL. Mildly oxidized LDL plays a role in monocyte recruitment by inducing the expression of adhesive cell-surface glycoproteins in the endothelium such as: P-selectin, E-selectin, vascular cell adhesion molecule-1 (VCAM-1), or intercellular adhesion molecule-1 (ICAM-1)[43,44]. Numerous molecules within the intravascular space, such as monocyte chemotactic protein 1 (MCP-1), transforming growth factor ß (TGF-ß), and colony -stimulating factors (CSF) attract and modify monocytes within the subendothelial space[16,45,46]. The subendothelial space becomes an environment rich in modified lipoproteins, cytokines, chemoattractants, and growth factors, all of which facilitate monocyte activation and differentiation into macrophages. The activated macrophage in turn also expresses several biologically active molecules. Some of these secretory products may serve as chemoattractants or growth promoting factors, amplifying monocyte recruitment, and promoting SMC migration and proliferation. Free radicals generated by macrophages not only act on cellular components of the atherosclerotic plaque but also can oxidize LDL present in the intima. Macrophages are also active phagocytes. The scavenger receptor implicated in the ingestion of modified LDL is expressed on the surface of macrophages[47]. Macrophages take up LDL via the LDL receptor at a very low rate without formation of cholesterol deposits. However, chemically modified oxLDL is taken up much more rapidly via the acetyl-LDL or scavenger receptor[48]. Lipid ingestion by macrophages results in their transformation into lipid-laden foam cells. Since the macrophage receptors for modified LDL are not auto-regulated, excessive intracellular accumulation of this lipoprotein eventually leads to the destruction of the cell with release of ox-LDL and abundant free radicals. This in turn maintains the cycle of cytotoxicity and extends the damage to the endothelium. The abundant lipid content released into the extracellular compartment favors the formation of a soft atheromatous core. The release of proteases by the dying macrophage leads to the digestion of extracellular matrix, further eroding the surrounding fibrous cap and contributing to its weakening[49-51].

Monocyte/macrophage recruitment into the arterial wall

Monocyte-derived macrophages are the predominant inflammatory cell in atherogenesis. Macrophages are ubiquitous throughout the stages of plaque formation. Among their numerous roles in plaque formation: They act as an antigen-presenting cell to T-lymphocytes; as a scavenger cell to remove lipoproteins and other noxious materials; and as a source of growth-regulatory molecules and cytokines[52].

The focal accumulation of monocytes/macrophages in atherogenesis likely involves the expression of specific adhesive glycoproteins on the endothelial surface, in addition to the generation of numerous chemoattractant factors by modified endothelial cells, lymphocytes and SMCs. As has already been mentioned several molecules are relevant to attracting monocytes to the subendothelial space, such as MCP-1, CSFs and TGF-β[16,53]. In more advanced and vulnerable plaques, thrombin, fibrin, fibronectin, elastin, and collagen degradation products may become predominant monocyte chemoattractants[54].

Macrophages are able to modify (oxidize) LDL via the formation of lipoxygenase[55]. This enzyme causes fatty acids to undergo peroxidation, and short chain aldehydes, ketones, and other substances are formed which can become covalently crosslinked to the apoprotein moiety of the LDL particle, permitting the ox-LDL to bind to the scavenger receptor of the macrophage[55].

In addition, the macrophages can form numerous molecules that have a significant effect on the surrounding environment. Activated macrophages form several matrix hydrolytic enzymes (metalloproteinases) such as collagenase, stromelysin, and elastase, all of which are esssential in plaque formation and in lesion stability as well as vessel remodeling[37].

Smooth muscle cells in atherosclerotic plaques:

The initial lipid and macrophage driven process is subsequently accompanied by SMC activation, migration, and proliferation, followed by extracellular matrix deposition and further lipid accumulation. This gives rise to a more mature and clinically significant atherosclerotic plaque (Stary type IV or V)[10]. Proliferation of SMCs has been established as a major event in the evolution of atherosclerosis. It was initially assumed that SMCs were a single uniform population of cells in atherosclerotic lesions. However, there is diversity in SMCs, such that some may be capable of replicating numerous times while others are capable of few doublings. In addition, during early development, SMCs are derived from different embryonic sources. Thus different SMCs may respond differently to various cyto-active proteins. At least two different phenotypes of SMCs have been described in atherosclerotic plaques[9,56]. The contractile phenotype is rich in myofilaments and contractile apparatus and respond to vasoactive agents such as endothelin, cathecholamines, prostacyclins, and NO to name a few. In contrast, synthetic phenotype cells are rich in endoplasmic reticulum and Golgi apparatus. In addition, they are capable of expressing genes for a number of growth-regulatory and cytokine receptors. They respond to these cellular medintors by activation, proliferation and synthesis of extracellular matrix[13].

SMCs are the principle source of connective tissue in the atherosclerotic lesion. The extracellular matrix synthethized by SMCs is made up of collagen, elastin and numerous proteoglycans. Collagen formation is the major contributor to the growth of atherosclerotic plaques (collagen type I and III are the primary components of the plaque). Proteoglycans and elastins are important in the binding of platelets, leukocytes and extracellular lipids to the subendothelial matrix[10,57].

Vasa vasorum

Over the last decades, pathologic studies have shown an increased number of vasa vasorum in advanced atherosclerotic lesions[58-61]. The process of neovascularization (angiogenesis), results in the formation of a dense plexus of thin-walled microvessels extending from the adventitia to the base of the plaque. A correlation between the extent of vasa vasorum neovascularisation and severity of atherosclerotic disease has been demonstrated in human coronary arteries. In addition, there is a close association between vasa vasorum neovascularisation and rupture of the internal elastica lamina in disrupted plaques. Therefore, this observation indicates that the vasa vasorum might play a role in atherogenesis as a regulator of plaque instability and disruption. However, whether neovascularisation precedes or follows plaque development is still not known. Transudation (edema) or small bleeds from these fragile vessels theoretically may increase the intraplaque pressure (compressive stress) sufficient to blow out the cap from the inside[62].

Apoptosis

The role of apoptosis in atherothrombosis can be described at two separate levels, at site of the plaque and in the circulation. Apoptosis in atherothrombotic disease involves all cell types[63]. Within and around the necrotic core, as well as in the fibrous cap, there is an accumulation of foam cells and nuclear fragments staining positive for TUNEL[64,65].

Despite the initiation of cell death process, apoptotic cells are involved in the inflammatory process through further recruitment of other inflammatory cells. For example the externalization of phosphatidylserine by apoptotic cells, which can be detected with Annexin V[66], has the immunogenic potential to activate neighboring cells for phagocytosis[67].

Mallat et al.[68] reported a clear association between apoptosis and inflammation. They demonstrated coexistence of inflammation and apoptotic cells in areas of plaque rupture resulting in exposure of a high fraction of apoptotic cells and debris to the circulation[69]. Besides the immunogenic and inflammatory characteristics, it is believed that apoptotic cells possess a highly thrombogenic potential[70,71] and therefore are postulated as one of the determinants of plaque thrombogenicity.

It has been demonstrated that apoptosis is coexistent with high levels of tissue factor (TF) expression within the atherosclerotic plaque[68]. TF is functional on the cell surface and its activity is highly dependent on presence of phosphatidylserine[72]. Since PS exposure is associated with apoptosis, it has been suggested that apoptosis may partly be responsible for TF activation within the plaque. Recently Hutter et al.[73] demonstrated the co-localization of TF and apoptosis in macrophages within lipid rich human atherosclerotic plaques and in addition, showed in vitro that a significant percentage of macrophages exposed to ox-LDL undergoing apoptosis expressed TF. There is further evidence that apoptosis in different cell types promotes procoagulant activity.

Interestingly, the prothrombotic potential of different apoptotic cells is not only confined locally to the atherosclerotic plaque, but is also present in the circulation. Mallat et al.[74] initially demonstrated the presence of high levels of shed membrane apoptotic particles in extracts from atherosclerotic plaques but not the underlying arterial wall. Later on, the same group showed the presence of high levels of endothelial membrane microparticles with procoagulant potential in the peripheral circulating blood of patients with acute coronary syndromes, inferring that they might participate in the generation and perpetuation of intracoronary thrombi[69]. This indicates a major role of apoptosis in atherothrombosis following plaque rupture.

CD 40 ligand

Over the last few years, a particular cytokine known as CD154 (or familiarly CD40 ligand) has captured attention. CD40 ligation of endothelial cells can induce adhesion molecules, such as VCAM-1[75]. However, work over the last few years has revealed that there is a broader role for CD40 ligand and its receptor CD40. T lymphocytes in human plaque were known to stain positively for CD40L. The role of CD40L in lesion progression and thrombosis was established through gene-targeting studies utilizing murine knockout models. In a LDL deficient knockout, treatment with an anti-CD40L monoclonal antibody significantly reduced atherosclerotic lesion size and macrophage, T lymphocyte, and lipid content[76]. Furthermore, Schonbeck et al. utilizing the same murine model in a temporally-longer, randomized study not only demonstrated that anti-CD40L monoclonal antibody limited atherosclerotic disease evolution, but also conferred stable plaque characteristics[77]. Moreover, CD40L deficiency was shown to protect against microvascular thrombus formation, while recombinant soluble CD40L (sCD40L) restored normal thrombosis[78]. Recently, much attention has been focused on CD40L's cryptic existence in platelets and its potential role in mediating platelet-dependent inflammatory response associated with the atherothrombotic state. Pioneering work has shown platelet-associated CD40L to elicit an inflammatory response from endothelial cells [75] and induce human monocytic[79], endothelial[80,81] and vascular SMC[82] TF expression in a CD40/CD40L-dependent manner. Furthermore, Henn et al. have demonstrated that upon platelet stimulation, CD40L is expressed on the surface and then subsequently cleaved to generate a soluble, trimeric fragment, sCD40L[83]. Though no definitive data identifies platelets as the sole source of sCD40L found in circulation[83,84], platelet counts[85] and platelet activation[86] have been shown to correlate with sCD40L. Additionally, sCD40L is able to ligate platelet glycoprotein (GP) IIb/IIIa complex confering a thrombogenic proclivity, and through this mechanism, may play a role in high shear dependent platelet aggregation[78].

Based on this hypothesis, and using a strategy of antibody neutralization of CD40 signaling in vivo in an atherosclerosis-susceptible mouse, the hypothesis that CD40 signaling participates in the initiation and progression of atherosclerosis was tested. Inhibition of CD40 signaling by the administration of a neutralizing antibody reduced surface area and thickness of atheroma in these mice[77]. Administration of irrelevant antibody or of saline solution did not do this. In addition to lesion size, functional characteristics of lesions also have great importance. Interfering with CD40 ligand signaling also reduced arterial levels of VCAM-1, a useful gauge of inflammatory activation.

Although this strategy of interfering with a primordial inflammatory mediator blocked the initiation of atherosclerosis, it was unknown whether interruption of CD40 function could affect the progression of established lesions. The question remained whether this strategy could arrest lesion progression, cause its regression, or if it would be too late if therapy began only after lesion initiation. In fact, the administration of neutralizing antibody after formation of initial lesions did stem lesion evolution; although lesions did not regress, they progressed much more slowly[87]. More importantly, not only did interruption of CD40 signaling stop lesion progression, but it also changed the character of the lesion (eg, there were fewer inflammatory cells, more SMCs, and more collagen). These experiments proved that interfering with inflammatory pathways could change the character of the plaque in a way that should confer stability in terms of human disease. Overall, blocking the action of CD40 ligand in mice inhibits formation of atherosclerotic lesions, prevents evolution of established atheroma, and fosters features of the plaque that are associated with its stability. Others working with double-knockout animals have subsequently confirmed these observations[78].

Next, it was important to test whether the laboratory findings extended to the clinic. CD40 ligand, which is a cell surface molecule, can be shed and measured in the circulation[75]. A nested case-control study tested the hypothesis that soluble CD40 ligand might prospectively predict cardiovascular risk in apparently healthy women. Indeed, although most of the individuals in this population had low levels of soluble CD40 measured in plasma, those with high levels had an increased incidence of cardiovascular events[81].

More recently, Heeschen et al. reported on the value of CD40 ligand in the management of acute coronary syndromes[86]. The major objective of the study was to investigate the predictive value of serum levels of CD40 ligand with respect to cardiac events and the effect of the glycoprotein IIb/IIIa inhibitor abciximab in patients with acute coronary syndromes who were enrolled in the c7E3 Fab Anti-Platelet Therapy in Unstable Refractory Angina (CAPTURE) trial. The combined primary endpoint was death or nonfatal MI during 30 days and 6 months follow up. In a subgroup of 161 patients, they found a strong correlation between monocytes-platelet aggregates (marker of platelet activation) and soluble CD40 ligand. Similar results were obtained for P-selectin expression (another marker of activated platelets) on platelets. It was concluded that soluble CD40 ligand is a powerful biochemical marker of inflammatory and thrombotic activity in patients with acute coronary syndromes.

Progression of atherosclerosis

Atherogenesis and lesion progression may be expected to be linear with time. The severity of coronary artery stenosis and the number of diseased vessels are known markers for future cardiac events. However, angiographic studies show that progression of coronary artery disease in humans is neither linear nor predictable[88-91] (*Figure 5*). New high-grade lesions often appear in segments of artery that appeared normal or near normal on previous angiographic examinations[88]. Almost three-quarters of the culprit lesions responsible for unstable angina or MI were only mildly to moderately stenotic on prior angiograms. Giroud and colleagues[92] demonstrated that over three-quarters of MIs were in areas supplied by mildly stenosed (<50%) coronary arteries on a previous angiogram. Ambrose et al. [88] found that on the initial angiogram, the lesion responsible for a MI had a less than 50% luminal stenosis in one half of cases and less than 70% in over two thirds of them. Little and colleagues[93] further supported these observations by showing that the average degree of stenosis in lesions progressing to a later MI was mildly stenotic (<50%) on the first angiogram in two thirds of patients and less than 70% in the majority of them. It is now generally accepted that that coronary artery lesions presumably responsible for an acute ischemic event (unstable angina, MI) appear only moderately stenotic in a great number of patients at the time of their initial angiogram.

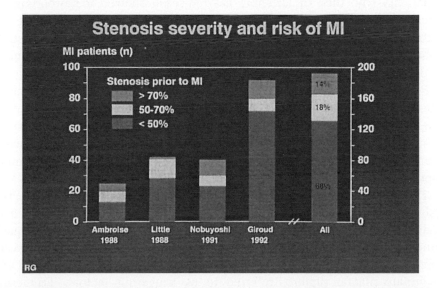

Figure 5. **Different angiographic studies performed demonstrating lesion characteristics of disrupted atherosclerotic plaques.**

Progression of early atherosclerotic lesions to larger or disrupted, clinically significant, lesions is variable and poorly understood. However, in persons at risk for coronary artery disease, this progression appears more rapid[94]. The extent of atherosclerotic lesions or overall plaque burden found at autopsy was found to correlate well to age, male sex, hypercholesterolemia, diabetes, hypertension, and smoking[95]. Diabetes, proximal or midvessel lesion location, hypercholesterolemia, time from MI, and complex lesion morphology (calcified, and ulcerated lesions or plaques with overhanging edges) were identified as predictors of angiographic progression in the Coronary Artery Surgery Study (CASS)[96]. However, with the exception of data suggesting more extracellular oxidized lipids in smokers, no relation of specific risk factors to plaque composition has been convincingly identified.

Plaque disruption

Rupture of the fibrous cap overlying an atheromatous core allows dissection into the intima by blood exposing the thrombogenic gruel[3,54,57]. A mass of platelet-rich thrombus forms within the intima, leading to plaque expansion. Ultimately the intraluminal thrombus may grow to become totally occlusive or is lysed and the plaque fissure seals, becoming incorporated within the atheromatous plaque. Analysis of the coronary tree in patients who died of ischemic heart disease showed a morphological appearance consistent with previously healed fissures with different stages of thrombosis and thrombus organization. This suggests that most fissures probably reseal with incorporation of thrombus without clinical manifestations[28].

Plaque disruption is clinically important. Early work by Constantinides revealed that thrombi causing myocardial infarction, (reconstructed from serial sections of coronary arteries) could be traced to cracks or fissures within the fibrous cap of an atheromatous plaque. Further work by Davies et al. and Falk has shown that plaque rupture underlies the majority of thrombi responsible (about 75%) of acute coronary syndromes[97-100].

The risk of plaque disruption is essentially a function of two factors. The first reflects the inherent biological and physical properties of a plaque, predisposing it to disruption, collectively referred to as plaque's vulnerability to rupture. The second is a sum of all external physical, hemodynamic and pathophysiological forces acting on plaques, which can precipitate plaque rupture, referred to as triggering factors. Triggering factors are not a cause of plaque disruption unless the plaque is intrinsically weakened and primed for rupture[1].

Vulnerability of atherosclerotic plaques

Size of the atheromatous core

Coronary plaques are predominantly sclerotic, and collagen-rich (constitutes over 70% of its mass)[3]. However, the size and consistency of the atheromatous core determine their stability. By studying postmortem aortic plaques, several investigators have demonstrated that the greater the atheromatous core size, the more vulnerable the plaque. This early work has established an atheromatous core occupying more than 40% of total plaque area as a threshold above which the plaque was considered particularly at high risk for subsequent rupture and thrombosis[19,99].

The atheromatous core is extremely rich in plasma-derived lipid, predominantly free cholesterol and its esters[100]. Cholesterol esters are less viscous at body temperature and will soften plaques, whereas crystalline cholesterol has an opposite effect[57]. Lipid-lowering therapy in humans is beneficial for reducing cardiovascular events. Presumably, they tilt the balance towards greater crystalline cholesterol, and lesser free cholesterol ester content of plaques, thus stabilizing the lesion and ultimately decreasing the incidence of plaque rupture.

Fibrous cap

Cap structure and strength are important determinants of plaque stability[101]. The fibrous cap is histologically the result of SMC activation, proliferation and extracellular matrix deposition. It is initially formed as a defense mechanism to protect the vessel wall from the underlying atheromatous process.

Fibrous caps vary widely in thickness, cellularity, strength and stiffness. Additionally, there are no blood vessels within the cap and all nutrients must be acquired by diffusion, a less efficient process[102]. Fibrous caps are thinnest at the shoulder area of the atherosclerotic lesion (the junction of the fibrous cap with adjacent more normal intima)[4]. This region is often heavily infiltrated by macrophages and foam cells[4,103]. As the atherosclerotic lesion progresses, there is a steady decline in the presence of SMCs[97]. In fact, apoptosis contributes to SMCs disappearance[104-106]. Lee and colleagues[107] have shown that cellular and calcified caps were two to five times stiffer than hypocellular caps. Ruptured caps have reduced mechanical strength. They contain less collagen, and glycosaminoglycans, more extracellular lipids, less SMCs and significantly more macrophages[103].

Inflammation

Infiltration of disrupted fibrous caps by activated macrophage and foam cells has been known for some time[108]. The shoulder regions of eccentric plaques are sites of predilection for macrophage infiltration and plaque rupture. In vitro studies have also confirmed that foam cell infiltration reduces the tensile strength of fibrous caps[109]. Richardson and colleagues[19] found that 75% of rupture sites were infiltrated with foam cells. van der Wal et al.[109] identified significant macrophage infiltration in plaques beneath all coronary thrombi examined. Furthermore immunohistochemistry confirmed the presence of activated macrophages, and T lymphocytes, both markers of ongoing inflammation at rupture sites. Moreno and colleagues[103] demonstrated that culprit lesions responsible for acute coronary syndromes (unstable angina, non-Q-wave MI) contained significantly more macrophages than lesions associated with stable angina (14% versus 3% of plaque tissue occupied by macrophages, respectively).

Progressive extracellular lipid accumulation and macrophage infiltration destabilizes plaques by destroying intimal tissue and fibrous caps[16]. Macrophage and foam cell recruitment is associated with progressive tissue destruction eroding into and through surrounding tissue. The internal elastic membrane at the base of an atherosclerotic plaque is often disrupted, and the adjacent media is frequently atrophic and occasionally destroyed. Likewise, the fibrous cap may be eroded from beneath thinning and weakening it. Macrophages, and/or foam cells within the atheromatous core and fibrous cap are capable of degrading extracellular matrix by direct phagocytosis or by secreting numerous proteolytic enzymes such as plasminogen activators and a variety of matrix metalloproteinases (MMPs: collagenases, elastases, gelatinases, and stromelysins). Together with the generation of toxic products (free radicals, products of lipid oxidation), they facilitate vessel wall damage and contribute to plaque instability.

MMPs are secreted in a proenzyme form requiring extracellular activation[110]. The nature of this activator is unknown at this time. MMPs are capable of degrading practically all components of the extracellular matrix. Additionally, MMPs are co-secreted with their natural inhibitors referred to collectively as tissue inhibitors of metalloproteinases (TIMPs). These inhibitors have been identified as participants in cell migration, tumor invasion, wound healing, inflammation, and vascular remodeling. Macrophages, monocytes, and SMCs have been shown to secrete MMPs. Shah and colleagues have recently shown that human monocyte-derived macrophages grown in culture may express interstitial collagenase (MMP-1) and degrade collagen of aortic fibrous caps during incubation[51]. Stromelysin, and other MMPs capable of degrading extracellular matrix components has been identified in macrophages of human atherosclerotic plaques and lipid-laden foam cells[111].

Mast cells and neutrophils are also found in disrupted plaques[112]. Mast cells are present in the shoulder regions of intact atherosclerotic plaques but at relatively low densities. They can secrete very powerful proteolytic enzymes such as tryptase and chymase which subsequently activate the pro-enzymatic form of MMPs. The role of neutrophils is less clear. Their role in tissue destruction especially in inflammatory diseases is well established[113]. However, they are rare in intact atherosclerotic plaques. It is postulated that they enter plaques shortly after disruption. The precise role of neutrophils in the progression of the atherosclerotic plaque and their contribution to plaque disruption has not been widely elucidated.

Cap fatigue

Any physical object exposed to a steady repeated loading and unloading will show signs of fatigue at particular stress points. The cyclic stretching, compression, bending, flexing, shear and pressure fluctuations encountered in a normal cardiac cycle may in themselves eventually weaken a fibrous cap leading to spontaneous rupture[114]. In theory, lowering the number (heart rate), and magnitude (pressure) of the repetitive load should postpone the time to rupture. Reducing the physical strain on plaques could be one way by which ß-blockers reduce the rate of reinfarctions.

Extrinsic triggers of plaque disruption

In many cases, acute coronary syndromes are not random events. Nearly 50% of patients with an acute MI report a triggering event[115,116]. Muller and colleagues introduced the concept of an atherosclerotic plaque that may have been progressively weakened by prior internal processes, becoming susceptible to even minor every day stresses. They also noticed that most MIs occurred with increased frequency in the morning particularly within the first hour after awakening. They referred to this phenomenon as circadian-triggering. Additional clinical observations indicate that the incidence of MIs is higher on Mondays, during cold days, especially during the winter months, and during emotional stress, and physical exercise, especially if sedentary[115].

Extrinsic physical forces (Figure 6)

Atherosclerotic plaques rupture when the sum of external forces acting on the plaque exceed its intrinsic tensile strength[54]. Normally, blood pressure exerts two forces on the surrounding vessel wall. The first is a circumferential wall stress exerted to all components around the vessel wall (**tensile stress**). The second is a radial force exerted across the vessel wall (**compressive stress**). The vessel wall is not immune from the basic laws of physics; in order for the vessel wall to remain intact both these forces must be counteracted by an equal and opposite force. In the case of plaque rupture, circumferential stress appears to be the predominant disruptive force[1].

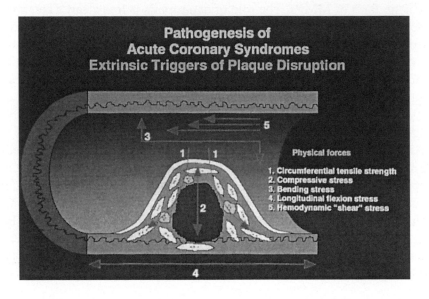

Figure 6. **The different physical forces exerted on an atherosclerotic plaque**. See text for details.

Circumferential wall stress is described by Laplace's law which relates luminal pressure and radius to wall tension: $\sigma = p \cdot r/h$, where σ = circumferential well stress; p = pressure differential; r = vessel radius; and h = wall thickness. Accordingly, the larger the vessel, or the higher the blood pressure, or the thinner the vessel wall, the greater will be the force exerted on the vessel wall[102]. Similarly, applying this same rule, the tension created in fibrous caps of mildly or moderately stenotic plaques is greater than that created in caps of severely stenotic plaques if the pressure and cap thickness are similar.

Circumferential forces are redistributed to those areas most capable of bearing the imposed forces, resulting in focal concentrations of circumferential stress at certain critical points within a plaque. Since the soft atheromatous gruel of a vulnerable plaque has almost no tensile strength, all the stress that should normally be borne by that region is displaced to the overlying fibrous cap. Using computer modeling and taking into account the physical properties of atherosclerotic plaque components, both Richardson et al.[19] and Cheng et al.[117] showed high concentrations of circumferential stress at the shoulder areas of atherosclerotic plaque caps. In addition, these forces appeared maximal when the atheromatous gruel exceeded 45% of the vessel circumference. The thickness of the fibrous cap is also an important determinant of tensile strength. Using computer modeling, Loree and colleagues[101] demonstrated a fourfold increase in wall stress as plaque thickness was reduced from 250µm to 50µm, for a constant vessel stenosis.

Circumferential tensile stress is the predominant force exerted on an atherosclerotic plaque. However, it is not the only one. Compressive stresses exert their pressure from the plaque out into the lumen. High-velocity jets or turbulent eddy currents caused by blood flowing through very tight stenoses can result in negative transmural pressures. The constant and repetitive buckling and deformation of the vessel wall through each cardiac cycle results in highly concentrated compressive stresses within the plaque; compounded by the negative transluminal pressures, the fibrous cap may blow-up out into the lumen.

Coronary arteries cyclically undergo changes in size and shape during each cardiac cycle. A normal coronary artery may vary as much as 10% in diameter throughout a cardiac cycle. The transmitted pulse pressure causes changes in the size and shape of atheromatous plaques, resulting in deformation and circumferential bending. Sudden accentuation of this bending may be a trigger for plaque rupture, especially at the junction between the more flexible normal vessel wall and the stiffer atherosclerotic plaque. Long-term repetitive bending may result in tissue fatigue with a similar outcome.

Similar to circumferential bending, coronary arteries undergo longitudinal or axial bending and stretching during each cardiac cycle. In an interesting angiographic study performed by Stein and colleagues[114] the angle of flexing correlated with subsequent lesion progression, however, the coefficient of correlation was rather low.

Finally, hemodynamic forces do not appear to be as important as the physical forces imposed on the plaque by blood pressure and pulse pressure. In normal coronary arteries, the response to increased shear stress is to dilate. Since the overlying endothelium is dysfunctional, compensatory endothelium-dependent vasodilation does not occur in atherosclerotic segments[118]. Shear stress can cause superficial endothelial damage[119]. Whether this damage is sufficient to provoke plaque rupture is unlikely. If shear stress was a major factor in plaque rupture, we would expect to see more severely stenotic lesions rupture more frequently. However, as already mentioned, numerous angiographic studies do not prove this to be the case. Theoretically, shear stress may also contribute indirectly to plaque rupture by modulating the influx of monocytes/macrophages, and plasma proteins, into an atherosclerotic lesion[37].

Thrombosis

Variables that determine the thrombotic response of a disrupted plaque include, the quantity (fissure size), and quality (plaque composition) of the substrate exposed, and the rheology of blood flow. Systemic factors such as the fibrinolytic system, cathecholamines, and lipoproteins also modulate thrombosis[120-122].

The thrombotic response to plaque rupture is influenced by the various components of the atherosclerotic plaque exposed to flowing blood following rupture[123]. Our group has demonstrated that the most thrombogenic component of the atherosclerotic plaque is the atheromatous gruel[99]. The lipid core exposed in the atheromatous plaque resulted in thrombus formation four to six times greater than other plaque components. Therefore, lipid-rich plaques are not only the most vulnerable but also appear to be the most thrombogenic. The atheromatous core is a rich source of *tissue factor*[124]. The origin of this tissue factor appears to be disintegrating macrophages, or produced de-novo by activated SMCs, macrophages/monocytes, and possibly activated endothelial cells[124]. Moreno and colleagues[103] have shown that atherosclerotic plaques taken by directional atherectomy from patients with unstable angina were rich in macrophages. Furthermore, by using an *ex vivo* perfusion system, it has recently been shown that platelet thrombus formation is greatest in those plaques that were rich in tissue factor[125].

Fresh thrombus on a disrupted plaque or residual thrombus on a chronic lesion is also a very thrombogenic substrate[126]. Thrombus is a rich source of thrombin, and activated factor X (Xa). It also contains numerous natural inhibitors to heparins such as platelet-factor 4, and fibrin monomer II, and a source of plasminogen activator inhibitor - 1 (PAI-1). Residual thrombus also protrudes into the vessel lumen, obstructing flow and decreasing the lumen diameter, increasing shear stress and platelet deposition. Thrombin, present in high concentrations at sites of arterial thrombosis, has been shown to share many growth-related signals with mitogens such as platelet-derived growth factor (PDGF). Furthermore, thrombin induces a significant increase in protein synthesis that induces growth promoting activity for vascular SMCs.

The acute thrombotic response following plaque disruption also depends on the degree of stenosis and sudden geometric changes following rupture. The greater the geometric deformation, the greater the shear stress. Platelet deposition increases directly with shear stress[127]. Blood flowing through a vessel is accelerated as it passes through the stenosis or disrupted and deformed plaque. Blood also undergoes deceleration distal to the stenosis. This acceleration/deceleration of blood induces flow separations and vortices downstream from the stenosis. With higher shear forces, circulating red blood cells displace platelets, monocytes, fibrinogen and other plasma proteins to the periphery and enhance their deposition. The low shear rate area distal to the stenosis induces fibrinogen deposition, leading to a thrombus with a platelet-rich head, and a fibrin-rich tail[128,129].

Systemic thrombogenic risk factors

Recent experimental and clinical evidence suggests that a primary hypercoagulable or thrombogenic state of circulation can favor thrombosis. Catecholamines enhance platelet activation and the generation of thrombin[130]. This may be of major clinical significance since it may link emotional stress, physical exercise, cigarette smoking, and circadian variations to arterial thrombosis[131,132]. Patients with coronary artery disease may have increased blood viscosity, and elevated fibrinogen levels. Fibrinogen is the major plasma determinant of blood viscosity and red cell aggregation. Fibrinogen and factor VII are recognized as major independent risk factors for coronary artery disease. As a further note, plasma fibrinogen levels and blood viscosity are highest in the morning.

Enhanced sympathetic tone can also stimulate alpha-receptors, promoting platelet aggregation and vasoconstriction. Heart rate, mean arterial pressure, and norepinephrine levels are all at a minimum at approximately six am and rise sharply to a maximum around nine am. Furthermore the low plasma norepinephrine levels present during sleep induce an up-regulation of ß-adrenergic receptors. Therefore upon awakening, the increased catecholamine levels combine with an increased responsiveness of receptors. Accordingly, aspirin blocks the morning increase in platelet activity, and like ß-blockers, blunts the morning increase in plaque rupture-associated events[133]. Thus the circadian variation in thrombogenic factors parallels variations in the sympathetic and catecholamine levels.

Platelet activation and generation of thrombin may also be enhanced by hypercholesterolemia, hyperhomocysteinemia, diabetes, and cigarette smoking[122]. Increased levels of lipoprotein (a), Lp(a), have been identified as a risk factor for coronary artery disease. Lp(a) has close structural homology to plasminogen. This structural similarity may result in competetive inhibition of the fibrinolytic properties of plasminogen[134].

Vasoconstriction

Plaque disruption and vasoconstriction do frequently coexist, but spasm is not necessarily the causative factor[8]. Atherosclerotic arteries have abnormal vasodilator function related to a deficiency in the production and release of endothelium-derived relaxing factors[118,135]. Acetylcholine administered directly into the coronary arteries of patients with early and advanced atherosclerosis results in vasoconstriction. Animal experiments have shown that damaged endothelium responds abnormally to vasoactive substances[136]. Vessels with even early atherosclerosis have increased vasoconstrictor response to serotonin and thromboxane A_2, as well as impaired vasodilatory responses to adenosine. These data suggest that atherosclerosis is associated with an abnormal vasodilatory function, or exaggerated vasoconstrictor response, perhaps due to loss of endothelium-derived growth factor[137].

Proponents of vasospasm as a trigger of plaque rupture suggest that vessel constriction will result in compression of an atheromatous core resulting in rupture of the fibrous cap into the lumen[138,139]. However, spasm has been provoked in many patients with severely diseased coronary arteries, without serious complications. Furthermore spasmolytic agents (such as calcium antagonists) have not been proven effective in the prevention of MIs. In a study by Nobuyoshi and colleagues[140], a positive correlation between ergonovine-induced vasospasm and plaque progression was found, but it was not clear whether this resulted in an increase in the incidence of MIs[140].

Clinical consequences of atherosclerotic

Plaque growth and rupture

Clinical manifestations of atherosclerotic plaques depend on several factors including: the degree and suddenness of blood flow obstruction, the duration of decreased myocardial perfusion and the myocardial oxygen demand at the time of blood flow obstruction. The importance of the thrombotic response to the disrupted plaque is also a major determinant. Plaque rupture is accompanied by hemorrhage into the plaque and is accompanied by various amounts of luminal thrombosis. If the thrombus is small, plaque rupture probably proceeds unnoticed; if on the other hand, the thrombus is large, compromising blood flow to the myocardium, the individual may experience an acute ischemic syndrome.

Plaque disruption is a common event, and in the majority of cases is clinically silent[141] (*Figure 7*). Plaque growth is also usually unpronounced and the result of both the atherosclerotic process and thrombus deposition. Most coronary thrombi (> 80%) have a layered structure indicating an episodic growth by repeated mural deposits[142]. A ruptured plaque is found beneath almost all coronary thrombi (90%), and displaced plaque fragments are frequently found buried deep within the thrombus[143]. Autopsy data indicates that 9% of healthy persons dying of non-cardiovascular deaths have asymptomatic disrupted plaques in their coronary arteries. Interestingly, this number increases to 22% in patients with diabetes mellitus or hypertension[97].

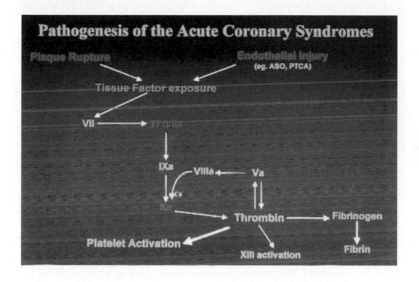

Figure 7. **Tissue Factor is the physiologic initiator and principal modulator of the coagulation cascade in arterial thrombosis.**

In *unstable angina*, a smaller fissure or disruption leads to an acute change in plaque structure, thrombus formation, and a reduction of blood flow resulting in exacerbation of angina. Transient episodes of vessel occlusion or near occlusion by thrombus at the site of plaque injury may occur, leading to angina at rest. The thrombus may be labile and result in temporary obstruction to flow, perhaps lasting minutes. Release of vasoactive substances by platelets (serotonin, thromboxane), and vasoconstriction secondary to endothelial vasodilator dysfunction, contribute to further reduction of blood flow[144]. The process may be sufficiently severe to cause total occlusion and MI. Collateral vessels, however may modify the outcome of a sudden coronary occlusion[145]. Chronic ischemia, may promote collateral development, permitting a severe stenosis to occlude silently[146]. A total occlusion is found in 10% of patients with unstable angina (*Figure 8*)[90].

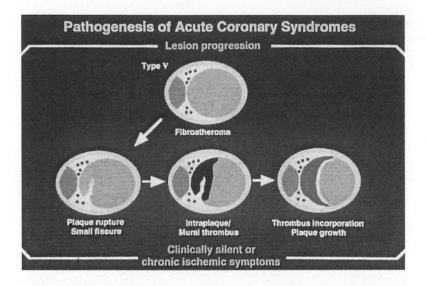

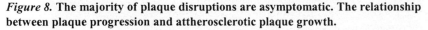

Figure 8. **The majority of plaque disruptions are asymptomatic. The relationship between plaque progression and attherosclerotic plaque growth.**

In *Non-Q wave MI*, the angiographic form of the responsible lesion is similar to that seen in unstable angina[90]. More severe plaque damage results in more persistent, transient, perhaps lasting up to one hour, thrombotic occlusion. At early angiography, about 25% of patients with non-Q-wave MI have an infarct-related vessel that is completely occluded, with the distal territory usually supplied by collaterals[146]. During the evolution of a coronary thrombus, its growth alternates with fragmentation and peripheral embolization. It is likely that platelet aggregates or floating thrombus that forms beyond the stenosis has a high propensity towards embolization. Arterial thrombi forming within and distal to a ruptured atherosclerotic plaque are dynamic, waxing and waning in size over a period of hours or even days. Spontaneous thrombolysis, the resolution of arterial spasm, and the presence of collaterals limit the duration and extent of myocardial ischemia and prevents Q-wave MI and more permanent damage (*Figure 9*)[147,148].

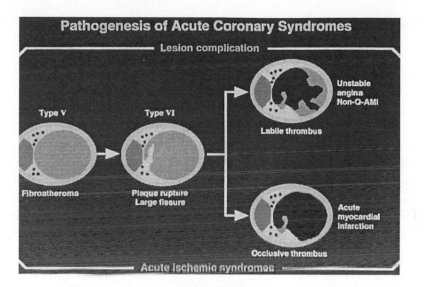

Figure 9. The pathogenesis of an acute ischemic syndrome. The relationship between plaque progression and the acute coronary syndromes.

In *Q-wave MI*, a larger plaque disruption may be associated with deep arterial injury or ulceration, resulting in the formation of a fixed and persistent thrombus. This leads to an abrupt cessation of myocardial perfusion often for more than one hour and subsequent transmural necrosis of the involved myocardium. One study by DeWood et al.[149] demonstrated that occlusive thrombosis is an early event in more than 80% of transmural infarcts. In patients with long standing coronary artery disease and severe coronary stenosis, the presence of well-developed collaterals can prevent or reduce the extent of MI. In a minority of patients, coronary thrombosis results from superficial injury or blood stasis in areas of high-grade stenosis. Impaired mechanisms of fibrinolysis, states of increased platelet aggregability, activation of the coagulation system and increased fibrinogen levels may be contributing factors in this situation.

Sudden death, related to ischemia probably involves the disruption of a plaque that is rapidly obstructive resulting in acute occlusion generating a polymorphic arrhythmia[28]. Absence of collateral flow, vasoconstriction or platelet microthrombi to the microcirculation may contribute[146]. However the more frequent fatal ventricular arrhythmias are common in patients after extensive MI or other forms of cardiomyopathy, where a substrate for the generation and maintance of ventricular tachycardia or fibrillation exists.

Although a substantial proportion of episodes of unstable angina and MI are caused by plaque rupture with superimposed thrombosis (over two-thirds), other mechanisms that alter the balance between myocardial oxygen supply and demand need to be considered. By transiently decreasing myocardial oxygen supply coronary spasm contributes to the pathogenesis of unstable angina and MI. In addition, chronic progression of the atherosclerotic plaque resulting in complete occlusion of an artery with insufficient collateral supply can result in an ischemic syndrome independently of plaque disruption.

In patients with stable angina, coronary blood flow does not meet the myocardial oxygen demand. Usually the luminal stenosis is a >50% reduction in diameter. The atherosclerotic lesions can be of any type, but are predominantly advanced fibrolipoid plaques (Stary type VI), or fibrotic lesion (Stary type VII). There is usually no plaque ulceration or thrombosis, but signs of previous plaque rupture with intraplaque hemorrhage or luminal thrombosis incorporated in the plaque are observed. The pattern of angina is not proportional to the severity of the underlying disease, mild or infrequent angina does not imply insignificant disease. Prognosis in stable angina is most accurately predicted by the extent and severity of individual obstructions, and by left ventricular function.

References

1. Corti R, Fuster V, Badimon JJ. Pathogenetic concepts of acute coronary syndromes. J Am Coll Cardiol 2003;41:7S-14S.
2. Davies MJ. A macro and micro view of coronary vascular insult in ischemic heart disease. Circulation 1990;82:II38-46.
3. Falk E, Shah PK, Fuster V. Coronary plaque disruption. Circulation 1995;92:657-71.
4. Falk E. Why do plaques rupture? Circulation 1992;86:III30-42.
5. Ross R, Glomset JA. Atherosclerosis and the arterial smooth muscle cell: Proliferation of smooth muscle is a key event in the genesis of the lesions of atherosclerosis. Science 1973;180:1332-9.
6. Ross R. Atherosclerosis--an inflammatory disease. N Engl J Med 1999;340:115-26.
7. Corti R, Farkouh ME, Badimon JJ. The vulnerable plaque and acute coronary syndromes. Am J Med 2002;113:668-80.
8. Fuster V, Corti R, Fayad ZA, Schwitter J, Badimon JJ. Integration of vascular biology and magnetic resonance imaging in the understanding of atherothrombosis and acute coronary syndromes. J Thromb Haemost 2003;1:1410-21.
9. Stary HC, Chandler AB, Dinsmore RE, et al. A definition of advanced types of atherosclerotic lesions and a histological classification of atherosclerosis. A report from the Committee on Vascular Lesions of the Council on Arteriosclerosis, American Heart Association. Arterioscler Thromb Vasc Biol 1995;15:1512-31.
10. Stary HC. Natural history and histological classification of atherosclerotic lesions: an update. Arterioscler Thromb Vasc Biol 2000;20:1177-8.
11. Stary HC. Macrophage foam cells in the coronary artery intima of human infants. Ann N Y Acad Sci 1985;454:5-8.
12. Stary HC, Blankenhorn DH, Chandler AB, et al. A definition of the intima of human arteries and of its atherosclerosis-prone regions. A report from the Committee on Vascular Lesions of the Council on Arteriosclerosis, American Heart Association. Circulation 1992;85:391-405.
13. Stary HC. The sequence of cell and matrix changes in atherosclerotic lesions of coronary arteries in the first forty years of life. Eur Heart J 1990;11 Suppl E:3-19.
14. Stary HC, Chandler AB, Dinsmore RE, et al. A definition of advanced types of atherosclerotic lesions and a histological classification of atherosclerosis. A report from the Committee on Vascular Lesions of the Council on Arteriosclerosis, American Heart Association. Circulation 1995;92:1355-74.
15. Katz SS, Shipley GG, Small DM. Physical chemistry of the lipids of human atherosclerotic lesions. Demonstration of a lesion intermediate between fatty streaks and advanced plaques. J Clin Invest 1976;58:200-11.
16. Faxon DP, Fuster V, Libby P, et al. Atherosclerotic vascular disease conference: Writing Group III: pathophysiology. Circulation 2004;109:2617-25.
17. Kolodgie FD, Gold HK, Burke AP, et al. Intraplaque hemorrhage and progression of coronary atheroma. N Engl J Med 2003;349:2316-25.

18. Stary HC. The development of calcium deposits in atherosclerotic lesions and their persistence after lipid regression. Am J Cardiol 2001;88:16E-19E.

19. Richardson PD, Davies MJ, Born GV. Influence of plaque configuration and stress distribution on fissuring of coronary atherosclerotic plaques. Lancet 1989;2:941-4.

20. Reidy MA, Bowyer DE. Scanning electron microscopy of arteries. The morphology of aortic endothelium in haemodynamically stressed areas associated with branches. Atherosclerosis 1977;26:181-94.

21. Glagov S. Hemodynamic factors in localisation of atherosclerosis. Acta Cardiol 1965:Suppl 11:311+.

22. Glagov S, Zarins C, Giddens DP, Ku DN. Hemodynamics and atherosclerosis. Insights and perspectives gained from studies of human arteries. Arch Pathol Lab Med 1988;112:1018-31.

23. Davies MJ, Woolf N, Rowles PM, Pepper J. Morphology of the endothelium over atherosclerotic plaques in human coronary arteries. Br Heart J 1988;60:459-64.

24. Behrendt D, Ganz P. Endothelial function. From vascular biology to clinical applications. Am J Cardiol 2002;90:40L-48L.

25. Weiss N, Keller C, Hoffmann U, Loscalzo J. Endothelial dysfunction and atherothrombosis in mild hyperhomocysteinemia. Vasc Med 2002;7:227-39.

26. Callow AD. Endothelial dysfunction in atherosclerosis. Vascul Pharmacol 2002;38:257-8.

27. Malek AM, Alper SL, Izumo S. Hemodynamic shear stress and its role in atherosclerosis. JAMA 1999;282:2035-42.

28. Virmani R, Kolodgie FD, Burke AP, Farb A, Schwartz SM. Lessons from sudden coronary death: a comprehensive morphological classification scheme for atherosclerotic lesions. Arterioscler Thromb Vasc Biol 2000;20:1262-75.

29. Chester AH, O'Neil GS, Moncada S, Tadjkarimi S, Yacoub MH. Low basal and stimulated release of nitric oxide in atherosclerotic epicardial coronary arteries. Lancet 1990;336:897-900.

30. Golino P, Piscione F, Willerson JT, et al. Divergent effects of serotonin on coronary-artery dimensions and blood flow in patients with coronary atherosclerosis and control patients. N Engl J Med 1991;324:641-8.

31. Yang ZH, Richard V, von Segesser L, et al. Threshold concentrations of endothelin-1 potentiate contractions to norepinephrine and serotonin in human arteries. A new mechanism of vasospasm? Circulation 1990;82:188-95.

32. Lerman A, Holmes DR, Jr., Bell MR, Garratt KN, Nishimura RA, Burnett JC, Jr. Endothelin in coronary endothelial dysfunction and early atherosclerosis in humans. Circulation 1995;92:2426-31.

33. Zeiher AM, Goebel H, Schachinger V, Ihling C. Tissue endothelin-1 immunoreactivity in the active coronary atherosclerotic plaque. A clue to the mechanism of increased vasoreactivity of the culprit lesion in unstable angina. Circulation 1995;91:941-7.

34. Tomasian D, Keaney JF, Vita JA. Antioxidants and the bioactivity of endothelium-derived nitric oxide. Cardiovasc Res 2000;47:426-35.

35. Cai H, Harrison DG. Endothelial dysfunction in cardiovascular diseases: the role of oxidant stress. Circ Res 2000;87:840-4.

36. Davignon J, Ganz P. Role of endothelial dysfunction in atherosclerosis. Circulation 2004;109:III27-32.

37. Libby P. Inflammation in atherosclerosis. Nature 2002;420:868-74.

38. Libby P, Ridker PM, Maseri A. Inflammation and atherosclerosis. Circulation 2002;105:1135-43.

39. Steinberg D. Atherogenesis in perspective: hypercholesterolemia and inflammation as partners in crime. Nat Med 2002;8:1211-7.

40. Griendling KK, FitzGerald GA. Oxidative stress and cardiovascular injury: Part I: basic mechanisms and in vivo monitoring of ROS. Circulation 2003;108:1912-6.

41. Griendling KK, FitzGerald GA. Oxidative stress and cardiovascular injury: Part II: animal and human studies. Circulation 2003;108:2034-40.

42. Khatri JJ, Johnson C, Magid R, et al. Vascular oxidant stress enhances progression and angiogenesis of experimental atheroma. Circulation 2004;109:520-5.

43. Zeiffer U, Schober A, Lietz M, et al. Neointimal smooth muscle cells display a proinflammatory phenotype resulting in increased leukocyte recruitment mediated by P-selectin and chemokines. Circ Res 2004;94:776-84.

44. Navab M, Hama SY, Nguyen TB, Fogelman AM. Monocyte adhesion and transmigration in atherosclerosis. Coron Artery Dis 1994;5:198-204.

45. Pan JH, Sukhova GK, Yang JT, et al. Macrophage migration inhibitory factor deficiency impairs atherosclerosis in low-density lipoprotein receptor-deficient mice. Circulation 2004.

46. Libby P, Ridker PM. Inflammation and atherosclerosis: role of C-reactive protein in risk assessment. Am J Med 2004;116 Suppl 6A:9S-16S.

47. Boullier A, Bird DA, Chang MK, et al. Scavenger receptors, oxidized LDL, and atherosclerosis. Ann N Y Acad Sci 2001;947:214-22; discussion 222-3.

48. Goldstein JL, Ho YK, Basu SK, Brown MS. Binding site on macrophages that mediates uptake and degradation of acetylated low density lipoprotein, producing massive cholesterol deposition. Proc Natl Acad Sci U S A 1979;76:333-7.

49. Orbe J, Rodriguez JA, Arias R, et al. Antioxidant vitamins increase the collagen content and reduce MMP-1 in a porcine model of atherosclerosis: implications for plaque stabilization. Atherosclerosis 2003;167:45-53.

50. Schafers M, Riemann B, Kopka K, et al. Scintigraphic imaging of matrix metalloproteinase activity in the arterial wall in vivo. Circulation 2004;109:2554-9.

51. Shah PK, Falk E, Badimon JJ, et al. Human monocyte-derived macrophages induce collagen breakdown in fibrous caps of atherosclerotic plaques. Potential role of matrix-degrading metalloproteinases and implications for plaque rupture. Circulation 1995;92:1565-9.

52. Ross R. Atherosclerosis is an inflammatory disease. Am Heart J 1999;138:S419-20.

53. Libby P. Vascular biology of atherosclerosis: overview and state of the art. Am J Cardiol 2003;91:3A-6A.

54.   Maseri A, Fuster V. Is there a vulnerable plaque? Circulation 2003;107:2068-71.

55.   Dwyer JH, Allayee H, Dwyer KM, et al. Arachidonate 5-lipoxygenase promoter genotype, dietary arachidonic acid, and atherosclerosis. N Engl J Med 2004;350:29-37.

56.   Schwartz SM, Heimark RL, Majesky MW. Developmental mechanisms underlying pathology of arteries. Physiol Rev 1990;70:1177-209.

57.   Fuster V, Stein B, Ambrose JA, Badimon L, Badimon JJ, Chesebro JH. Atherosclerotic plaque rupture and thrombosis. Evolving concepts. Circulation 1990;82:II47-59.

58.   Herrmann J, Lerman LO, Rodriguez-Porcel M, et al. Coronary vasa vasorum neovascularization precedes epicardial endothelial dysfunction in experimental hypercholesterolemia. Cardiovasc Res 2001;51:762-6.

59.   Kwon HM, Sangiorgi G, Ritman EL, et al. Adventitial vasa vasorum in balloon-injured coronary arteries: visualization and quantitation by a microscopic three-dimensional computed tomography technique. J Am Coll Cardiol 1998;32:2072-9.

60.   Kwon HM, Sangiorgi G, Spagnoli LG, et al. Experimental hypercholesterolemia induces ultrastructural changes in the internal elastic lamina of porcine coronary arteries. Atherosclerosis 1998;139:283-9.

61.   Kwon HM, Sangiorgi G, Ritman EL, et al. Enhanced coronary vasa vasorum neovascularization in experimental hypercholesterolemia. J Clin Invest 1998;101:1551-6.

62.   Badimon L, Steele P, Badimon JJ, Bowie EJ, Fuster V. Aortic atherosclerosis in pigs with heterozygous von Willebrand disease. Comparison with homozygous von Willebrand and normal pigs. Arteriosclerosis 1985;5:366-70.

63.   Cai W, Devaux B, Schaper W, Schaper J. The role of Fas/APO 1 and apoptosis in the development of human atherosclerotic lesions. Atherosclerosis 1997;131:177-86.

64.   Kockx MM, De Meyer GR, Buyssens N, Knaapen MW, Bult H, Herman AG. Cell composition, replication, and apoptosis in atherosclerotic plaques after 6 months of cholesterol withdrawal. Circ Res 1998;83:378-87.

65.   Kockx MM, Herman AG. Apoptosis in atherogenesis: implications for plaque destabilization. Eur Heart J 1998;19 Suppl G:G23-8.

66.   Martin SJ, Reutelingsperger CP, McGahon AJ, et al. Early redistribution of plasma membrane phosphatidylserine is a general feature of apoptosis regardless of the initiating stimulus: inhibition by overexpression of Bcl-2 and Abl. J Exp Med 1995;182:1545-56.

67.   Fadok VA, Bratton DL, Frasch SC, Warner ML, Henson PM. The role of phosphatidylserine in recognition of apoptotic cells by phagocytes. Cell Death Differ 1998;5:551-62.

68.   Mallat Z, Tedgui A. Current perspective on the role of apoptosis in atherothrombotic disease. Circ Res 2001;88:998-1003.

69.   Mallat Z, Benamer H, Hugel B, et al. Elevated levels of shed membrane microparticles with procoagulant potential in the peripheral circulating blood of patients with acute coronary syndromes. Circulation 2000;101:841-3.

70. Bombeli T, Karsan A, Tait JF, Harlan JM. Apoptotic vascular endothelial cells become procoagulant. Blood 1997;89:2429-42.

71. Flynn PD, Byrne CD, Baglin TP, Weissberg PL, Bennett MR. Thrombin generation by apoptotic vascular smooth muscle cells. Blood 1997;89:4378-84.

72. Rauch U, Nemerson Y. Circulating tissue factor and thrombosis. Curr Opin Hematol 2000;7:273-7.

73. Hutter R, Valdiviezo C, Sauter BV, et al. Caspase-3 and tissue factor expression in lipid-rich plaque macrophages: evidence for apoptosis as link between inflammation and atherothrombosis. Circulation 2004;109:2001-8.

74. Mallat Z, Hugel B, Ohan J, Leseche G, Freyssinet JM, Tedgui A. Shed membrane microparticles with procoagulant potential in human atherosclerotic plaques: a role for apoptosis in plaque thrombogenicity. Circulation 1999;99:348-53.

75. Henn V, Slupsky JR, Grafe M, Anagnostopoulos I, Forster R, Muller-Berghaus G, Kroczek RA. CD40 ligand on activated platelets triggers an inflammatory reaction of endothelial cells. Nature 1998;391:591-4.

76. Mach F, Schonbeck U, Sukhova GK, Atkinson E, Libby P. Reduction of atherosclerosis in mice by inhibition of CD40 signalling. Nature 1998;394:200-3.

77. Schonbeck U, Sukhova GK, Shimizu K, Mach F, Libby P. Inhibition of CD40 signaling limits evolution of established atherosclerosis in mice. Proc Natl Acad Sci U S A 2000;97:7458-63.

78. Andre P, Prasad KS, Denis CV, et al. CD40L stabilizes arterial thrombi by a beta3 integrin--dependent mechanism. Nat Med 2002;8:247-52.

79. Lindmark E, Tenno T, Siegbahn A. Role of platelet P-selectin and CD40 ligand in the induction of monocytic tissue factor expression. Arterioscler Thromb Vasc Biol 2000;20:2322-8.

80. Slupsky JR, Kalbas M, Willuweit A, Henn V, Kroczek RA, Muller-Berghaus G. Activated platelets induce tissue factor expression on human umbilical vein endothelial cells by ligation of CD40. Thromb Haemost 1998;80:1008-14.

81. Bavendiek U, Libby P, Kilbride M, Reynolds R, Mackman N, Schonbeck U. Induction of tissue factor expression in human endothelial cells by CD40 ligand is mediated via activator protein 1, nuclear factor kappa B, and Egr-1. J Biol Chem 2002;277:25032-9.

82. Schonbeck U, Mach F, Sukhova GK, et al. CD40 ligation induces tissue factor expression in human vascular smooth muscle cells. Am J Pathol 2000;156:7-14.

83. Henn V, Steinbach S, Buchner K, Presek P, Kroczek RA. The inflammatory action of CD40 ligand (CD154) expressed on activated human platelets is temporally limited by coexpressed CD40. Blood 2001;98:1047-54.

84. Aukrust P, Muller F, Ueland T, et al. Enhanced levels of soluble and membrane-bound CD40 ligand in patients with unstable angina. Possible reflection of T lymphocyte and platelet involvement in the pathogenesis of acute coronary syndromes. Circulation 1999;100:614-20.

85.   Viallard JF, Solanilla A, Gauthier B, et al. Increased soluble and platelet-associated CD40 ligand in essential thrombocythemia and reactive thrombocytosis. Blood 2002;99:2612-4.

86.   Heeschen C, Dimmeler S, Hamm CW, et al. Soluble CD40 ligand in acute coronary syndromes. N Engl J Med 2003;348:1104-11.

87.   Lutgens E, Gorelik L, Daemen MJ, et al. Requirement for CD154 in the progression of atherosclerosis. Nat Med 1999;5:1313-6.

88.   Ambrose JA, Tannenbaum MA, Alexopoulos D, et al. Angiographic progression of coronary artery disease and the development of myocardial infarction. J Am Coll Cardiol 1988;12:56-62.

89.   Fuster V, Badimon L, Cohen M, Ambrose JA, Badimon JJ, Chesebro J. Insights into the pathogenesis of acute ischemic syndromes. Circulation 1988;77:1213-20.

90.   Ambrose JA, Hjemdahl-Monsen CE, Borrico S, Gorlin R, Fuster V. Angiographic demonstration of a common link between unstable angina pectoris and non-Q-wave acute myocardial infarction. Am J Cardiol 1988;61:244-7.

91.   Moise A, Lesperance J, Theroux P, Taeymans Y, Goulet C, Bourassa MG. Clinical and angiographic predictors of new total coronary occlusion in coronary artery disease: analysis of 313 nonoperated patients. Am J Cardiol 1984;54:1176-81.

92.   Giroud D, Li JM, Urban P, Meier B, Rutishauer W. Relation of the site of acute myocardial infarction to the most severe coronary arterial stenosis at prior angiography. Am J Cardiol 1992;69:729-32.

93.   Little WC, Constantinescu M, Applegate RJ, et al. Can coronary angiography predict the site of a subsequent myocardial infarction in patients with mild-to-moderate coronary artery disease? Circulation 1988;78:1157-66.

94.   Fuster V, Fayad ZA, Badimon JJ. Acute coronary syndromes: biology. Lancet 1999;353 Suppl 2:SII5-9.

95.   Solberg LA, Strong JP. Risk factors and atherosclerotic lesions. A review of autopsy studies. Arteriosclerosis 1983;3:187-98.

96.   Alderman EL, Corley SD, Fisher LD, et al. Five-year angiographic follow-up of factors associated with progression of coronary artery disease in the Coronary Artery Surgery Study (CASS). CASS Participating Investigators and Staff. J Am Coll Cardiol 1993;22:1141-54.

97.   Davies MJ, Richardson PD, Woolf N, Katz DR, Mann J. Risk of thrombosis in human atherosclerotic plaques: role of extracellular lipid, macrophage, and smooth muscle cell content. Br Heart J 1993;69:377-81.

98.   Davies MJ, Thomas AC. Plaque fissuring--the cause of acute myocardial infarction, sudden ischaemic death, and crescendo angina. Br Heart J 1985;53:363-73.

99.   Fernandez-Ortiz A, Badimon JJ, Falk E, et al. Characterization of the relative thrombogenicity of atherosclerotic plaque components: implications for consequences of plaque rupture. J Am Coll Cardiol 1994;23:1562-9.

100. Falk E. Coronary thrombosis: pathogenesis and clinical manifestations. Am J Cardiol 1991;68:28B-35B.

101. Loree HM, Kamm RD, Stringfellow RG, Lee RT. Effects of fibrous cap thickness on peak circumferential stress in model atherosclerotic vessels. Circ Res 1992;71:850-8.

102. Lee RT, Schoen FJ, Loree HM, Lark MW, Libby P. Circumferential stress and matrix metalloproteinase 1 in human coronary atherosclerosis. Implications for plaque rupture. Arterioscler Thromb Vasc Biol 1996;16:1070-3.

103. Moreno PR, Falk E, Palacios IF, Newell JB, Fuster V, Fallon JT. Macrophage infiltration in acute coronary syndromes. Implications for plaque rupture. Circulation 1994;90:775-8.

104. Geng YJ, Libby P. Progression of atheroma: a struggle between death and procreation. Arterioscler Thromb Vasc Biol 2002;22:1370-80.

105. Geng YJ, Libby P. Evidence for apoptosis in advanced human atheroma. Colocalization with interleukin-1 beta-converting enzyme. Am J Pathol 1995;147:251-66.

106. Isner JM, Kearney M, Bortman S, Passeri J. Apoptosis in human atherosclerosis and restenosis. Circulation 1995;91:2703-11.

107. Lee RT, Grodzinsky AJ, Frank EH, Kamm RD, Schoen FJ. Structure-dependent dynamic mechanical behavior of fibrous caps from human atherosclerotic plaques. Circulation 1991;83:1764-70.

108. Lendon CL, Davies MJ, Born GV, Richardson PD. Atherosclerotic plaque caps are locally weakened when macrophages density is increased. Atherosclerosis 1991;87:87-90.

109. van der Wal AC, Becker AE, van der Loos CM, Das PK. Site of intimal rupture or erosion of thrombosed coronary atherosclerotic plaques is characterized by an inflammatory process irrespective of the dominant plaque morphology. Circulation 1994;89:36-44.

110. Matrisian LM. The matrix-degrading metalloproteinases. Bioessays 1992;14:455-63.

111. Henney AM, Wakeley PR, Davies MJ, et al. Localization of stromelysin gene expression in atherosclerotic plaques by in situ hybridization. Proc Natl Acad Sci U S A 1991;88:8154-8.

112. Kaartinen M, Penttila A, Kovanen PT. Accumulation of activated mast cells in the shoulder region of human coronary atheroma, the predilection site of atheromatous rupture. Circulation 1994;90:1669-78.

113. Weiss SJ. Tissue destruction by neutrophils. N Engl J Med 1989;320:365-76.

114. Stein PD, Hamid MS, Shivkumar K, Davis TP, Khaja F, Henry JW. Effects of cyclic flexion of coronary arteries on progression of atherosclerosis. Am J Cardiol 1994;73:431-7.

115. Muller JE, Tofler GH, Stone PH. Circadian variation and triggers of onset of acute cardiovascular disease. Circulation 1989;79:733-43.

116. Tofler GH, Stone PH, Maclure M, et al. Analysis of possible triggers of acute myocardial infarction (the MILIS study). Am J Cardiol 1990;66:22-7.

117. Cheng GC, Loree HM, Kamm RD, Fishbein MC, Lee RT. Distribution of circumferential stress in ruptured and stable atherosclerotic lesions. A structural analysis with histopathological correlation. Circulation 1993;87:1179-87.

118. Rubanyi GM, Romero JC, Vanhoutte PM. Flow-induced release of endothelium-derived relaxing factor. Am J Physiol 1986;250:H1145-9.

119. Gertz SD, Uretsky G, Wajnberg RS, Navot N, Gotsman MS. Endothelial cell damage and thrombus formation after partial arterial constriction: relevance to the role of coronary artery spasm in the pathogenesis of myocardial infarction. Circulation 1981;63:476-86.

120. Osende JI, Badimon JJ, Fuster V, et al. Blood thrombogenicity in type 2 diabetes mellitus patients is associated with glycemic control. J Am Coll Cardiol 2001;38:1307-12.

121. Rauch U, Crandall J, Osende JI, et al. Increased thrombus formation relates to ambient blood glucose and leukocyte count in diabetes mellitus type 2. Am J Cardiol 2000;86:246-9.

122. Sambola A, Osende J, Hathcock J, et al. Role of risk factors in the modulation of tissue factor activity and blood thrombogenicity. Circulation 2003;107:973-7.

123. Badimon L, Chesebro JH, Badimon JJ. Thrombus formation on ruptured atherosclerotic plaques and rethrombosis on evolving thrombi. Circulation 1992;86:III74-85.

124. Wilcox JN, Smith KM, Schwartz SM, Gordon D. Localization of tissue factor in the normal vessel wall and in the atherosclerotic plaque. Proc Natl Acad Sci U S A 1989;86:2839-43.

125. Toschi V, Gallo R, Lettino M, et al. Tissue factor modulates the thrombogenicity of human atherosclerotic plaques. Circulation 1997;95:594-9.

126. Viles-Gonzalez JF, Badimon JJ. Atherothrombosis: the role of tissue factor. Int J Biochem Cell Biol 2004;36:25-30.

127. Lassila R, Badimon JJ, Vallabhajosula S, Badimon L. Dynamic monitoring of platelet deposition on severely damaged vessel wall in flowing blood. Effects of different stenoses on thrombus growth. Arteriosclerosis 1990;10:306-15.

128. Badimon L, Badimon JJ, Turitto VT, Vallabhajosula S, Fuster V. Platelet thrombus formation on collagen type I. A model of deep vessel injury. Influence of blood rheology, von Willebrand factor, and blood coagulation. Circulation 1988;78:1431-42.

129. Fuster V, Badimon L, Badimon JJ, Ip JH, Chesebro JH. The porcine model for the understanding of thrombogenesis and atherogenesis. Mayo Clin Proc 1991;66:818-31.

130. Larsson PT, Wallen NH, Hjemdahl P. Norepinephrine-induced human platelet activation in vivo is only partly counteracted by aspirin. Circulation 1994;89:1951-7.

131. Willich SN, Linderer T, Wegscheider K, Leizorovicz A, Alamercery I, Schroder R. Increased morning incidence of myocardial infarction in the ISAM Study: absence with prior beta-adrenergic blockade. ISAM Study Group. Circulation 1989;80:853-8.

132. Gelernt MD, Hochman JS. Acute myocardial infarction triggered by emotional stress. Am J Cardiol 1992;69:1512-3.

133. Ridker PM, Manson JE, Buring JE, Muller JE, Hennekens CH. Circadian variation of acute myocardial infarction and the effect of low-dose aspirin in a randomized trial of physicians. Circulation 1990;82:897-902.

134. Loscalzo J. Lipoprotein(a). A unique risk factor for atherothrombotic disease. Arteriosclerosis 1990;10:672-9.

135. Ridker PM, Hennekens CH, Stampfer MJ. A prospective study of lipoprotein(a) and the risk of myocardial infarction. Jama 1993;270:2195-9.

136. Lerman A, Webster MW, Chesebro JH, et al. Circulating and tissue endothelin immunoreactivity in hypercholesterolemic pigs. Circulation 1993;88:2923-8.

137. Bogaty P, Hackett D, Davies G, Maseri A. Vasoreactivity of the culprit lesion in unstable angina. Circulation 1994;90:5-11.

138. Leary T. The genesis of coronary sclerosis. N Engl J Med 1951;245:397-402.

139. Etsuda H, Mizuno K, Arakawa K, Satomura K, Shibuya T, Isojima K. Angioscopy in variant angina: coronary artery spasm and intimal injury. Lancet 1993;342:1322-4.

140. Nobuyoshi M, Tanaka M, Nosaka H, et al. Progression of coronary atherosclerosis: is coronary spasm related to progression? J Am Coll Cardiol 1991;18:904-10.

141. Fuster V. 50th anniversary historical article. Acute coronary syndromes: the degree and morphology of coronary stenoses. J Am Coll Cardiol 2000;35:52B-54B.

142. Falk E. Unstable angina with fatal outcome: dynamic coronary thrombosis leading to infarction and/or sudden death. Autopsy evidence of recurrent mural thrombosis with peripheral embolization culminating in total vascular occlusion. Circulation 1985;71:699-708.

143. Fuster V, Fallon JT, Badimon JJ, Nemerson Y. The unstable atherosclerotic plaque: clinical significance and therapeutic intervention. Thromb Haemost 1997;78:247-55.

144. Fuster V, Badimon L, Badimon JJ, Chesebro JH. The pathogenesis of coronary artery disease and the acute coronary syndromes (2). N Engl J Med 1992;326:310-8.

145. Cohen M, Sherman W, Rentrop KP, Gorlin R. Determinants of collateral filling observed during sudden controlled coronary artery occlusion in human subjects. J Am Coll Cardiol 1989;13:297-303.

146. Fuster V, Frye RL, Kennedy MA, Connolly DC, Mankin HT. The role of collateral circulation in the various coronary syndromes. Circulation 1979;59:1137-44.

147. Braunwald E, Antman EM, Beasley JW, et al. ACC/AHA guideline update for the management of patients with unstable angina and non-ST-segment elevation myocardial infarction--2002: summary article: a report of the American College of Cardiology/American Heart Association Task Force on Practice Guidelines (Committee on the Management of Patients With Unstable Angina). Circulation 2002;106:1893-900.

148. Braunwald E. Application of current guidelines to the management of unstable angina and non-ST-elevation myocardial infarction. Circulation 2003;108:III28-37.

149. DeWood MA, Stifter WF, Simpson CS, et al. Coronary arteriographic findings soon after non-Q-wave myocardial infarction. N Engl J Med 1986;315:417-23.

Chapter 4

THE ANTIOXIDANT HYPOTHESIS

Charlene Bierl, Marc Forgione, and Joseph Loscalzo
Boston University School of Medicine, Whitaker Cardiovascular Institute, and Evans Department of Medicine, Boston, MA

Introduction

Recent studies suggest that oxidative stress plays a significant role in the pathogenesis of atherosclerosis. This process serves as the basis for the oxidative-modification hypothesis of atherosclerosis. Several risk factors for atherothrombotic disease, such as hypercholesterolemia, hypertension, diabetes mellitus, cigarette smoking, and hyperhomocysteinemia, promote oxidative reactions in the vasculature. Oxidant stress adversely modifies low-density-lipoprotein (LDL), attracts and activates leukocytes, and stimulates platelets. Oxygen radicals, while harmful, are also produced as byproducts of the general metabolic activity of the cell. In order to combat factors promoting oxidative stress, mammals have evolved several antioxidant defenses to limit oxidant injury. These defenses, which include water-soluble antioxidants (e.g., glutathione, ascorbate), lipid soluble antioxidants (e.g., α-tocopherol), and antioxidant enzymes (e.g., glutathione peroxidases) in the vasculature and extracellular space, offset the effects of reactive oxygen species (ROS). A disruption of this balance, by increased production of ROS or decreased antioxidant defenses, results in elevated levels of ROS, or oxidative stress. The antioxidant hypothesis derives from this limitation of endogenous antioxidant defenses, and posits that inadequate endogenous antioxidants promote, and antioxidant supplementation prevents, atherothrombosis. The results of the Heart Outcomes Prevention Evaluation (HOPE) Study[1] have failed to show a protective effect of α-tocopherol, challenging the underlying principles of this hypothesis. As will be discussed further, however, evidence suggests damage to the vascular wall represents an accumulation of multiple levels of imbalance in oxidative and reductive potentials over long periods of time, limiting the potential benefits of short-term antioxidant therapy.

Oxidative reactions

Free radicals generated under conditions of oxidant stress induce significant tissue damage and modification of lipids and proteins in the vasculature. A free radical is a molecule with one unpaired electron, and is, therefore, chemically unstable, seeking to donate this electron or acquire another electron. Importantly, when a free radical donates or accepts an electron, it often generates another species with an unpaired electron, i.e., another free radical.

Several free radicals are of central importance in the oxidative reactions occurring in the vasculature. At the beginning of the cascade lies superoxide anion (O_2^-). Superoxide anion is well established as a toxic oxygen radical produced by NADPH oxidase, nitric oxide synthases, and xanthine oxidase, as well as a byproduct of mitochondrial electron transport. All of these enzymes have also been identified in the vascular wall. Macrophages utilize NADPH oxidase-dependent superoxide production during inflammatory and innate immune responses to foreign antigens. Simultaneously, O_2^- is released by these activated leukocytes into the local environment, including the vascular wall. NADPH oxidase is also activated by angiotensin II, suggesting a physiological role in addition to host defense[2]. Xanthine oxidase is commonly recognized for its role in the metabolism of adenylate monophosphate to uric acid for excretion. Inhibition of xanthine oxidase, has been found to decrease vasodilation in patients with atherosclerosis[3], suggesting a physiologic role of the enzyme in the vascular space. Nitric oxide synthases (NOS), while necessary for the production of nitric oxide, have been found to produce O_2^-, as well, when either the substrate L-arginine or the cofactor tetrahydrobiopterin are absent[4-6] in a process termed, "uncoupling."

Once produced, O_2^- can directly damage neighboring tissue, or can be converted by superoxide dismutase (SOD) into H_2O_2. Hydrogen peroxide can, in turn, lead to the formation of hydroperoxide (OH-) and hydroxyl radical (OH$^-$) in the presence of iron or copper ions and another superoxide anion via the Haber-Weiss reaction[7]:

$$H_2O_2 + O_2^-. \rightarrow \quad O_2 + OH^- + OH^-$$

or directly by the Fenton reaction[8]:

$$H_2O_2 + Fe^{+2} \rightarrow Fe^{+3} + OH^- + OH^-$$

The hydroxyl radical formed is highly reactive toward the nearest available relative positive charge, including lipid, RNA, DNA or proteins. The hydroxide anion, the more stable byproduct, lowers the pH of its microenvironment, resulting in alkaline tissue damage.

Recently, ozone and its derivatives have surfaced as additional ROS with a potential role in the pathogenesis of atherosclerosis. Wentworth and colleagues initially identified ozone production by neutrophils via an antibody catalyzed conversion of water to hydrogen peroxide as part of an inflammatory reaction and nonspecific bactericidal activity[9,10]. More recently, they have documented the production of ozone within an atherosclerotic plaque, both through the presence of signature byproducts of ozone based reactions and through direct production in isolated lesions[11]. They hypothesize that leukocyte activation, and subsequently ozone production, within a plaque is critical to the pathogenesis of atherosclerosis[11]. The complex reaction involves the formation of a trioxygen species, dihydrogen trioxide (H_2O_3), from singlet oxygen ($^1O_2^*$) and water, and the subsequent production of ozone and hydrogen peroxide. The ozone then reacts with the hydrogen peroxide to yield the hydrotrioxy radical, which disproportionates into triplet oxygen and the hydroxyl radical[12]:

$$^1O_2^* + H_2O \rightarrow H_2O_3$$

$$H_2O_3 + {}^1O_2^* \rightarrow O_3 + H_2O_2 \rightarrow [O_3HO_2H]$$

$$\cdot O_3H \rightarrow {}^3O_2 + \cdot OH$$

This mechanism, if proven correct, would offer a means of generating hydoxyl radicals independent of the presence of transition metals[12].

Of central importance to the oxidative modification hypothesis is lipid peroxidation and, in particular, the generation of oxidized low-density lipoprotein (oxLDL). LDL is a complex particle composed of lipid and protein components. The protein portion comprises exclusively apolipoprotein B-100 (apo-B); lipid moieties include phospholipids, fatty acids, triglycerides, cholesterol, cholesteryl ester[13], and lipid-soluble antioxidants. The fatty acids are either unsaturated or saturated, and the polyunsaturated fatty acids (PUFAs) have varying numbers of carbon-carbon double bonds. The most common PUFAs in LDL are lineolenic (18:3) and arachidonic acids (20:4)[14]. The important antioxidants present in LDL are shown in *Figure 1*[15].

Generation of oxidized LDL

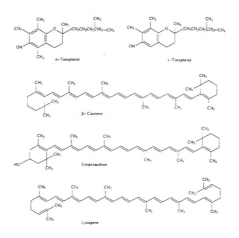

Figure 1. **Structures of common antioxidants found in LDL** (Reproduced with permission from reference 15).

Reactive oxygen species are generated in an area of high oxidant stress. When OH˙ comes into contact with PUFA, it initiates ROS formation by abstracting a H˙ radical from a carbon-carbon double bond. This reaction forms a stable oxygen species (H₂O) and a PUFA radical, as shown in the following equation where LH represents a PUFA:

$$OH˙ + LH \rightarrow H_2O + L$$

The PUFA radical then rearranges to form a conjugated diene that reacts with molecular O₂ to form a PUFA-peroxyl radical:

XC==CXCX

|

O

|

O   (4)

⊣

The newly formed radical then abstracts an H· radical from another PUFA (L'H) forming a lipid hydroperoxide:

$$LOO· + L'H \rightarrow LOOH + L'$$

These processes define the propagation phase of lipid peroxidation. As unstable compounds (free radicals) are generated in this phase, the reactions occur as chain reactions and end with a termination reaction. Concomitant with the oxidation of PUFAs, oxidation of the apo-B portion of LDL also occurs, principally at lysine residues[16].

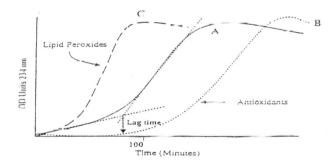

Figure 2. **LDL oxidation by copper.** A) Copper-induced LDL oxidation. B) Inhibition of oxidation with antioxidants. C) Lipid peroxides potentiate the oxidation of LDL. (Reproduced with permission from reference 15).

The rate of PUFA oxidization is dependent on several factors. The number of carbon-carbon double bonds represents the number of abstractable hydrogens, and an increase in the degree of unsaturation of a PUFA will increase the rate at which it is oxidized. Lipid-soluble antioxidants in LDL, such as α-tocopherol, become oxidized prior to the PUFA in the particle and delay the propagation phase of the process. This delay defines the lag phase, the difference in PUFA oxidation as a result of the presence of antioxidants, and is demonstrated in *Figure 2*[17]. Thus, lipid soluble antioxidants protect LDL from oxidative damage as they become oxidized before (i.e., are more readily oxidized than) the PUFAs in the LDL particle.

Oxidative stress damages proteins as well as lipids. The oxidation of the apo-B subfraction of LDL induces derivatization of lysine residues that neutralize the positively charged ϵ-amino group[18]. Malondialdehyde (MDA)- and 4-hydroxynonenal (HNE)-modified lysine residues of apo-B formed concomitantly during lipid peroxidation are immunogenic and localize to atherosclerotic lesions[19]. Aldehyde-modified bovine serum albumin is phagocytosed by murine periotoneal macrophages through a scavenger-receptor mechanism[20]. Oxidized apo-B may also play an important role in the induction of macrophage activation[21].

Oxidized LDL (OxLDL) has a short half-life in plasma; thus, the generation of oxLDL important for atherogenesis likely occurs elsewhere, possibly in the subendothelial space. Importantly, LDL and oxLDL entry into macrophages in the subendothelial space occurs through the LDL receptor and through the scavenger receptor pathways, respectively. Uptake of LDL by its receptor is feedback-inhibited, while uptake of oxLDL by the scavenger receptor is not. Plasma LDL diffuses into the subendothelial space and becomes mildly oxidized, initially termed minimally oxidized (MM-LDL). As MM-LDL is not recognized by the scavenger receptor, it can be assumed to have a plasma half-life similar to that of native LDL[22]. Further modification of LDL results in oxLDL. These two particles stimulate the activity of leukocytes and platelets, potentiating their role in atherothrombosis. Importantly, these actions can be impaired by antioxidants.

Consequences of oxidative reactions in the vasculature

The mechanisms underlying the pathological effects of oxLDL has been extensively studied. MM-LDL stimulates the release of monocyte chemotactic protein 1 (MCP-1) and macrophage colony-stimulating factor (M-CSF)[23] from the endothelium, attracting monocytes to the vessel wall and promoting their differentiation into tissue macrophages. OxLDL also directly attracts macrophages, and stimulates the release of M-CSF and MCP-1[24] from endothelial cells and interleukin-1 release from macrophages[25]. Alpha-tocopherol prevents the consequences of OxLDL, in part, by decreasing the ability of monocytes to bind to endothelial cells[26,27]. Endothelial cells express certain adhesion molecules, for example, the selectins that are recognized by monocytes, promoting their adhesion and entry into the subendothelial space. E-selectin is important in the development of atherothrombosis, and its expression on the endothelium is decreased by α-tocopherol[26].

The pathology of an atherosclerotic plaque suggests roles for activated platelets and for remodeling of the vascular wall, including apoptosis and migration of endothelial and smooth muscle cells. The presence of oxLDL leads to increased platelet adhesion in vascular preparations in a process prevented by SOD and catalase[28]. MM-LDL induces apoptosis in coronary endothelial and smooth muscle cells[29], and does so through a Fas-ligand-based mechanism in vascular endothelial cells[30]. LDL also stimulates smooth muscle cell proliferation[31], utilizing the MAPK pathway[32], PI3 kinase, EGF receptor[33], and spingomyelin pathways[34].

Antioxidant defenses

Owing to the prevalence and toxicity of these ROS, cells have evolved extensive mechanisms to inactivate them. Three different forms of superoxide dismutase (manganese, copper/zinc, extracellular) metabolize O_2 to hydrogen peroxide. Catalase and at least four isoforms of glutathione peroxidase then convert H_2O_2 into water. The overexpression of catalase protects vascular smooth muscle cells from the cytotoxic effected of oxidized lipids[35]. In addition, the presence of lipid peroxides appears to stimulate the expression of catalase[36]. While catalase expression could not be directly tied to the progression of an atherosclerotic lesion, there does appear to be an intense increase in expression within migrating smooth muscle cells and macrophages[37]. Considering the evidence previously mentioned for the role of oxLDL in smooth muscle cell migration and macrophage recruitment, a parallel increase in oxidative defenses in these cells is not surprising.

If SOD activity outpaces the activity of peroxidases, then there arises a danger of accumulating hydrogen peroxide. Extracellular SOD (ecSOD) is produced by vascular smooth muscle cells and not endothelial cells[38, 39], and localizes in highest concentrations between the endothelium and vascular smooth muscle cells[40]. Recent work has also found that the expression of this enzyme is induced by nitric oxide (NO)[41]. These later findings raise the possibility that its function is to protect the bioavailability of NO released by endothelial cells. Increased expression and activity of ecSOD have also been found in macrophage-rich atherosclerotic lesions[42,43]. Whether or not this activity is the result of increased stimulation by oxLDL or the cause of an excess of hydrogen peroxide production that then leads to increased oxidant stress and atherogenesis[38] remains unclear.

Nitric oxide as an antioxidant

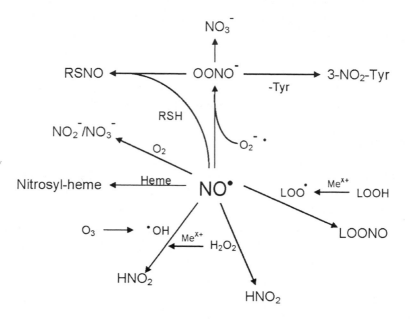

Figure 3. **Reactive oxygen species and NO.** NO can undergo several fates within platelets, including oxidative inactivation to nitrite (NO_2^-) and nitrate (NO_3^-) and react with superoxide anion to form peroxynitrite ($OONO^-$). Peroxynitrite can react with tyrosyl residues in proteins to form 3-nitrosyl residues, and with thiols to form S-nitrosothiols (RSNO); the latter can also form by the reaction of NO with thiols in the presence of oxygen via an N_2O_3 intermediate. By reacting with heme iron, nitrosyl-heme charge transfer complexes can form, accounting for the biological activation of guanylyl cyclase by NO. Lipid peroxides (LOOH) can yield lipid peroxyl radicals (LOO•), which can react with NO to form lipid peroxynitrites (LOONO), and hydrogen peroxide can react with NO or with hydroxyl radical formed from ozone, to form nitrous acid (HNO_2). Each of these reactions and the reactants that engage in them are present in platelets and in the extracellular microenvironment of activated platelets. (Modified with permission from reference 44).

Many of the adverse vascular effects of ROS are inhibited by NO. Biochemically, NO itself reacts directly with superoxide anion to form peroxynitrite[44] with hydrogen peroxide to form nitrite and hydroxyl radical[45], and with lipid peroxides to form lipid peroxynitrite[46] (*Figure 3*). When NO reacts with ROS, its biologic activity, such as platelet inhibition and vasodilation, is eliminated. Thus, an excess of ROS, either due to a deficiency in enzyme defenses or increased production, can result in consumption of bioavailable NO. As previously mentioned, inactivation of

NO by radicals generated by enzymes, such as myeloperoxidase, may also have a physiological role in regulating vasodilation[47].

Glutathione peroxidase family

There are four well-characterized isoforms of glutathione peroxidase (GPx), including extracellular or plasma, phospholipid, gastrointestinal, and cellular. These enzymes are unique because they contain a redox-active selenocysteine residue in the active site of the enzyme. Selenium deficiency, which results in deficiencies of the GPx enzymes, is clinically recognized as Keshan disease and is manifest by cardiomyopathy and vascular disease[48]. This disease was only seen in the Dechang area of China, and has now been eradicated through dietary supplementation with selenium, which raised both serum selenium concentrations and GPx activity[49]. Since this original observation, three other studies have evaluated the relationship among selenium, glutathione peroxidase, and cardiovascular disease. One study, a five year risk evaluation in rural Finland, found that a low serum selenium level was significantly associated with stroke mortality[50]. A later prospective cohort study in Denmark showed an increased risk of ischemic heart disease with a low serum selenium level[51]. A recent, large, prospective cohort study showed an inverse association between cellular glutathione peroxidases (GPx-1) activity and risk of cardiovascular events, while SOD had no association in this study cohort[52].

The GPxs catalyze the reduction of lipid and hydrogen peroxides to their corresponding alcohols at the expense of oxidizing two reduced glutathione molecules. Each isoform has a slightly different spectrum of substrates upon which it is active. The plasma isoform reduces phospholipid-derived hydroperoxides, but not cholesteryl hydroperoxides[53], in the extracellular environment. In contrast, phospholipid GPx (GPx-4) is localized to the cytosolic and intracellular membrane compartments, including the mitochondrial surface[54], and catalyzes the reduction of longer fatty acyl peroxides. Cellular GPx (GPx-1) has very similar structure and properties to the extracellular isoform, the major difference being its intracellular localization. Overexpression of GPx-4 was found to inhibit hydroperoxide-induced oxidation, NFkB activation, and apoptosis in rabbit aortic smooth muscle cells[55].

Previously, our laboratory has published studies on the platelets of two brothers with a cerebral arterial thrombotic disorder of unknown etiology[56]. Their platelets were found to be hyperreactive; thrombin-induced aggregation was inhibited by prostacyclin, as expected, but was not inhibited by NO. When patient platelets were isolated and resuspended in plasma from an unaffected control, the platelet response to NO was restored. Similarly, when platelets isolated from a control individual were resuspended in plasma from the patients, the response to NO was eliminated. These results suggest that NO was being inactivated by the patients' plasma. Levels of hydrogen peroxide were found to be elevated in the patients' plasma, which could interact with and inactive NO. To further this investigation, patient antioxidant defenses were measured. Plasma GPx (GPx-3) levels were found to be lower in patient plasma than controls, and the addition of cGPx to the patient plasma restored the inhibitory effect of NO[56]. Subsequent work on the GPx-3 promoter has demonstrated hypoxia-sensitive promoter activity[57]. This finding led to the identification of seven linked polymorphisms in the promoter of the GPx3 gene that correlated with reduced induction of GPx-3 under the same hypoxic conditions, and an association with a significant increase in the risk of arterial ischemic stroke in young adults[58]. This combination of findings, in context with the previous work, provides further evidence that a reduction in the expression of antioxidant defenses (such as GPx3) in response to oxidative stress, results in decreased bioavailable NO, decreased platelet inhibition, and increased risk of arterial thrombosis.

Further evidence of the connection between GPx and cardiovascular disease lies in the mechanism of action of homocysteine, an established risk factor for atherosclerosis[59,60]. Homocysteine is a sulfur-containing amino acid that undergoes auto-oxidation in plasma to produce $OH^.$, OH^-, and H_2O_2. While the mechanism underlying risk is not entirely understood, several proposals have been offered, all of which have a common denominator of decreasing levels of bioavailable NO. The ROS generated from the auto-oxidation of homocysteine enter the endothelium and are detoxified by GPx-1[61]; however, elevated concentration of homocysteine overwhelm this crucial defense, principally by decreasing expression of cellular GPx-1[62]. Restoration of GPx-1 activity, through overexpression, rescued vasodilator function to normal levels in mouse models[63]. Thus, increased levels of homocysteine would directly result in decreased inactivation of peroxides and decreased bioavailable NO.

Myeloperoxidase, another oxidative enzyme, is classically known for its release by activated monocytes and neutrophils as part of the host defense system. This enzyme is a heme-containing protein secreted by phagocytes that converts hydrogen peroxide to hypochlorite and other free radical intermediates[64, 65]. Increased expression of myeloperoxidase has been found in atherosclerotic lesions[66], and one of its byproducts, hypochlorite, oxidizes a lysine residue in apo-B[16], leading to high-uptake of this oxidized LDL by macrophages[16]. More recent work suggests that it may also modulate vascular dysfunction in inflammation by catalytic consumption of NO through the generation of reactive intermediates[47]. In addition, a recent study of emergency room patients presenting with chest pain has shown that a single initial measurement of plasma activity of myeloperoxidase independently predicted the risk of early myocardial infarction as well as the risk of major adverse cardiac events in the ensuing 30 days and six months[67].

Endothelial dysfunction

There is a significant amount of evidence correlating a loss of the balance between ROS and antioxidant potential to the progression of atherosclerotic disease, including early changes in endothelial function. An important determinant of endothelial function affected by the imbalance of these forces is NO. Evidence suggesting impaired NO production, as well as increased oxidative inactivation, has been correlated with reduced vasodilation, enhanced platelet activation, and increased vascular smooth muscle migration and proliferation, all of which define the phenotype of endothelial dysfunction.

References

1. Yusuf S, Dagenais G, Pogue J, Bosch J, Sleight P. Vitamin E supplementation and cardiovascular events in high-risk patients. The Heart Outcomes Prevention Evaluation Study Investigators. N Engl J Med 2000;342:154-60.
2. Griendling KK, Minieri CA, Ollerenshaw JD, Alexander RW. Angiotensin II stimulates NADH and NADPH oxidase activity in cultured vascular smooth muscle cells. Circ Res 1994;74:1141-8.
3. Cardillo C, Kilcoyne CM, Cannon RO, III, Quyyumi AA, Panza JA. Xanthine oxidase inhibition with oxypurinol improves endothelial vasodilator function in hypercholesterolemic but not in hypertensive patients. Hypertension 1997;30:57-63.
4. Heinzel B, John M, Klatt P, Bohme E, Mayer B. Ca2+/calmodulin-dependent formation of hydrogen peroxide by brain nitric oxide synthase. Biochem J 1992;281:627-30.
5. Pou S, Pou WS, Bredt DS, Snyder SH, Rosen GM. Generation of superoxide by purified brain nitric oxide synthase. J Biol Chem 1992;267:24173-6.
6. Vasquez-Vivar J, Kalyanaraman B, Martasek P, et al. Superoxide generation by endothelial nitric oxide synthase: the influence of cofactors. Proc Natl Acad Sci U S A 1998;95:9220-5.
7. Haber F, Weiss J. The catalytic decomposition of hydrogen peroxide by iron salts. Proc R Soc Lond 1934;147:332-52.
8. Fenton J. Oxidation of tartaric acid in the presence of iron. J Chem Soc Trans 1894;65:899-910.
9. Wentworth P, Jr., McDunn JE, Wentworth AD, et al. Evidence for antibody-catalyzed ozone formation in bacterial killing and inflammation. Science 2002;298:2195-9.
10. Babior BM, Takeuchi C, Ruedi J, Gutierrez A, Wentworth P, Jr. Investigating antibody-catalyzed ozone generation by human neutrophils. Proc Natl Acad Sci U S A 2003;100:3031-4.
11. Wentworth P, Jr., Nieva J, Takeuchi C, et al. Evidence for ozone formation in human atherosclerotic arteries. Science 2003;302:1053-6.
12. Loscalzo J. Ozone--from environmental pollutant to atherogenic determinant. N Engl J Med 2004;350:834-5.
13. Patrono C, FitzGerald G. Isoprostanes: potential markers of oxidant stress in atherothrombotic disease. Atheroscler Thromb Vasc Biol 1997;17:2309-15.
14. Esterbauer H, Jurgens G, Quehenberger O, Koller E. Autoxidation of human low density lipoprotein: loss of polyunsaturated fatty acids and vitamin E and generation of aldehydes. J Lipid Res 1987;28:495-509.
15. Frei B. Natural Antioxidants in Human Health and Disease. Academic Press, 1994.
16. Hazell LJ, Stocker R. Oxidation of low-density lipoprotein with hypochlorite causes transformation of the lipoprotein into a high-uptake form for macrophages. Biochem J 1993;290:165-72.
17. Parthasarathy S, Auge N, Santanam N. Implications of lag time concept in the oxidation of LDL. Free Radic Res 1998;28:583-91.
18. Steinberg D. Low density lipoprotein oxidation and its pathobiological significance. J Biol Chem 1997;272:20963-6.
19. Steinbrecher UP. Oxidation of human low density lipoprotein results in derivatization of lysine residues of apolipoprotein B by lipid peroxide decomposition products. J Biol Chem 1987;262:3603-8.
20. Haberland ME, Fong D, Cheng L. Malondialdehyde-altered protein occurs in atheroma of Watanabe heritable hyperlipidemic rabbits. Science 1988;241:215-8.

21. Beppu M, Fukata Y, Kikugawa K. Interaction of malondialdehyde-modified bovine serum albumin and mouse peritoneal macrophages. Chem Pharm Bull (Tokyo) 1988;36:4519-26.

22. Napoli C, D'Armiento F, Mancini F, et al. Removal of mild oxidized lipoprotein(a) by rat hepatic Kupffer cells. Circulation 1996;94 (suppl II):104.

23. Henriksen T, Mahoney EM, Steinberg D. Interactions of plasma lipoproteins with endothelial cells. Ann N Y Acad Sci 1982;401:102-16.

24. Quinn MT, Parthasarathy S, Fong LG, Steinberg D. Oxidatively modified low density lipoproteins: a potential role in recruitment and retention of monocyte/macrophages during atherogenesis. Proc Natl Acad Sci U S A 1987;84:2995-8.

25. Thomas CE, Jackson RL, Ohlweiler DF, Ku G. Multiple lipid oxidation products in low density lipoproteins induce interleukin-1 beta release from human blood mononuclear cells. J Lipid Res 1994;35:417-27.

26. Faruqi R, de la Motte C, DiCorleto PE. Alpha-tocopherol inhibits agonist-induced monocytic cell adhesion to cultured human endothelial cells. J Clin Invest 1994;94:592-600.

27. Devaraj S, Li D, Jialal I. The effects of alpha tocopherol supplementation on monocyte function. Decreased lipid oxidation, interleukin 1 beta secretion, and monocyte adhesion to endothelium. J Clin Invest 1996;98:756-63.

28. Vink H, Constantinescu AA, Spaan JAE. Oxidized lipoproteins degrade the endothelial surface layer: implications for platelet-endothelial cell adhesion. Circulation 2000;101:1500-2.

29. Napoli C, Quehenberger O, De Nigris F, Abete P, Glass CK, Palinski W. Mildly oxidized low density lipoprotein activates multiple apoptotic signaling pathways in human coronary cells. FASEB J. 2000;14:1996-2007.

30. Sata M, Walsh K. Oxidized LDL activates Fas-mediated endothelial cell apoptosis. J Clin Invest 1998;102:1682-9.

31. Resink TJ, Bochkov VN, Hahn AW, Philippova MP, Buhler FR, Tkachuk VA. Low- and high-density lipoproteins as mitogenic factors for vascular smooth muscle cells: individual, additive and synergistic effects. J Vasc Res 1995;32:328-38.

32. Kusuhara M, Chait A, Cader A, Berk BC. Oxidized LDL stimulates mitogen-activated protein kinases in smooth muscle cells and macrophages. Arterioscler Thromb Vasc Biol 1997;17:141-8.

33. Auge N, Garcia V, Maupas-Schwalm F, Levade T, Salvayre R, Negre-Salvayre A. Oxidized LDL-induced smooth muscle cell proliferation involves the EGF receptor/PI-3 kinase/Akt and the sphingolipid signaling pathways. Arterioscler Thromb Vasc Biol 2002;22:1990-5.

34. Auge N, Nikolova-Karakashian M, Carpentier S, et al. Role of sphingosine 1-phosphate in the mitogenesis induced by oxidized low density lipoprotein in smooth muscle cells via activation of sphingomyelinase, ceramidase, and sphingosine kinase. J. Biol. Chem. 1999;274:21533-8.

35. Santanam N, Auge N, Zhou M, Keshava C, Parthasarathy S. Overexpression of human catalase gene decreases oxidized lipid-induced cytotoxicity in vascular smooth muscle cells. Arterioscler Thromb Vasc Biol 1999;19:1912-7.

36. Meilhac O, Zhou M, Santanam N, Parthasarathy S. Lipid peroxides induce expression of catalase in cultured vascular cells. J Lipid Res 2000;41:1205-13.

37. Kobayashi S, Inoue N, Azumi H, et al. Expressional changes of the vascular antioxidant system in atherosclerotic coronary arteries. J Atheroscler Thromb 2002;9:184-90.

38. Fukai T, Folz RJ, Landmesser U, Harrison DG. Extracellular superoxide dismutase and cardiovascular disease. Cardiovasc Res 2002;55:239-49.

39. Stralin P, Karlsson K, Johansson BO, Marklund SL. The interstitium of the human arterial wall contains very large amounts of extracellular superoxide dismutase. Arterioscler Thromb Vasc Biol 1995;15:2032-6.

40. Oury TD, Day BJ, Crapo JD. Extracellular superoxide dismutase: a regulator of nitric oxide bioavailability. Lab Invest 1996;75:617-36.

41. Fukai T, Siegfried MR, Ushio-Fukai M, Cheng Y, Kojda G, Harrison DG. Regulation of the vascular extracellular superoxide dismutase by nitric oxide and exercise training. J Clin Invest 2000;105:1631-9.

42. Luoma JS, Stralin P, Marklund SL, Hiltunen TP, Sarkioja T, Yla-Herttuala S. Expression of extracellular SOD and iNOS in macrophages and smooth muscle cells in human and rabbit atherosclerotic lesions: colocalization with epitopes characteristic of oxidized LDL and peroxynitrite-modified proteins. Arterioscler Thromb Vasc Biol 1998;18:157-67.

43. Fukai T, Siegfried MR, Ushio-Fukai M, Griendling KK, Harrison DG. Modulation of extracellular superoxide dismutase expression by angiotensin II and hypertension. Circ Res 1999;85:23-8.

44. Loscalzo J. Nitric oxide insufficiency, platelet activation, and arterial thrombosis. Circ Res 2001;88:756-62.

45. Nappi AJ, Vass E. Hydroxyl radical formation resulting from the interaction of nitric oxide and hydrogen peroxide. Biochim Biophys Acta 1998;1380:55-63.

46. Loscalzo J. Nitric oxide and the cardiovascular system. In: Loscalzo J, Vita J, eds. Contemporary Cardiology. Volume 4. Totowa NJ: Humana Press Inc, 2000.

47. Eiserich JP, Baldus S, Brennan ML, et al. Myeloperoxidase, a leukocyte-derived vascular NO oxidase. Science 2002;296:2391-4.

48. Litov RE, Combs GF, Jr. Selenium in pediatric nutrition. Pediatrics 1991;87:339-51.

49. Xia YM, Hill KE, Burk RF. Biochemical studies of a selenium-deficient population in China: measurement of selenium, glutathione peroxidase and other oxidant defense indices in blood. J Nutr 1989;119:1318-26.

50. Virtamo J, Valkeila E, Alfthan G, Punsar S, Huttunen JK, Karvonen MJ. Serum selenium and the risk of coronary heart disease and stroke. Am J Epidemiol 1985;122:276-82.

51. Chang CY, Lai YC, Cheng TJ, Lau MT, Hu ML. Plasma levels of antioxidant vitamins, selenium, total sulfhydryl groups and oxidative products in ischemic-stroke patients as compared to matched controls in Taiwan. Free Radic Res 1998;28:15-24.

52. Blankenberg S, Rupprecht HJ, Bickel C, et al. Glutathione peroxidase 1 activity and cardiovascular events in patients with coronary artery disease. N Engl J Med 2003;349:1605-13.

53. Yamamoto Y, Takahashi K. Glutathione peroxidase isolated from plasma reduces phospholipid hydroperoxides. Arch Biochem Biophys 1993;305:541-5.

54. Pushpa-Rekha TR, Burdsall AL, Oleksa LM, Chisolm GM, Driscoll DM. Rat phospholipid-hydroperoxide glutathione peroxidase. cDNA cloning and identification of multiple transcription and translation start sites. J Biol Chem 1995;270:26993-9.

55. Brigelius-Flohe R, Maurer S, Lotzer K, et al. Overexpression of PHGPx inhibits hydroperoxide-induced oxidation, NFkappaB activation and apoptosis and affects oxLDL-mediated proliferation of rabbit aortic smooth muscle cells. Atherosclerosis 2000;152:307-16.

56. Freedman JE, Loscalzo J, Benoit SE, Valeri CR, Barnard MR, Michelson AD. Decreased platelet inhibition by nitric oxide in two brothers with a history of arterial thrombosis. J Clin Invest 1996;97:979-87.

57. Bierl C, Voetsch B, Jin RC, Handy DE, Loscalzo J. Determinants of human plasma glutathione peroxidase (GPx-3) expression. J Biol Chem 2004;279:26839-45.
58. Voetsch B, Bierl C, Handy D, Loscalzo J. Adverse functional consequences of promoter polymorphisms in the plasma glutathione peroxidase gene. American Heart Association, Scientific Sessions 2003, manuscript in preparation.
59. Stampfer MJ, Malinow MR, Willett WC, et al. A prospective study of plasma homocyst(e)ine and risk of myocardial infarction in US physicians. JAMA 1992;268:877-81.
60. Selhub J, Jacques PF, Bostom AG, et al. Association between plasma homocysteine concentrations and extracranial carotid-artery stenosis. N Engl J Med 1995;332:286-91.
61. Welch GN, Upchurch GR, Jr., Loscalzo J. Homocysteine, oxidative stress, and vascular disease. Hosp Pract (Off Ed) 1997;32:81-2, 85, 88-92.
62. Upchurch GR, Jr., Welch GN, Fabian AJ, et al. Homocyst(e)ine decreases bioavailable nitric oxide by a mechanism involving glutathione peroxidase. J Biol Chem 1997;272:17012-7.
63. Weiss N, Zhang YY, Heydrick S, Bierl C, Loscalzo J. Overexpression of cellular glutathione peroxidase rescues homocyst(e)ine-induced endothelial dysfunction. Proc Natl Acad Sci U S A 2001;98:12503-8.
64. Winterbourn CC, Vissers MC, Kettle AJ. Myeloperoxidase. Curr Opin Hematol 2000;7:53-8.
65. Carr AC, McCall MR, Frei B. Oxidation of LDL by myeloperoxidase and reactive nitrogen species: reaction pathways and antioxidant protection. Arterioscler Thromb Vasc Biol 2000;20:1716-23.
66. Daugherty A, Dunn JL, Rateri DL, Heinecke JW. Myeloperoxidase, a catalyst for lipoprotein oxidation, is expressed in human atherosclerotic lesions. J Clin Invest 1994;94:437-44.
67. Brennan ML, Penn MS, Van Lente F, et al. Prognostic value of myeloperoxidase in patients with chest pain. N Engl J Med 2003;349:1595-604.

Chapter 5

REACTIVE OXYGEN SPECIES AS MEDIATORS OF SIGNAL TRANSDUCTION IN CARDIOVASCULAR DISEASES

Charles Kunsch and Xilin Chen
AtheroGenics Inc, Alpharetta, GA

Introduction

The generation of reactive oxygen species (ROS) is an inevitable consequence of life in an aerobic environment. ROS are a family of molecules derived from oxygen and characterized by their high chemical reactivity and ability to act as oxidants in redox reactions. They include both free radicals (species with one or more unpaired electrons such as the superoxide anion radical ($O2^-$), hydroxyl radical ($^.OH$), and lipid radicals ($LO^.$, LOO)), and hydrogen peroxide (H_2O_2), peroxynitrite ($ONOO$) and hypochlorous acid ($HOCl$) which are not free radicals, but can act as oxidizing agents that effect biological processes. There is a balance between ROS generation and the activity of enzymatic (i.e., superoxide dismutase, catalase, glutathione peroxidase) and non-enzymatic (glutathione, α-tocopherol, ascorbate, thioredoxin) antioxidant systems that scavenge or reduce ROS concentrations. In biological systems, redox imbalance, caused by an overall net increase in ROS production or a decrease in antioxidant capacity, leads to a generalized condition referred to as oxidative stress.

Historically, oxidative stress has been considered harmful and toxic due to free radical-induced oxidation and damage to biomolecules such as lipids, DNA and proteins[1,2]. Such damage can lead to membrane oxidation and instability, irreversible protein modifications and DNA mutagenesis and instability. ROS-mediated cellular damage has been thought to be associated with the pathogenesis of many diseases including Alzheimer, rheumatoid arthritis, asthma, diabetes as well as myocardial ischemia-reperfusion injury, atherosclerosis and restenosis.

It has become well accepted in the past decade that oxidative stress also exerts more subtle effects on cellular function. In a mechanism commonly referred to as "redox signaling", it is now apparent that the tightly regulated homeostatic control of ROS influences the activity of diverse intracellular molecules and signaling pathways. Therefore, ROS are not only toxic agents, but also mediators of physiological function by serving as second messengers. The net effect of redox signaling is the modulation of highly specific changes in gene expression and cellular phenotype[3,4]. Teleologically, the notion of ROS as signaling molecules helps explain the ubiquitous nature of ROS in biological systems, even in conditions of health.

The purpose of this review is to discuss the influence of ROS and oxidative stress on components of key signal transduction pathways in cardiovascular disease. Because there is a plethora of literature pertinent to this subject, we will limit our discussion to known ROS-sensitive signaling pathways as they relate primarily to coronary artery disease (CAD). The role of ROS-mediated signaling pathways in the pathogenesis of conditions such as congestive heart failure, ischemia/reperfusion injury, angiogenesis and vascular remodeling. has been reviewed in detail elsewhere[5-7]. We will briefly discuss the enzymatic sources and physiological mechanisms for generation of ROS in the vasculature followed by a more detailed discussion of the signaling pathways that are regulated by ROS. Finally, we will briefly discuss the biological impact of redox signaling and how it relates to regulation of gene expression in CAD.

ROS as signaling molecules

A general schematic overview of the production of key ROS is shown in *Figure 1*. The formation of ROS often begins with a one-electron reduction of molecular oxygen to superoxide anion (O_2^-) by several oxidases which are discussed later. The cell's endogenous defense against high levels of O_2^- is dismutation of O_2^- by superoxide dismutase (SOD), forming hydrogen peroxide (H_2O_2) and molecular oxygen. In the presence of nitric oxide (NO), O_2^- reacts more rapidly with NO than with SOD to peroxynitrite ($ONOO^-$), one of the most reactive and toxic ROS species. Hydrogen peroxide is much less reactive than O_2^-, and is metabolized by catalase to form oxygen and water. H_2O_2 can further be reduced by iron-containing molecules (i.e. the Fenton reaction) to yield the highly reactive hydroxyl radical ($^.OH$).

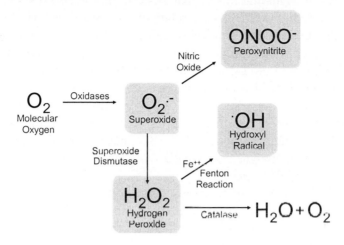

Figure 1. **Pathways for generation of key reactive oxygen species (ROS).** Major ROS implicated in signaling are indicated by a grey box. Single electron reduction of molecular oxygen, catalyzed by several oxidases (discussed in the text), generates superoxide. Reaction of superoxide with nitric oxide yields the reactive species peroxynitrite. Alternatively dismutation of superoxide via superoxide dismutase yields hydrogen peroxide which can be converted into hydroxyl radical by metal ion-dependent reactions such as the Fenton reaction (9). Modified from reference[23]with permission.

The physicochemical nature of each ROS is quite distinct and has important implications when considering ROS as signaling molecules. For example, both O_2^- and $\cdot OH$ are single-electron oxidants that are extremely short-lived in biological systems. Therefore, their ability to interact with targets at any significant distance from their site of production is limited by their short half-life. O_2^- is charged and, thus, crosses biological membranes primarily through anion channels[8], thus limiting its potential role as a paracrine signaling mediator. $\cdot OH$ does not exist in large amounts under normal conditions; however, in the presence of excess iron, the Fenton reaction may occur resulting in elevated levels of $\cdot OH$ from H_2O_2[9]. $\cdot OH$ is the key initiating ROS in lipid peroxidation which impairs cell membrane function, resulting in loss of normal ionic homeostasis, membrane permeability and receptor function. Lipid peroxides can also be formed by the action of cellular lipoxygenases on polyunsaturated fatty acids to yield biologically active lipid peroxides. Lipid peroxides have been shown to act as potent biological mediators. For example, they are implicated in the induction of NF-κB and cell adhesion molecules expression in endothelial cells (ECs) and in signaling in vascular smooth muscle cells (VSMCs)[10-13]. In contrast to ·OH and O_2^-, H_2O_2 is a relatively stable species with biological diffusion properties that are similar to H_2O and NO[8]. Thus, in many ways, H_2O_2 is well suited for a signaling role. First, H_2O_2 has a much longer half-life than other ROS in biological systems and, therefore, is able to reach its cellular target prior to it either reacting or being catalyzed[14]. Secondly, H_2O_2 reacts with protein thiol moieties to produce a variety of sulfur oxidation states including disulfides, sulfenic (-SOH), sulfinic (-SO$_2$H) or sulfonic (-SO$_3$H) acid products[15,16]. As has been demonstrated in bacteria[17], these different thiol oxidation states have the potential to produce distinct cellular responses.

The notion that ROS may mediate specific cellular events is not new. For example, ROS have well established roles in nature ranging from the fertilization of sea urchin eggs[18], to inflammation[19, 20] and thyroid hormone synthesis[21]. Furthermore, it has been known for decades that adipocytes possess an insulin-stimulated, NAD(P)H oxidase that has been implicated in the propagation of the insulin signal[22]. Thus, there is considerable precedence for ROS in mediating specific cellular functions. A number of physiological and pathophysiological stimuli induce phenotypic changes in vascular cell types as a function of ROS-mediated signal transduction[23-25]. Hyperlipidemia, diabetes, age, hypertension, physical inactivity and smoking are well-established risk factors for the development of atherosclerosis and all have an underlying commonality in their ability to impart oxidative stress to the vasculature. Some of the specific biological factors that mediate the increase in ROS via these diverse risk factors include oxidatively modified low-density lipoprotein (oxLDL), advanced glycation end products (AGE), angiotensin II (Ang II), inflammatory cytokines, and endothelial shear stress. It is now well-established that modulation of the expression of vascular gene products by intracellular oxidative signals may provide a molecular mechanism linking these seemingly diverse risk factors with the early pathogenesis of atherosclerosis[26,27]. These ROS then behave as second messenger molecules that transmit extracellular signals to modulate the expression of gene products involved in vascular disease such as adhesion molecules, proliferative genes, cytokines, and matrix-degrading enzymes (*Figure 2*). Before we discuss the specific signaling pathways that are modulated by ROS in the vasculature, we will discuss the sources of ROS and mechanisms that control the redox homeostasis in the vasculature.

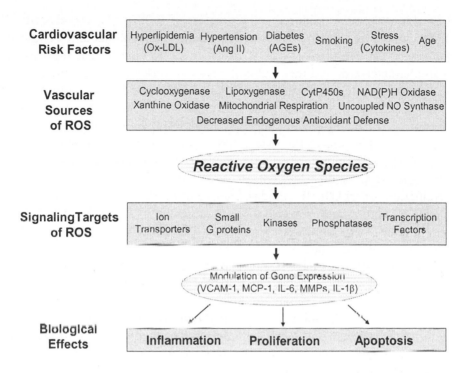

Figure 2. **Sources of reactive oxygen species (ROS) and their effects on signaling systems in cardiovascular disease.** Diverse risk factors for CAD include diabetes, hypertension, hyperlipidemia, smoking, age and stress. Mediators produced in response to these risk factors, including advanced glycation end-products (AGEs), low-density lipoproteins (LDL) and oxidized LDL (oxLDL), angiotensin II (Ang II), and cytokines such as TNF-a induce the formation of ROS in the vasculature by a variety of enzymatic and non-enzymatic sources. These ROS influence the activity of a variety of cellular signaling pathways ultimately leading to changes in the expression of redox-sensitive genes that regulate cellular processes involved in the pathogenesis of CAD.

Sources of ROS in the vasculature

Several excellent reviews have discussed the mechanism of production of ROS in cardiovascular disease[28-30]. Therefore, we will only briefly highlight key areas. Xanthine oxidase[31,32], cyclooxygenase[33-35], lipoxygenase [36], mitochondrial respiration[37-41], cytochrome P450[42] and uncoupled NO synthases[43-45] have all been identified as sources of ROS in cell types of the vasculature. All of these sources may contribute to ROS formation; however, their relative involvement likely depends on cell type, cellular activation state, and disease context. Recently, it has been shown that NAD(P)H oxidoreductase systems, expressed in most cell types of the vasculature, are the predominant generators of ROS in the vessel wall[46-49]. These enzymes, like the neutrophil oxidases, are multisubunit complexes. However, the vascular NAD(P)H oxidases are unique in that they are less well characterized, and their subunit compositions differ from one cell type to another. Recent excitement has surrounded the cloning and characterization of the Nox family of proteins[50-53]; these are homologs of the catalytic subunit of the phagocyte oxidase (gp91^{phox}). The Nox proteins are expressed in cells of the vasculature although there appear to be cell-type differences in expression patterns. Despite the fact that animal models of atherosclerosis and hypertension are characterized by an increased production of NAD(P)H oxidase activity, production of ROS[54-56], and elevated expression of some of the Nox isoforms[50,57], solid evidence for the role of the Nox family of proteins in the underlying pathology of the diseases is lacking. Clearly, this will be an exciting area for future research.

Numerous studies have shown that various physiological stimuli relevant to the pathogenesis of vascular disease can induce the formation of ROS. For example, a variety of agents, including vasoactive agents such as Ang II, endothelin-1 and thrombin, have been shown to activate NAD(P)H oxidase activity. Treatment of VSMCs with Ang II causes an increase in expression of, as well as increased ROS generation by, NAD(P)H[58,59], cytokines (IL-1β, TNF-α), growth factors (platelet-derived growth factor (PDGF), transforming growth factor–β) and hemodynamic forces (shear stress and cyclic stretch), which impart a pro-atherogenic, pro-inflammatory, or pro-proliferative phenotype, and regulate the expression and/or activity of the vascular NAD(P)H oxidase[60-64]. One mechanism by which these stresses exert their pathophysiological effects is via increased expression of ROS in the vessel wall, which consequently activates numerous signaling cascades (see below) and modulates the cellular phenotype.

The specificity that is essential for biological signaling may derive at least in part from the properties and regulation of the ROS sources. A major requisite of a signaling molecule is that its expression/production and cellular localization is highly regulated. Each active source of ROS production within a subcellular compartment contributes to the local levels of each species. In addition, the transport of individual ROS across cellular compartments is often possible when the capacity of the antioxidant scavenging system is exceeded. Thus, in any consideration of ROS as signaling molecules, one must keep in mind both the temporal as well as spatial regulation of these transient species.

Interaction of ROS with signaling systems

Signal transduction proceeds from the cell surface through the plasma membrane to generate second messengers that transmit the signal to intracellular mediators in both the cytoplasm and the nucleus. ROS participate in signal transduction by generating classic second-messengers (eg. calcium and lipid mediators) or by themselves, acting as second messengers to influence the activity of signaling proteins. ROS are elaborated in response to a variety of host stimuli. Experiments over-expressing antioxidant enzymes or using exogenously added antioxidants to identify redox-sensitive signaling pathways, changes in gene expression, or cellular phenotype have confirmed that ROS are an integral component of signal transduction. However, less is known about the precise components targeted by ROS. In the following section, we review several signal transduction pathways that have been revealed to be targets of ROS-mediated signaling.

ROS-sensitive ion transport systems

Intracellular calcium (Ca^{2+}) and potassium channels play major roles in vascular constriction and hyperpolarization-elicited relaxation, respectively. Ca^{2+} is a widely used second messenger that regulates a variety of biological processes including gene expression, neurotransmission, cell motility, and cell growth. In response to physiological stimuli at the cell surface, the intracellular level of Ca^{2+} rises and elicits the activation of Ca^{2+}-dependent proteins such as protein kinase C, Ca^{2+}-calmodulin kinases, and calmodulin-dependent protein phosphatases (calcineurin). Oxidants stimulate Ca^{2+} signaling by increasing cytosolic Ca^{2+} concentration [3] suggesting a possible physiological role of ROS in the regulation of Ca^{2+}-induced signaling in the vasculature. Increases in intracellular Ca^{2+} were detected in response to H_2O_2 treatment of VSMCs[65] and ECs with hypoxanthine and hypoxanthine oxidase (a physiological oxidant-generating enzyme system)[66] and H_2O_2[67] showed a transient release of Ca^{2+} from intracellular stores. Similarly, in rabbit aortic ECs, treatment with linoleic acid hydroperoxide resulted in a transient increase in intracellular Ca^{2+}[68]. Although the exact molecular targets of oxidant-mediated Ca^{2+} signaling are not known, the ability of various oxidants to inhibit the activity of an ATP-dependent Ca^{2+}-pump[69, 70] suggests that direct modification of Ca^{2+}-pumps by oxidants may be one mechanism of oxidant-mediated Ca^{2+} signaling. Enhanced Ca^{2+}-transport through Ca^{2+} channels is another potential target since the Ca^{2+} channel blocker, Ni^{2+}, partially inhibited H_2O_2-mediated increases in intracellular Ca^{2+} in ECs[67]. Plasma membrane potassium channels in VSMCs that control a hyperpolarization-elicited relaxation appear to be opened by mechanisms associated with thiol oxidation by ROS[71]. Thus, evidence exists to suggest the potential involvement of ROS-mediated ion flux in early signaling pathways; however the exact mechanisms remain to be elucidated.

Small G proteins in ROS signaling

Small guanine nucleotide binding proteins (G proteins), including Ras, Rac and Rho, a family of proteins that exert GTPase activity, have been proposed as mediators of ROS signaling[23,72]. Rac is fairly well defined as a mediator of oxidant-induced signaling [61,73]. It has been shown to be a target for H_2O_2, O_2^- and NO [23]. Rac1 is a regulatory component of the vascular NAD(P)H oxidase and its functional association is required for O_2^- generation by a variety of stimuli. In addition, the expression of several endothelial inflammatory genes such as VCAM-1, E-selectin, ICAM-1 and MCP-1 is inhibited by expression of a dominant-negative Rac in ECs[74,75]. Rho is important in cell cycle progression and proliferation in VSMCs. Expression of a dominant-negative Rho in ECs negatively regulated eNOS expression[76]. Likewise, Ras has also been implicated in ROS-mediated signaling. Expression of a dominant-negative Ras or treatment with agents that block farnesylation inhibited oxidant-stress induced (i.e. H_2O_2) activation of ERK and NF-κB signaling[77]. In addition, direct activation of Ras by ROS was demonstrated by stimulation of guanine nucleotide exchange. Given their hierarchy in the cellular signaling, G proteins are likely key sensors of redox homeostasis. However, more than 70 small G proteins exist in mammals and their involvement in redox signaling is only beginning to be understood.

Kinases as mediators of redox-sensitive signal transduction

Modulation of the phosphorylation state of biological substrates is a major point of regulation in cellular signaling. The function of multiple components of protein phosphorylation systems are altered by ROS[78]. Although many studies describe effects of ROS on a particular kinase pathway, these studies do not always distinguish between direct modifications of the kinase by ROS, or by alterations in the function and/or activity of an independent signaling system (i.e. calcium, cGMP or phosphatase) indirectly influencing the activity of the kinase. For example, signaling through cGMP-dependent protein kinases is likely to be highly regulated by ROS and the redox status because of their influence on the activity of guanylate cyclase.

Tyrosine kinases

A common theme in signaling is that growth factor-mediated responses in the vasculature involve ROS generation as a component of their signaling. For example, considerable data links both PDGF and epidermal growth factor (EGF) signaling to ROS production[60, 62]. Not only is there a link in growth factor ligand-dependent production of ROS, but also emerging data indicate that receptor tyrosine kinases (RTKs) are themselves a target of ROS signaling through a process known as receptor "transactivation" that involves ligand-independent stimulation of receptor kinase activity.

In ECs, H_2O_2 activation of c-jun kinase (JNK) and eNOS activity has been attributed to EGF receptor transactivation[79, 80]. Likewise, in VSMCs, Ang II-mediated activation of the MAP kinase ERK involves activation of NAD(P)H oxidase and H_2O_2-mediated EGF receptor transactivation[81]. There is also evidence for transactivation of the PDGF receptor by ROS. For example, H_2O_2 (in mesangial cells and fibroblasts) and Ang II (in VSMCs) stimulate tyrosine phosphorylation of the PDGFβ receptor[82-84]. The activation of tyrosine phosphorylation by Ang II is inhibited by antioxidants suggesting a role for ROS in this process[85]. H_2O_2-induced transactivation of EGFr and PDGFr may be due to inactivation of tyrosine phosphatases[86]. EGF and PDGFβ receptor transactivation is distinct from ligand-dependent activation in that the tyrosine phosphorylation sites in the receptor are different between these two modes of activation[79]. Interestingly, the mode of activation (e.g. ligand-dependent vs ligand-independent) of these receptor tyrosine kinases has mechanistic implications. Ligand-dependent activation of the EGF receptor is regulated via receptor internalization and degradation, whereas H_2O_2-mediated transactivation is not.

Although ligand-dependent phosphorylation of EGF receptors does not appear to involve ROS, phosphorylation of the EGF receptor by Ang II (i.e. transactivation) is redox sensitive. Several investigators have implicated the non-receptor tyrosine kinase Src in EGF receptor transactivation. Src is an important signaling molecule with multiple functions: it phosphorylates phospholipase C-gamma, forms complexes with the EGFr, paxillin and Janus kinase (JAK)-2, and mediates activation of MAPK[87]. Src is activated directly by H_2O_2 in fibroblasts[88] and Ang II-stimulated VSMCs, and cardiac fibroblasts induces the phosphorylation of Src which is inhibited by antioxidants[81, 89]. These results indicate that the activation of Src by Ang II is mediated by NAD(P)H oxidase-derived ROS. In addition to c-Src, other Src family member tyrosine kinases, including Lck and Fyn[90], are activated by ROS. Berk's group has proposed that the tyrosine kinases Src and Fyn confer a level of specificity on downstream targets in response to activation by ROS. They found that c-Src, but not Fyn, is required for H_2O_2-mediated BMK1/ERK5 and JNK activation; whereas Fyn, but not c-Src, is required for H_2O_2-mediated ERK1/2 activation[91]. These results suggest that c-Src and Fyn have separate and distinct roles in ROS-mediated signal transduction.

Some evidence is beginning to emerge implicating the Janus kinase (JAK) family of tyrosine kinases in ROS-mediated signaling. The JAKs were originally described in cytokine signaling where dimerization of the cytokine receptors leads to JAK autophosphorylation and activation of the downstream Signal Transducer and Activator of Transcription (STATs). Ang II activation of JAK2 has been reported in VSMCs[92] and cardiac myocytes[93]. Involvement of ROS in this process was demonstrated by inhibition of Ang II-mediated JAK2 activation by the NAD(P)H oxidase inhibitor DPI and neutralizing antisera against the p47phox subunit of NAD(P)H oxidase[94]. These studies suggest that superoxide production via the NAD(P)H oxidase is important for Ang II-mediated activation of JAK2.

It is not yet clear whether ROS cause direct activation of tyrosine kinase activity or whether the observed increases in tyrosine phosphorylation are due to inhibition of a tyrosine phosphatase activity by oxidant-mediated signals. Since all tyrosine phosphatases have reactive cysteine residues in their active site, inhibition of tyrosine phosphatase activity by oxidants may account for the mechanisms of stimulation of tyrosine phosphorylation by oxidant stimuli[3]. In this regard, it has been reported that oxidizing agents phenylarsine oxide[95] and H_2O_2[96, 97] inhibit tyrosine phosphatase activity. Similarly, PKC-mediated serine/threonine phosphorylation in response to oxidative stress may be the result of inhibition of protein phosphatase 1 and 2A activity since thiol oxidation in these phosphatases has been shown to inhibit the enzyme activity[3].

Mitogen-activated protein kinase (MAPK) pathways

MAPKs are serine and threonine protein kinases that are activated by a wide variety of stimuli. These so-called dual-specificity kinases, because they are activated on both threonine and tyrosine, are grouped based on the primary amino acid sequence of their activation motif. Of the mammalian MAPKs, ERK1/2, p38, JNK (also called stress-activated protein kinase, SAPK) and big MAP kinase (BMK1, also called ERK5) are the most well studied. MAPKs are the downstream-most kinase components of the MAPK signaling cascade; their activation most commonly leads to phosphorylation of specific transcription factors that regulate the expression of specific sets of genes. MAPKs are themselves activated by phosphorylation by upstream members of the MEK (MAPK and ERK kinase) protein kinase family. The MEKs in turn, are activated by the MEKK (MEK kinase) family of protein kinases such as ASK1 (see below). For an excellent overview of MAPK signaling, refer to a recent review by Johnson and Lapadat[98]. The specificity of activation within the MAPK family is determined by specific pairing of downstream substrates for each kinase member. Although there appears to be somewhat discrete linear "pathways" in this activation cascade, there is significant cross-talk and multiple protein: protein interactions within the pathways. ROS mediated activation of MAPK in cell types of the vasculature is well documented[87,99]. It is likely that modulation of MAPK activity by ROS (either directly or indirectly) in the vasculature is a primary determinant of redox-mediated gene regulation that governs the pathogenesis of many vascular diseases.

Various physiological agents believed to play a role in vascular dysfunction, including oxLDL,[100] Ang II,[101] lactosylceramide,[102] and linoleic acid and its metabolites,[68] have been shown to activate MAPK activity in VSMCs via the generation of intracellular ROS. H_2O_2 has been shown to activate p38[91,101], JNK[91] and ERK5[103] in VSMCs. The effect of H_2O_2 on ERK activation are somewhat controversial; with investigators showing both activation and inhibition of ERK activation[91,101,104-108]. In one of the studies that demonstrated ROS-mediated activation of ERK, only O_2^{-}, but not H_2O_2, activated ERK[105]. With respect to ROS-mediated, agonist-induced activation of these enzymes, the activation of p38 and JNK by Ang II is inhibited by the antioxidants N-acetylcysteine (NAC) and diphenylene iodonium (DPI), overexpression of catalase, and antisense inhibition of the p22phox subunit of NADPH[101,107]. In ECs, the involvement of ROS in MAPK activation has been demonstrated by showing that H_2O_2 activated p38 and its downstream targets[109,110] and shear stress activation of ERK was inhibited by cotreatment with antioxidants[111].

Apoptosis signal-regulating kinase-1 (ASK1) is a MEKK that plays a role in stress-induced apoptosis[112]. Berk's laboratory has shown both in cultured ECs and isolated intact vessels that steady laminar shear stress inhibits TNF-α-induced activation of the ASK1/JNK pathway[113, 114]. This is of interest because shear stress is known to modulate redox homeostasis[64]. It has been shown that thioredoxin (an endogenous antioxidant protein that exhibits ROS-scavenging properties) binds directly to ASK1 and inhibits ASK1 activity[115]. This interaction is regulated by redox status as the interaction is only observed under reducing conditions and not with a redox-inactive mutant of thioredoxin. In addition, a recently identified protein termed vitamin D-upregulated protein 1 (VDUP1) binds to the catalytic site of thioredoxin and inhibits its activity. In cultured ECs, RNA inhibition of VDUP1 increases thioredoxin binding to ASK1 and inhibits TNF-α stimulation of JNK, p38 and VCAM-1[116]. Therefore, endogenous proteins that modulate redox status such as thioredoxin may have direct effects on MAPK signaling and gene expression. Given the enormous complexity of the MAPK signaling cascade, we are far from a complete understanding of how ROS modulate this pathway. Nonetheless, regulation of the MAPK pathways by ROS is likely to be dependent on the cell type, stimuli, and nature of the ROS species.

Akt/protein kinase B (PKB)

Akt/PKB is a serine/threonine kinase, which lies downstream of the phosphoinositide 3-kinase and plays a role in apoptosis regulation and protein synthesis. Akt/PKB is activated in a redox-dependent manner. In VSMCs, Akt/PKB is activated by H_2O_2 and Ang II. DPI (an inhibitor of NAD(P)H oxidase), overexpression of catalase, and antisense inhibition of Nox-1 block the Ang II-mediated activation of Akt/PKB in VSMCs[117, 118]. In ECs, Akt/PKB is activated by shear stress; however, whether this is a result of an alteration in shear-dependent redox state is not known. These results indicate that ROS production is critical for Akt/PKB activation in both ECs and VSMCs.

ROS modulation of transcription factor activity and gene expression

Transcription factors are central to any discussion of signal transduction, as they are the nuclear components and ultimate targets modulated by upstream signaling events. By nature of their ability to interact with very specific DNA sequences (which are unique to each transcription factor) in the regulatory regions of target genes, they modulate not only the magnitude of gene expression, but also the specificity of the signal. Redox-sensitive modulation of transcription factor activity can occur via direct oxidative modification of the transcription factor by intracellular ROS, or via posttranslational modifications (i.e., phosphorylation/dephosphorylation) by upstream redox-regulated intracellular signaling cascades. Either mechanism potentially affects various aspects of transcription factor activity such as subcellular localization, DNA binding properties, protein: protein interactions, and inherent transcriptional activity. Several excellent reviews have provided an in-depth discussion of redox-sensitive transcription factors in general[14,119,120] as well as the role of redox-sensitive transcription factors and gene expression in relationship to cardiovascular disease[6,121,122]. Therefore, we will only briefly mention a few of the most well examined redox-sensitive transcription factors that have relevance to cardiovascular disease.

AP-1

The transcription factor AP-1 is composed of dimers of members of the Fos and Jun transcription factor families and has been implicated in transcriptional regulation of a wide range of genes involved in cellular inflammatory responses, growth control and cardiovascular disease. AP-1 behaves as a redox-sensitive transcription factor in several cell types and is activated under pro-oxidant conditions generated by treatment with agents such as superoxide, H_2O_2, ultraviolet light, γ irradiation and cytokines [123-126]. In ECs, agents such as H_2O_2[127], LDL[128], and oxLDL[129] activate AP-1 DNA binding activity. In VSMCs, oxLDL[130], H_2O_2[131] and the lipid peroxidation product 4-hydroxy-2-nonenal [132] increase AP-1 expression or DNA binding activity. Furthermore, regulation of the vascular inflammatory genes MCP-1 and ICAM-1 by H_2O_2 is mediated by AP-1 binding elements in the promoters of these genes[133, 134]. Little information is known about the exact mechanisms underlying ROS-mediated AP-1 activation; however, roles of phospholipase A2, arachidonic acid, lipoxygenases, and protein kinase C have been proposed for H_2O_2 induction of c-Fos[135] and c-Jun[131] expression in VSMCs. In addition, H_2O_2-induced AP-1 activation in ECs requires both tyrosine and serine/threonine phosphorylation[136] and AP-1 activation under oxidative conditions may be, at least in part, mediated by phosphorylation of Jun proteins[137]. Therefore, posttranslational modifications following oxidative stress may be central to modulating AP-1 activity.

NF-κB

NF-κB is an inducible transcription factor complex composed of homo- or heterodimeric complexes of the Rel family of transcriptional activators. NF-κB controls the expression of a multitude of genes involved in the pathogenesis of cardiovascular disease such as cytokines, adhesion molecules, and proliferative genes. Numerous studies have documented a role of NF-κB in the pathogenesis of disorders of the vasculature including restenosis[138] and atherosclerosis[139]. A substantial body of evidence indicates that activation of NF-κB in vascular cells may be controlled by the redox status of the cell[140]. In fact, NF-κB was the first eukaryotic transcription factor shown to respond directly to oxidative stress[141]. A common step in the activation mechanisms which lead to degradation of IκB (the inhibitor of NF-κB) probably involves ROS[140,142,143]. This conclusion was reached based upon the inhibition of NF-κB activation by several chemically distinct antioxidants including NAC, dithiocarbamates, vitamin E derivatives, glutathione peroxidase activators and various metal chelators.

The precise target molecules that are subject to redox regulation during NF-κB activation remain unknown. It is unlikely that the NF-κB subunits themselves are directly activated by oxidation because only the reduced form of NF-κB binds to DNA *in vitro*[144], and attempts to activate isolated NF-κB by oxidation *in vitro* were unsuccessful[140]. Direct oxidative inactivation of IκB is also not likely to be involved in the redox-regulation of NF-κB since treatment of isolated NF-κB/IκB complexes with H_2O_2 *in vitro* failed to dissociate IκB or lead to NF-κB DNA binding[140,145]. Most evidence suggests that oxidative stresses induce, and antioxidants prevent, the cytoplasmic-nuclear translocation of NF-κB. Therefore, the most likely scenario is that the signaling cascade leading to the phosphorylation and subsequent degradation of IκB is regulated by redox processes[146,147]. However, not all antioxidants block the nuclear translocation of NF-κB. For example, despite the fact that the antioxidant compounds apigenin[148], PD098063[149], and AGI-1067[150] have all been reported to inhibit inducible endothelial gene expression, none of these compounds interferes with the TNF-α-induced nuclear translocation of NF-κB. ROS may also modulate the activity of NF-κB by regulating post-translational modifications of the NF-κB subunits themselves or of other transcriptional cofactors which influence the transcriptional activity of NF-κB. In support of this, NAC has been shown to inhibit TNF-α-induced phosphorylation of the p65(RelA) subunit of NF-κB[151].

Nrf2/antioxidant response element (ARE) pathway

The ARE is a *cis*-acting sequence that mediates transcriptional activation of genes in cells exposed to oxidative stress[152-154]. The ARE is present in the 5' flanking regions of genes encoding phase II detoxification enzymes and cellular antioxidant proteins including glutathione-S-transferase (GST)[155], NAD(P)H:quinone oxidoreductase (NQO1)[156], glucuronosyltransferase[155], heme oxygenase-1[157] and ferritin[158]. Nrf2 (NF-E2-related factor-2) is the transcription factor that, upon activation by oxidative stress, binds to the ARE and activates transcription of ARE-regulated genes[159,160]. In vascular cells, the ARE pathway is activated by oxLDL[161,162] and exposure to NO[163]. We recently reported that when ECs were exposed to prolonged laminar flow, there is a marked increase in the expression of ARE-mediated genes such as GST, NQO1, HO-1 and ferritin through Nrf2-dependent mechanism[164]. Whether or not this activation is due to shear-induced modulation of the redox status[64] is not known. In non-activated cells, Nrf2 is retained in the cytosol bound to an inhibitor protein, KEAP-1. Upon exposure to oxidative stress, Nrf2 dissociates from KEAP-1, translocates to the nucleus and activates transcription[165]. Several protein kinases have been implicated in ROS activation of Nrf2 including the MAPKs, protein kinase C and PI3-kinase[166-169]. It is believed that these kinases phosphorylate a critical serine on Nrf2. Alternatively, a direct role of ROS in activation of the Nrf2/Keap pathway has been proposed through a direct attack by ROS on reactive cysteines in KEAP-1[165]. Therefore, KEAP-1 and/or Nrf2 may constitute a sensitive oxygen-sensing mechanism in mammalian cells to activate a coordinate set of cellular protective and antioxidant genes in response to oxidative stress.

We have recently demonstrated that the Nrf2/ARE pathway is important in regulating redox-sensitive gene expression in ECs[164,170]. By using adenoviral-mediated expression of Nrf2 or addition of sulforaphane, a naturally occurring isothiocyanate and an activator of Nrf2, we demonstrated that activation of the Nrf2/ARE pathway suppresses TNF-α-induced VCAM-1, MCP-1, but not ICAM-1, expression in ECs and protected ECs from H_2O_2-mediated cytotoxicity. These observations demonstrate an important role for the Nrf2/ARE pathway in modulating redox-sensitive gene expression in ECs and protection from oxidant-induced toxicity. Because the involvement of the Nrf2/ARE pathway in vascular oxidant-mediated signaling has been described only recently, more research into this pathway may uncover novel roles for redox-mediated signaling in the vascular system.

Regulation of gene expression by ROS

As discussed above, subtle alterations in the cellular redox status are "sensed" by a variety of cell signaling components that ultimately lead to modulation of transcription factor activity. The net result is alteration of gene expression. Because multiple physiological factors that participate in the pathogenesis of CAD alter ROS levels and activities of key components in their signaling pathways, it is not surprising that many genes involved in CAD are redox-sensitive[24]. Genes such as adhesion molecules, chemotactic factors, antioxidant enzymes and growth factors are all regulated by ROS. Induction of some of these, such as the antioxidant proteins, SOD, HO-1 and catalase are a compensatory inductive responses to the increase in ROS [171]. Genes including MCP-1[172,173], VCAM-1[174,175], E-selectin[176], PDGF[177], VEGF[178], MCSF[172] and MMPs[179] have either been shown to be induced by externally applied oxidant stress or their expression in response to known inducers of ROS is inhibited by antioxidants. Regulation of gene expression could occur at several levels, through either modulation of upstream signaling or through direct effects of ROS on binding or activity of transcription factors that regulate the expression of these genes.

Concluding remarks

Given the ubiquitous nature of ROS in biological systems and the numerous cellular proteins that maintain the redox balance, it is not surprising that modulation of signal transduction, and ultimately gene expression, as a result of alterations in cellular redox homeostasis is now a well-recognized signaling mechanism throughout biology. Oxidative stress is a key contributor to the pathogenesis of nearly all chronic inflammatory diseases, especially cardiovascular disease. In atherosclerosis, although oxidative stress contributes to the generation of oxLDL which plays a critical role in initiating the inflammatory events [180], redox-signaling, in response to subtle changes in intracellular ROS levels, also contributes to the underlying pathogenesis of the disease. A strong body of evidence supports the notion that ROS, generated locally in the vasculature in response to environmental risk factors and biological mediators, modulate signal transduction events and gene expression changes regulating processes such as smooth muscle cell hypertrophy, apoptosis, endothelial dysfunction, inflammatory responses and matrix remodeling. Mechanistically, this suggests that the observed therapeutic benefit of some antioxidants in cardiovascular disease is in large part attributable to modulation in the molecular signaling pathways and gene expression alterations in endothelial, smooth muscle and inflammatory cells. Most dietary antioxidants have only modest physiological effects because they seem to protect against the consequences of lipid peroxidation (i.e., $^{\cdot}$OH and ONOO^{-} generation) but the intracellular concentrations of these antioxidants are likely to have only minimal effect on $O_2^{\cdot-}$, H_2O_2, NO and thiol redox processes[8]. Therefore, pharmacological agents that act as intracellular antioxidants, target specific ROS, or that modulate specific enzyme systems involved in oxidant signaling may offer a unique approach for modulating ROS species inside the cell and offer greater potential for therapeutic efficacy in patients with CAD. Hopefully, elucidation of the precise redox-regulated signaling pathways will encourage the exploration of novel treatment modalities targeting these redox-sensitive pathways.

References

1. Freeman BA, Capro JD. Free radicals and tissue injury. Lab Invest 1982;46:412-26.
2. Halliwell B, Gutteridge JM. The importance of free radicals and catalytic metal ions in human diseases. Mol Aspects Med 1985;8:89-193.
3. Suzuki YJ, Forman HJ, Sevanian A. Oxidants as stimulators of signal transduction. Free Radic Biol Med 1997;22:269-85.
4. Finkel T. Signal transduction by reactive oxygen species in non-phagocytic cells. J Leukoc Biol 1999;65:337-40.
5. Maulik N, Das DK. Potentiation of angiogenic response by ischemic and hypoxic preconditioning of the heart. J Cell Mol Med 2002;6:13-24.
6. Maulik N, Das DK. Redox signaling in vascular angiogenesis. Free Radic Biol Med 2002;33:1047-60.
7. Lelkes Pl, Hahn KL, Sukovich DA, Karmiol S, Schmidt DH. On the possible role of reactive oxygen species in angiogenesis. Adv Exp Med Biol 1998;454:295-310.
8. Wolin MS. Interactions of oxidants with vascular signaling systems. Arterioscler Thromb Vasc Biol 2000;20:1430-42.
9. Lynch SM, Frei B. Mechanisms of copper- and iron-dependent oxidative modification of human low density lipoprotein. J Lipid Res 1993;34:1745-53.
10. Khan BV, Parthasarathy SS, Alexander RW, Medford RM. Modified low density lipoprotein and its constituents augment cytokine-activated vascular cell adhesion molecule-1 gene expression in human vascular endothelial cells J Clin Invest 1995;95:1262-70.
11. Reddy MA, Thimmalapura PR, Lanting L, Nadler JL, Fatima S, Natarajan R. The oxidized lipid and lipoxygenase product 12(S)-hydroxyeicosatetraenoic acid induces hypertrophy and fibronectin transcription in vascular smooth muscle cells via p38 MAPK and cAMP response element-binding protein activation. Mediation of angiotensin II effects. J Biol Chem 2002;277:9920-8.
12. Natarajan R, Reddy MA, Malik KU, Fatima S, Khan BV. Signaling mechanisms of nuclear factor-kappab-mediated activation of inflammatory genes by 13-hydroperoxyoctadecadienoic acid in cultured vascular smooth muscle cells. Arterioscler Thromb Vasc Biol 2001;21:1408-13.
13. Sultana C, Shen Y, Rattan V, Kalra VK. Lipoxygenase metabolites induced expression of adhesion molecules and transendothelial migration of monocyte-like HL-60 cells is linked to protein kinase C activation. J Cell Physiol 1996;167:477-87.
14. Chen K, Thomas SR, Keaney J, J.F. Beyond LDL oxidation: ROS in vascular signal transduction. Free Radic Biol Med 2003;35:117-32.
15. Denu JM, Tanner KG. Specific and reversible inactivation of protein tyrosine phosphatases by hydrogen peroxide: evidence for a sulfenic acid intermediate and implications for redox regulation. Biochemistry 1998;37:5633-42.
16. Claiborne A, Miller H, Parsonage D, Ross RP. Protein-sulfenic acid stabilization and function in enzyme catalysis and gene regulation. FASEB J 1993;7:1483-90.

17. Kim SO, Merchant K, Nudelman R, et al. OxyR: a molecular code for redox-related signaling. Cell 2002;109:383-96.

18. Heinecke JW, Shapiro BM. Respiratory burst oxidase of fertilization. Proc Natl Acad Sci U S A. 1989;86:1259-63.

19. Babior BM, Curnutte JT, McMurrich BJ. The particulate superoxide-forming system from human neutrophils. Properties of the system and further evidence supporting its participation in the respiratory burst. J Clin Invest 1976;58:989-96.

20. Verweij CL, Gringhuis SI. Oxidants and tyrosine phosphorylation: role of acute and chronic oxidative stress in T-and B-lymphocyte signaling. Antiox Redox Signal 2002;4:543-51.

21. Ekholm R. Biosynthesis of thyroid hormones. Int Rev Cytol 1990;120:243-88.

22. Krieger-Brauer HI, Kather H. Human fat cells possess a plasma membrane-bound H_2O_2-generating system that is activated by insulin via a mechanism bypassing the receptor kinase. J Clin Invest 1992;89:1006-13.

23. Abe J, Berk BC. Reactive oxygen species as mediators of signal transduction in cardiovascular disease. In:Antioxidants and Cardiovascular Disease, edited by J.-C. Tardif and M. Bourassa (Kluwer Academic Publishers, 2000), pp. 57-70.

24. Kunsch C, Medford RM. Oxidation-sensitive transcription and gene expression in atherosclerosis. In: Oxidative Stress and Vascular Disease, edited by J.F. Keaney (Kluwer Academic Publishers, 1999), pp. 135-54.

25. Chen X, Medford RM. Oxidation-reduction sensitive regulation of inflammatory gene expression in the vasculature. In: Vascular adhesion molecules and inflammation, edited by Pearson JD (Birkhauser Press, 1999) pp. 161-78.

26. Gibbons GH, Dzau VJ. Molecular therapies for vascular diseases. Science 1996;272:689-93.

27. Ross R. Cell biology of atherosclerosis. Annu Rev Physiol 1995;57:791-804.

28. Souza HP, Cardounel AJ, Zweier JL. Mechanisms of free radical production in the vascular wall. Coron Artery Dis 2003;14:101-7.

29. Hanna IR, Taniyama Y, Szocs K, Rocic P, Griendling KK. NAD(P)H oxidase-derived reactive oxygen species as mediators of angiotensin II signaling. Antiox Redox Signal 2002;4:899-914.

30. Heinecke J. Sources of vascular oxidative stress. In: Oxidative Stress and Vascular Disease, edited by J.F. Keaney (Kluwer Academic Publishers, 1999), pp. p 9-26.

31. Phan SH, Gannon DE, Varani J, Ryan US, Ward PA. Xanthine oxidase activity in rat pulmonary artery endothelial cells and its alteration by activated neutrophils. Am J Pathol 1989;134:1201-11.

32. Ratych RE, Chuknyiska RS, Bulkley GB. The primary localization of free radical generation after anoxia/reoxygenation in isolated endothelial cells. Surgery 1987;102:122-31.

33. Holland JAP, K.A., Pappolla MA, Wolin MS, Rogers NJ, Stemerman MB. Bradykinin induces superoxide anion release from human endothelial cells. J Cell Physiol 1990;143:21-5.

34. Tesfamariam B, Cohen RA. Role of superoxide anion and endothelium in vasoconstrictoraction of prostaglandin endoperoxide. Am J Physiol 1992;262:H1915-9.

35. Kukreja RC, Kontos HA, Hess ML, Ellis EF. PGH synthetase and lipoxygenase generate superoxide in the presence of NADH or NADPH. Circ Res 1986;59:612-9.

36. Hsieh CC, Yen MH, Yen CH, Lau YT. Oxidized low density lipoprotein induces apoptosis via generation of reactive oxygen species in vascular smooth muscle cells. Cardiovasc Res 2001;49:135-45.

37. Sanders SP, Zweier JL, Kuppusamy P, Harrison SJ, Bassett DJ, Gabrielson E. Hyperoxic sheep pulmonary microvascular endothelial cells generate free radicals via mitochondrial electron transport. J Clin Invest 1993;91:46-52.

38. Ballinger SW, Patterson C, Knight-Lozano CA, et al. Mitochondrial integrity and function in atherogenesis. Circulation 2002;106:544-9.

39. Cadenas E, Davies KJ. Mitochondrial free radical generation, oxidative stress, and aging. Free Radic Biol Med 2000;29:222-30.

40. Ishida I, Kubo H, Suzuki S, et al. Hypoxia diminishes toll-like receptor 4 expression through reactive oxygen species generated by mitochondria in endothelial cells. J Immunol 2002;169:2069-75.

41. Nishikawa T, Edelstein D, Du XL, et al. Normalizing mitochondrial superoxide production blocks three pathways of hyperglycemic damage. Nature 2000;404:787-90.

42. Fleming I, Michaelis UR, Bredenkotter D, Fisslthaler B, F. D, Brandes RP, Busse R. Endothelium-derived hyperpolarizing factor synthase (cytochrome P450 2C9) is a functionally significant source of reactive oxygen species in coronary arteries. Circ Res 2001;88:44-51.

43. Vasquez-Vivar J, Kalyanaraman B, Martasek P, et al. Superoxide generation by endothelial nitric oxide synthase: the influence of cofactors. Proc Natl Acad Sci U S A 1998;95:9220-5.

44. Xia Y, Tsai AL, Berka V, Zweier JL. Superoxide generation from endothelial nitric oxide synthase. A Ca2+/calmodulin-dependent and tetrahydrobiopterin regulatory process. J Biol Chem 1998;273:25804-8.

45. Harrison DG. Cellular and molecular mechanisms of endothelial cell dysfunction. J Clin Invest 1997;100:2153-7.

46. Griendling KK, Sorescu D, Ushio-Fukai M. NAD(P)H oxidase: role in cardiovascular biology and disease. Circ Res 2000;86:494-501.

47. Mohazzab KM, Kaminski PM, Wolin MS. NADH oxidoreductase is a major source of superoxide anion in bovine coronary artery endothelium. Am J Physiol 1994;266:H2568-72.

48. Pagano PJ, Tornheim K, Cohen RA. Superoxide anion production by rabbit thoracic aorta: effect of endothelium-derived nitric oxide. Am J Physiol 1993;265:H707-12.

49. Mohazzab KM, Wolin MS. Sites of superoxide anion production detected by lucigenin in calf pulmonary artery smooth muscle. Am J Physiol 1994;267:L815-22.

50. Sorescu D, Weiss D, Lassegue B, et al. Superoxide production and expression of nox family proteins in human atherosclerosis. Circulation 2002;105:1429-35.

51. Cheng G, Cao Z, Xu X, van Meir EG, Lambeth JD. Homologs of gp91phox: cloning and tissue expression of Nox3, Nox4, and Nox5. Gene 2001;269:131-40.

52. Suh YA, Arnold RS, Lassegue B, et al. Cell transformation by the superoxide-generating oxidase Mox1. Nature 1999;401:79-82.

53. Griendling KK. Novel NAD(P)H oxidases in the cardiovascular system. Heart 2004;90:491-3.

54. Rajagopalan S, Kurz S, Munzel T, et al. Angiotensin II mediated hypertension in the rat increases vascular superoxide production via membrane NADH/NADPH oxidase activation: Contribution to alterations of vasomotor tone. J Clin Invest 1996;97:1916-0193.

55. Warnholtz A, Nickenig G, Schulz E, et al. Increased NADH-oxidase-mediated superoxide production in the early stages of atherosclerosis: evidence for involvement of the renin-angiotensin system. Circulation 1999;99:2027-33.

56. Fukui T, Ishizaka N, Rajagopalan S, et al. p22phox mRNA expression and NADPH oxidase activity are increased in aortas from hypertensive rats. Circ Res 1997;80:45-51.

57. Kalinina N, Agrotis A, Tararak E, et al. Cytochrome b558-dependent NAD(P)H oxidase-phox units in smooth muscle and macrophages of atherosclerotic lesions. Arterioscler Thromb Vasc Biol 2002;22:2037-43.

58. Ushio-Fukai M, Zafari AM, Fukui T, Ishizaka N, Griendling KK. p22phox is a critical component of the superoxide-generating NADH/NADPH oxidase system and regulates angiotensin II induced hypertrophy in vascular smooth muscle cells. J. Biol. Chem. 1996;271:23317-21.

59. Zafari AM, Ushio-Fukai M, Akers M, et al. Role of NADH/NADPH oxidase-derived H_2O_2 in angiotensin II-induced vascular hypertrophy. Hypertension 1998;32:488-95.

60. Sundaresan M, Yu ZX, Ferrans VJ, Irani K, Finkel T. Requirement for generation of H_2O_2 for platelet-derived growth factor signal transduction. Science 1995;270:296-9.

61. Irani K, Xia Y, Zweier JL, et al. Mitogenic signaling mediated by oxidants in Ras-transformed fibroblasts. Science 1997;275:1649-52.

62. Bae YS, Kang SW, Seo MS, et al. Epidermal growth factor (EGF)-induced generation of hydrogen peroxide. Role in EGF receptor-mediated tyrosine phosphorylation. J Biol Chem 1997;272:217-21.

63. Ohba M, Shibanuma M, Kuroki T, Nose K. Production of hydrogen peroxide by transforming growth factor-beta 1 and its involvement in induction of egr-1 in mouse osteoblastic cells. J Cell Biol 1994;126:1079-88.

64. De Keulenaer GW, Chappell DC, Ishizaka N, Nerem RM, Alexander RW, Griendling KK. Oscillatory and steady laminar shear stress differentially affect human endothelial redox state: role of a superoxide-producing NADH oxidase. Circ Res 1998;82:1094-101.

65. Roveri A, Coassin M, Maiorino M, et al. Effect of hydrogen peroxide on calcium homeostasis in smooth muscle cells. Arch Biochem Biophys 1992;297:265-70.

66. Dreher D, Jornot L, Junod AF. Effects of hypoxanthine xanthine oxidase on Ca2+ stores and protein synthesis in human endothelial cells. Circ Res 1995;76:388-95.

67.   Doan TN, Gentry DL, Taylor AA, Elliott SJ. Hydrogen peroxide activates agonist-sensitive CA2+-flux pathways in canine venous endothelial cells. Biochem J 1994;297:209-15.

68.   Rao GN, Alexander RW, Runge MS. Linoleic acid and its metabolites, hydroperoxyoctadecadienoic acids, stimulate c-Fos, c-Jun, and c-Myc mRNA expression, mitogen-activated protein kinase activation, and growth in rat aortic smooth muscle cells. J Clin Invest 1995;96:842-7.

69.   Grover AK, Samson SE. Effect of superoxide radical on Ca2+ pumps of coronary artery. Am J Physiol 1988;255:C297-303.

70.   Grover AK, Samson SE, Fomin VP. Peroxide inactivates calcium pump in pig coronary artery. Am J Phyisol 1992;263:H537-43.

71.   Weir EK, Archer SL. The mechanism of acute hypoxic pulmonary vasoconstriction: the tale of two channels. FASEB J 1995;9:183-9.

72.   Spitaler MM, Graier WF. Vascular targets of redox signaling in diabetes mellitus. Diabetologia 2002;45:476-94.

73.   Sundaresan M, Yu ZX, Ferrans VJ, et al. Regulation of reactive-oxygen-species generation in fibroblasts by Rac1. Biochem J 1996;318:379-82.

74.   Chen XL, Zhang Q, Zhao R, et al. Rac1 and Superoxide are required for the expression of cell adhesion molecules induced by tumor necrosis factor-alpha in endothelial cells. J Pharmacol Exp Ther 2003;305:573-80.

75.   Chen XL, Zhang Q, Zhao R, Medford RM. TNF-alpha-induced MCP-1 expression is activated by the Rac1 and NADPH oxidase-dependent pathways in endothelial cells: Role of superoxide and hydrogen peroxide. 4th Annual Arteriosclerosis Thrombosis and Vascular Biology 2003:p311.

76.   Laufs U, Liao JK. Targeting Rho in cardiovascular disease. Circ Res 2000;87:526-8.

77.   Lander HM, Ogiste JS, Teng KK, Novogrodsky A. p21ras as a common signaling target of reactive free radicals and cellular redox stress. J Biol Chem 1995;270:21195-8.

78.   Berk BC. Protein kinases that mediate redox-sensitive signal transduction. In: Oxidative Stress and Vascular Disease, edited by J.F. Keaney (Kluwer Academic Publishers, 1999), pp. 335-48.

79.   Chen K, Vita JA, Berk BC, Keaney JF, Jr. c-Jun N-terminal kinase activation by hydrogen peroxide in endothelial cells involves SRC-dependent epidermal growth factor receptor transactivation. J Biol Chem 2001;276:16045-50.

80.   Thomas SR, Chen K, Keaney JF, Jr. Hydrogen peroxide activates endothelial nitric-oxide synthase through coordinated phosphorylation and dephosphorylation via a phosphoinositide 3-kinase-dependent signaling pathway. J Biol Chem 2002;277:6017-24.

81.   Ushio-Fukai M, Griendling KK, Becker PL, Hilenski L, Halleran S, Alexander RW. Epidermal growth factor receptor transactivation by angiotensin II requires reactive oxygen species in vascular smooth muscle cells. Arterioscler Thromb Vasc Biol 2001;21:489-95.

82. Gonzalez-Rubio M, Voit S, Rodriguez-Puyol D, Weber M, Marx M. Oxidative stress induces tyrosine phosphorylation of PDGF alpha-and beta-receptors and pp60c-src in mesangial cells. Kidney Int 1996;50:164-73.

83. Min DS, Kim EG, Exton JH. Involvement of tyrosine phosphorylation and protein kinase C in the activation of phospholipase D by H2O2 in Swiss 3T3 fibroblasts. J Biol Chem 1998;273:29986-94.

84. Linseman DA, Benjamin CW, Jones DA. Convergence of angiotensin II and platelet-derived growth factor receptor signaling cascades in vascular smooth muscle cells. J Biol Chem 1995;270:12563-8.

85. Heeneman S, Haendeler J, Saito Y, Ishida M, Berk BC. Angiotensin II induces transactivation of two different populations of the platelet-derived growth factor beta receptor. Key role for the p66 adaptor protein Shc. J Biol Chem 2000;275:15926-32.

86. Touyz RM. Recent advances in intracellular signaling in hypertension. Current Opinion in Nephrology and Hypertension 2003;12:165-74.

87. Griendling KK, Sorescu D, Lassegue B, Ushio-Fukai M. Modulation of protein kinase activity and gene expression by reactive oxygen species and their role in vascular physiology and pathophysiology. Arterioscler Thromb Vasc Biol 2000;20:2175-83.

88. Abe J, Takahashi M, Ishida M, Lee JD, Berk BC. c-Src is required for oxidative stress-mediated activation of big mitogen-activated protein kinase 1. J Biol Chem 1997;272:20389-94.

89. Wang D, Yu X, Cohen RA, Brecher P. Distinct effects of N-acetylcysteine and nitric oxide on angiotensin II-induced epidermal growth factor receptor phosphorylation and intracellular Ca(2+) levels. J Biol Chem 2000;275:12223-30.

90. Berk BC. Redox signals that regulate the vascular response to injury. Thromb Haemost 1999;82:810-7.

91. Yoshizumi M, Abe J, Haendeler J, Huang Q, Berk BC. Src and Cas mediate JNK activation but not ERK1/2 and p38 kinases by reactive oxygen species. J Biol Chem 2000;275:11706-12.

92. Marrero MB, Schieffer B, Paxton WG, et al. Direct stimulation of Jak/STAT pathway by the angiotensin II AT1 receptor. Nature 1995;375:247-50.

93. McWhinney CD, Dostal D, Baker K. Angiotensin II activates Stat5 through Jak2 kinase in cardiac myocytes. J Mol Cell Cardiol 1998;30:751-61.

94. Schieffer B, Luchtefeld M, Braun S, Hilfiker A, Hilfiker-Kleiner D, Drexler H. Role of NAD(P)H oxidase in angiotensin II-induced JAK/STAT signaling and cytokine induction. Circ Res 2000;87:1195-201.

95. Garcia-Morales P, Minami Y, Luong E, Klausner RD, Samelson LE. Tyrosine phosphorylation in T cells is regulated by phosphatase activity: Studies with phenylarsine oxide. Proc Natl Acad Sci. U S A. 1990;87:9255-9.

96. Hadari YR, Geiger B, Nadiv O, et al. Hepatic tyrosine-phosphorylated proteins identified and localized following in vivo inhibition of protein tyrosine phosphatases: Effects of H2O2 and vanadate administration into rat livers. Mol Cell Endocrinol 1993;97:9-17.

97. Sullivan SG, Chiu DT-Y, Errasfa M, Wang JM, Qi J-S, Stern A. Effects of H2O2 on protein tyrosine phosphatase activity in HER14 cells. Free Radic Biol Med 1994;16:399-403.

98. Johnson GL, Lapadat R. Mitogen-activated protein kinase pathways mediated by ERK, JNK, and p38 protein kinases. Science 2002;298:1911-2.

99. Yoshizumi M, Tsuchiya K, Tamaki T. Signal transduction of reactive oxygen species and mitogen-activated protein kinases in cardiovascular disease. J Med Invest 2001;48:11-24.

100. Auge N, Escargueil-Blanc I, Lajoie-Mazenc I, et al. Potential role for ceramide in mitogen-activated protein kinase activation and proliferation of vascular smooth muscle cells induced by oxidized low density lipoprotein. J Biol Chem 1998:12893-900.

101. Ushio-Fukai M, Alexander RW, Akers M, Griendling KK. p38 Mitogen-activated protein kinase is a critical component of the redox-sensitive signaling pathways activated by angiotensin II. Role in vascular smooth muscle cell hypertrophy. J Biol Chem 1998;273:15022-9.

102. Bhunia AK, Han H, Snowden A, Chatterjee S. Redox-regulated signaling by lactosylceramide in the proliferation of human aortic smooth muscle cells. Biol Chem 1997;272:15642-9.

103. Abe J, Kusuhara M, Ulevitch RJ, Berk BC, Lee JD. Big mitogen-activated protein kinase 1 (BMK1) is a redox-sensitive kinase. J Biol Chem 1996;271:16586-90.

104. Zhang J, Jin N, Liu Y, Rhoades RA. Hydrogen peroxide stimulates extracellular signal-regulated protein kinases in pulmonary arterial smooth muscle cells. Am J Respir Cell Mol Biol 1998;19:324-32.

105. Baas AS, Berk BC. Differential activation of mitogen-activated protein kinases by H_2O_2 and O_2- in vascular smooth muscle cells. Circ Res 1995;77:29-36.

106. Touyz RM, Cruzado M, Tabet F, Yao G, Salomon S, Schiffrin EL. Redox-dependent MAP kinase signaling by Ang II in vascular smooth muscle cells: role of receptor tyrosine kinase transactivation. Can J Physiol Pharmacol 2003;81:159-67.

107. Viedt C, Soto U, Krieger-Brauer HI, et al. Differential activation of mitogen-activated protein kinases in smooth muscle cells by angiotensin II: involvement of p22phox and reactive oxygen species. Arterioscler Thromb Vasc Biol 2000;20:940-8.

108. Frank GD, Eguchi S, Inagami T, Motley ED. N-acetylcysteine inhibits angiotensin II-mediated activation of extracellular signal-regulated kinase and epidermal growth factor receptor. Biochem Biophys Res Commun 2001;280:1116-9.

109. Huot J, Houle F, Rousseau S, Deschesnes RG, Shah GM, Landry J. SAPK2/p38-dependent F-actin reorganization regulates early membrane blebbing during stress-induced apoptosis. J Cell Biol 1998;143:1361-73.

110. Huot J, Houle F, Marceau F, Landry J. Oxidative stress-induced actin reorganization mediated by the p38 mitogen-activated protein kinase/heat shock protein 27 pathway in vascular endothelial cells. Circ Res 1997;80:383-92.

111. Yeh LH, Park YJ, Hansalia RJ, et al. Shear-induced tyrosine phosphorylation in endothelial cells requires Rac1-dependent production of ROS. Am J Physiol 1999;276:C838-47.

112. Ichijo H, Nishida E, Irie K, et al. Induction of apoptosis by ASK1, a mammalian MAPKKK that activates SAPK/JNK and p38 signaling pathways. Science 1997;275:90-4.

113. Surapisitchat J, Hoefen RJ, Pi X, Yoshizumi M, Yan C, Berk BC. Fluid shear stress inhibits TNF-alpha activation of JNK but not ERK1/2 or p38 in human umbilical vein endothelial cells: Inhibitory crosstalk among MAPK family members. Proc Natl Acad Sci U S A 2001;98:6476-81.

114. Yamawaki H, Lehoux S, Berk BC. Chronic physiological shear stress inhibits tumor necrosis factor-induced proinflammatory responses in rabbit aorta perfused ex vivo. Circulation 2003;108:1619-25.

115. Saitoh M, Nishitoh H, Fujii M, et al. Mammalian thioredoxin is a direct inhibitor of apoptosis signal-regulating kinase (ASK) 1. Embo J 1998;17:2596-606.

116. Yamawaki H, Haendeler J, Berk BC. Thioredoxin: a key regulator of cardiovascular homeostasis. Circ Res 2003;93:1029-33.

117. Lassegue B, Sorescu D, Szocs K, et al. Novel gp91(phox) homologues in vascular smooth muscle cells: nox1 mediates angiotensin II-induced superoxide formation and redox-sensitive signaling pathways. Circ Res 2001;88:888-94.

118. Ushio-Fukai M, Alexander RW, Akers M, et al. Reactive oxygen species mediate the activation of Akt/protein kinase B by angiotensin II in vascular smooth muscle cells. J Biol Chem 1999;274:22699-704.

119. Haddad JJ. Antioxidant and prooxidant mechanisms in the regulation of redox-sensitive transcription factors. Cell Signal 2002;14:879-97.

120. Haddad JJ. Science review: redox and oxygen-sensitive transcription factors in the regulation of oxidant-mediated lung injury: role for hypoxia-inducible factor-1alpha. Crit Care 2003;7:47-54.

121. de Nigris F, Lerman LO, Napoli C. New insights in the transcriptional activity and coregulator molecules in the arterial wall. Int J Cardiol 2002;86:153-68.

122. Kunsch C, Medford RM. Oxidative stress as a regulator of gene expression in the vasculature. Circ Res 1999;85:753-66.

123. Crawford K, Zbinden I, Amstad P, Cerutti P. Oxidant stress induces the proto-oncogenes c-fos and c-myc in mouse epidermal cells. Oncogene 1988;3:27-32.

124. Devary Y, Gottlieb RA, Lau LF, Karin M. Rapid and preferential activation of the c-jun gene during the mammalian UV response. Mol Cell Biol 1991;11:2804-11.

125. Nose K, Shibanuma M, Kikuchi K, Kageyama H, Sakiyama S, Kuroki T. Transcriptional activation of early-response genes by hydrogen peroxide in a mouse osteoblastic cell line. Eur J Biochem 1991;201:99-106.

126. Collart FR, Horio M, Huberman E. Heterogeneity in c-jun gene expression in normal and malignant cells exposed to either ionizing radiation or hydrogen peroxide. Radiat Res 1995;142:188-96.

127. Shono T, Ono M, Izumi H, et al. Involvement of the transcription factor NF-kB in tubular morphogenesis of human microvascular endothelial cells by oxidative stress. Mol Cell Biol 1996;16:4231-9.

128. Lin JH, Zhu Y, Liao HL, Kobari Y, Groszek L, Stemerman MB. Induction of vascular cell adhesion molecule-1 by low-density lipoprotein. Atherosclerosis 1996;127:185-94.

129. Maziere C, Kjavaheri-Mergny M, Frye-Fressart V, Kelattre J, Maziere JC. Copper and cell-oxidized low-density lipoprotein induces activator protein 1 in fibroblasts, endothelial and smooth muscle cells. FEBS Lett 1997;409:351-6.

130. Ares MP, Kallin B, Eriksson P, Nilsson J. Oxidized LDL induces transcription factor activator protein-1 but inhibits activation of nuclear factor-kB in human vascular smooth muscle cells. Arterioscler Thromb Vasc Biol 1995;15:1584-90.

131. Rao GN, Lassegue B, Griendling KK, Alexander RW. Hydrogen peroxide stimulates transcription of c-jun in vascular smooth muscle cells: role of arachidonic acid. Oncogene 1993;8.2759-64.

132. Ruef J, Rao GN, Li F, et al. Induction of rat aortic smooth muscle cell growth by the lipid peroxidation product 4-hydroxy-2-nonenal. Circulation 1998;97:1071-8.

133. Wung BS, Cheng JJ, Hsieh HJ, Shyy YJ, Wang DL. Cyclic strain-induced monocyte chemotactic protein-1 gene expression in endothelial cells involves reactive oxygen species activation of activator protein 1. Circ Res 1997;81:1-7.

134. Roebuck KA, Rahman A, Lakshminarayanan V, Janakidevi K, Malik AB. H_2O_2 and tumor necrosis factor-alpha activate intercellular adhesion molecule 1 (ICAM-1) gene transcription through distinct cis-regulatory elements within the ICAM-1 promoter. J Biol Chem 1995;270:18966-74.

135. Rao GN, Lassegue B, Griendling KK, Alexander RW, Berk BC. Hydrogen peroxide-induced c-fos expression is mediated by arachidonic acid release: role of protein kinase C. Nucleic Acids Res 1993;21:1259-63.

136. Barchowsky A, Munro SR, Morana SJ, Vincenti MP, Treadwell M. Oxidant-sensitive and phosphorylation-dependent activation of NF-kappa B and AP-1 in endothelial cells. Am J Physiol 1995;269:L829-36.

137. Del Arco PG, Martinez-Martinez S, Calvo V, Armesilla AL, Redondo JM. Antioxidants and AP-1 activation: A brief overview. Immunobiol 1997;198:273-8.

138. Maruyama I, Shigeta K, Miyahara H, et al. Thrombin activates NF-kappa B through thrombin receptor and results in proliferation of vascular smooth muscle cells: role of thrombin in atherosclerosis and restenosis. Ann N Y Acad of Sci 1997;811:429-36.

139. Brand K, Page S, Rogler G, et al. Activated transcription factor nuclear factor-kappa B is present in the atherosclerotic lesion. J Clin Invest 1996;97:1715-22.

140. Schreck R, Rieber P, Baeuerle PA. Reactive oxygen intermediates as apparently widely used messengers in the activation of the NF-kappa B transcription factor and HIV-1. EMBO J. 1991;10:2247-58.

141. Schreck R, Albermann K, Baeuerle PA. Nuclear factor kappa B: an oxidative stress-responsive transcription factor of eukaryotic cells. Free Radic Res. Commun. 1992;17:221-37.

142. Suzuki YJ, Packer L. Inhibition of NF-kB activation by vitamin E derivatives. Biochem Biophys Res Commun 1993;193:227-83.

143. Kretz-Remy C, Mehlen P, Mirault ME, Arrigo AP. Inhibition of I kappa B-alpha phosphorylation and degradation and subsequent NF-kappa B activation by glutathione peroxidase overexpression. J Cell Biol 1996;133:1083-93.

144. Hayashi T, Ueno Y, Okamoto T. Oxidoreductive regulation of nuclear factor kappa B. Involvement of a cellular reducing catalyst thioredoxin. J Biol Chem 1993;268:11380-8.

145. Grimm S, Baeuerle PA. The inducible transcription factor NF-kB: Structure-function relationship of its protein subunits. Biochem J 1993;290:297-308.

146. Chan MM. Inhibition of tumor necrosis factor by curcumin, a phytochemical. Biochem Pharmacol 1995;49:1551-6.

147. Pierce JW, Read MA, Ding H, Luscinskas FW, Collins T. Salicylates inhibit I kappa B-alpha phosphorylation, endothelial-leukocyte adhesion molecule expression, and neutrophil transmigration. J Immunol 1996;156:3961-9.

148. Gerritsen ME, Carley WW, Ranges GE, et al. Flavonoids inhibit cytokine-induced endothelial cell adhesion protein gene expression. Am J Pathol 1995;147:278-92.

149. Wolle J, Hill RR, Ferguson E, et al. Selective inhibition of tumor necrosis factor-induced vascular cell adhesion molecule-1 gene expression by a novel flavonoid. Lack of effect on transcription factor NF-kappa B. Arterioscler Thromb Vasc Biol 1996;16:1501-8.

150. Kunsch C LJ, Grey JY, Olliff LK, et al. Selective inhibition of endothelial and monocyte redox-sensitive genes by AGI-1067: a novel antioxidant and anti-inflammatory agent. J of Pharmacol and Exp Ther 2004;308:820-9.

151. Schubert SY, Neeman I, Resnick N. A novel mechanism for the inhibition of NF-kappaB activation in vascular endothelial cells by natural antioxidants. FASEB J 2002;16:1931-3.

152. Chen XL, Kunsch C. Induction of cytoprotective genes through Nrf2/antioxidant response element pathway: a new therapeutic approach for the treatment of inflammatory diseases. Curr Pharm Des 2004;10:879-91.

153. Rushmore TH, Morton MR, Pickett CB. The antioxidant responsive element. Activation by oxidative stress and identification of the DNA consensus sequence required for functional activity. J Biol Chem 1991;266:11632-9.

154. Wasserman WW, Fahl WE. Functional antioxidant responsive elements. Proc Natl Acad Sci U S A 1997;94:5361-6.

155. Prestera T, Talalay P. Electrophile and antioxidant regulation of enzymes that detoxify carcinogens. Proc Natl Acad Sci U S A 1995;92:8965-9.

156. Jaiswal AK. Regulation of genes encoding NAD(P)H:quinone oxidoreductases. Free Radic Biol Med 2000;29:254-62.

157. Alam J, Stewart D, Touchard C, Boinapally S, Choi AM, Cook JL. Nrf2, a Cap'n'Collar transcription factor, regulates induction of the heme oxygenase-1 gene. J Biol Chem 1999;274:26071-8.

158. Tsuji Y, Ayaki H, Whitman SP, Morrow CS, Torti SV, Torti FM. Coordinate transcriptional and translational regulation of ferritin in response to oxidative stress. Mol Cel Biol 2000;20:5818-27.

159. Itoh K, Chiba T, Takahashi S, et al. An Nrf2/small Maf heterodimer mediates the induction of phase II detoxifying enzyme genes through antioxidant response elements. Biochem Biophys Res Commun 1997;236:313-22.

160. Chan K, Kan YW. Nrf2 is essential for protection against acute pulmonary injury in mice. Proc Natl Acad Sci U S A 1999;96:12731-6.

161. Bea F, Hudson FN, Chait A, Kavanagh TJ, Rosenfeld ME. Induction of glutathione synthesis in macrophages by oxidized low-density lipoproteins is mediated by consensus antioxidant response elements. Circ Res 2003;92:386-93.

162. Ishii T, Itoh K, Ruiz E, et al. Role of Nrf2 in the regulation of CD36 and stress protein expression in murine macrophages: activation by oxidatively modified LDL and 4-hydroxynonenal. Circ Res 2004;94:609-16.

163. Buckley BJ, Marshall ZM, Whorton AR. Nitric oxide stimulates Nrf2 nuclear translocation in vascular endothelium. Biochem Biophys Res Commun 2003;307:973-9.

164. Chen XL, Varner SE, Rao AS, et al. Laminar flow induction of antioxidant response element-mediated genes in endothelial cells. A novel anti-inflammatory mechanism. J Biol Chem 2003;278:703-11.

165. Itoh K, Tong KI, Yamamoto M. Molecular mechanism activating Nrf2-Keap1 pathway in regulation of adaptive response to electrophiles. Free Radic Biol Med 2004;36:1208-13.

166. Nguyen T, Sherratt PJ, Pickett CB. Regulatory mechanisms controlling gene expression mediated by the antioxidant response element. Annu Rev Pharmacol Toxicol 2003;43:233-60.

167. Kong AN, Owuor E, Yu R, et al. Induction of xenobiotic enzymes by the MAP kinase pathway and the antioxidant or electrophile response element (ARE/EpRE). Drug Metab Rev 2001;33:255-71.

168. Huang HC, Nguyen T, Pickett CB. Phosphorylation of Nrf2 at Ser-40 by protein kinase C regulates antioxidant response element-mediated transcription. J Biol Chem 2002;277:42769-74.

169. Numazawa S, Ishikawa M, Yoshida A, Tanaka S, Yoshida T. Atypical protein kinase C mediates activation of NF-E2-related factor 2 in response to oxidative stress. Am J Physiol Cell Physiol 2003;285:C334-42.

170. Chen XL, Thomas S, Wasserman MA, Kunsch C. Activation of the Nrf2/Antioxidant response element pathway protects endothelial cells from oxidant Injury and Inhibits redox-sensitive inflammatory gene expression: A novel vascular protective pathway. Circulation 2003;108:IV-304.

171. Lu D, Maulik N, Moraru, II, Kreutzer DL, Das DK. Molecular adaptation of vascular endothelial cells to oxidative stress. Am J Physiol 1993;264:C715-22.

172. Satriano JA, Shuldiner M, Hora K, Xing Y, Shan Z, Schlondorff D. Oxygen radicals as second messengers for expression of the monocyte chemoattractant protein, JE/MCP-1, and the monocyte colony-stimulating factor, CSF-1, in response to tumor necrosis factor-alpha and immunoglobulin G. Evidence for involvement of reduced nicotinamide adenine dinucleotide phosphate (NADPH)-dependent oxidase. J Clin Invest 1993;92:1564-71.

173. Chen XL, Tummala PE, Obrych M, Alexander RW, Medford RM. Angiotensin II induces monocyte chemoattractant protein-1 gene expression in vascular smooth muscle cells. Circ Res 1998;83:952-9.

174. Marui N, Offermann MK, Swerlick R, et al. Vascular cell adhesion molecule-1 (VCAM-1) gene transcription and expression are regulated through an antioxidant-sensitive mechanism in human vascular endothelial cells. J Clin Invest 1993;92:1866-74.

175. Weber C, Erl W, Pietsch A, Strobel M, Ziegler-Heitbrock H, Weber P. Antioxidants inhibit monocyte adhesion by suppressing nuclear factor-kB mobilization and induction of vascular cell adhesion molecule-1 in endothelial cells stimulated to generate radicals. Arterio Thromb 1994;14:1665-73.

176. Spiecker M, Darius H, Kaboth K, Hubner F, Liao JK. Differential regulation of endothelial cell adhesion molecule expression by nitric oxide donors and antioxidants. J Leukoc Biol 1998;63:732-9.

177. Weber DS, Taniyama Y, Rocic P, et al. Phosphoinositide-dependent kinase 1 and p21-activated protein kinase mediate reactive oxygen species-dependent regulation of platelet-derived growth factor-induced smooth muscle cell migration. Circ Res 2004;94:1219-26.

178. Chua CC, Hamdy RC, Chua BH. Upregulation of vascular endothelial growth factor by H_2O_2 in rat heart endothelial cells. Free Radic Biol Med 1998;25:891-7.

179. Galis ZS, Asanuma K, Godin D, Meng X. N-acetyl-cysteine decreases the matrix-degrading capacity of macrophage-derived foam cells: new target for antioxidant therapy. Circulation 1998;97:2445-53.

180. Witztum JL, Steinberg D. Role of oxidized low density lipoprotein in atherogenesis. J Clin Invest 1991;88:1785-92.

Chapter 6

BIOMARKERS OF OXIDANT STRESS IN VIVO: OXIDATIVE MODIFICATIONS OF LIPIDS, PROTEINS AND DNA

Ian A. Blair[1-5], John A Lawson[1,2], Harry Ischiropoulos[2,3] and Garret A. FitzGerald[1,2]

[1]The Institute for Translational Medicine and Therapeutics, Departments of [2]Pharmacology, [3]Pediatrics and [4]Chemistry, and [5]The Center for Cancer Pharmacology, University of Pennsylvania, Philadelphia, PA

Introduction

Oxidative stress (OS) has been widely implicated in physiological processes, such as aging and in disease pathogenesis, ranging from carcinogenesis through the aetiology of Alzheimer's disease to atherogenesis. However, until recently our ability to interrogate integrated systems, such as model organisms and humans, has been restricted by the lack of availability of quantitiative indices of oxidant stress *in vivo*. Indeed, the failure to identify benefit from antioxidants in clinical trials thus far may reflect, in part, the absence of such biomarkers to identify susceptible patients and to guide drug response[1,2]. This review focuses on developments in the analytical biochemistry of oxidant stress. Particular emphasis is placed on the still emerging technologies to study oxidative damage to DNA *in vivo*. The emergence of these new technologies promises to elucidate the role of this process in human disease and to afford a necessary adjunct to the development of novel antioxidant therapeutic strategies[3].

Oxidative modification of lipids

Methodology for the direct observation of free radicals *in vivo* has been elusive, requiring reliance for quantitation on compounds secondary to the attack of free radicals on biomolecules. The primary components of mammalian cell membranes are phospholipids (PLs), and approximately half of the lipid components of the PLs are polyunsaturated fatty acids (PUFAs), notably arachidonic acid. The methylene hydrogens of arachidonic acid or other PUFAs are susceptible to abstraction by a free radical and the ensuing PUFA free radical can spontaneously rearrange and/or attack one or more molecules of molecular oxygen. The ensuing lipid peroxides (LPOs) may dehydrate to form conjugated dienes, fragment to form aldehydes or alkanes, or rearrange to form isoeicosanoids — compounds that are isomeric to naturally occurring enzymatic products such as prostaglandins (PGs). The proximity to other PUFAs allows a chain reaction to occur, in which a free radical can attack and alter a succession of PUFA molecules, until it is quenched. Although these products may have physiological and/or pathological significance locally through perturbation of membrane function or distally through receptor mediated effects, these considerations will not be the focus of this chapter which rather, will deal with their utility as indices of OS. All of the above LPO products have been proposed to be markers of OS and each has its strengths and weaknesses. No single method encompassing all the characteristics required of a reliable marker of OS has been developed. These include non-invasive sample acquisition, sensitivity, specificity, facile sample preparation, accuracy, reproducibility, and affordability. Some methods have been in use for decades and have been thoroughly discussed in print. We will attempt to summarize their various strengths and drawbacks, but we will place emphasis on methods applicable to OS research in humans, including some recent innovations. For an introduction to the chemistry of lipid peroxidation, see Porter[4]. Gutterdge and Halliwell published an excellent review of methods for detection of LPO related compounds[5].

Lipid peroxides

Quantitation of LPOs is attractive as an approach, as it focuses on primary products of lipid peroxidation, as opposed to degradation products. Some general characteristics warrant comment; hydroperoxides are relatively unstable, so susceptibility to degradation before and after sample collection must be minimized, e.g. separation from, or inactivation of, tissue and circulating peroxidases, including albumin, which has substantial peroxidase activity[6,7]. Taking an extracted sample to dryness may result in loss of hydroperoxides[8]. Holley and Slater documented a "large and rapid loss" of hydroperoxide from plasma at 0^0C or 27^0C[9]. Artifactual production of LPOs can occur both by enzymatic (e.g. cyclooxygenases (COXs), lipoxygenases (LOXs) or by autooxidative mechanisms. This can be minimized by freezing, pH alteration, or extraction into organic solvents to halt enzymatic activity and/or by inclusion of a free radical scavenger, such as butylated hydroxytoluene (BHT) to inhibit free radical reactions. A limitation of LPO assays in general is their lack of applicability to urine samples.

A frequently used method is based on the ability of LPOs to convert ferrous ions to ferric, which complex with thiocyanate to form a chromophore that can be measured by ultraviolet (UV) absorption[8]. Lipid extraction is required, since amino acid hydroperoxides, hydrogen peroxide[8] or endogenous ferric ions may be a source of error. In some versions, xylenol orange is substituted for thiocyanate. A similar method utilizes the ability of LPOs to convert iodide to triiodide (I_3^-), which can be measured spectrophotometrically. In this assay, enzymatic hydrolysis of cholesterol esters, triglycerides, and phospholipids is required, followed by extraction into ethyl acetate. In a recent study, which compared several potential biomarkers in plasma and urine from a rat model of OS[10], neither of these methods yielded reliable data.

Other methods utilize chromatography to resolve individual molecular species. An interesting approach by Miyazawa et al[11] bypasses the hydrolysis steps in the above methods, and measures phospholipid hydroperoxides (PLPOs) directly. After extraction from plasma, they are subjected to high-performance liquid chromatography (HPLC) with a method of chemiluminescence detection that is specific for hydroperoxides[12]. Spickett et al have recently published a method using a similar extraction followed by HPLC, with detection by mass spectrometry (MS), instead of chemiluminescence[9,13]. This worked well for lipids from oxidatively stressed cells in culture, but it is not clear if the technique will be sensitive enough to monitor PLPOs in plasma. The difficulty in absolute identification of oxidized species makes a clear call for transfer of the method to a tandem MS detector with analysis patterned after the seminal work of Khaselev and Murphy[14]. Although they obtained and interpreted the negative ion MS/MS spectrum of some PLPOs, the method has not, to our knowledge, been configured as a quantitative tool for PLPO analysis.

Short chain hydrocarbons

Several short chain hydrocarbons are generated from the omega end of autooxidizing PUFAs[15,16,17]. Thus, ω-3 fatty acids, such as linolenic acid, evolve ethane, and ω-6 PUFAs, such as arachidonic acid, evolve mainly pentane. The quantitation of evolved hydrocarbons is fraught with technical problems, such as high background levels (from environmental pollution or from intestinal flora), difficulties in sample handling and storage, sensitivity to oxygen concentration[18]. In spite of these drawbacks, pentane evolution has been correlated with physiology and pathology in humans[19-27]. Since it is the only method for obtaining lipid peroxidation data noninvasively in vivo, a major value of the method is in the study of small animals in a controlled atmosphere.

Conjugated dienes

An early event in the peroxidation of unsaturated lipids with at least two methylene-interrupted double bonds is the formation of a conjugated diene (CD) system[4]. Since the diene remains after the associated peroxide has degraded, quantitation of CDs negates one of the criticisms of peroxide quantitation[9]. The UV absorption at 234 nm is used as a basis for quantitation. Since the CD absorption is overlaid on the spectrum of the PUFAs, the height and exact wavelength of the absorption maximum are often difficult to quantitate. The introduction of derivative spectroscopy lessened these problems[28]. This assay has been utilized mainly with tissue extracts, but its application in human plasma[29,30] makes it a potentially important tool in OS research. CDs from dietary sources, such as those from milk products can obfuscate the measurement of autooxidative products. A noteworthy application is the quantitation of baseline diene conjugation (BDC) in circulating low-density lipoproteins (LDLs)[31]. This method is not applicable to urine.

Aldehydes

In addition to alkanes, LPOs degrade spontaneously into an array of carbonyls[18,32], many of which are toxic. Although some have been used as indices of OS[33], malondialdehyde (MDA) has seen by far the most use, and has been the most popular method for measuring OS for decades, in spite of many caveats associated with the technique[18,34,35]. The most common way of measuring MDA is the simple, but non-specific thiobarbituric acid (TBA) test, in which TBA reacts with MDA at low pH to form a chromophore that absorbs UV light at 532 nm. Since several other compounds react with TBA, this is more correctly referred to as the TBA reactive substances (TBARS) assay. Many of the problems associated with MDA quantitation in crude samples have been addressed by utilizing the more specific HPLC or GC/MS methods which are able to separate the authentic (TBA)$_2$-MDA adduct. This assay has been commonly used, but any researcher considering its use should thoroughly study its limitations. In the above-mentioned study comparing biomarkers of OS in a rat model[10], three variations of the TBARS method and a GC/MS version failed to yield informative data from plasma when compared with other more specific methods. Further, an HPLC method for measuring MDA in urine also failed to yield useful data.

In recent years, the toxicity of 4-hydroxynonenal (HNE) has been recognized, and it has consequently become a target for quantitation[36]. HNE is able to diffuse throughout cells and to pass through membranes, and mediates toxicity through direct effects and through the modification of nucleophilic sites on proteins[32]. HNE-protein adducts have been quantitated immunologically and by mass spectrometry[37], while free HNE has been measured in serum[38], using a method in which HPLC with fluorescence detection is used to measure the product of the reaction of HNE with 1,3-cyclohexanedione. Measurement of aldehydes is accomplished in plasma by GC/MS of the oxime-tert-butyldimethylsilyl derivatives. The use of the O-pentafluorobenzyl (O-PFB) trimethylsilyl ether and GC/negative ion electron capture MS techniques with a labeled internal standard increased the sensitivity of the method[39], and Luo et al. expanded the method to measure 22 saturated an unsaturated aldehydes, including HNE[40]. HNE has also been measured in urine by a similar method[41]. The biological significance of HNE and the ability to measure it in plasma and in urine make it likely that this compound will see further use as a marker for OS. Caveats to its use include its volatility and reactivity toward proteins.

Isoprostanes

Isoprostanes (iPs) are autooxidized lipids that resemble enzymatically-derived prostaglandins. Since their first description by Morrow et al.[42], iPs have been postulated to be excellent biomarkers of OS. Although many general types of iPs are formed[43], the F_2-iPs — named for their structural similarity to PGF_2 — have garnered the most attention, due to their chemical stability, involatility, excellent chromatographic characteristics and relatively high concentration in urine.

Hydrogen abstraction from one of the three methylene carbons of AA can initiate a series of intramolecular rearrangements and attack of molecular oxygen resulting in four types of F_2-iPs[43]. Due to the plethora of iP isomers, a systematic nomenclature is imperative. Two systems have been proposed[44,45]; we will use that of Rokach et al. in the following discussion[45].

Type III iPs, those most similar to PGF_2, were the first to be investigated, due to their more familiar analytical characteristics and, significantly, the fact that a likely isomer, 8-iso-$PGF_{2\alpha}$ (i$PF_{2\alpha}$-III) had been previously synthesized and was available for experimentation. This particular isomer can be enzymatically produced by COX-1[46] and COX-2[47], although this route of formation appears to contribute undetectably to iP concentrations in urine[48]. The highly sensitive GC/EC/NI/MS method, well-proven for the analysis of PFB esters of eicosanoids[49] was immediately applied to iP analysis[42], and this method, with minor modifications, has been extensively used for iP analysis. A major improvement came with the availability of a stable isotope labeled internal standard for i$PF_{2\alpha}$-III[46,50]. Later, immunologic methods were developed such as enzyme immunoassays (EIA) and radio immunoassays (RIA). EIA use has eclipsed RIA.

Almost all iP EIA research has targeted $iPF_{2\alpha}$-III. Simplicity and affordability are attractions of the method, and several commercial kits are offered (e.g. Cayman, Assay Design, Oxis). Results must be considered to be semi-quantitative, for several considerations, e.g., cross-reactivity of the antibody with other iP species and, if urine or plasma are being used, with iP metabolites. Also, problems with non-specific binding dictate that most samples must undergo a purification step, which can lead to loss of analyte. A method for controlling for these losses has been published, with results that correlated well with GC/MS measurement[51], but the added steps and the need for radioactive standards kept the method from wide use. Bearing these considerations in mind, EIA analysis of iPs can be a valuable tool for researchers without access to complex and expensive MS facilities.

As mentioned, GC/EC/NI/MS methods have predominated in the instrumental analysis of iPs, due to the inherent sensitivity of the method. However, serious drawbacks exist, among them a tedious sample preparation protocol (usually involving one or two solid phase extraction (SPE) steps, two TLC steps, two derivatization steps, and all the associated extraction, transfer, and evaporation steps). It may take a technician two days to prepare a dozen samples, and recoveries may be in the 5% range. Autosampler and capillary column considerations may limit the injection to 5-10% of the remaining sample. The sensitivity of the method and the availability of stable isotope-labeled internal standards, e.g. tetradeuterated $iPF_{2\alpha}$-III, which traverse the sample preparation steps with losses proportional to those of the endogenous iP are able to compensate for the losses incurred during workup. Another detraction is the inability of the GC completely to separate the myriad isomers, which include up to 64 F_2-iPs and at least two enzymatic products, $PGF_{2\alpha}$ and 11_β-PGF_2, that are potentially present. Since electron capture ionization method is very "gentle", and the PFB ester is a good leaving group, the spectrum of iPs consists, in large part, to a single ion, M-PFB (M-181). This means that all F_2-iPs look the same to the MS. It is these factors that necessitate the extensive sample preparation regimen outlined above. It is clear that GC/MS peaks are often composed of two or more co-eluting isomers. When the medium assayed is urine, its complex and variable nature further complicate the picture. These caveats have not prevented the method from yielding valuable data from tissue homogenates, cell culture medium, urine, plasma, synovial fluid, spinal fluid, and other sources, and it has served as the "gold standard" against which other methods must be proven[52].

Recent advances in MS technology, namely tandem MS (MS/MS) with sample purification by HPLC followed by introduction via an electrospray

(ES) interface (LC/ES/MS/MS), have enabled the development of a dramatically streamlined method for the analysis of urinary iPs[53,54]. Since the iPs do not have to survive volatilization for gas-phase chromatography, they do not require derivatization, and since they are chromatographed above their pKa, they are delivered to the MS as preformed anions. The tandem MS uses the first MS to filter all but the parent ions, which are then fragmented by collision with an inert gas before entering the second MS, which selects for a characteristic product ion. This technique is termed selected reaction monitoring (SRM), and is specific enough that a urine sample can be analyzed after a single SPE step. In fact, by selecting the proper product ions, the four types of F_2-iPs can be analyzed in a mutually-exclusive manner[54]. Added to the ability of reverse phase HPLC to separate the various isomers, a powerful tool for iP quantitation is made available. Using this technique, it was demonstrated that a pair of stereoisomers - 8,12 *iso*-iPF$_{2\alpha}$-VI and 5-cpi-8,12-*iso* iPF$_{2\alpha}$-VI - are the prevalent F_2-iPs in human urine, - present at approximately 20 times the concentration of iPF$_{2\alpha}$-III[55]. When used with a tetradeuterated analog, the former is an excellent indicator of OS in urine[10,54], but the method does not have enough sensitivity to measure iPs in plasma or other matrices where the levels are low. These samples must still be analyzed by GC/MS.

A recent innovation in sample ionization technique has the potential of combining the best aspects of GC/EC/NI/MS (sensitivity) and LC/ES/MS/MS (specificity). EC ionization of PFB esters in an atmospheric pressure chemical ionization source (APCI) may enhance LC/MS/MS sensitivity in a manner analogous to that of GC/EC/NI/MS while retaining the intrinsic specificity of the method[56]. Time will tell whether this technique will revolutionize LC/MS/MS analysis of iPs as it did for GC/EC/NI/MS.

Finally, another aspect of F_2-iP analysis is quantitation of urinary metabolites. One rationale for looking at a metabolite is artifactual ex vivo production of iPs from arachidonic acid in plasma. At present, the only iP where metabolism has been documented to any extent is iPF$_{2\alpha}$-III, which is metabolized to 2,3-dinor-iPF$_{2\alpha}$-III[57] and 2,3-dinor-5,6-dihydro-iPF$_{2\alpha}$-III[58]. Quantitation of 2,3-dinor-5,6-dihydro-iPF$_{2\alpha}$-III is complicated by the fact that this compound also originates as a primary iP formed by the autooxidation of γ-linolenic acid[59].

To summarize, there exists no perfect tool for measuring lipid markers of OS. Every technique fails to incorporate at least one of the requirements listed above. As a rule of thumb, the more general the assay - those with no or minimal sample purification - are the cheapest and simplest, but also the most susceptible to obfuscation by artefacts. The most specific and sensitive methods are also the most expensive and technologically challenging.

Complex and expensive, LC/ES/MS/MS, is able to meet the requirements for non-invasive sample acquisition, facile sample preparation, specificity, accuracy, and reproducibility, but lacks the sensitivity of GC/EC/NI/MS and remains out of the reach of many laboratories. Analysis of urinary iPs by EIA offers the best combination of characteristics of the less expensive methods, but in order to obtain reliable data, the researcher must systematically address the potential drawbacks associated with the method.

Oxidative modification of proteins

Commensurate with developments in assessment of lipid peroxidation, quantitative approaches to assessing oxidatively modified proteins has developed apace. Certain amino acids within proteins, such as cysteine, methionine, histidine, lysine, tyrosine, tryptophan and phenylalanine are modified by reactive species or by electrophiles generated from the oxidation of polyunsaturated lipids[60-67]. The unusual amino acids generated provide unique signature markers that indicate the formation and reactivity of oxidants and potentially diagnostic biomarkers for disease risk assessment. Furthermore, the formation of post-translationally modified amino acids in proteins could be responsible for cellular dysfunction provided that these oxidative modifications induce alterations in protein function. A prototypical protein target for oxidants in cardiovascular disease is the LDL and oxidation of LDL has been considered as an important mechanism for the development of atherosclerosis[62-65]. There follows a brief review of the principal chemistry, the methods of detection and studies that have evaluated two prevalent oxidant-mediated protein modifications, protein carbonylation and protein tyrosine nitration, as biomarkers in cardiovascular disease.

Protein carbonylation
Protein carbonylation reflects several oxidizing pathways. The formation of reactive carbonyls on proteins could result from at least three distinct biochemical pathways[60]: 1) Direct oxidation of amino acid residues such as arginine, histidine and proline. Inappropriate binding of redox active metals in the vicinity of these amino acids could facilitate the direct oxidation. 2) Michael-type addition to lysine, histidine or reduced cysteine of reactive bi-functional aldehydes such as MDA and 4-HNE, generated by oxidation of polyunsaturated fatty acids. Several studies have indicated that the unsaturated C3 carbon in 4-HNE reacts with nucleophiles such as lysine, histidine, and cysteine residues in proteins[61]. The most common product generated is the156 Da Michael adduct, although Schiff base additions resulting in a 138 Da modifications of lysine residues have also been

noted[61]. The carbonyl carbon C1 and the hydroxy carbon C4 are also reactive and can cross-link proteins together via lysine residues. 3) Alternatively, Schiff base formation and Amidori rearrangement of an oxidized sugar could give rise to reactive aldehydes in proteins. All these biochemical pathways indicate either a direct amino acid oxidation or indirect oxidation and thus a potential direct correlation with the magnitude of oxidative stress. *In vitro* data has revealed that plasma protein carbonylation is rather specific because only a few proteins, i.e., fibrinogen, transferrin, IgG and albumin (in the order of mol of carbonyls per mole of protein), were modified after exposure to oxidants[68]. This initially unexpected selectivity was ascribed to the presence of specific residues in these proteins that were more accessible and/or more reactive to oxidants. The selective oxidation of specific proteins was clearly independent of the protein concentration and might be related to the ability of these proteins to bind divalent metals[68], or to other currently undefined restrictive mechanisms.

Protein carbonylation is most often quantified by detection of the reactive aldehydes after derivatization with 2,4 dinitrophenylhydrazine (DNPH). Quantification can be achieved by direct spectrophotometric determination of DNPH or by the employment of antibodies against DNPH[68-71]. A limited number of specific proteins modified by carbonylation have been reported in human diseases, but the number of specific proteins modified *in vivo* is expected to grow as proteomic approaches are becoming available[72-74].

Several studies have identified LDL modified on lysine residues by MDA or 4-HNE in atherosclerotic lesions[62-65]. Despite the increased interest in the oxidation of LDL in foam cell formation and other processes that result in the formation of atherosclerotic lesions, the quantification of these adducts has not been evaluated in individuals with coronary artery disease (CAD) or in individuals with other known risk factors for atherosclerosis[62-65].

Protein tyrosine nitration

Endogenous nitration of tyrosine residues in proteins is mediated by nitric oxide-derived reactive nitrogen species[66]. Nitrating agents can be generated *in vivo* by at least three different chemistries: 1) oxidation of nitrite, one of the stable products of nitric oxide metabolism, by peroxidases and H_2O_2. Several recently published reports have placed myeloperoxidase, the predominant peroxidase of neutrophils and monocytes, as one of the critical peroxidases for catalyzing the nitration of tyrosine residues in proteins[75]. 2) Formation of nitrous acid (HNO_2) by the acidification of nitrite, which then slowly (typically over 18 hours under typical in vitro conditions) will nitrate tyrosine residues. 3) Protein tyrosine nitration is derived by the rapid, (second order rate constant 10^{10} M^{-1} s^{-1}) reaction of nitric oxide with superoxide forming peroxynitrite. The likely proximal species for peroxynitrite mediated protein nitration is the nitrocarbonate $(ONO(O)CO_2^-)$ intermediate, which is formed by the reaction of peroxynitrite with CO_2.

Both immunohistochemical and analytical methodologies have been developed for the localization and quantification of proteins modified by tyrosine nitration[66,67]. Although major concerns with the artificial formation of 3-nitrotyrosine during tissue processing have been raised, recently developed methodologies incorporate appropriate controls to eliminate these concerns. Specifically, the analytical methodologies employ a stable isotope dilution liquid chromatography-electrospray ionization tandem mass spectrometry (LC-ESI/MS/MS) method. Synthetic 3-nitro-[$^{13}C_6$] nitrotyrosine as well as an isotope of L-tyrosine, [$^{13}C_9$$^{15}N_1$] tyrosine, as internal standard and as a monitor of artificial generation of 3-nitrotyrosine are included in the analysis[75,76].

Despite the reactive nature of the nitrating agents, protein tyrosine nitration is a rather selective and specific process, as nitrated proteins are localized only at sites of injury and only few proteins within the injured tissue are modified in human diseases[66,67]. This well documented selectivity and specificity is derived by the conformation and structure of proteins and more significantly by the local electrostatic environment and location of certain tyrosine residues in proteins[77]. These requirements appear to hold true for several nitrating species (either chemically or enzymatically generated) and indicate that the reactivity of tyrosine residues within proteins is the major determinant for both the yield and the selectivity of protein tyrosine nitration *in vivo*.

Unlike protein carbonylation, a case-control study of 208 individuals (100 cases and 108 controls) with documented CAD and peripheral arterial disease evaluated the utility of plasma protein 3-nitrotyrosine as a biomarker for the prevalence of CAD[78]. In the same publication an interventional study in 35 patients examined the effect of hydroxymethylglutaryl coenzyme-A-reductase (statin) on the levels of 3-nitrotyrosine. The data revealed that the protein 3-nitrotyrosine levels measured by the validated LC-ESI/MS/MS method were significantly higher in CAD patients than controls. Moreover, the patients with the highest values, classified in the upper quartile, had a higher odds ratio of CAD even after multivariate model adjustment for other risk factors and biomarkers such as C-reactive protein was applied[78]. Statin therapy significantly reduced the levels of plasma protein 3-nitrotyrosine[78]. Interestingly, recent studies have indicated that quantification of 3-nitrotyrosine levels in specific proteins may reveal more robust associations between protein nitration and cardiovascular disease. For example, the median levels of 3-nitrotyrosine, expressed as mmol per mol of tyrosine, in apolipoprotein B-100 and apolipoprotein A-I recovered from atherosclerotic lesions were 2- and 20-fold higher, respectively, than the median 3-nitrotyrosine level in total protein[78]. Similarly the median level of 3-nitrotyrosine in circulating fibrinogen in CAD patients was 4-fold higher than the median level of the total plasma protein[79]. These data indicate that quantification of 3-nitrotyrosine in specific proteins may be a robust biomarker for cardiovascular disease. Proteomic approaches should facilitate the discovery of additional protein targets, which in addition to existing proteins could provide sound and well-validated biomarkers for cardiovascular disease risk assessment.

Oxidative modification of DNA

DNA damage can occur during OS directly from reactive oxygen species (ROS)[80,81] and reactive nitrogen species (RNS)[82,83]. It can also occur from the breakdown of lipid-hydroperoxides that are formed during OS from ROS, COXs, or LOXs[80,84,85]. The analysis of DNA-adducts is very attractive for framing hypotheses, for molecular epidemiology studies, and for monitoring treatment options because they can provide insight into the amount of genotoxin that has reached the DNA in the tissue under study[86,87]. The action of DNA-repair enzymes results in the excretion of DNA-adducts in the urine. This makes it possible to use non-invasive techniques to monitor urinary DNA-adducts. Until recently, less specific methodology such as ELISA and ^{32}P-postlabeling has used to monitor urinary adducts[87]. The availability of new sensitive MS instrumentation, together with the implementation of routine immunoaffinity purification procedures[88-92], suggests that MS-based methodologies for the analysis of urinary adducts will become the methods of choice in the near future. For example, it was reported recently that immunoaffinity purification in combination with LC/MS could be used to analyze the MDA adduct of 2'-deoxyguanosine (M_1G) in human urine[92].

ROS-mediated formation of lipid hydroperoxides involves the initial abstraction of a bis-allylic methylene hydrogen atom from a PUFA (*Figure 1*)[93]. This is followed by a propagation step, which involves the addition of molecular oxygen. A second (rate-limiting) propagation step then occurs to generate the lipid hydroperoxide with concomitant generation of another radical species. In the case of linoleic acid, this results in the formation of two 13-hydroperoxyoctadecadienoic acid (HPODE) isomers and two 9-HPODE isomers, each of which exists as a mixture of R- and S-enantiomers. They are subsequently reduced to the corresponding hydroxyoctadecadienoic acids (HODEs). ROS-mediated peroxidation of arachidonic acid results in the formation of a complex mixture hydroperoxyeicosatetraenoic acids (HPETEs) that are reduced to racemic hydroxyeicosatetraenoic acids (HETEs) including 15(R)- and 15-(S)-HETE[93].

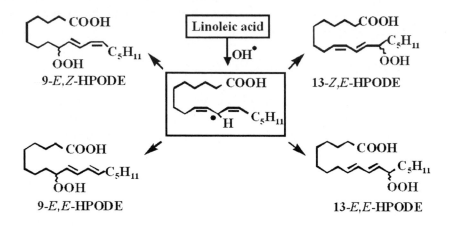

Figure 1: **ROS-mediated formation of lipid hydroperoxides derived from linoleic acid.**

Lipid hydroperoxides can also be formed by the action of LOXs[94] and COXs[95] on PUFAs (*Figure 2*). The enzymatic pathways result in a much simpler profile of HPODEs than the free radical pathways. Linoleic acid is converted primarily to 13(S)-HPODE) by human 15-LOX-1[96] and 15-LOX-2[97] (*Figure 2*). COX-1 and COX-2 produce mainly 9(R)-HPODE and 13(S)-HPODE from linoleic acid[98]. The HPODEs are subsequently reduced to the corresponding 9(R)- and 13(S)-HODEs by intracellular peroxide reducing enzymes[99]. With arachidonic acid as substrate, COX-1 and COX-2 both produce 15-HPETE (*Figure 2*). The 15-HPETE is subsequently reduced to 15-HETE through the peroxidase activity of the COXs or by GSH-dependent peroxidases that are present in the cellular milieu[99] (*Figure 3*). There is a subtle difference in the HETEs that are formed. COX-1 produces 15-HETE that is almost racemic (33 % R; 67 % S)[100,101]; whereas, COX-2 forms mainly 15(S)-HETE (14 % R; 86 % S)[101]. Arachidonic is also an excellent substrate for 15-LOX-1[96] and 15-LOX-2[97]. 15-LOX-1 and 2 both produce exclusively 15(S)-HPETE; whereas, 5-LOX produces exclusively 5(S)-HPETE. The HPETEs are subsequently reduced to the corresponding HETEs[99].

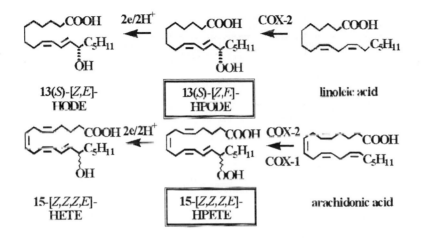

Figure 2: Lipid hydroperoxides derived from COX and LOX enzymes.

LOX and COX-mediated pathways of PUFA metabolism can potentially provide a rich source of lipid hydroperoxide-derived genotoxins. DNA-adducts formed through these pathways are normally repaired in order to maintain fidelity of the DNA. If the lesions are not repaired, subsequent DNA replication can lead to mutations[80,84,85,102,103]. Mutations in protooncogenes and tumour suppressor genes have been directly implicated in human cancer. The resulting genetic modifications can initiate a series of events, which cause cells to proliferate beyond their normal constraints. Therefore, DNA-adducts formed as a consequence of LOX- and COX-mediated lipid peroxidation could contribute to the multiple steps involved in carcinogenesis. The ability to quantify such lesions in DNA could potentially provide powerful dosimeters of exposure to endogenous genotoxins.

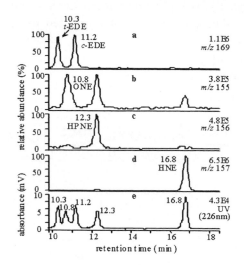

Figure 3

***Figure 3*:LC/MS/UV analysis of authentic standards (200 ng): trans-EDE (1.2 nmol), ONE (1.3 nmol), cis-EDE (1.2 nmol), HPNE (1.2 nmol), HNE (1.3 nmol). (a) Ion chromatograms (m/z 169) for the protonated molecular ion (MH+) of trans-EDE and cis-EDE. (b) Ion chromatogram (m/z 155) for MH+ of ONE. (c) Ion chromatogram (m/z 156) for (MH-OH)+ of HPNE. (d) Ion chromatogram (m/z 157) for MH+ of HNE. (e) UV chromatogram monitoring at 226 nm.**

Genotoxic bifunctional electrophiles

Three of the genotoxic bifunctional electrophiles that are formed from lipid hydroperoxides trans-4,5-epoxy-2(E)-decenal (EDE), cis-EDE, and 4-oxo-2(E)-nonenal (ONE) are poorly ionized under electrospray ionization (ESI) conditions. Furthermore, they are difficult to separate from each other and from other bifunctional electrophiles, such as 4-hydroperoxy-2(E)-nonenal (HPNE) and HNE using reversed-phase solvents. It is possible to derivatize the bifunctional electrophiles as oxime derivatives to improve their reversed phase LC/MS characteristics. However, this leads to the formation of complex mixtures of syn- and anti-oxime isomers that make the chromatograms extremely complex[104]. It was also reasoned that some of the electrophiles would be unstable (particularly HPNE) if GC/MS was used. Therefore, in order to quantify the products of homolytic lipid hydroperoxide decomposition, methodology based on normal phase LC coupled with atmospheric pressure chemical ionization (APCI)/MS was developed[105]. Individual synthetic bifunctional electrophiles revealed a protonated molecule (MH^+) for trans-EDE, cis-EDE, ONE and HNE at m/z 169, 169, 155, and 157, respectively. Product ion spectra of individual bifunctional electrophiles were used to confirm their identity during LC/MS analysis[105]. The bifunctional electrophiles were all separated under normal phase LC conditions (*Figure 3*). Quantitation was performed using selected ion monitoring (SIM) analysis of the most intense ions present in the APCI mass spectra. HNE was more readily ionized than the other bifunctional electrophiles so that its APCI response was almost an order of magnitude more intense than the signals from the other bifunctional electrophiles (*Figure 3d*).

HPNE, EDE, and ONE were the major products of the reaction between 13(S)-HPODE and FeII as evidenced by normal phase LC/APCI/MS analysis (*Figure 4a,b,c*) and the UV response (*Figure 4e*). There was lower amount of HNE (*Figure 4d,e*), and cis-EDE was barely detectable (*Figure 4b,e*). When the concentration of FeII was increased, the HPNE completely disappeared and increased concentrations of EDE, ONE, and HNE were observed. However, the ratio of ONE to HNE remained at 2:1. The increased formation of ONE and HNE at high concentrations of FeII suggested that this was arising from FeII-mediated decomposition of HPNE. The possible formation of ONE and HNE from HPNE was confirmed by treating HPNE with increasing concentrations of FeII[105]. The addition of vitamin C at low FeII incubations resulted in an additive effect. This implied that vitamin C might be able to induce homolytic decomposition of 13(S)-HPODE rather than simply causing a 1-electron reduction to the corresponding 13(S)-HODE. In order to test this possibility, 13(S)-HPODE was treated with transition metal ion-free solutions containing vitamin C[106]. At low vitamin C concentrations, the major products were trans-EDE, HPNE and ONE. As the vitamin C concentration increased, HNE levels decreased with a concomitant increase in trans- and cis-EDE, ONE, and HNE. Maximal yields of ONE, 4,5-EDE, and HNE were obtained with an excess of vitamin C. It was found to more than twice as efficient at initiating the decomposition of 13-HPODE to bifunctional electrophiles than transition metal ions.

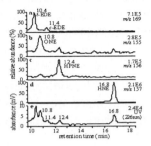

***Figure 4*: LC/MS/UV analysis of reaction between 13-HPODE (400 mM) and FeII (50 mM) in transition metal ion-free Mops buffer (100 mM) containing NaCl (150 mM) at pH 7.0 and 37 oC for 2-h.** Legends as in Figure 3.

The initial formation of HNE from 13-HPODE at low vitamin C concentrations and its subsequent decline at higher concentrations suggested that it was a precursor to ONE and HNE. To test this possibility, authentic HPNE was treated with increasing concentrations of vitamin C[106]. As the concentration of vitamin C increased, there was a decline in HNE with a concomitant increase in ONE and HNE. When the vitamin C was in excess, no residual HNE was observed. Stoichiometric amounts of ONE and HNE were formed in a ratio that was identical with that from the reaction of 13-HPODE with vitamin C. This confirmed that HPNE was indeed a major precursor to ONE and HNE as was found with transition metal ions.

The LC/APCI/MS methodology was also used to determine whether vitamin C-mediated decomposition of 15(S)-HPETE resulted in formation of the same bifunctional electrophiles that were detected from the decomposition of 13-(S)-HPODE. HPNE, trans-EDE, and ONE were the major products of the reaction as evidenced by the APCI/MS response and the LC/UV response[107]. Minor amounts of HNE and cis-EDE were produced. When the concentration of vitamin C was increased to 2 mM, the amount of HPNE was decreased markedly. There was a concomitant increase in the amount of trans-EDE and ONE. In contrast to what was observed with 13-HPODE[104,105], the concentration of trans-EDE was always greater than the ONE. At concentrations > 250 µM vitamin C, there was a decline in HPNE with a concomitant increase in the amounts of ONE and HNE[107]. This is directly analogous to what was observed with 13-HPODE and is due to the conversion of HPNE to ONE and HNE[105,106].

Lipid hydroperoxide-mediated DNA damage

DNA-adducts are formed from the well-known lipid hydroperoxide-derived bifunctional electrophiles MDA[89,92,108,109], HNE[110-113], and trans,trans-2,4-decadienal (DDE)[114,115]. DNA-adducts have also been found to arise from the more recently discovered lipid hydroperoxide-derived bifunctional electrophiles, HPNE, ONE, EDE, and 9,12- dioxo-10(E)-dodecenoic acid (DODE). The reaction between 13-HPODE and 2'-deoxyguanosine (dGuo) was shown by LC/MS to result in the formation of three products that contained 9-carbon units of the starting fatty acid[116]. The initially formed etheno adducts (A) all dehydrated to give a single DNA-adduct (B). Collision induced dissociation (CID) and tandem mass spectrometry (MS/MS) suggested that the dehydrated DNA-adduct was derived from the novel bifunctional electrophile, ONE. 2D-NMR data provided a heptanone-etheno-dGuo structure for the adduct. Subsequently, it was unequivocally demonstrated that ONE was indeed a major product of homolytic 13-HPODE decomposition (*Figure 5*)[104]. Three DNA-adducts were detected in the reaction between 2'-deoxyadenosine (dAdo) and 13-HPODE[117]. The rate of formation of these adducts was increased in the presence of Fe^{II}, indicating that they were formed through a homolytic process. The two initially formed etheno adducts subsequently dehydrated to give a single heptanone etheno-dAdo adduct (*Figure 5*). Heptanone-etheno-dGuo and dAdo adducts were formed in high yield when calf thymus DNA was treated with ONE[118].

Analysis of the reaction between ONE and 2'-deoxycytidine (dCyd) revealed the presence of three major products[119]. The initially formed unstable adducts were shown by LC/MS to be a mixture of substituted etheno-dCyd adduct diastereomers (*Figures 5 and 6*). They subsequently dehydrated to a heptanone-etheno-dCyd adduct, which was identified by a combination of LC/MS (*Figures 5 and 7*) and NMR spectroscopy. In acidic conditions, the etheno adducts were transformed primarily the stable heptanone-etheno-dCyd adduct. Under basic conditions, however, the etheno adducts were hydrolyzed primarily to dCyd most likely by a retro-aldol reaction.

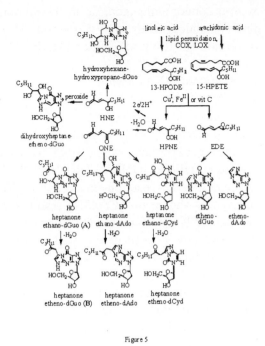

Figure 5

Figure 5: Formation of lipid hydroperoxide-derived bifunctional electrophiles and subsequent formation of DNA-adducts.

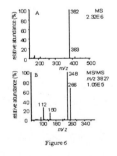

Figure 6

Figure 6: LC/MS/MS analysis of the heptanone- ethano-dCyd adducts using the ESI mode. The spectrum for (A) Full scan mass spectrum; (B) MS/MS spectrum.

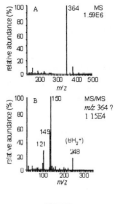

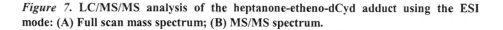

Figure 7

Figure 7. LC/MS/MS analysis of the heptanone-etheno-dCyd adduct using the ESI mode: (A) Full scan mass spectrum; (B) MS/MS spectrum.

Unsubstituted etheno adducts are highly mutagenic in mammalian cells due to error prone translesion DNA synthesis by the atypical polymerases pol eta and pol kappa[120,121]. Sodum and Chung suggested that unsubstituted etheno adducts can arise from intracellular epoxidation of HNE by lipid hydroperoxides[111-113]. Subsequently, it was suggested that this reaction was unlikely to occur in cells due to the relatively high pKa of the lipid hydroperoxides[121]. Unsubstituted etheno adducts are also formed from the reaction lipid hydroperoxide-derived DDE with dAdo or dGuo in the presence of peroxides[114,115]. This pathway would require the unlikely possibility that intracellular epoxidation of DDE could occur more rapidly than its detoxification by glutathione transferases and aldo-keto reductases.

Unsubstituted etheno adducts were formed when DNA bases were treated with EDE (*Figure 5*)[123]. As the epoxide is formed directly by homolytic decomposition of lipid hydroperoxides (*Figure 5*), no additional intracellular activation is required and this seemed to be a more likely candidate as the precursor to unsubstituted etheno adduct formation. In separate studies, it was shown that lipid hydroperoxide-derived HPNE is the precursor to the formation of HNE and the DNA-reactive bifunctional electrophile, ONE[105-107]. A recent study has now demonstrated that HPNE can also react with DNA-bases to form etheno-dGuo and heptanone-etheno-dGuo adducts (*Figure 5*)[124]. Furthermore, HPNE was much more reactive to dGuo than EDE. Based on this increased reactivity, it appears that HPNE is the major lipid hydroperoxide-derived bifunctional electrophile responsible for the formation of unsubstituted etheno-adducts[124]. The action of DNA repair enzymes in vivo results in the presence of unsubstituted etheno-DNA-adducts in biological fluids such as urine. Therefore, the analysis of these DNA-adducts in tissue DNA and in urine will provide dosimeters of exposure to lipid hydroperoxide-derived genotoxins. It is anticipated that modern methods of LC/MS in combination with immmunoaffinity purification or immunoprecipitation will play a vital role in conducting such studies.

It has been proposed that 13-HPODE-mediated formation of HNE requires a Hock rearrangement through the intermediate formation of 9-HPODE (*Figure 8*)[125,126]. However, a direct Hock rearrangement of 13-HPODE would lead to the intermediate formation of 12-oxo-9(Z)-dodecenoic acid, a carboxylate analog of 3(Z)-nonenal[127]. 3(Z)-nonenal is known to rapidly form HPNE[127], which in turn is converted to ONE and HNE[105-107]. Therefore, the ONE-related molecule, DODE could also be formed from 13-HPODE through the intermediate formation of 12-oxo-9(Z)-dodecenoic acid and 9-hydroperoxy-12-oxo-10(E)-dodecenoic acid (HPODD) (*Figure 8*). This raised the possibility that a novel bifunctional electrophile could result from linoleic acid peroxidation, which could modify DNA and proteins in a similar manner to ONE. DODE as its 10(Z)-isomer was detected as a linoleic acid peroxidation product from lentil seeds[128]. It was presumed to arise through intermediate formation of 9-HPODE. Reactions of 13(S)-HPODE with enzyme preparations of both soybean and alfalfa seedlings resulted in the formation of 9-hydroxy-12-oxo-10(E)-dodecenoic acid (HODD) (*Figure 8*). The formation of HODD implies that there was an intermediate formation of HPODD. Reduction of HPODD in a similar manner to HPNE[105-107] would lead to the formation of HODD; whereas, dehydration would lead to DODE. Further evidence for the intermediate formation of HPODD comes from the detection of HODD in trace amounts during the autoxidation of linoleic acid[129,130]. A recent report has described the formation of DODE-derived-etheno adducts when 13-HPODE was allowed to decompose in the presence of 2'-deoxynucleosides or DNA[131].

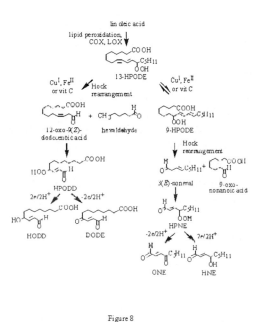

Figure 8

***Figure 8*: Proposed mechanism for formation of DODE.**

DODE was synthesized in order to determine whether it was the lipid hydroperoxide-derived bifunctional electrophile responsible for the formation of carboxylate containing DNA-adducts[132]. Extensive LC/MS and nuclear magnetic resonance (NMR) studies showed that a single carboxynonanone-etheno-dGuo regioisomer was formed. Methylation of the carboxynonanone-etheno-dGuo improved its MS ionization characteristics by a factor of approximately when compared with the free carboxylate. This derivatization procedure revealed that approximately equimolar amounts of heptanone-etheno-dGuo and carboxynonanone-etheno-dGuo were formed when 13(S)-HPODE underwent homolytic decomposition in the presence of dGuo[132]. Therefore, DODE is an important product of 13(S)-HPODE decomposition. In contrast, homolytic decomposition of 15(S)-HPETE in the presence of dGuo produced no detectable carboxynonanone-etheno-dGuo. This is consistent with the proposed intermediate formation of HPODD from 13(S)-HPODE and its subsequent oxidation to DODE as is observed in the oxidation of HPNE to ONE (*Figure 5*). This cannot occur with 15(S)-HPETE.

Covalent modifications to DNA in vivo from lipid hydroperoxide-derived genotoxins

Substantial efforts have been made over the last two decade to develop MS methodology for the quantification of DNA lesions formed in vivo through covalent binding of lipid hydroperoxide-derived bifunctional electrophiles[80,84,85,87-89,92,103,108,109,122,133-143]. MDA is one of the most intensively studied lipid-derived endogenous genotoxins (*Figure 5*). The cyclic DNA-adduct it forms with dGuo (M_1G) can also be formed from base propenals by treatment of DNA with calicheamicin or bleomycin[143]. M_1G has been detected in mammalian DNA[108,109] and in circulating human leukocytes[141]. Using sensitive and specific gas chromatography/electron capture negative chemical ionization (GC/ECNCI/)MS, levels in the range of 4.8 $M_1G/10^8$ to 2.0 $M_1G/10^7$ normal bases were observed[108,109,141]. The levels of M_1G in human leukocyte DNA were less than one-tenth the level found in human liver DNA[141]. This was ascribed to the fact that leukocytes are relatively short-lived cells, and may not be expected to accumulate high levels of adduct during their lifetime. On the other hand, leukocytes have active COX- and LOX- enzymes, which could have given rise to significant MDA production. Therefore, it was expected that higher M_1G levels would have been observed. The leukocytes from several smokers were examined and no striking differences were observed with age, or between smokers and non-smokers in the study. A small difference was observed between the M_1G levels of male and female donors, although there were insufficient samples to draw any firm conclusions from this study[141].

Chen et al. employed stable isotope dilution GC/ECNCI/MS methodology to determine the levels of etheno-adenine (Ade) adducts in human placental DNA. They found that the adducts were present at a level of 2-4 adducts/10^6 Ade[140]. This was an order of magnitude higher than M_1G levels in liver and leukocyte DNA. Liquid chromatography (LC)/MS/MS was used to confirm the structural assignment but did not have sufficient sensitivity for quantitative studies. A subsequent study reported the development of an LC/MS/MS technique in which there was a considerable improvement in sensitivity[137]. The use of LC/MS made it possible to analyze the intact DNA-adduct without having to remove the 2'-deoxyribose sugar or having to prepare an electron-capturing derivative. Using this sensitive and specific LC/MS/MS methodology Doerge et al. were able to show that etheno-dAdo adducts were present at levels of 1.1 etheno dAdo/10^8 normal bases in human placental DNA. These levels are much closer to those found for M_1G in human leukocytes[141]. The discrepancy between the GC/ECNCI/MS and LC/MS/MS studies was suggested to result from artifactual formation of etheno dAdo during the isolation and derivatization procedure. This serves to highlight the difficulties associated with high sensitivity determinations of lipid hydroperoxide-derived DNA-adducts in human tissue samples.

Direct ROS-mediated oxidative DNA damage

The direct reaction of ROS with DNA-bases is complex and dependent upon the system used. The most widely accepted index of ROS-mediated DNA damage involves quantitation of 7,8-dihydro-8-oxo-2'-deoxyguanosine (8-oxo-dGuo). This is most likely because of the high sensitivity with which it can be analyzed using electrochemical detection. A comprehensive study of oxidative damage to 2'-deoxyguanosine was conducted using hydrogen peroxide and Fe[III]. In this system, 8-oxo-dGuo was a minor product and at least ten other covalent modifications to dGuo were characterized[80,145]. Mixtures of ascorbic acid, hydrogen peroxide, and Cu[II] have also been used to generate oxidized DNA-bases. Under carefully controlled conditions, yields in excess of 25 % of 8-oxo-dGuo can be obtained. The currently accepted mechanism for the formation of 8-oxo-dGuo from hydroxyl radicals involves initial attack at C-8 with concomitant formation of a nitrogen-centered radical at N-7 and a carbon-centered radical located primarily at C-4[80]. A one-electron reduction gives the formamidopyrimidine (FAPY) derivative; whereas, a one-electron oxidation yields 8-oxo-dGuo. Singlet oxygen generated from N,N'-di(2,3-dihydroxypropyl)-1,4-naphthalenedipropanamide (1,4-endoperoxide of DHPNO$_2$) also results in the formation of 8-oxo-dGuo[146]. ROS-derived modifications to other DNA-bases include: 5,6-dihydroxy-5,6-dihydro-thymidine, 5-hydroxy-2'-deoxyuridine, 5-hydroxymethyl-2'-deoxyuridine, 7,8-dihydro-8-oxo- -2'-deoxyadenosine (8-oxo-dAdo), 4,6-diamino-5-formado-pyrimidine, and 2,6-diamino-4-hydroxy-5-formadopyrimidine[80].

Substantial efforts have been made over the last decade to develop methodology for the quantification of DNA lesions formed in vivo from direct reaction with ROS. The measurement of oxidative damage has relied heavily on the analysis of 8-oxo-dGuo in DNA or urine[80,147]. These measurements have been extremely controversial because of the ease with which adventitious oxidation can occur during DNA-hydrolysis and derivatization of the resulting DNA-bases. It has been demonstrated that biological buffers normally contain at least 500 nM of transition metal ions. Molecular oxygen undergoes a transition metal ion-mediated one-electron reduction to superoxide radical anion, which dismutates into hydrogen peroxide and oxygen. Further transition metal ion-mediated reduction of the hydrogen peroxide to hydroxyl radicals can then occur by Fenton chemistry.

High concentrations of unmodified bases are present in DNA hydrolysates and so a significant amount of hydroxyl radical-mediated oxidation can then occur. This provides artificially increased concentrations of oxidized bases, which has led to erroneous quantitative results in a number of studies[148]. Oxidation of DNA bases during derivatization reactions for GC/MS analyses can be minimized by the use of antioxidants. Unfortunately, there is still no consensus on the analysis of urinary 8-oxo-dGuo. Therefore any reported values should be viewed with extreme caution.

Accurate measurement of low levels of 8-oxod-Guo in DNA is hampered by the ease with which guanine is oxidized during preparation of DNA for analysis. The formamidopyrimidine DNA glycosylase (FPG)-based methods seem to be less prone to the artefact of additional oxidation[148]. Although they can be used quantitatively, they require careful calibration and standardization if they are to be used in human biomonitoring. The background level of DNA oxidation in normal human cells was suggested to be approximately 0.3-4.2 8-oxo-guanine (Gua) per 10^6 Gua bases by the European Standards Committee on Oxidative DNA Damage (ESCODD), a consortium of mainly European laboratories, has attempted to minimize this artefact and to provide standard, reliable protocols for sample preparation and analysis. ESCODD has recently analyzed 8-oxo-dGuo in the DNA of lymphocytes isolated from venous blood from healthy young male volunteers in several European countries[149]. Two approaches were used. Analysis of 8-oxo-dGuo by HPLC with electrochemical detection was performed on lymphocytes from 10 groups of volunteers, in eight countries. The alternative enzymic approach was based on digestion of DNA with FPG to convert 8-oxo-Gua to apurinic sites, subsequently measured as DNA breaks using the comet assay (7 groups of volunteers in six countries). The median concentration of 8-oxo-dGuo in lymphocyte DNA, calculated from the mean values of each group of subjects as determined by HPLC, was 4.24 per 10^6 Gua. The median concentration of FPG-sensitive sites, measured with the comet assay, was 0.34 per 10^6 Gua. Identical samples of HeLa cells were supplied to all participants as a reference standard. The median values for 8-oxo-dGuo in HeLa cells were 2.78 per 10^6 Gua (by HPLC) and 0.50 per 10^6 Gua (by enzymic methods). The discrepancy between chromatographic and FPG-based approaches may reflect overestimation by HPLC (if spurious oxidation is still not completely controlled) or underestimation by the enzymic method Meanwhile, it is clear that the true background level of base oxidation in DNA is orders of magnitude lower than has often been claimed in the past[149].

Careful purification of buffers by Chelex treatment coupled with the use of deferoxamine to chelete transition metal ions, chaotropic sodium iodide DNA extraction methods, and immunoaffinity purification can prevent most of the artifactual oxidation during DNA-adduct. The current state-of-the art involves the isolation of DNA-bases using these methods coupled with stable isotope dilution LC/MS/MS analysis[91]. The level of 8-oxo-dGuo in control calf thymus DNA was determined to be 28.8 ± 1.2 8-oxo-dGuo per 10^6 unmodified nucleotides (n=5) using 5 μg of digested DNA. The limit of detection of the LC/MS/MS was determined to be 25 fmol on-column with a signal-to-noise ratio of 3.5. However, rigorous validation of 8-oxo-dGuo in human urine tissue samples for this method has not yet been reported.

Summary

Considerable progress has been made in developing quantitative approaches to assessing oxidant stress in vivo. Mass spectrometry has afforded a precision and sensitivity in analyte assessment, which has been missing from many of the earlier methodologies. However, the approach is still one that is essentially indirect, based on analysis of chemically stable targets of free radical catalyzed modifications. Furthermore, while studies of lipid peroxidation and protein modification have been reasonably well validated, it is still unusual to find both deployed together in the characterization of syndromes of oxidant stress. There are few data, which characterize dose response relationships of putative antioxidant strategies using either, never mind both approaches. Oddly, large scale clinical trials of antioxidants have yet to incorporate such measures either in patient selection or in determination of drug response. It is hardly surprising that they have failed to yield a clear picture in any disease to date. Finally, approaches to measuring oxidative modification of DNA are at perhaps an even earlier stage of development and acceptance. However, the painstaking approach to anylate selection detailed in this chapter, coupled with the rapid evolution of MS technology suggests that such analyses will shortly complement the more mature technologies already noted.

Acknowledgements

Ian Blair is the A.N. Richards Professor of Pharmacology and Garret A. FitzGerald is the Elmer Bobst Professor of Pharmacology. We acknowledge the support of NIH grants RR0040, HL70128, HL62250, CA91016, CA95586, and HL54926.

References

1. Griendling KK, FitzGerald GA. Oxidative stress and cardiovascular injury. Part I: Basic mechanisms and *in vivo* monitoring of ROS. Circulation 2003;108:1912-6.

2. Griendling KK, FitzGerald GA. Oxidative stress and cardiovascular injury. Part II: Animal and human studies. Circulation 2003;108: 2034-40.

3. Meagher EA, Barry OP, Lawson JA, Rokach J, FitzGerald GA. Effects of vitamin E on lipid peroxidation in healthy persons. JAMA 2001;285:1178-82.

4. Porter NA. Chemistry of lipid peroxidation. Methods Enzymol 1984;105:273-82.

5. Gutteridge JM, Halliwell B, The measurement and mechanism of lipid peroxidation in biological systems. Trends in Biochemical Sciences 1990;15:129-35.

6. Pirisino R, Di Simplicio P, Ignesti G, Bianchi G, Barbera P. Sulfhydryl groups and peroxidase-like activity of albumin as scavenger of organic peroxides. Pharmacol Res Commun 1988;20:545-52.

7. Hurst R, Bao Y, Ridley S, Williamson G. Phospholipid hydroperoxide cysteine peroxidase activity of human serum albumin. Biochem J 1999; 338:723-8.

8. Mihaljevic B, Katusin-Razem B, Razem D. The reevaluation of the ferric thiocyanate assay for lipid hydroperoxides with special considerations of the mechanistic aspects of the response. Free Radic Biol Med 1996;21:53-63.

9. Holley AE, Slater TF. Measurement of lipid hydroperoxides in normal human blood plasma using HPLC-chemiluminescence linked to a diode array detector for measuring conjugated dienes. Free Radic Res Commun 1991;15:51-63.

10. Kadiiska MB, Gladen BC, Baird DD, et al. Biomarkers of oxidative stress study II. Are oxidation products of lipids, proteins, and DNA markers of CCl_4 poisoning? Free Radic Biol Med 2005;38:698–710.

11. Miyazawa T, Suzuki T, Fujimoto K, Yasuda K. Chemiluminescent simultaneous determination of phosphatidylcholine hydroperoxide and phosphatidylethanolamine hydroperoxide in the liver and brain of the rat. J Lipid Res 1992;33:1051-9.

12. Yamamoto Y, Frei B, Ames BN. Assay of lipid hydroperoxides using high-performance liquid chromatography with isoluminal chemiluminescence detection. Methods Enzymol 1990;186:371-80.

13. Spickett CM, Rennie N, Winter H, et al. Detection of phospholipid oxidation in oxidatively stressed cells by reversed-phase HPLC coupled with positive-ionization electrospray [correction of electroscopy] MS.[erratum appears in Biochem J 2001 Aug 1;357 Pt 3:911].Biochem J 2001;355:449-57.

14. Khaselev N, Murphy RC. Structural characterization of oxidized phospholipid products derived from arachidonate-containing plasmenyl glycerophosphocholine. J Biol Chem 1994;269:20437-40.

15. Horvat RJ, Lane WG, Ng H, Shepherd AD. Saturated hydrocarbons from autoxidizing methyl linoleate. Nature 1964;203: 523-4.

16. Riely CA, Cohen G, Lieberman M. Ethane evolution: a new index of lipid peroxidation. Science 1974;183:208-10.

17. Kivits GA, Ganguli-Swarttouw MA, Christ EJ. The composition of alkanes in exhaled air of rats as a result of lipid peroxidation *in vivo*. Effects of dietary fatty acids, vitamin E and selenium. Biochim Biophys Acta 1981;665:559-70.

18. de Zwart LL, Meerman JH, Commandeur JN, Vermeulen NP. Biomarkers of free radical damage applications in experimental animals and in humans. Free Radic Biol Med 1999;26:202-26.

19. Drury JA, Nycyk JA, Cooke RW. Pentane measurement in ventilated infants using a commercially available system. Free Radic Biol Med 1997;22:895-900.

20. Olopade CO, Christon JA, Zakkar M, et al. Exhaled pentane and nitric oxide levels in patients with obstructive sleep apnea. Chest 1997;111:1500-4.

21. Olopade CO, Zakkar M, Swedler WI, Rubinstein I. Exhaled pentane levels in acute asthma. Chest 1997;111:862-5.

22. Mendis S, Sobotka PA, Leja FL, Euler DE. Breath pentane and plasma lipid peroxides in ischemic heart disease. Free Radic Biol Med 1995;19:679-84.

23. Kokoszka J, Nelson RL, Swedler WI, Skosey J, Abcarian H. Determination of inflammatory bowel disease activity by breath pentane analysis. Dis Colon Rectum 1993;36:597-601.

24. Zarling EJ, Mobarhan S, Bowen P, Kamath S. Pulmonary pentane excretion increases with age in healthy subjects. Mech Ageing Dev 1993;67:141-7.

25. Weitz ZW, Birnbaum AJ, Sobotka PA, Zarling EJ, Skosey JL. High breath pentane concentrations during acute myocardial infarction. Lancet 1991;337:933-5.

26. Humad S, Zarling E, Clapper M, Skosey JL. Breath pentane excretion as a marker of disease activity in rheumatoid arthritis. Free Radic Res Commun 1988;5:101-6.

27. Moscarella S, Caramelli L, Mannaioni PF, Gentilini P. Effect of alcoholic cirrhosis on ethane and pentane levels in breath. Boll Soc Ital Biol Sper 1984;60:529-33.

28. Corongiu FP, Milia A. An improved and simple method for determining diene conjugation in autoxidized polyunsaturated fatty acids. Chem Biol Interact 1983;44:289-97.

29. Situnayake RD, Crump BJ, Zezulka AV, Davis M, McConkey B, Thurnham DI. Measurement of conjugated diene lipids by derivative spectroscopy in heptane extracts of plasma. Ann Clin Biochem 1990;27:258-66.

30. Corongiu FP, Milia A. An improved and simple method for determining diene conjugation in autoxidized polyunsaturated fatty acids. Chem Biol Interact 1983;44:289-97.

31. Ahotupa M, Asankari TJ. Baseline diene conjugation in LDL lipids: an indicator of circulating oxidized LDL. Free Radic Biol Med 1999;27:1141-50.

32. Esterbauer H, Schaur RJ, Zollner H. Chemistry and biochemistry of 4-hydroxynonenal, malonaldehyde and related aldehydes. Free Radic Biol Med 1991;11:81-128.

33. de Zwart LL, Hermanns RC, Meerman JH, Commandeur JN. Salemink PJ, Vermeulen NP. Evaluation of urinary biomarkers for radical-induced liver damage in rats treated with carbon tetrachloride. Toxicol Appl Pharmacol 1998;148:71-82.

34. Halliwell B, Grootveld M. The measurement of free radical reactions in humans. Some thoughts for future experimentation. FEBS Lett 1987;213:9-14.

35. Janero DR. Malondialdehyde and thiobarbituric acid-reactivity as diagnostic indices of lipid peroxidation and peroxidative tissue injury. Free Radic Biol Med 1990;9:515-40.

36. Zarkovic N. 4-hydroxynonenal as a bioactive marker of pathophysiological processes. Mol Aspects Med 2003;24:281-91.

37. Carini M, Aldini G, Facino RM. Mass spectrometry for detection of 4-hydroxy-trans-2-nonenal (HNE) adducts with peptides and proteins. Mass Spectrom Rev 2004;23:281-305.

38. Simpson EP, Henry YK, Henkel JS, Smith RG, Appel SH. Increased lipid peroxidation in sera of ALS patients: a potential biomarker of disease burden. Neurology 2004;62:1758-65.

39. Selley ML, Bartlett MR, McGuiness JA, Hapel AJ, Ardlie NG. Determination of the lipid peroxidation product trans-4-hydroxy-2-nonenal in biological samples by high-performance liquid chromatography and combined capillary column gas chromatography-negative-ion chemical ionisation mass spectrometry. J Chromatogr 1989;488:329-40.

40. Luo XP, Yazdanpanah M, Bhooi N, Lehotay DC. Determination of aldehydes and other lipid peroxidation products in biological samples by gas chromatography-mass spectrometry. Anal Biochem 1995;228:294-8.

41. Meagher EA, Barry OP, Burke A, et al. Alcohol-induced generation of lipid peroxidation products in humans. J Clin Invest 1999;104:805-13.

42. Morrow JD, Hill KE, Burk RF, Nammour TM, Badr KF, Roberts LJ 2nd. A series of prostaglandin F2-like compounds are produced in vivo in humans by a non-cyclooxygenase, free radical-catalyzed mechanism. Proc Natl Acad Sci U S A 1990;87:9383-7.

43. Rokach J, Khanapure SP, Hwang SW, Adiyaman M, Lawson JA, FitzGerald GA. The isoprostanes: a perspective. Prostaglandins 1997;54:823-51.

44. Taber DF, Morrow JD, Roberts LJ 2nd. A nomenclature system for the isoprostanes. Prostaglandins 1997;53:63-7.

45. Rokach J, Khanapure SP, Hwang SW, Adiyaman M, Lawson JA, FitzGerald GA. Nomenclature of isoprostanes: a proposal. Prostaglandins 1997;54:853-73.

46. Pratico D, Lawson JA, FitzGerald GA. Cyclooxygenase-dependent formation of the isoprostane, 8-epi prostaglandin $F_{2\alpha}$. J Biol Chem 1995;270:9800-8.

47. Pratico D, FitzGerald GA. Generation of 8-epi prostaglandin $F_{2\alpha}$ by human monocytes. J Biol Chem 1996;271:8919-8924.

48. Reilly M, Delanty N, Lawson JA, FitzGerald GA. Modulation of oxidant stress in vivo in chronic cigarette smokers. Circulation 1996;94:19-25.

49. Blair IA, Barrow SE, Waddell KA, Lewis PJ, Dollery CT. Prostacyclin is not a circulating hormone in man. Prostaglandins 1982;23:579-89.

50. Roberts LJ 2nd, Morrow JD. The generation and actions of isoprostanes. Biochim Biophys Acta 1997;1345:121-35.

51. Wang Z, Ciabattoni G, Creminon C, et al. Immunological characterization of urinary 8-epi-prostaglandin $F_{2\alpha}$ excretion in man. J Pharmacol Exp Ther 1995;275:94-100.

52. Morrow JD. Quantification of isoprostanes as indices of oxidant stress and the risk of atherosclerosis in humans. Arterioscler Thromb Vasc Biol 2005;25:279-86.

53. Waugh RJ, Morrow JD, Roberts LJ 2nd, Murphy RC. Identification and relative quantitation of F2-isoprostane regioisomers formed *in vivo* in the rat. Free Radic Biol Med 1997;23:943-54.

54. Li H, Lawson JA, Reilly M, et al. Quantitative high performance liquid chromatography/tandem mass spectrometric analysis of the four classes of F_2-isoprostanes in human urine. Proc Natl Acad Sci U S A 1999;96:13381-6.

55. Lawson JA, Li H, Rokach J, et al. Identification of two major F2 isoprostanes, 8,12-*iso*-and 5-epi-8, 12-*iso*-isoprostane $F_{2\alpha}$-VI, in human urine. J Biol Chem 1998;273:29295-301.

56. Singh G, Gutierrez A, Xu K, Blair IA. Liquid chromatography/electron capture atmospheric pressure chemical ionization/mass spectrometry: analysis of pentafluorobenzyl derivatives of biomolecules and drugs in the attomole range. Anal Chem 2000;72:3007-13.

57. Chiabrando C, Rivalta C, Bagnati R, et al. Identification of metabolites from type III F2-isoprostane diastereoisomers by mass spectrometry. J Lipid Res 2992;43:495-509.

58. Roberts LJ 2nd, Moore KP, Zackert WE, Oates JA, Morrow JD. Identification of the major urinary metabolite of the F2-isoprostane 8-iso-prostaglandin F2alpha in humans. J Biol Chem 1996;271:20617-20.

59. Burke A, Lawson JA, Meagher, EA, Rokach J, FitzGerald GA. Specific analysis in plasma and urine of 2,3-dinor-5, 6-dihydro-isoprostane $F_{2\alpha}$-III, a metabolite of isoprostane $F_{2\alpha}$-III and an oxidation product of γ-linolenic acid. J Biol Chem 2000;275:2499-504.

60. Stadtman ER. Protein oxidation and aging. Science 1992;257:1220-4.

61. Marnett LJ, Riggins JN, West JD. Endogenous generation of reactive oxidants and electrophiles and their reactions with DNA and protein. J Clin Invest 2003;111:583-93.

62. Heinecke JW. Oxidized amino acids: Culprits in human atherosclerosis and indicators of oxidative stress. Free Radic Biol Med 2002;32:1090-101.

63. Brennan ML, Hazen SL. Amino acid and protein oxidation in cardiovascular disease. Amino Acids 2003;25:365-74.

64. Heinecke JW. Oxidative stress: new approaches to diagnosis and prognosis in atherosclerosis. Am J Cardiol 2003;91:12A-16A.

65. Shishehbor MH, Hazen SL. Inflammatory and oxidative markers in atherosclerosis: relationship to outcome. Curr Atheroscler Rep 2004;6:243-50.

66. Ischiropoulos H. Biological tyrosine nitration: a pathophysiological function of nitric oxide and reactive oxygen species. Arch Biochem Biophys 1998;356:1-11.

67. Turko IV. Murad F. Protein nitration in cardiovascular diseases. Pharmacol Rev 2002;54:619-34.

68. Shacter E, Williams JA, Lim M, Levine RL. Differential susceptibility of plasma proteins to oxidative modification: Examination by western blot immunoassay. Free Radic Biol Med 1994;17: 429-37.

69. Headlam HA, Davies MJ. Markers of protein oxidation: different oxidants give rise to variable yields of bound and released carbonyl products. Free Radic Biol Med 2004;36:1175-84.

70. Gladstone IM Jr, Levine RL. Oxidation of proteins in neonatal lungs. Pediatrics 1994;93:764-8.

71. Winterbourn CC, Chan T, Buss IH, Inder TE, Mogridge N, Darlow BA. Protein carbonyls and lipid peroxidation products as oxidation markers in preterm infant plasma: associations with chronic lung disease and retinopathy and effects of selenium supplementation. Pediatr Res 2000;48:84-90.

72. Poon HF, Castegna A, Farr SA, et al. Quantitative proteomics analysis of specific protein expression and oxidative modification in aged senescence-accelerated-prone mice brain. Neuroscience 2004;126:915-26.

73. Hollyfield JG, Salomon RG, Crabb JW. Proteomic approaches to understanding age-related macular degeneration. Adv Exp Med Biol 2003;533:83-9.

74. Ghezzi P, Bonetto V. Redox proteomics: identification of oxidatively modified proteins. Proteomics 2003;3:1145-53.

75. Brennan ML, Wu W, Fu X, et al. A tale of two controversies: i) Defining the role of peroxidases in nitrotyrosine formation in vivo using eosinophil peroxidase and myeloperoxidase deficient mice; and ii) Defining the nature of peroxidase-generated reactive nitrogen species. J Biol Chem 2002;277:17415-27.

76. Shishehbor MH, Aviles RJ, Brennan ML, et al. Association of nitrotyrosine levels with cardiovascular disease and modulation by statin therapy. JAMA 2003;289:1675-80.

77. Souza JM, Daikhin E, Yudkoff M, Raman CS, Ischiropoulos H. Factors determining the selectivity of protein tyrosine nitration. Arch Biochem Biophys 1999;371:169-78.

78. Zheng L, Nukuna B, Brennan ML, et al. Apolipoprotein A-I is a selective target for myeloperoxidase-catalyzed oxidation and functional impairment in subjects with cardiovascular disease. J Clin Invest 2004;114:529-41.

79. Vadseth C, Souza JM, Thomson L, et al. Pro-thrombotic state induced by post translational modification of fibrinogen by reactive nitrogen species. J Biol Chem 2004;279:8820-6.

80. Lee SH, Blair IA. Oxidative DNA damage and cardiovascular disease. Trends Cardiovasc Med 2001;11:148-55.

81. Evans MD, Dizdaroglu M, Cooke MS. Oxidative DNA damage and disease: induction, repair and significance. Mutat Res 2004;567:1-61.

82. Dedon PC, Tannenbaum SR. Reactive nitrogen species in the chemical biology of inflammation. Arch Biochem Biophys 2004;423:12-22.

83. Singer II, Kawka DW, Scott S, et al. Expression of inducible nitric oxide synthase and nitrotyrosine in colonic epithelium in inflammatory bowel disease. Gastroenterology 1996;111:871-85.

84. Blair IA. Lipid hydroperoxide-mediated DNA damage. Exp Geronto. 2001;36:1473-81.

85. Marnett LJ. Oxy radicals, lipid peroxidation and DNA damage. Toxicology 2002;181-182:219-22.

86. Kensler TW, Qian GS, Chen JG, Groopman JD. Translational strategies for cancer prevention in liver. Nat Rev Cancer 2003;3:321-9.

87. Farmer PB, Singh R, Kaur B, et al. Molecular epidemiology studies of carcinogenic environmental pollutants. Effects of polycyclic aromatic hydrocarbons (PAHs) in environmental pollution on exogenous and oxidative DNA damage. Mutat Res 2003;544:397-402.

88. Yen TY, Holt S, Sangaiah R, Gold A, Swenberg JA. Quantitation of 1,N[6]-ethenoadenine in rat urine by immunoaffinity extraction combined with liquid chromatography/electrospray ionization mass spectrometry. Chem Res Toxicol 1998;11.810-5.

89. Otteneder M, Scott Daniels J, Voehler M, Marnett LJ. Development of a method for determination of the malondialdehyde-deoxyguanosine adduct in urine using liquid chromatography-tandem mass spectrometry. Anal Biochem 2003;315:147-51.

90. Roberts DW, Churchwell MI, Beland FA, Fang JL, Doerge DR. Quantitative analysis of etheno-2'-deoxycytidine DNA adducts using on-line immunoaffinity chromatography coupled with LC/ES-MS/MS detection. Anal Chem 2001;73:303-9.

91. Singh R, McEwan M, Lamb JH, Santella RM, Farmer PB. An improved liquid chromatography/tandem mass spectrometry method for the determination of 8-oxo-7,8-dihydro-2'-deoxyguanosine in DNA samples using immunoaffinity column purification. Rapid Commun Mass Spectrom 2003;17:126-34.

92. Hoberg AM, Otteneder M, Marnett LJ, Poulsen HE. Measurement of the malondialdehyde-2'-deoxyguanosine adduct in human urine by immuno-extraction and liquid chromatography/atmospheric pressure chemical ionization tandem mass spectrometry. J Mass Spectrom 2004;39:38-42.

93. Porter NA, Caldwell SE, Mills KA. Mechanisms of free radical oxidation of unsaturated lipids. Lipids 1995;30:277-90.

94. Brash AR. Lipoxygenases: occurrence, functions, catalysis, and acquisition of substrate. J Biol Chem 1999;274:23679-82.

95. Laneuville O, Breuer D, K, Xu N, et al. Fatty acid substrate specificities of human prostaglandin-endoperoxide H synthase-1 and -2. Formation of 12-hydroxy-(9Z, 13E/Z, 15Z)- octadecatrienoic acids from alpha-linolenic acid. J Biol Chem 1995;270:19330-6.

96. Ikawa H, Kamitani H, Calvo BF, Foley JF, Eling TE. Expression of 15-lipoxygenase-1 in human colorectal cancer. Cancer Res 1999;59:360-366.

97. Brash AR, Boeglin WE, Chang MS. Discovery of a second 15S-lipoxygenase in humans. Proc Natl Acad Sc U S A 1997;94:6148-52.

98. Hamberg M. Stereochemistry of oxygenation of linoleic acid catalyzed by prostaglandin endoperoxide H synthase-2. Arch Biochem Biophys 1998;349:376-80.

99. Kuhn H, Borchert A. Regulation of enzymatic lipid peroxidation: the interplay of peroxidizing and peroxide reducing enzymes. Free Radic Biol Med 2002;33:154-72.

100. Thuresson ED, Lakkides KM, Smith WL. Different catalytically competent arrangements of arachidonic acid within the cyclooxygenase active site of prostaglandin endoperoxide H synthase-1 lead to the formation of different oxygenated products. J Biol Chem 2000;275:8501-7.

101. Schneider C, Boeglin WE, Prusakiewicz JJ, et al. Control of prostaglandin stereochemistry at the 15-carbon by cyclooxygenases-1 and -2. A critical role for serine 530 and valine 349. J Biol Chem 2002;277:478-85.

102. Burcham PC. Internal hazards: baseline DNA damage by endogenous products of normal metabolism. Mutat Res 1999;443:11-36.

103. Marnett LJ. Oxyradicals and DNA damage. Carcinogenesis 2000;21:361-70.

104. Lee SH, Blair IA. Characterization of 4-oxo-2-nonenal as a novel product of lipid peroxidation. Chem Res Toxicol 2000;13:698-702.

105. Lee SH, Oe T, Arora JS, Blair IA. Analysis of FeII-mediated decomposition of linoleic acid-derived lipid hydroperoxide by lipid chromatography/mass spectrometry. J Mass Spectrom 2005, Web Release Date:28-Oct-2004; DOI: 10.1002/jms.838.

106. Lee SH, Oe T, Blair IA. Vitamin C-induced decomposition of lipid hydroperoxides to endogenous genotoxins. Science 2001;292:2083-6.

107. Williams MV, Lee SH, Blair IA. Liquid chromatography/mass spectrometry analysis of bifunctional electrophiles and DNA adducts from vitamin C mediated decomposition of 15-hydroperoxyeicosatetraenoic acid. Rapid Commun Mass Spectrom 2005;19:849-58.

108. Chaudhary AK, Nokubo M, Marnett LJ, Blair IA. Analysis of the malondialdehyde-2'-deoxyguanosine adduct in rat liver DNA by gas chromatography/electron capture negative chemical ionization mass spectrometry. Biol Mass Spectrom 1994;23:457-64.

109. Chaudhary AK, Nokubo M, Reddy GR, et al. Detection of endogenous malondialdehyde-deoxyguanosine adducts in human liver. Science 1994;265:1580-2.

110. Winter CK, Segall HJ, Haddon WF. Formation of cyclic adducts of deoxyguanosine with the aldehydes trans-4-hydroxy-2-hexenal and trans-4-hydroxy-2-nonenal *in vitro*. Cancer Res 1986;46:5682-6.

111. Sodum RS, Chung FL. Structural characterization of adducts formed in the reaction of 2,3-epoxy-4-hydroxynonanal with deoxyguanosine. Chem Res Toxicol 1989;2:23-8.

112. Sodum RS, Chung FL. Stereoselective formation of in vitro nucleic acid adducts by 2,3-epoxy-4-hydroxynonanal. Cancer Res 1991;51:137-43.

113. Chen HJC, Chung FL. Epoxidation of trans-4-hydroxy-2-nonenal by fatty acid hydroperoxides and hydrogen peroxide. Chem Res Toxicol 1996;9:306-12.

114. Carvalho VM, Asahara F, Di Mascio P, de Arruda Campos IP, Cadet J, Medeiros MHG. Novel 1,N[6]-etheno-2'-deoxyadenosine adducts from lipid peroxidation products. Chem Res Toxicol 2000;13:397-405.

115. Loureiro AP, Di Mascio P, Gomes OF, Medeiros MH. trans,trans-2,4-Decadienal-induced 1,N[2]-etheno-2'-deoxyguanosine adduct formation. Chem Res Toxicol 2000;13:601-9.

116. Rindgen D, Nakajima M, Wehrli S, Blair IA. Covalent modification of 2'-deoxyguanosine by products of lipid peroxidation. Chem Res Toxicol 1999;12:1195-204.

117. Rindgen D, Lee SH, Nakajima M, Blair IA. Formation of a substituted $1,N^6$-etheno-2'-deoxyadenosine adduct by lipid hydroperoxide-mediated generation of 4-oxo-2-nonenal. Chem Res Toxicol 2000;13:846-52.

118. Lee SH, Rindgen D, Bible RH Jr, Hajdu E, Blair IA. Characterization of 2'-deoxyadenosine adducts derived from 4-oxo-2-nonenal, a novel product of lipid peroxidation. Chem Res Toxicol 2000;13:565-74.

119. Pollack M, Oe T, Lee SH, Elipe MV, Arison BH, Blair IA. Characterization of 2'-deoxycytidine adducts derived from 4-oxo-2-nonenal, a novel lipid peroxidation product. Chem Res Toxicol 2003;16:893-900.

120. Levine RL, Yang IY, Hossain M, Pandya G, Grollman AP, Moriya M. Mutagenesis induced by a single $1,N^6$-ethenodeoxyadenosine adduct in human cells. Cancer Res 2000;60:4098-104.

121. Levine RL, Miller H, Grollman A, et al. Translesion DNA synthesis catalyzed by human pol eta and pol kappa across 1,N6-ethenodeoxyadenosine. J Biol Chem 2001;276:18717-21.

122. Douki T, Odin F, Caillat S, Favier A, Cadet J. Predominance of the 1,N2-propano 2'-deoxyguanosine adduct among 4-hydroxy-2-nonenal-induced DNA lesions. Free Rad Biol Med 2004;37:62-70.

123. Lee SH, Oe T, Blair IA. 4,5-Epoxy-2(E)-decenal-induced formation of $1,N^6$-etheno-2'-deoxyadenosine and $1,N^2$-etheno-2'-deoxyguanosine adducts. Chem Res Toxicol 2002;15:300-4.

124. Lee SH, Arora JS, Oe T, Blair IA. 4-Hydroperoxy-2-nonenal-induced formation of $1,N^2$-etheno-2'-deoxyguanosine adducts. Chem Res Toxicol 2005;In press.

125. Schneider C, Tallman KA, Porter NA, Brash AR. Two distinct pathways of formation of 4-hydroxynonenal. Mechanisms of nonenzymatic transformation of the 9- and 13-hydroperoxides of linoleic acid to 4-hydroxyalkenals. J Biol Chem 2001;276:20831-8.

126. Uchida K. 4-Hydroxy-2-nonenal: a product and mediator of oxidative stress. Prog Lipid Res 2003;42:318-43.

127. Gardner HW, Hamberg M. Oxygenation of 3(Z)-nonenal to 2(E)-4-hydroxy-2-nonenal in the broad bean (Vicia faba L). J Biol Chem 1993;268:6971-7.

128. Gallasch BAW, Spiteller G. Synthesis of 9,12-di-oxo-10(Z)-dodecanoic acid, a new fatty acid metabolite derived from 9-hydroperoxy-10,12-octadecadienoic acid in lentil seed (Lens culinaris Medik). Lipids 2000;35:953-60.

129. Loidl-Stahlhofen A, Hannemann K, Spiteller G. Generation of □-hydroxyaldehydic compounds in the course of lipid peroxidation. Biochim Biophys Acta 1994;1213:140-8.

130. Mlakar A, Spiteller G. Reinvestigation of lipid peroxidation of linolenic acid. Biochim Biophys Acta 1994;1214:209-20.

131. Kawai Y, Uchida K, Osawa T. 2'-deoxycytidine in free nucleosides and double-stranded DNA as the major target of lipid peroxidation products. Free Radic Biol Med 2004;36:529-41.

132. Lee SH, Silva Elipe MV, Arora JS. Blair IA. Dioxododecenoic acid: a lipid hydroperoxide-derived bifunctional electrophile responsible for etheno DNA-adduct formation. Chem. Res. Toxicol. Web Release Date: 22-Feb-2005; DOI: 10.1021/tx049693d.

133. Farmer PB. Exposure biomarkers for the study of toxicological impact on carcinogenic processes. IARC Sci Publ 2004;157:71-90.

134. Sharma RA, Farmer PB. Biological relevance of adduct detection to the chemoprevention of cancer. Clin Cancer Res 2004;10:4901-12.

135. Chaudhary AK, Nokubo M, Oglesby TD, Marnett LJ, Blair IA. Characterization of endogenous DNA adducts by liquid chromatography/electrospray ionization tandem mass spectrometry. J Mass Spectrom 1995;30:1157-66.

136. Chaudhary AK, Reddy GR, Blair IA, Marnett LJ. Characterization of an N^6-oxopropenyl-2'-deoxyadenosine adduct in malondialdehyde-modified DNA using liquid chromatography/electrospray ionization tandem mass spectrometry. Carcinogenesis 1996;17:1167-70.

137. Doerge DR, Churchwell MI, Fang JL, Beland FA. Quantification of etheno DNA adducts using liquid chromatography, on-line sample processing, and electrospray tandem mass spectrometry. Chem Res Toxicol 2000;13:1259-64.

138. Nath RG, Chung FL. Detection of exocyclic 1,N2-propanodeoxyguanosine adducts as common DNA lesions in rodents and humans. Proc Natl Acad Sci U S A 1994;91:7491-5.

139. Nath RG, Ocando JE, Guttenplan JB, Chung FL. 1,N2-propanodeoxyguanosine adducts: potential new biomarkers of smoking-induced DNA damage in human oral tissue. Cancer Res 1998;581:581-4.

140. Chen HJC, Chiang LC, Tseng MC, Zhang LL, Ni J, Chung FL. Detection and quantification of 1,N^6-ethenoadenine in human placental DNA by mass spectrometry. Chem Res Toxicol 1999;12:1119-26.

141. Rouzer CA, Chaudhary AK, Nokubo M, Ferguson DM, Blair IA, Marnett LJ. Analysis of the malondialdehyde-2'-deoxyguanosine adduct pyrimidopurinone in human leukocyte DNA by gas chromatography/electron capture/negative chemical ionization/mass spectrometry. Chem Res Toxicol 1997;10:181-8.

142. Chen HJ, Chang CM. Quantification of urinary excretion of 1,N6-ethenoadenine, a potential biomarker of lipid peroxidation, in humans by stable isotope dilution liquid chromatography-electrospray ionization-tandem mass spectrometry: comparison with gas chromatography-mass spectrometry. Chem Res Toxicol 2004;17:963-71.

143. Chen HJ, Wu CF, Hong CL, Chang CM. Urinary excretion of 3,N4-etheno-2'-deoxycytidine in humans as a biomarker of oxidative stress: association with cigarette smoking. Chem Res Toxicol 2004;17:896-903.

144. Dedon PC, Plastaras JP, Rouzer CA, Marnett LJ. Indirect mutagenesis by oxidative DNA damage: formation of the pyrimidopurinone adduct of deoxyguanosine by base propenal. Proc Natl Acad Sci U S A 1998;95:11113-6.

145. Churchwell MI Beland FA Doerge DR. Quantification of multiple DNA adducts formed through oxidative stress using liquid chromatography and electrospray tandem mass spectrometry. Chem Res Toxicol 2002;15:1295-301.

146. Ravanat JL, Di Mascio P, Medeiros MHG, et al. Singlet oxygen induces oxidation of cellular DNA. J Biol Chem 2000;275:40601-4.

147. Guetens G, De Boeck G, Highley M, van Oosterom AT, de Bruijn EA. Oxidative DNA damage: biological significance and methods of analysis. Crit Rev Clin Lab Sci 2002;39:331-457.

148. Collins A., Cadet J, Moller L, Poulsen HE, Vina J. Are we sure we know how to measure 8-oxo-7,8-dihydroguanine in DNA from human cells? Arch Biochem Biophys 2004;423:57-65.

149. Gedik CM, Collins A. ESCODD (European Standards Committee on Oxidative DNA Damage). Establishing the background level of base oxidation in human lymphocyte DNA: results of an interlaboratory validation study. FASEB J 2005;19:82-4.

Chapter 7

PHARMACOLOGICAL COMPOUNDS WITH ANTIOXIDANT ACTIVITY

Sergey Dikalov and David G. Harrison
Division of Cardiology, Department of Medicine, Emory University School of Medicine, Atlanta, GA

Introduction

Before entering into a discussion about various potential antioxidants, their pharmacological actions and their reactivity, there are several caveats that should be considered about this general field. The major caveat is that most prospective large clinical trials have shown that simple administration of what seems to be an antioxidant have failed to show any reduction in hard endpoints. This is particularly true in the area of cardiovascular disease. Despite the fact that retrospective analyses have clearly shown a lower rate of cardiovascular events in humans that consume diets rich in antioxidant vitamins, several large clinical trials have failed to show benefit of traditional antioxidants in patients with established coronary artery disease. As an example, vitamin E was not effective in reducing cardiovascular events in the Heart Outcome Prevention Evaluation (HOPE) trial[1], and a combination of vitamin E, vitamin C, and beta carotene proved no better than placebo in the recently completed Heart Protection Study[2]. Surprisingly, beta carotene actually increased the incidence of lung cancer in a study of smokers[3]. One interpretation of these clinical trials is that oxidant stress plays either no role or a minimal role in the pathogenesis of atherosclerosis and coronary artery disease, however it is possible the antioxidants employed were ineffective, have been used incorrectly, or have been given to the wrong subjects. One problem with these studies is that there have been no measures employed to allow identification of subjects with oxidant stress or to allow monitoring of therapeutic effectiveness. In this regard, the antioxidants vitamin E and N-acetylcysteine have proven effective in reducing cardiovascular events in humans with chronic renal failure, a population particularly predisposed to oxidant stress[4,5]. A second problem is that most studies have been performed in subjects with advanced atherosclerosis, and it is conceivable that antioxidant therapy would be more effective when used earlier in the disease. This might explain the retrospective observations demonstrating that a long-term diet rich in antioxidant vitamins is associated with reductions in cardiovascular events. Subjects that consume such diets likely do so throughout their lives, allowing the antioxidant agents to have an impact at the very earliest stages of disease. Finally, the agents employed need to be targeted to the proper component of the cell and must be efficacious in scavenging or reducing the offending reactive oxygen species (ROS). For instance, vitamin E, commonly used in many studies, is highly lipophilic and unlikely to have effects on oxidative events that occur in the cytoplasm or interstitial spaces. In this regard, agents that specifically scavenge radicals or prevent their formation in hydro- and lipophilic compartments of the cell could prove useful in specific diseases, and their use could be guided by markers of oxidative stress specific to these compartments. As an example, iso-s have proven to be useful markers of lipid oxidation, while the ratio of oxidized to reduced glutathione might reflect oxidation within non-lipid compartments[6,7]. Subjects with evidence of lipid oxidation might respond to vitamin E, while subjects with evidence of cytoplasmic oxidation might require a water-soluble antioxidant.

Another issue related to the subject of antioxidant therapy is that one should not lump all ROS together when considering how they cause disease. While this seems obvious, this fact seems to have escaped many who plan clinical trials. As shown in *figure 1*, superoxide in many respects is a "progenitor radical", which can serve as the source for formation of other reactive oxygen species. For example, reactions of superoxide with NO lead to formation of peroxynitrite, and superoxide can either spontaneously dismutate or be dismutated to hydrogen peroxide by one of the superoxide dismutases. There is accumulating evidence that hydrogen peroxide (H_2O_2) plays a major role in the genesis of atherosclerosis and hypertension. There is no reaction between vitamin E or vitamin C and hydrogen peroxide, and in fact, when these agents react with superoxide, hydrogen peroxide is formed. Thus, the administration of such antioxidants can in fact worsen matters rather than prove helpful.

Finally, and related to the above considerations, it will likely prove to be more effective to prevent the formation of ROS rather than to try to scavenge them after they are formed. Efforts should be made to understand the enzymatic source of radicals, to gain insight into how these sources are activated, and to find agents that reduce their activity. In this regard, the HMG CoA reductase inhibitors have been reported to reduce activity of the

NADPH oxidases, and this property could contribute to some of their therapeutic benefits. In this chapter, we will consider current knowledge regarding pharmacological agents with antioxidant properties, particularly in context of the above considerations.

Membrane targeted and PEG-modified SOD and catalase

Superoxide and hydrogen peroxide (H_2O_2) are primary ROS (*Figure 1*), which participate in cellular redox signaling and initiate cascades of oxidative damage leading to a myriad of pathophysiological conditions. The superoxide dismutases (SODs) are the first line of defense against superoxide. SODs have a transition metal at their active center (Cu^{2+}, Fe^{3+} or Mn^{3+}), which undergoes cycles of reduction and reoxidation by superoxide[8]. This leads to the catalytic scavenging of superoxide and ultimate formation of H_2O_2, which is subsequently decomposed by catalase and glutathione peroxidases to water and oxygen[9]. Glutathione peroxidase is more efficient than catalase in this latter step, but its enzymatic function is coupled with oxidation of glutathione. Because catalase directly decomposes H_2O_2 and preserves reduced glutathione, SOD and catalase provide a near ideal antioxidant combination. The problem, however, is that both SOD and catalase are large proteins that do not enter cells and are rapidly cleared from the blood if injected intravenously. For this reason, efforts have been made to increase tissue uptake of SOD and catalase. A particularly useful modification has been the conjugation to polyethylene glycol (PEG) via a reaction in which the hydroxyl group of PEG is linked to the ε-amino groups of lysine[10]. Up to 15 or 20 such lysines are modified by PEG, increasing the molecular weight from 32 to approximately 100 kDa. The bulk of this modified molecule reduces its immunogenecity, decreases renal clearance, and more importantly promotes cellular uptake by pinocytotoic-like mechanisms. Because of this several hours of incubation with PEG-SOD or PEG catalase are required to increase tissue levels of SOD or catalase; however several hours of exposure can increase SOD and catalase activities by more than five-fold[10]. PEG-SOD can be administered in vivo, and has been used to reduce ischemic myocardial and renal injury[11,12], improve endothelial function[13], limit lung injury in sepsis and decrease oxidant damage in cerebral ischemia[14,15]. In one rather small human trial of subjects with severe head trauma, bolus injection of PEG-SOD reduced vegetative state and death by half compared to placebo treatment[16]. Despite the fact that PEG-SOD and PEG-catalase have been recognized as useful agents for more than a decade, the development of these agents for human therapy has not progressed[17]. These agents are widely used in experimental studies of cultured cells and animals to probe the role of ROS in various pathophysiological states and signaling pathways.

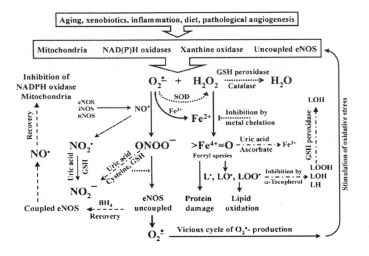

Figure 1: **Antioxidants in action: prevention, defense and repair.**

Other modifications of SOD have been employed with some success. One is incorporation of SOD into liposomes, which promotes membrane uptake[18]. The problem with this approach is that the liposomes need to be prepared shortly after administration, and the liposomes themselves may have non-specific effects. Yet another approach has been to genetically incorporate a heparin-binding domain into SOD, mimicking the extracellular superoxide dismutase[19]. This allows membrane-targeting of SOD, and has proven effective in lowering blood pressure in hypertensive animals[1], improving endothelium-dependent vasodilatation[20], and reducing myocardial ischemic insult[21]. Very recently, Muzykantov and co-workers have conjugated SOD and catalase to anti-PECAM and anti-ICAM antibodies, allowing very specific delivery to the endothelium where they are incorporated by endocytosis[22]. These modifications have not been used in humans.

Metalloporphyrin based compounds

Several small molecules with SOD-like activity have been developed in which a transition metal has been incorporated into a porphyrin ring[23]. The transition metals are thought to react catalytically with superoxide in a fashion similar to the transition metals of the superoxide dismutases. Most commonly manganese has been used as the active metal, resulting in molecules such as Mn(III)tetrakis(1-methyl-4-pyridyl)porphyrin (MnTMPyP) and Mn (III) tetrakis (4-benzoic acid) porphyrin (MnTBAP)[24,25]. Ferrous iron has also been used in production of Fe-porhyrins[26]. While metalloporphyrins were initially proposed to be SOD mimetics, they have been shown to have peroxidase-like activity and to be able to inhibit peroxynitrite mediated damage and peroxynitrite-induced protein oxidation and nitration[27]. These effects are likely due not only to their SOD-like activity but also due to other structural characteristics that allow them to act as electron acceptors from a variety of ROS. Among other uses, metalloporphyrins have proven effective in reducing experimentally-induced inflammatory bowel disease[28], reduction in hypoxic brain injury[29], to prevent lung injury in response to radiation[30] and to improve cardiac function after peroxynitrite mediated injury attending cytokine exposure or chemotherapy[31,32]. Because of their SOD-like activity, one would anticipate that these agents would modulate vasodilatation; however studies with these compounds have yielded conflicting results. In a model of subarachnoid hemorrhage, vasospasm has been improved by MnTBAP[33]. Some have also been shown to lower blood pressure in rats, although this seems related to stimulation of histamine release[34]. In contrast, in studies of isolated vessels, MnTMPyp has proven only partly effective in restoring endothelium-dependent vasodilatation caused by oxidant stress[35]. There is some evidence that these compounds can have pro-oxidant effects under some circumstances[36]. Their reaction with superoxide yields hydrogen peroxide, which in turn can react with their metal center to form the hydroxyl radical. Comparison of water-soluble and lipophilic derivatives suggests that the catalytic properties of these antioxidants may involve auto-oxidation of metals or peroxidase-like properties of metalloporphyrins which may cause pro-oxidant effects[37,38]. To date, these agents have not been employed in human studies.

Vitamin C

Vitamin C (ascorbic acid) (*figure 2*), is a cofactor for proline and lysine hydroxylase and is essential for connective tissue formation. It also has antioxidant properties, which are mediated by hydrogen donation from one of the two enol groups, leading to formation of the ascorbyl radical which in turn disproportionates to dehydroascorbate and ascorbate[39]. Ascorbate is particularly effective in scavenging superoxide, leading to formation of hydrogen peroxide. Ascorbate has been also implicated in protection from peroxynitrite (ONOO⁻)-mediated oxidative damage[40], likely due to its ability to scavenge superoxide, thus preventing peroxynitrite formation[41]. In addition, ascorbate may reduce free radicals formed as a result of oxidation by peroxynitrite. For example, as shown in *figure 3*, peroxynitrite oxidizes tetrahydrobiopterin (BH_4) to the trihydrobiopterin radical ($BH_3^{\bullet}$), which can be reduced back to BH_4 by ascorbate[42]. In this regard, it has recently been shown that ascorbate increases endothelial cell nitric oxide (NO) synthesis and tetrahydrobiopterin levels[43,44], likely via this interaction with the $BH_3^{\bullet}$ radical. The $BH_3^{\bullet}$ radical is formed during formation of NO by the nitric oxide synthases, and the ability of ascorbate to regenerate BH_4 from the $BH_3^{\bullet}$ radical is likely very important in supporting NO production. In addition, ascorbate may act as a "free radical sink" scavenging organic radicals $R^{\bullet}$ and reducing them to RH[45], reactions which are likely important in scavenging of various protein, lipid, and antioxidant radicals. For example, ascorbate is responsible for recycling of one-electron oxidized vitamin E and glutathione by reduction of α-tocopheryl and glutathiyl radicals.

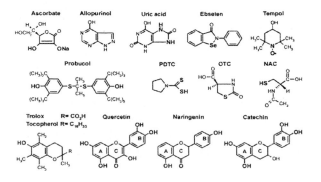

Figure 2: **Chemical structures of antioxidants (active groups marked bold).**

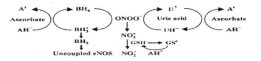

***Figure 3*: Interactions of ONOO⁻, urate, ascorbate and cysteine.**

The antioxidant properties of ascorbate have some important limitations. First, ascorbate is not as effective as superoxide dismutase in scavenging $O_2^{\bullet-}$ as its rate constant for reaction with superoxide is 10^5 M⁻¹c⁻¹ vs. 10^9 M⁻¹c⁻¹ for the superoxide dismutases[46]. Likewise, the rate constant of the reaction of $O_2^{\bullet-}$ with NO is much more rapid than that of ascorbic acid with $O_2^{\bullet-}$ [47]. Because of this, high concentrations of ascorbate (50 μM and higher) are needed to supplement the endogenous superoxide scavenging capacities. This is made difficult in vivo, because excess amounts of vitamin C are eliminated in the urine, so that extremely high levels of ascorbate are not achieved via oral treatment. Second, scavenging of superoxide by ascorbate produces H_2O_2 which in turn affects redox cell signaling, mediates protein and lipid oxidation and serves as a substrate for peroxidase mediated oxidation and nitrosation events. Third, ascorbate's antioxidant action is limited to hydrophilic compartments and it is not effective in lipid membranes. Finally, high concentrations of ascorbate may have pro-oxidant effects. For example, it has been shown that ascorbate can stimulate lipid peroxidation via reduction of redox active ferric and cupric ions[48]. These limitations may explain the failure of vitamin C to reduce cardiovascular events in humans with established coronary artery disease.

Vitamin E and water-soluble analog trolox

Lipid peroxidation, a classical free radical chain reaction, has been implicated in a variety of pathophysiological processes, including atherosclerosis[49], autoimmune disorders[50], alcoholic liver disease[51], neurodegenerative processes[52], osteoarthritis and infectious processes[53,54].

Given this, there is substantial interest in limiting lipid peroxidation via agents that promote decomposition of peroxides, chelation of metals or scavenging of lipid peroxyl radicals (*Figure 1*).

Under normal circumstances, the tocopherols generically referred to as Vitamin E, provide protection against lipid peroxidation by scavenging peroxyl radicals. Vitamin E is actually composed of several tocopherols, classified as α, β, γ, and δ based on their side chain composition (*Figure 2*). The predominant forms in humans are α and γ-tocopherol, and most antioxidant trials have preferentially employed α-tocopherol. The tocopherols, like other phenolic antioxidants, donate a hydrogen from the hydroxyl portion of their chroman ring moiety to the radical target, leaving behind a tocopheroxyl radical, which can be recovered back to vitamin E by ascorbate or thiols such as dihydrolipoic acid[55]. The antioxidant properties of vitamin E have been reviewed extensively[56], and will not be covered in this review, except to mention a few very important caveats that affect its utility as an antioxidant. One major concern is that the tocopheroxyl radical generated when vitamin E donates its hydrogen, is not completely harmless, and has been shown to contribute to lipid peroxidation under some circumstances[57,58]. Secondly, as mentioned above, most studies have only employed α-tocopherol, and this is well known to lead to depletion of γ-tocopherol[59]. The consequences of this are not clear, but could lead to a worsening of peroxynitrite-mediated oxidation[60]. Finally, as mentioned above, none of the large clinical trials have attempted to monitor the effectiveness of therapy to assure that sufficient doses of vitamin E are given. Recently, Morrow and co-workers have shown that at least 800 U/day is required to lower plasma isoprostanes[61]. In this regard, an important recent study demonstrated that this dose of vitamin E markedly lowered cardiovascular events in hemodialysis patients[5]. It is conceivable that vitamin E would prove useful when directed toward a population that truly has oxidant stress, such as individuals with renal failure, and also when used in the correct doses.

As discussed above, vitamin E is lipid soluble, and highly concentrated in lipid bilayers and LDL particles. A water soluble form of vitamin E, trolox (*Figure 2*), has been created by replacement of the phytyl tail with carboxylic acid[62]. The antioxidant reactions of trolox are similar to those of vitamin E, utilizing hydrogen donation, and formation of a phenoxy radical, which can be regenerated by ascorbic acid. Trolox seems to be effective in scavenging of peroxynitrite and protecting against protein oxidation by strong oxidants like peroxynitrite and the hydroxyl-like species[63,64]. In experimental animal models trolox has been shown to reduce myocardial infarct size[65], decrease ischemia-induced arrhythmias[66], reduce chemical-mediated central nervous system damage[67], and to prevent hepatotoxicity caused by ischemia/reperfusion[68]. To our knowledge, trolox has never been used in human clinical trials, and its clinical utility remains unclear.

Probucol and related compounds

Initially developed as a cholesterol-lowering agent, probucol was subsequently recognized to have potent antioxidant properties, based almost certainly on its bis-phenolic structure (*Figure 2*). Probucol is concentrated into LDL particles, and potently inhibits LDL oxidation. In animal models, probucol has been shown to inhibit atherosclerosis, improve endothelium-dependent vasodilatation and lower vascular superoxide production in cholesterol-fed rabbits[69-71]. In contrast, probucol has been shown to increase atherosclerosis in Apo(E)-deficient mice[72]. Historically, probucol was found to be ineffective in altering femoral artery atherosclerosis, as assessed by measurements of lumen diameter, in the Probucol Quantitative Regression Swedish Trial (PQRST) trial[73]. Given what is now known about remodeling of blood vessels in active atherosclerosis, endpoints such as this are not any longer used. In more recent clinical studies performed in Japan and Canada, probucol has been shown to reduce restenosis following balloon angioplasty[74,75], and to cause regression of carotid atherosclerosis as assessed by ultrasound[76]. Probucol lowers low-density lipoprotein (LDL) cholesterol by about 10 to 20%, but also lowers high-density lipoprotein (HDL)-cholesterol by as much as 30%[77]. Given the beneficial effects of HDL cholesterol, this has alarmed clinicians. In addition, probucol prolongs the QT interval of the electrocardiogram. Such a change in QT interval has been associated with malignant arrhythmias in the case of other drugs, and this has further dampened enthusiasm for the clinical use of probucol in the US.

More recently, a mono-succinic acid ester of probucol, referred to as AGI-1067, has been developed and is being studied in phase III clinical trials. This agent, unlike probucol, is hydrophilic and is more cell permeable than probucol. AGI 1067 potently inhibits LDL oxidation, lowers cellular superoxide production, and inhibits activation of nuclear factor kappa B[78]. AGI 1067 has potently inhibited atherosclerosis development in both murine and primate animal models[79]. In a recent clinical trial, the Canadian Antioxidant Restenosis Trial (CART I), AGI 1067 reduced restenosis following angioplasty, and at an intermediate dose, seemed to cause regression of "reference" lesions, those not intervened upon[80]. Larger clinical trials of this agent are underway. Importantly, AGI 1067 does not prolong the QT interval or lower HDL as much as probucol.

Carvedilol

Carvedilol is a widely used non-selective beta-adrenergic antagonist, which contains an aromatic ring connected to a cabazole structure by a methoxyphenoxyethyl) amino)-2-propanol chain. In addition to its beta-blocking activities, carvedilol has weak alpha-adrenergic antagonist properties[81]. Very early studies with this compound indicated that it much more potently inhibited production of the hydroxyl radical than other beta-adrenergic antagonists[82], and that it was capable of preventing lipid oxidation[83]. The antioxidant effect has been attributed largely to the carbazole structure, and hydroxylated metabolites have increased antioxidant activities compared to the parent compound[82]. The antioxidant potency of carvedilol may be related to its ability to bind Fe^{3+} and Cu^{2+}, which prevents lipid, protein and LDL oxidation mediated by these metals. Crystal studies have revealed that carvedilol chelates Cu^{2+} ions via the N and O atoms belonging to the amino and propanol moiety (*Figure 2*)[84]. In addition, carvedilol's lipophilic nature enhances its concentration in lipid membranes and LDL, providing site specific antioxidant protection[85].

Numerous studies in experimental animals have shown that carvedilol prevents apoptosis[86], ischemia reperfusion injury[87], experimental nephrosclerosis[88], nitrate tolerance (which is at least in part mediated by oxidative stress)[89], and endothelial dysfunction[90,91]. Carvedilol is widely used to treat human heart failure and has been proven effective in numerous clinical trials[92-94]. In head to head comparisons among subjects with heart failure, carvedilol seems slightly superior to other beta-adrenergic antagonists in prolonging life and reducing clinical events[92,93,95]. The mechanism for its superiority remains undefined, but may be related to its antioxidant effects.

Flavonoids and other polyphenol antioxidants

The flavonoids are class of plant aromatic polyphenol derivatives of flavones (naringenin), isoflavones, flavonols (quercetin) and anthocyanins (*Figure 2*). Additional structural modifications such as hydroxylation, glycosylation, acylation and alkylation give rise to a huge variety of flavonoids[96]. It has been generally assumed that phenolic groups are responsible for the antioxidant properties of flavonoids. Flavonoids are thought to have numerous pharmacological effects, which have been attributed to radical scavenging, metal chelation, inhibition of calcium influx, regulation of cell signaling, and modification of gene expression[97].

There are a few popular misconceptions about flavonoids and other polyphenols. These compounds have been reported to be scavengers of the hydroxyl radical ($^{\bullet}$OH)[98,99]. The $^{\bullet}$OH-radical, however, reacts rapidly with all organic compounds and there are no true specific $^{\bullet}$OH-radical scavengers. Flavonoids, like many other antioxidants, may also have pro-oxidant action, particularly, when partially oxidized[100]. A one-electron oxidation of these compounds may lead to formation of flavonoid-derived phenoxy-radicals, which can stimulate lipid oxidation. In addition, a two-electron oxidation of flavonoids leads to formation of quinone-containing structures, which are capable of futile redox cycling and generation of large amounts of superoxide radicals.

Flavonoids have been reported to be active for treatment of disorders of the peripheral circulation and flavonoid-based herbal medicines are used as anti-inflammatory, antispasmodic, antiallergic, and antiviral remedies[101]. Several retrospective analyses of dietary intake has supported the concept that intake of flavonoids and related compounds are beneficial in preventing cardiovascular disease, dementia and cancer. In particular, some of the benefits of red wine have been attributed to quercetin and related compounds. Despite this, there are no prospective studies of flavonoid treatments that have shown benefit in any large clinical trials.

Thiol based compounds NAC, PDTC and OTC, Mesna

Thiol containing compounds, such as cysteine, N-acetyl cysteine, glutathione and thiol precursors such as OTC (*Figure 2*) have several potential antioxidant effects. These agents can directly scavenge radicals via hydrogen donation from their SH group, resulting in formation of a thiyl (S) radical. In addition, many of these agents bolster intracellular glutathione which in turn plays crucial role in removal of intracellular peroxides via its reaction with the glutathione peroxidases and by maintenance of the intracellular redox potential (predominantly affected by the GSH/GSSG ratio). Glutathione also scavenges peroxynitrite, $^{\bullet}$NO$_2$, and recycles the tocopheroxyl radical back to tocopherol. Glutathione cannot be effectively administered orally, because it is broken down by intestinal peptidases to its individual amino acids and is not taken up by cells. In contrast, cysteine and N-acetyl cysteine (NAC) have proven effective in supplementing intracellular levels of glutathione. Upon entering the cell, NAC is hydrolyzed to cysteine which is rapidly incorporated into glutathione. An enormous literature has shown that NAC is beneficial in a variety of pathophysiological states in both the experimental setting and in human studies. NAC improves mitochondria respiration, endothelial function, protect lungs from oxidative injury, and prevents acetaminophen toxicity. In the case of acetaminophen toxicity, NAC is the major clinical tool used to treat this condition. In addition, NAC has been used extensively to prevent contrast-induced nephrotoxicity in humans with renal insufficiency, and several meta-analyses have illustrated its efficacy[102]. This condition is thought in part to be mediated by oxidative stress caused by the contrast agents used. A recent clinical trial showed that NAC dramatically reduced cardiovascular events in patients on hemodialysis[4]. This study is in keeping with the previous study of Boaz et al, supporting the concept that antioxidants may be useful when employed in a population that truly has oxidant stress[5].

L-2-oxothiazolidine-4-carboxylate (OTC) has also been used to supply cysteine for intracellular GSH synthesis (*Figure 2*). OTC is converted intracellularly to cysteine by the 5-L-oxoprolinase[103] and markedly enhances cellular GSH concentration[104]. OTC has also been shown effective in animal models of diverse diseases including amyotrophic lateral sclerosis, Parkinson's disease, lipopolysaccharide-induced peritonitis, diabetes and cancer. In humans with angiographically proven coronary artery disease, OTC has been shown to significantly improve flow-mediated dilation[105], suggesting that improved action or synthesis of endothelium-derived nitric oxide can be obtained by increasing intracellular thiols.

Supplementation with 2-mercaptoethane sulfonate (Mesna) seems to preserve intracellular GSH due to direct reduction of GSSG and via direct antioxidant properties. Mesna is used extensively to prevent cystitis that often complicates chemotherapy. Mesna has also been shown to be beneficial in preventing ischemic renal failure in animals[106]. In small clinical studies, Mesna has reduced contrast induced nephrotoxicity[107,108].

Dithiocarbamate pyrrolidine dithiocarbamate (PDTC) increases de novo synthesis of intracellular GSH[109] and has been used as a thiol antioxidant, although many of its actions are quite likely related to its ability to act as a metal chelator. PDTC has been used as an inhibitor of NFκB, and it inhibits endothelial expression of vascular cell adhesion molecule-1 (VCAM-1)[110]. This effect is likely not via an antioxidant effect, as it seems to interfere with the IκB-ubiquitin ligase activity involved in activation of NFκB in a redox insensitive fashion[111]. While PDTC has been used in a variety of animal and cell culture studies, there have been no clinical studies using this compound.

Tempol

Tempol contains a nitroxide group ($>N-O^\bullet$) which undergoes cycles of oxidation and reduction and conveys an antioxidant property to the molecule (*Figure 2*). In the reduced state, tempol can contribute its electron to superoxide leading to formation of hydrogen peroxide, and therefore has SOD mimetic like properties. It has also been described as a peroxynitrite scavenger but the role of this reaction in vivo is not clear. Tempol has been reported to be an inhibitor of metal catalyzed oxidation, an interaction that may be of crucial importance. Tempol oxidizes ferrous ions to ferric form, and therefore prevents reactions of ferrous iron with peroxides. This interaction can inhibit lipid peroxidation, protein and DNA modifications mediated by transition metals. In experimental animals, tempol has been shown to lower blood pressure in several models of hypertension[112,113], to improve endothelium-dependent vasodilatation[35], to reduce severity of stroke[35,114].

The use of tempol as an antioxidant is complicated by several factors. The concentration of tempol achieved in vivo is usually in the micromolar range and at these concentrations, its scavenging capacity is not as great as vitamin C or SOD. Indeed recent data suggest that tempol can inhibit catecholamine release in vivo, and this, rather than antioxidant effects, may explain its ability to lower blood pressure[115]. The reaction of tempol with superoxide or peroxynitrite produces an oxoammonium cation of tempol, which is a strong oxidant that is recycled to tempol in vitro by reaction with a second molecule of superoxide or peroxynitrite. This oxoammonium cation can oxidize thiols and lipid molecules and may therefore have pro-oxidant effects. Tempol also impairs mitochondrial function and augments glucose transport in vascular endothelial and smooth muscle cells[116]. These effects need further evaluation. Recent data have suggested that bioreduction of high concentrations of tempol by the hexose monophosphate shunt can lead to cytotoxicity, although the in vivo significance of this is unclear.

Ebselen

Ebselen (*Figure 2*) is a selenium containing compound that has been reviewed extensively in prior publications, and its chemical reactions have been studied in depth[117,118]. As a glutathione peroxidase mimetic, it undergoes cycles in which H_2O_2 oxidizes selenium, which is later recycled by reduced glutathione. It also reacts with lipid hydroperoxides (LOOH) via a similar reaction, and can act as a scavenger of peroxynitrite, catalyzing its decomposition to nitrite. The selenium center, via various redox reactions, can undergo transition to various oxidation states, including seleninic acid, selenol, and diselinide. In vitro, ebselen has been shown to be an inhibitor of 15-lipoxygenase, NO synthase, protein kinase C, NADPH oxidase and cytochrome P-450 reductases. These reactions are largely inhibited by glutathione and other thiols, and thus in vivo it is unlikely that these enzymes are effectively inhibited by ebselen[117]. Ebselen has been shown to have numerous beneficial effects in experimental studies by preventing cellular apoptosis, protecting peroxynitrite mediated mitochondrial function, preventing neuronal cell death and reducing the severity of embolic stroke.

Recently, ebselen has been shown to reduce endothelial cell damage and nephropathy in rats with experimentally induced diabetes[119,120]. We have also found that ebselen was effective in blunting the hypertension caused by angiotensin II infusion in mice. In this study, the effect of angiotensin II on blood pressure was augmented in mice with overexpression of the NADPH oxidase, and that this was prevented by concomitant administration of ebselen[121]. In several studies in Japan, ebselen has been used to treat humans with stroke and subarachnoid hemorrhage with mixed results[122-124]. In most of these studies, only marginal improvements in outcome were observed. One difficulty with studies such as this is that treatment is often delayed until after neurological damage is permanent. Given the experimental evidence that ebselen can improve lipid peroxidation, ameliorate diabetes and improve hypertension, it would seem that prospective clinical studies of this drug in these conditions are warranted.

Uric acid and inosine

Uric acid is an effective scavenger of peroxynitrite and nitrogen dioxide (*Figures 2 and 3*), and is considered to be an important endogenous antioxidant. As such, urate is not a drug, but there has been interest in either manipulating its concentration or using analogs that mimic its effect as a means of treating various diseases. Comparison of $ONOO^-$ scavenging by various purine derivatives has revealed a unique reactivity of urate, which was shared with xanthine and to a lesser extent by histamine but not other analogs. These results indicate that the 5-membered ring of the purine structure likely plays a major role in the $ONOO^-$ scavenging. Epidemiological studies have demonstrated a positive correlation between plasma urate levels and the risk of cardiovascular diseases[125,126]; however, this might be due to increased activity of xanthine oxidase[127] or co-morbid conditions such as obesity and diabetes, which are associated with hyperuricemia and gout, rather than untoward properties of urate itself. We have shown that increasing uric acid levels in hypercholesterolemic mice prevents oxidative inactivation of the Cu/Zn-containing superoxide dismutases[128]. Moreover, administration of urate to humans has been shown to prevent the increase in plasma isoprostanes caused by exercise[129]. Recently it has been suggested that the neuro-protective effect of urate is due to $ONOO^-$ scavenging[130]. Several clinical studies have shown that administration of urate or its precursor inosine can hinder multiple sclerosis progression[131]. It is now well established that numerous common diseases such as hypercholesterolemia, hypertension, diabetes and heart failure are associated with a loss of $NO^\bullet$ production by the endothelium, a condition commonly referred to as endothelial dysfunction[132]. In many of these conditions, eNOS uncoupling by $ONOO^-$ or similar oxidants seems to be present, leading to an increase in endothelial cell $O_2^{\bullet-}$ production and a decrease in $NO^{\bullet}$ production. It is interesting to speculate that increasing urate levels in vivo would prove protective against $ONOO^-$ mediated disorders.

Angiotensin receptor antagonists and angiotensin I converting enzyme inhibitors

A growing body of evidence has supported a critical role of the NAD(P)H oxidases in the pathogenesis of cardiovascular diseases[133]. Recently, these enzymes, also referred to as the Nox enzymes for their catalytic subunits, have been implicated in numerous disorders including cancer[134], bone resorption[135] and Alzheimer's disease[136]. In cardiovascular cells, a major stimulus for activation of the NADPH oxidases is angiotensin II (*Figure 4*), and over the long term, angiotensin II increases expression of several of the NADPH oxidase subunits. Given this, it is not surprising that angiotensin I converting enzyme (ACE) inhibitors, which prevent production of angiotensin II, and antagonists of the angiotensin AT1 receptor reduce activity of these enzymes in a variety of pathophysiological conditions. In control rabbits and rats, we have found that the AT1 receptor antagonists reduce activity of the vascular NADPH oxidase, and prevent increased vascular superoxide production caused by conditions such as hypertension, diabetes, and atherosclerosis[137-139]. Simply exposing vessels to high pressure seems to stimulate ACE activity and induce NADPH oxidase activity, and this can be prevented by ACE inhibitors[140]. In humans with the metabolic syndrome, the ACE inhibitor quinapril has been shown to decrease markers of oxidative stress[141]. Thus, the ACE inhibitors and angiotensin receptor antagonists have an antioxidant effect not via scavenging of ROS, but by preventing their formation (*Figure 4*). This property might in part explain the beneficial effect of these agents in several large clinical trials.

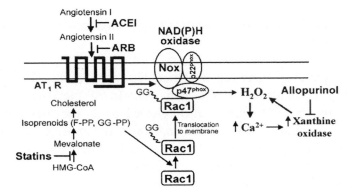

Figure 4: Inhibitors of NAD(P)H oxidases and xanthine oxidase.

HMG CoA reductase inhibitors

The HMG CoA reductase inhibitors (statins) have become a cornerstone of therapy for cardiovascular disease. In addition to their potent cholesterol-lowering properties, these agents seem to have effects that cannot be accounted for by altering lipid levels. These so-called "pleiotropic effects" of the statins are very likely related to the fact that they not only block cholesterol formation, but also prevent formation of a variety of isoprenoid intermediates[142]. One important pleiotropic effect relates to the effect of the small g-proteins Ras, Rac, Rho and Cdc42 which depend on isoprenoid attachment for membrane association and signaling. In the case of the NADPH oxidase, the association of the Rac to the membrane complex is dependent on geranylgeranyl pyrophosphate (*Figure 4*). Thus, atorvastatin inhibits Rac-1 membrane association in response to angiotensin II and the epidermal growth factor[143,144]. In addition, atorvastatin reduces expression of the NADPH oxidase expression Nox1. In failing human myocardium, both Rac1 membrane association and cellular superoxide production is increased, and this can be corrected by pretreatment with statins[145]. Statin therapy has been shown to diminish plasma markers of oxidative and nitrosative stress hypercholesterolemic humans[146]. Thus, like the ACE inhibitors and angiotensin receptor antagonists, the statins have antioxidant effect via preventing activation of the NADPH oxidase subunits.

Xanthine oxidase inhibitors

An important source of ROS in mammalian cells is the xanthine oxidoreductase (XOR). XOR exists in two forms, as xanthine dehydrogenase (XDH), and as xanthine oxidase (XO)[147]. XDH utilizes NAD+ to receive electrons from hypoxanthine and xanthine yielding NADH and uric acid. In contrast, XO utilizes oxygen as an electron acceptor from these same substrates to form superoxide and hydrogen peroxide. The ratio of XO to XDH in the cell is therefore critical to determine the amount of ROS produced by these enzymes. Conversion of XDH to XO is stimulated by inflammatory cytokines like TNFα, and also by oxidation of critical cysteine residues by oxidants such as peroxynitrite[148,149]. Recently, we have shown in bovine and mouse aortic endothelial cells that the relative levels of these is markedly altered by the presence of a functioning NADPH oxidase, such that in cells with an absence of the NADPH oxidase, the levels of XO are extremely low[150]. Xanthine oxidase is an important source of ROS in a variety of pathophysiological states, including hypertension, atherosclerosis, ischemia reperfusion and heart failure. In humans with heart failure and in subjects with CAD, the endothelial levels of xanthine oxidase are increased and correlate with the degree of impairment in endothelium-dependent vasodilatation[127]. Because of this, there has been substantial interest in using allopurinol or its active metabolite oxypurinol to reduce production of ROS in these conditions (*Figures 2 and 4*). Allopurinol has been shown to improve endothelial function in humans with atherosclerosis and heart failure[151]. Surprisingly, there have been no long-term studies of allopurinol in the treatment of humans with diseases thought related to oxidative stress however there currently is an ongoing study to examine the effect of oxypurinol in humans with heart failure[152].

Conclusion

During oxidative stress, the endogenous antioxidant defenses become overwhelmed and pharmacological interventions, at least theoretically, should be beneficial. Despite this line of reasoning, the promising effects of antioxidants observed in in vitro systems and in animal models of disease have not always been borne out in clinical studies or in large clinical trials. Despite an enormous body of prior research, we still lack a complete understanding of the complex roles of the endogenous antioxidants, their interactions and how they are affected by exogenous pharmacological interventions. Gaining greater insight into these interactions may help overcome the failure of some antioxidant treatments. As discussed above, many antioxidants fail to protect against hydrogen peroxide and in fact promote its formation. A major issue is that ROS have important redox signaling effects that are just being defined. For example, H_2O_2 is required for wound healing and angiogenesis and is important for cell growth. H_2O_2 has also been implicated as an endothelium-dependent hyperpolarizing factor and is involved in apoptosis, which is an important cellular housekeeping function and required for immune modulation and killing of cancer cells. Modulating the excessive, deleterious production of ROS while not interfering with these beneficial effects remains an elusive therapeutic target.

References

1. Yusuf S, Dagenais G, Pogue J, Bosch J, Sleight P. Vitamin E supplementation and cardiovascular events in high-risk patients. The Heart Outcomes Prevention Evaluation Study Investigators. N Engl J Med 2000;342:154-60.
2. MRC/BHF Heart Protection Study of antioxidant vitamin supplementation in 20,536 high-risk individuals: a randomised placebo-controlled trial. Lancet 2002;360:23-33.
3. Albanes D, Heinonen OP, Taylor PR, et al. Alpha-Tocopherol and beta-carotene supplements and lung cancer incidence in the alpha-tocopherol, beta-carotene cancer prevention study: effects of baseline characteristics and study compliance. J Natl Cancer Inst 1996;88:1560-70.
4. Tepel M, van der Giet M, Statz M, Jankowski J, Zidek W. The antioxidant acetylcysteine reduces cardiovascular events in patients with end-stage renal failure: a randomized, controlled trial Circulation 2003,107:992-5.
5. Boaz M, Smetana S, Weinstein T, et al. Secondary prevention with antioxidants of cardiovascular disease in endstage renal disease (SPACE): randomised placebo-controlled trial. Lancet 2000;356:1213-8.
6. Jones DP, Carlson JL, Mody VC, Cai J, Lynn MJ, Sternberg P. Redox state of glutathione in human plasma. Free Radic Biol Med 2000;28:625-35.
7. Liu TZ, Stern A, Morrow JD. The isoprostanes: unique bioactive products of lipid peroxidation. An overview. J Biomed Sci 1998;5:415-20.
8. Brunori M, Rotilio G. Biochemistry of oxygen radical species. Methods Enzymol 1984;105:22-35.
9. Jaeschke H, Mitchell JR. Use of isolated perfused organs in hypoxia and ischemia/reperfusion oxidant stress. Methods Enzymol 1990;186:752-9.
10. Liu TH, Beckman JS, Freeman BA, Hogan EL, Hsu CY. Polyethylene glycol-conjugated superoxide dismutase and catalase reduce ischemic brain injury. Am J Physiol 1989;256:H589-93.
11. Bennett JF, Bry WI, Collins GM, Halasz NA. The effects of oxygen free radicals on the preserved kidney. Cryobiology 1987;24:264-9.
12. Tamura Y, Chi LG, Driscoll EM Jr, et al. Superoxide dismutase conjugated to polyethylene glycol provides sustained protection against myocardial ischemia/reperfusion injury in canine heart. Circ Res 1988;63:944-59.
13. Mugge A, Elwell JH, Peterson TE, Hofmeyer TG, Heistad DD, Harrison DG. Chronic treatment with polyethylene-glycolated superoxide dismutase partially restores endothelium-dependent vascular relaxations in cholesterol-fed rabbits. Circ Res 1991;69:1293-300.
14. Matsumiya N, Koehler RC, Kirsch JR, Traystman RJ. Conjugated superoxide dismutase reduces extent of caudate injury after transient focal ischemia in cats. Stroke 1991;22:1193-200.
15. Suzuki Y, Tanigaki T, Heimer D, et al. Polyethylene glycol-conjugated superoxide dismutase attenuates septic lung injury in guinea pigs. Am Rev Respir Dis 1992;145:388-93.

16.   Muizelaar JP, Marmarou A, Young HF, et al. Improving the outcome of severe head injury with the oxygen radical scavenger polyethylene glycol-conjugated superoxide dismutase: a phase II trial. J Neurosurg 1993;78:375-82.

17.   Veronese FM, Caliceti P, Schiavon O, Sergi M. Polyethylene glycol-superoxide dismutase, a conjugate in search of exploitation. Adv Drug Deliv Rev 2002;54:587-606.

18.   Laursen JB, Rajagopalan S, Galis Z, Tarpey M, Freeman BA, Harrison DG. Role of superoxide in angiotensin II-induced but not catecholamine-induced hypertension. Circulation 1997;95:588-93.

19.   Stenlund P, Tibell LA. Chimeras of human extracellular and intracellular superoxide dismutases. Analysis of structure and function of the individual domains. Protein Eng 1999;12:319-25.

20.   Somers MJ, Mavromatis K, Galis ZS, Harrison DG. Vascular superoxide production and vasomotor function in hypertension induced by deoxycorticosterone acetate-salt. Circulation 2000;101:1722-8.

21.   Inoue M, Watanabe N, Utsumi T, Sasaki J. Targeting SOD by gene and protein engineering and inhibition of free radical injury. Free Radic Res Commun 1991;12-13:391-9.

22.   Christofidou-Solomidou M, Scherpereel A, Wiewrodt R, et al. PECAM-directed delivery of catalase to endothelium protects against pulmonary vascular oxidative stress. Am J Physiol Lung Cell Mol Physiol 2003;285:L283-92.

23.   Salvemini D, Riley DP, Cuzzocrea S. SOD mimetics are coming of age. Nat Rev Drug Discov 2002;1:367-74.

24.   Melov S. Therapeutics against mitochondrial oxidative stress in animal models of aging. Ann N Y Acad Sci 2002;959:330-40.

25.   Ferret PJ, Hammoud R, Tulliez M, et al. Detoxification of reactive oxygen species by a nonpeptidyl mimic of superoxide dismutase cures acetaminophen-induced acute liver failure in the mouse. Hepatology 2001;33:1173-80.

26.   Pasternack RF, Skowronek WR Jr. Catalysis of the disproportionation of superoxide by metalloporphyrins. J Inorg Biochem 1979;11:261-7.

27.   Bao F, DeWitt DS, Prough DS, Liu D. Peroxynitrite generated in the rat spinal cord induces oxidation and nitration of proteins: reduction by Mn (III) tetrakis (4-benzoic acid) porphyrin. J Neurosci Res 2003;71:220-7.

28.   Mabley JG, Liaudet L, Pacher P, et al. Part II: beneficial effects of the peroxynitrite decomposition catalyst FP15 in murine models of arthritis and colitis. Mol Med 2002;8:581-90.

29.   Panizzon KL, Dwyer BE, Nishimura RN, Wallis RA. Neuroprotection against CA1 injury with metalloporphyrins. Neuroreport 1996;7:662-6.

30.   Vujaskovic Z, Batinic-Haberle I, Rabbani ZN, et al. A small molecular weight catalytic metalloporphyrin antioxidant with superoxide dismutase (SOD) mimetic properties protects lungs from radiation-induced injury. Free Radic Biol Med 2002;33:857-63.

31.   Ferdinandy P, Danial H, Ambrus I, Rothery RA, Schulz R. Peroxynitrite is a major contributor to cytokine-induced myocardial contractile failure. Circ Res 2000;87:241-7.

32. Pacher P, Liaudet L, Bai P, et al. Potent metalloporphyrin peroxynitrite decomposition catalyst protects against the development of doxorubicin-induced cardiac dysfunction. Circulation 2003;107:896-904.

33. Aladag MA, Turkoz Y, Sahna E, Parlakpinar H, Gul M. The attenuation of vasospasm by using a sod mimetic after experimental subarachnoidal haemorrhage in rats. Acta Neurochir (Wien) 2003;145:673-7.

34. Ross AD, Sheng H, Warner DS, et al. Hemodynamic effects of metalloporphyrin catalytic antioxidants: structure-activity relationships and species specificity. Free Radic Biol Med 2002;33:1657-69.

35. MacKenzie A, Martin W. Loss of endothelium-derived nitric oxide in rabbit aorta by oxidant stress: restoration by superoxide dismutase mimetics. Br J Pharmacol 1998;124:719-28.

36. Perez MJ, Cederbaum AI. Antioxidant and pro-oxidant effects of a manganese porphyrin complex against CYP2E1-dependent toxicity. Free Radic Biol Med 2002;33:111-27.

37. Batinic-Haberle I. Manganese porphyrins and related compounds as mimics of superoxide dismutase. Methods Enzymol 2002;349:223-33.

38. Zhong W, Yan T, Webber MM, Oberley TD. Alteration of cellular phenotype and responses to oxidative stress by manganese superoxide dismutase and a superoxide dismutase mimic in RWPE-2 human prostate adenocarcinoma cells. Antioxid Redox Signal 2004;6:513-22.

39. Halliwell B. Vitamin C and genomic stability. Mutat Res 2001;475:29-35.

40. Warnholtz A, Tsilimingas N, Wendt M, Munzel T. Mechanisms underlying nitrate-induced endothelial dysfunction: insight from experimental and clinical studies. Heart Fail Rev 2002;7:335-45.

41. Dikalov S, Fink B, Skatchkov M, Bassenge E. Comparison of glyceryl trinitrate-induced with pentaerythrityl tetranitrate-induced in vivo formation of superoxide radicals: effect of vitamin C. Free Radic Biol Med 1999;27:170-6.

42. Kuzkaya N, Weissmann N, Harrison DG, Dikalov S. Interactions of peroxynitrite, tetrahydrobiopterin, ascorbic acid, and thiols: implications for uncoupling endothelial nitric-oxide synthase. J Biol Chem 2003;278:22546-54.

43. Heller R, Unbehaun A, Schellenberg B, Mayer B, Werner-Felmayer G, Werner ER. L-ascorbic acid potentiates endothelial nitric oxide synthesis via a chemical stabilization of tetrahydrobiopterin. J Biol Chem 2001;276:40-7.

44. Huang A, Vita JA, Venema RC, Keaney JF Jr. Ascorbic acid enhances endothelial nitric-oxide synthase activity by increasing intracellular tetrahydrobiopterin. J Biol Chem 2000;275:17399-406.

45. Patel KB, Stratford MR, Wardman P, Everett SA. Oxidation of tetrahydrobiopterin by biological radicals and scavenging of the trihydrobiopterin radical by ascorbate. Free Radic Biol Med 2002;32:203-11.

46. Gotoh N, Niki E. Rates of interactions of superoxide with vitamin E, vitamin C and related compounds as measured by chemiluminescence. Biochim Biophys Acta 1992;1115:201-7.

47. Huie RE, Padmaja S. The reaction of no with superoxide. Free Radic Res Commun 1993;18:195-9.

48. Buettner GR, Jurkiewicz BA. Catalytic metals, ascorbate and free radicals: combinations to avoid. Radiat Res 1996;145:532-41.

49. Parthasarathy S. Role of lipid peroxidation and antioxidants in atherogenesis. J Nutr Sci Vitaminol (Tokyo) 1992;Spec No:183-6.

50. Ames PR, Alves J, Murat I, Isenberg DA, Nourooz-Zadeh J. Oxidative stress in systemic lupus erythematosus and allied conditions with vascular involvement. Rheumatology (Oxford) 1999;38:529-34.

51. Albano E. Free radical mechanisms in immune reactions associated with alcoholic liver disease. Free Radic Biol Med 2002;32:110-4.

52. Montine TJ, Milatovic D, Gupta RC, Valyi-Nagy T, Morrow JD, Breyer RM. Neuronal oxidative damage from activated innate immunity is EP2 receptor-dependent. J Neurochem 2002;83:463-70.

53. Davi G, Neri M, Falco A, et al. Helicobacter pylori infection causes persistent platelet activation in vivo through enhanced lipid peroxidation. Arterioscler Thromb Vasc Biol 2004.

54. Grigolo B, Roseti L, Fiorini M, Facchini A. Enhanced lipid peroxidation in synoviocytes from patients with osteoarthritis. J Rheumatol 2003;30:345-7.

55. Thomas SR, Neuzil J, Mohr D, Stocker R. Coantioxidants make alpha-tocopherol an efficient antioxidant for low-density lipoprotein. Am J Clin Nutr 1995;62(Suppl):1357S-1364S.

56. Jiang Q, Christen S, Shigenaga MK, Ames BN. gamma-tocopherol, the major form of vitamin E in the US diet, deserves more attention. Am J Clin Nutr 2001;74:714-22.

57. Upston JM, Terentis AC, Stocker R. Tocopherol-mediated peroxidation of lipoproteins: implications for vitamin E as a potential antiatherogenic supplement. Faseb J 1999;13:977-94.

58. Santanam N, Parthasarathy S. Paradoxical actions of antioxidants in the oxidation of low density lipoprotein by peroxidases. J Clin Invest 1995;95:2594-600.

59. Handelman GJ, Epstein WL, Peerson J, Spiegelman D, Machlin LJ, Dratz EA. Human adipose alpha-tocopherol and gamma-tocopherol kinetics during and after 1 y of alpha-tocopherol supplementation. Am J Clin Nutr 1994;59:1025-32.

60. Frew MJ, Alden ER. Role of the pediatric nurse clinician in early identification of potential child abuse. Mil Med 1978;143:325-7.

61. Barany P, Stenvinkel P, Ottosson-Seeberger A, et al. Effect of 6 weeks of vitamin E administration on renal haemodynamic alterations following a single dose of neoral in healthy volunteers. Nephrol Dial Transplant 2001;16:580-4.

62. Davies MJ, Forni LG, Willson RL. Vitamin E analogue Trolox C. E.s.r. and pulse-radiolysis studies of free-radical reactions. Biochem J 1988;255:513-22.

63. Salgo MG, Pryor WA. Trolox inhibits peroxynitrite-mediated oxidative stress and apoptosis in rat thymocytes. Arch Biochem Biophys 1996;333:482-8.

64. Miura T, Muraoka S, Ogiso T. Inhibition of hydroxyl radical-induced protein damages by trolox. Biochem Mol Biol Int 1993;31:125-33.

65. Wu TW, Wu J, Zeng LH, Sugiyama H, Mickle DA, Au JX. Reduction of experimental myocardial infarct size by infusion of lactosylphenyl Trolox. Cardiovasc Res 1993;27:736-9.

66. Walker MK, Vergely C, Lecour S, Abadie C, Maupoil V, Rochette L. Vitamin E analogues reduce the incidence of ventricular fibrillations and scavenge free radicals. Fundam Clin Pharmacol 1998;12:164-72.

67. Chow HS, Lynch JJ 3rd, Rose K, Choi DW. Trolox attenuates cortical neuronal injury induced by iron, ultraviolet light, glucose deprivation, or AMPA. Brain Res 1994;639:102-8.

68. Wu TW, Hashimoto N, Au JX, Wu J, Mickle DA, Carey D. Trolox protects rat hepatocytes against oxyradical damage and the ischemic rat liver from reperfusion injury. Hepatology 1991;13:575-80.

69. Oshima R, Ikeda T, Watanabe K, Itakura H, Sugiyama N. Probucol treatment attenuates the aortic atherosclerosis in Watanabe heritable hyperlipidemic rabbits. Atherosclerosis 1998;137:13-22.

70. Keaney JF Jr, Xu A, Cunningham D, Jackson T, Frei B, Vita JA. Dietary probucol preserves endothelial function in cholesterol-fed rabbits by limiting vascular oxidative stress and superoxide generation. J Clin Invest 1995;95:2520-9.

71. Inoue N, Ohara Y, Fukai T, Harrison DG, Nishida K. Probucol improves endothelial-dependent relaxation and decreases vascular superoxide production in cholesterol-fed rabbits. Am J Med Sci 1998;315:242-7.

72. Bird DA, Tangirala RK, Fruebis J, Steinberg D, Witztum JL, Palinski W. Effect of probucol on LDL oxidation and atherosclerosis in LDL receptor-deficient mice. J Lipid Res 1998;39:1079-90.

73. Walldius G, Carlson LA, Erikson U, et al. Development of femoral atherosclerosis in hypercholesterolemic patients during treatment with cholestyramine and probucol/placebo: Probucol Quantitative Regression Swedish Trial (PQRST): a status report. Am J Cardiol 1988;62:37B-43B.

74. Tardif JC, Cote G, Lesperance J, et al. Probucol and multivitamins in the prevention of restenosis after coronary angioplasty. Multivitamins and Probucol Study Group. N Engl J Med 1997;337:365-72.

75. Daida H, Kuwabara Y, Yokoi H, et al. Effect of probucol on repeat revascularization rate after percutaneous transluminal coronary angioplasty (from the Probucol Angioplasty Restenosis Trial (PART)). Am J Cardiol 2000;86:550-2, A9.

76. Sawayama Y, Shimizu C, Maeda N, et al. Effects of probucol and pravastatin on common carotid atherosclerosis in patients with asymptomatic hypercholesterolemia. Fukuoka Atherosclerosis Trial (FAST). J Am Coll Cardiol 2002;39:610-6.

77. Franceschini G, Sirtori M, Vaccarino V, et al. Mechanisms of HDL reduction after probucol. Changes in HDL subfractions and increased reverse cholesteryl ester transfer. Arteriosclerosis 1989;9:462-9.

78. Wasserman MA, Sundell CL, Kunsch C, Edwards D, Meng CQ, Medford RM. Chemistry and pharmacology of vascular protectants: a novel approach to the treatment of atherosclerosis and coronary artery disease. Am J Cardiol 2003;91:34A-40A.

79. Sundell CL, Somers PK, Meng CQ, et al. AGI-1067: a multifunctional phenolic antioxidant, lipid modulator, anti-inflammatory and antiatherosclerotic agent. J Pharmacol Exp Ther 2003;305:1116-23.

80. Tardif JC, Gregoire J, Schwartz L, et al. Effects of AGI-1067 and probucol after percutaneous coronary interventions. Circulation 2003;107:552-8.

81. Feuerstein GZ, RR Ruffolo Jr. Carvedilol, a novel vasodilating beta-blocker with the potential for cardiovascular organ protection. Eur Heart J 1996;17(Suppl B):24-9.

82. Yue TL, Cheng HY, Lysko PG, et al. Carvedilol, a new vasodilator and beta adrenoceptor antagonist, is an antioxidant and free radical scavenger. J Pharmacol Exp Ther 1992;263:92-8.

83. Yue TL, McKenna PJ, Lysko PG, Ruffolo RR Jr, Feuerstein GZ. Carvedilol, a new antihypertensive, prevents oxidation of human low density lipoprotein by macrophages and copper. Atherosclerosis 1992;97:209-16.

84. Zoroddu MA, Grepioni F, Franconi F. Carvedilol, a beta adrenoceptor blocker with chelating properties. A copper 'superdimer' based on dimetal units. J Inorg Biochem 2003;95:315-20.

85. Tadolini B, Franconi F. Carvedilol inhibition of lipid peroxidation. A new antioxidative mechanism. Free Radic Res 1998;29:377-87.

86. Romeo F, Li D, Shi M, Mehta JL. Carvedilol prevents epinephrine-induced apoptosis in human coronary artery endothelial cells: modulation of Fas/Fas ligand and caspase-3 pathway. Cardiovasc Res 2000;45:788-94.

87. Feuerstein G, Liu GL, Yue TL, et al. Comparison of metoprolol and carvedilol pharmacology and cardioprotection in rabbit ischemia and reperfusion model. Eur J Pharmacol 1998;351:341-50.

88. Rodriguez-Perez JC, Losada A, Anabitarte A, et al. Effects of the novel multiple-action agent carvedilol on severe nephrosclerosis in renal ablated rats. J Pharmacol Exp Ther 1997;283:336-44.

89. Watanabe H, Kakihana M, Ohtsuka S, Sugishita Y. Randomized, double-blind, placebo-controlled study of carvedilol on the prevention of nitrate tolerance in patients with chronic heart failure. J Am Coll Cardiol 1998;32:1194-200.

90. Matsuda Y, Akita H, Terashima M, Shiga N, Kanazawa K, Yokoyama M. Carvedilol improves endothelium-dependent dilatation in patients with coronary artery disease. Am Heart J 2000;140:753-9.

91. Ma XL, Gao F, Nelson AH, et al. Oxidative inactivation of nitric oxide and endothelial dysfunction in stroke-prone spontaneous hypertensive rats. J Pharmacol Exp Ther 2001;298:879-85.

92. Sanderson JE, Chan SK, Yip G, et al. Beta-blockade in heart failure: a comparison of carvedilol with metoprolol. J Am Coll Cardiol 1999;34:1522-8.

93. Randomised, placebo-controlled trial of carvedilol in patients with congestive heart failure due to ischaemic heart disease. Australia/New Zealand Heart Failure Research Collaborative Group. Lancet, 1997;349:pp375-80.

94. Di Lenarda A, Sabbadini G, Salvatore L, et al. Long-term effects of carvedilol in idiopathic dilated cardiomyopathy with persistent left ventricular dysfunction despite chronic metoprolol. The Heart-Muscle Disease Study Group. J Am Coll Cardiol 1999;33:1926-34.

95. Poole-Wilson PA, Swedberg K, Cleland JG, et al. Carvedilol Or Metoprolol European Trial Investigators. Comparison of carvedilol and metoprolol on clinical outcomes in patients with chronic heart failure in the Carvedilol Or Metoprolol European Trial (COMET): randomised controlled trial. Lancet 2003;362:7-13.

96. Bloor SJ. Overview of methods for analysis and identification of flavonoids. Methods Enzymol 2001;335:3-14.

97. Kong AN, Owuor E, Yu R, et al. Induction of xenobiotic enzymes by the MAP kinase pathway and the antioxidant or electrophile response element (ARE/EpRE). Drug Metab Rev 2001;33:255-71.

98. Hanasaki Y, Ogawa S, Fukui S. The correlation between active oxygens scavenging and antioxidative effects of flavonoids. Free Radic Biol Med 1994;16:845-50.

99. Macrides TA, Shihata A, Kalafatis N, Wright PF. A comparison of the hydroxyl radical scavenging properties of the shark bile steroid 5 beta-scymnol and plant pycnogenols. Biochem Mol Biol Int 1997;42:1249-60.

100. Long LH, Halliwell B. Antioxidant and prooxidant abilities of foods and beverages. Methods Enzymol 2001;335:181-90.

101. Pietta P, Mauri P. Analysis of flavonoids in medicinal plants. Methods Enzymol 2001;335:26-45.

102. Birck R, Krzossok S, Markowetz F, Schnulle P, van der Woude FJ, Braun C. Acetylcysteine for prevention of contrast nephropathy: meta-analysis. Lancet 2003;362:598-603.

103. Williamson JM, Meister A. New substrates of 5-oxo-L-prolinase. J Biol Chem, 1982;257:12039-42.

104. Tsan MF, Danis EH, Del Vecchio PJ, Rosano CL. Enhancement of intracellular glutathione protects endothelial cells against oxidant damage. Biochem Biophys Res Commun 1985;127:270-6.

105. Vita JA, Frei B, Holbrook M, Gokce N, Leaf C, Keaney JF Jr. L-2-Oxothiazolidine-4-carboxylic acid reverses endothelial dysfunction in patients with coronary artery disease. J Clin Invest 1998;101:1408-14.

106. Kabasakal L, Sehirli AO, Cetinel S, Cikler E, Gedik N, Sener G. Mesna (2-mercaptoethane sulfonate) prevents ischemia/reperfusion induced renal oxidative damage in rats. Life Sci 2004;75:2329-40.

107. Mashiach E, Sela S, Weinstein T, Cohen HI, Shasha SM, Kristal B. Mesna: a novel renoprotective antioxidant in ischaemic acute renal failure. Nephrol Dial Transplant 2001;16:542-51.

108. Haeussler U, Riedel M, Keller F. Free reactive oxygen species and nephrotoxicity of contrast agents. Kidney Blood Press Res 2004;27:167-71.

109. Wild AC, Mulcahy RT. Pyrrolidine dithiocarbamate up-regulates the expression of the genes encoding the catalytic and regulatory subunits of gamma-glutamylcysteine synthetase and increases intracellular glutathione levels. Biochem J 1999;338:659-65.

110. Marui N, Offermann MK, Swerlick R, et al. Vascular cell adhesion molecule-1 (VCAM-1) gene transcription and expression are regulated through an antioxidant-sensitive mechanism in human vascular endothelial cells. J Clin Invest 1993;92:1866-74.

111. Hayakawa M, Miyashita H, Sakamoto I, et al. Evidence that reactive oxygen species do not mediate NF-kappaB activation. Embo J 2003;22:3356-66.

112. Onuma S, Nakanishi K. Superoxide dismustase mimetic tempol decreases blood pressure by increasing renal medullary blood flow in hyperinsulinemic-hypertensive rats. Metabolism 2004;53:1305-8.

113. Schnackenberg CG, Welch WJ, Wilcox CS. Normalization of blood pressure and renal vascular resistance in SHR with a membrane-permeable superoxide dismutase mimetic: role of nitric oxide. Hypertension 1998;32:59-64.

114. Rak R, Chao DL, Pluta RM, Mitchell JB, Oldfield EH, Watson JC. Neuroprotection by the stable nitroxide Tempol during reperfusion in a rat model of transient focal ischemia. J Neurosurg 2000;92:646-51.

115. Campese VM, Ye S, Zhong H, Yanamadala V, Ye Z, Chiu J. Reactive oxygen species stimulate central and peripheral sympathetic nervous system activity. Am J Physiol Heart Circ Physiol 2004;287:H695-703.

116. Alpert E, Altman H, Totary H, et al. 4-Hydroxy tempol-induced impairment of mitochondrial function and augmentation of glucose transport in vascular endothelial and smooth muscle cells. Biochem Pharmacol 2004;67:1985-95.

117. Schewe T. Molecular actions of ebselen--an antiinflammatory antioxidant. Gen Pharmacol 1995;26: 1153-69.

118. Sies H. Ebselen. Methods Enzymol 1995;252:341-2.

119. Chander PN, Gealekman O, Brodsky SV, et al. Nephropathy in Zucker diabetic fat rat is associated with oxidative and nitrosative stress: prevention by chronic therapy with a peroxynitrite scavenger ebselen. J Am Soc Nephrol 2004;15:2391-403.

120. Brodsky SV, Gealekman O, Chen J, et al. Prevention and reversal of premature endothelial cell senescence and vasculopathy in obesity-induced diabetes by ebselen. Circ Res 2004;94:377-84.

121. Weber DS, Rocic P, Mellis AM, et al. Angiotensin II-induced hypertrophy is potentiated in mice overexpressing p22phox in vascular smooth muscle. Am J Physiol Heart Circ Physiol 2004.

122. Yamaguchi T, Sano K, Takakura K, et al. Ebselen in acute ischemic stroke: a placebo-controlled, double-blind clinical trial. Ebselen Study Group. Stroke 1998;29:12-7.

123. Saito I, Asano T, Sano K, et al. Neuroprotective effect of an antioxidant, ebselen, in patients with delayed neurological deficits after aneurysmal subarachnoid hemorrhage. Neurosurgery 1998;42:269-77; discussion 277-8.

124. Ogawa A, Yoshimoto T, Kikuchi H, et al. Ebselen in acute middle cerebral artery occlusion: a placebo-controlled, double-blind clinical trial. Cerebrovasc Dis 1999;9:112-8.

125. Waring WS, Maxwell SR, Webb DJ. Uric acid concentrations and the mechanisms of cardiovascular disease. Eur Heart J 2002;23:1888-9.

126. Alderman MH. Serum uric acid as a cardiovascular risk factor for heart disease. Curr Hypertens Rep 2001;3:184-9.

127. Landmesser U, Spiekermann S, Dikalov S, et al. Vascular oxidative stress and endothelial dysfunction in patients with chronic heart failure: role of xanthine-oxidase and extracellular superoxide dismutase. Circulation 2002;106:3073-8.

128. Hink HU, Santanam N, Dikalov S, et al. Peroxidase properties of extracellular superoxide dismutase: role of uric acid in modulating in vivo activity. Arterioscler Thromb Vasc Biol 2002;22:1402-8.

129. Waring WS, Convery A, Mishra V, Shenkin A, Webb DJ, Maxwell SR. Uric acid reduces exercise-induced oxidative stress in healthy adults. Clin Sci (Lond) 2003;105:425-30.

130. Spitsin SV, Scott GS, Mikheeva T, et al. Comparison of uric acid and ascorbic acid in protection against EAE. Free Radic Biol Med 2002;33:1363-71.

131. Spitsin S, Hooper DC, Leist T, Streletz LJ, Mikheeva T, Koprowskil H. Inactivation of peroxynitrite in multiple sclerosis patients after oral administration of inosine may suggest possible approaches to therapy of the disease. Mult Scler 2001;7:313-9.

132. Zeiher AM, Drexler H, Saurbier B, Just H. Endothelium-mediated coronary blood flow modulation in humans. Effects of age, atherosclerosis, hypercholesterolemia, and hypertension. J Clin Invest 1993;92:652-62.

133. Cai H, Griendling KK, Harrison DG. The vascular NAD(P)H oxidases as therapeutic targets in cardiovascular diseases. Trends Pharmacol Sci 2003;24:471-8.

134. Suh YA, Arnold RS, Lassegue B, et al. Cell transformation by the superoxide-generating oxidase Mox1. Nature 1999;401:79-82.

135. Yang S, Madyastha P, Bingel S, Ries W, Key L. A new superoxide-generating oxidase in murine osteoclasts. J Biol Chem 2001;276:5452-8.

136. Shimohama S, Tanino H, Kawakami N, et al. Activation of NADPH oxidase in Alzheimer's disease brains. Biochem Biophys Res Commun 2000;273:5-9.

137. Warnholtz A, Nickenig G, Schulz E, et al. Increased NADH-oxidase-mediated superoxide production in the early stages of atherosclerosis: evidence for involvement of the renin-angiotensin system. Circulation 1999;99:2027-33.

138. Rajagopalan S, Kurz S, Munzel T, et al. Angiotensin II-mediated hypertension in the rat increases vascular superoxide production via membrane NADH/NADPH oxidase activation. Contribution to alterations of vasomotor tone. J Clin Invest 1996;97:1916-23.

139. Kurz S, Hink U, Nickenig G, Borthayre AB, Harrison DG, Munzel T. Evidence for a causal role of the renin-angiotensin system in nitrate tolerance. Circulation 1999;99:3181-7.

140. Ungvari Z, Csiszar A, Kaminski PM, Wolin MS, Koller A. Chronic high pressure-induced arterial oxidative stress: involvement of protein kinase C-dependent NAD(P)H oxidase and local renin-angiotensin system. Am J Pathol 2004;165:219-26.

141. Khan BV, Sola S, Lauten WB, et al. Quinapril, an ACE inhibitor, reduces markers of oxidative stress in the metabolic syndrome. Diabetes Care 2004;27:1712-5.

142. Laufs U, Liao JK. Isoprenoid metabolism and the pleiotropic effects of statins. Curr Atheroscler Rep 2003;5:372-8.

143. Wassmann S, Laufs U, Muller K, et al. Cellular antioxidant effects of atorvastatin in vitro and in vivo. Arterioscler Thromb Vasc Biol 2002;22:300-5.

144. Wagner AH, Kohler T, Ruckschloss U, Just I, Hecker M. Improvement of nitric oxide-dependent vasodilatation by HMG-CoA reductase inhibitors through attenuation of endothelial superoxide anion formation. Arterioscler Thromb Vasc Biol 2000;20:61-9.

145. Maack C, Kartes T, Kilter H, et al. Oxygen free radical release in human failing myocardium is associated with increased activity of rac1-GTPase and represents a target for statin treatment. Circulation 2003;108:1567-74.

146. Shishehbor MH, Brennan ML, Aviles RJ, et al. Statins promote potent systemic antioxidant effects through specific inflammatory pathways. Circulation 2003;108:426-31.

147. Cai H, Li Z, Dikalov S, et al. NAD(P)H oxidase-derived hydrogen peroxide mediates endothelial nitric oxide production in response to angiotensin II. J Biol Chem 2002;277:48311-7.

148. Sakuma S, Fujimoto Y, Sakamoto Y, et al. Peroxynitrite induces the conversion of xanthine dehydrogenase to oxidase in rabbit liver. Biochem Biophys Res Commun 1997;230:476-9.

149. Friedl HP, Till GO, Ryan US, Ward PA. Mediator-induced activation of xanthine oxidase in endothelial cells. Faseb J 1989;3:2512-8.

150. McNally JS, Davis ME, Giddens DP, et al. Role of xanthine oxidoreductase and NAD(P)H oxidase in endothelial superoxide production in response to oscillatory shear stress. Am J Physiol Heart Circ Physiol 2003;285:H2290-7.

151. Farquharson CA, Butler R, Hill A, Belch JJ, Struthers AD. Allopurinol improves endothelial dysfunction in chronic heart failure. Circulation 2002;106:221-6.

152. Freudenberger RS, Schwarz RP Jr, Brown J, et al. Rationale, design and organisation of an efficacy and safety study of oxypurinol added to standard therapy in patients with NYHA class III - IV congestive heart failure. Expert Opin Investig Drugs 2004;13:1509-16

Chapter 8

ANTIOXIDANT NUTRIENTS AND ANTIOXIDANT NUTRIENT-RICH FOODS AGAINST CORONARY HEART DISEASE

Michel de Lorgeril and Patricia Salen
Laboratoire Nutrition, Vieillissement et Maladies Cardiovasculaires (NVMCV), UFR de Médecine, Université Joseph Fourier, Grenoble, France

Introduction

Various foods are natural sources of antioxidant macro- and micro-nutrients (the latter being defined as any essential dietary components present in trace amounts). Antioxidant micronutrients have multiple roles as they both are involved in many metabolic processes throughout the body and counter the oxidative stress resulting from normal metabolism and daily exposure to environmental agents. The main antioxidant micronutrients are minerals (zinc and selenium) and vitamins (A, C and E). Macronutrients and non-nutrient food factors also have an antioxidant activity, to such an extent that they may actually be the major antioxidants in our diet. The influence of each specific natural antioxidant nutrient or non-nutrient factor in the development and complications of coronary heart disease (CHD) is poorly understood, and recent studies using some of them as supplements in the context of randomized trials have done little to clarify the situation. In this chapter, we will briefly summarize recent knowledge about a variety of natural antioxidants (*Table 1*).

Table 1: **Natural antioxidants**

Antioxidant nutrients	Antioxidant nutrient-rich foods

Minerals
    Zinc
    Selenium
Vitamins
    Vitamin A
        - Retinol and related compounds
        - Carotenoids
    Vitamin E
        - Alpha-tocopherol
        - Gamma-tocopherol
Vitamin C
Polyphenols
	Tea
	Wine
	Soy food
	Whole-grain foods
	Vegetables and fruit
	Garlic and onion
	Olive oil
	Ginseng
	Ginkgo Biloba
	Aromatic herbs
	Honey

Minerals

Zinc and selenium are the two main antioxidant minerals found in common foods.

Zinc

An adequate zinc intake is critical for good health, as shown in many clinical circumstances in children and in relation with infectious diseases[1]. Zinc deficiency affects immune cells, and alterations are noted even at an early stage of deficiency. The recommended daily allowance is ten mg but many people, in both developing and industrialized countries, do not find as much zinc in their diet. Zinc deficiency is biochemically defined as a serum concentration of less than nine μmol/L. However, serum zinc concentrations may not fully reflect an individual's physiological zinc status. Zinc is mainly absorbed through the duodenum and it is essentially reduced if the diet is low on proteins. It is a powerful site-specific antioxidant, and zinc deficiency leads to an increased oxidative stress[2]. However, in both clinical and experimental settings, there is no data suggesting that zinc deficiency may significantly affect CHD.

Selenium

Selenium, which is largely obtained from marine foods, meat and cereals, plays a vital part in many metabolic functions. In fact, it is a key component of a number of functional selenoproteins required for normal health[3]. The best known of these are the antioxidant glutathione peroxidase enzymes that remove hydrogen peroxide and the harmful lipid hydroperoxides generated in vivo by oxygen-derived species. Selenium also plays a role in the control of thyroid hormone metabolism and in protection against organic and inorganic mercury[4]. Selenium deficiency diseases, such as cardiomyopathy and deforming arthritis, have been described in areas where the soil is extremely poor in selenium. Less overt deficiencies have been shown in several studies to adversely affect the susceptibility to other disorders, in particular cancers[3] and chronic heart failure (CHF)[5]. However, there is no clear epidemiological or clinical data suggesting that selenium deficiency influences the development of CHD.

The incidence of CHF, the common end-result of most cardiac diseases, is increasing steadily in many countries despite improvements in the prevention and treatment of most types of heart disease[6,7]. Unidentified factors may contribute to the age-adjusted rise in the number of CHF patients. Increased oxidative stress has only recently been recognized as a possible factor in the pathogenesis of CHF[8,9]. In fact, clinical and experimental studies have suggested that CHF may be associated with increased free radical formation and reduced antioxidant defenses[10,11]. Selenium deficiency has been identified as a major factor in the etiology of certain non-ischemic CHF syndromes, especially in low-selenium soil areas such as Eastern China (Keshan disease) and Western Africa[12]. In Western countries, cases of congestive cardiomyopathy associated with low selenium have been reported in malnourished HIV-infected patients[13] and in subjects on chronic parenteral nutrition.

In a study of CHF patients, we found a strong positive correlation between blood selenium and exercise capacity[5]. However, the relation between selenium and peak VO2 in our patients was linear only for selenium levels below 70 µg/L. With levels higher than 70 µg/L, peak VO2 reached a plateau suggesting that there is a causal relationship between selenium and exercise capacity only (if at all) when selenium is low. CHF is now seen as a muscle disease, involving skeletal and respiratory muscles[14] and not only the heart muscle. Exercise and respiratory training actually result in significant improvements in peak VO2[15]. This means that while the lack of selenium accounts for the altered exercise capacity of these patients, this may be partly because of muscular deconditioning. As a matter of fact, we found no correlation between selenium and the left ventricular (LV) ejection fraction, which indicates that selenium is mostly involved in the symptoms of CHF (and peak VO$_2$) rather than in the development of the LV dysfunction itself. This hypothesis is also in line with the history of Keshan disease[16], probably the best illustration of the role of selenium in CHF. Ge and Yang have pointed out that selenium deficiency (which may have resulted in the mutation of the virus that is the primary cause of the disease) is an essential cause, but not the only reason, for the occurrence of Keshan disease, an endemic cardiomyopathy in low-selenium soil areas[12]. In the Keshan area, the selenium status is matched to the clinical severity rather than to the degree of LV dysfunction as assessed by echocardiographic studies. Other causes have been proposed but only selenium supplementation had a preventive effect in large trials and resulted in a reduced mortality rate[12,17]. In the endemic area, when the selenium levels of residents were raised to the typical levels in non-endemic areas, clinically latent cases were still found and the echocardiographic prevalence of the disease remained high. Selenium deficiency is therefore considered a predisposing (or aggravating) factor rather than a specific etiologic factor for the occurrence of Keshan disease. What we learn from Keshan disease is therefore that in patients with a known cause of CHF, even a mild deficiency in selenium may influence the clinical severity of the disease (in terms of exercise tolerance). In a recent study, a selenium intake of about 80 μg/day was required to obtain a blood concentration of 70 μg/L[5]. Beyond that point, higher blood levels were not associated with better exercise capacity. It is noteworthy that an intake of 80 μg/day is higher than the current recommendations for healthy adults (55 to 70 μg/day)[18] and also higher than the intake (40 μg/day) considered adequate for the prevention of Keshan disease in China[19]. Thus, in patients with CHF, dietary selenium requirements are probably higher than those recommended for the healthy population. This is a major practical point. The discrepancy between the symptoms of CHF and the degree of LV dysfunction is a major issue for the management of patients with CHF[20]. The pathophysiology underlying the symptoms of CHF (dyspnea and muscle fatigue) is poorly understood, and treatments aimed at correcting the hemodynamics of heart failure do not reliably reduce the symptoms[20]. What about selenium in that context?

Selenium is an essential trace element and has a variety of functions. The main one is its role as an antioxidant in the enzyme glutathione peroxidase (GP), the prime intracellular antioxidant. Selenium depletion results in a decrease of both GP activity and protein[21]. Until recently, studies on the function of selenium focused on GP. Recognition that several effects of selenium are not associated with GP has forced re-evaluation of its function. Another selenoprotein, named Selenoprotein P, has been discovered and is assumed to be a major extracellular antioxidant[22]. More recently, the selenium-dependent thioredoxin reductase system has been proposed to contribute in ascorbate regeneration[23]. Thus, selenium-dependent systems are crucial antioxidant defenses in humans. On the other hand, CHF is associated with peripheral vasoconstriction[24] and impaired skeletal muscle metabolism[25], both attributed to an impaired vascular endothelial function[26]. The correction of endothelial dysfunction results in a significant increase in exercise capacity[27], and can be achieved in these patients with vitamin C, which is thought to scavenge oxygen radicals and spare endogenous antioxidants from consumption[28]. The selenium-dependent systems act synergistically with vitamin C[29] to neutralize oxygen radicals and preserve endothelial function, which in turn may help to maintain exercise capacity.

Another question is whether the selenium status may play a role in the specific ability of the heart to withstand ischemic stress, at least in certain conditions. Our group has shown, using the Langendorff model and isolated rat hearts, that correction of selenium deficiency[30] or selenium supplementation in senescent rats[31], or supplementation in rats treated with the cardiotoxic adriamycin[32], decreases the sensibility of cardiac cells to ischemia and reperfusion. Although these data indicate that the heart is dependent on antioxidant defenses, in particular those related to the selenium status, further studies are needed to confirm the relevance of these data in the clinical setting.

Vitamins

The main antioxidant vitamins are vitamins C, E and A.

Vitamin A.
Vitamin A originates from two classes of compounds: preformed vitamin A (retinol and related compounds) and carotenoids. Retinol and related compounds are exclusively found in animal foods, whereas carotenoids are found in vegetable foods only. Most of the 700 carotenoids identified to date derive from two precursors: lycopene and beta-carotene. Those found in the human diet are essentially alpha- and beta-carotene, lycopene and beta-cryptoxanthine. Vitamin A is very important for a normal eyesight (retinol is a constituent of the retinal pigment rhodopsin) and gene expression (and cell differentiation), but the effects of vitamin A deficiency on CHD may result from a reduced antioxidant activity. However, there is no clinical study suggesting that vitamin A deficiency plays a role in the development and complications of CHD. Beta-carotene, a provitamin A carotenoid, performs the same functions as vitamin A after hydrolysis and also is a particularly effective antioxidant, capable of physically quenching reactive oxygen species (ROS) at a diffusion-controlled rate and inhibiting free radical chain

reaction and lipoxygenase activity[33]. In addition, observational studies have suggested an inverse association between certain carotenoids (namely lutein and zeaxanthin) and the risk of age-related eye maculopathy.

Plants synthesize carotenoids that are vitamin A precursors, but they do not directly synthesize retinol and retinoids. Humans and other animals convert carotenoids into retinol and its metabolites, but obtain preformed vitamin A from animal foods or dietary supplements. Common dietary sources of vitamin A are liver, dairy products (milk, cheese and butter) and fish oil. Common dietary sources of provitamin A carotenoids include carrots, dark green leafy vegetables, corn, tomatoes (lycopene), papayas, mangoes, and oranges[33]. Vitamin A deficiency still exists in parts of the developing world, especially in young children, but is extremely rare in developed countries. Hypervitaminosis A may result from an acute or chronic excessive intake of preformed vitamin A, but not from excess carotenoids. Its most important toxic effect is probably the teratogenic effect, and a high prevalence of spontaneous abortion and birth defects in fetuses was observed in women ingesting high doses of retinoic acid for skin diseases during the first trimester of pregnancy[33]. Beta-carotene has been used extensively as coloring in the food industry and in dietary supplements. Although associated with very low toxicity, it has been reported as the apparent cause of harmful effects in persons at high risk for cancer (smokers), which must be taken seriously[33].

Observational studies of the dietary intake and blood levels of natural antioxidants in humans point to preventive effects on CHD. In many studies, the protective effects were described only for a high consumption of antioxidant-rich foods (mainly fruit and vegetables), not for any single specific compound. A review reporting measures of association between CHD and fruit and vegetable intakes found that most studies reported significant protective effects[34]. In contrast, a review of published case-control studies focusing on specific antioxidants found significantly lower blood or tissue levels of carotenoids in cases in only five of eleven studies[35]. For instance, there was no difference between cases and controls for fatty tissue beta-carotene concentration in the large EURopean community multicenter study on Antioxidants, Myocardial Infarction and breast Cancer (EURAMIC)[36]. However, in the same study, the investigators reported that the strength of the inverse association between CHD and beta-carotene was actually dependent on polyunsaturated fatty acid (PUFA) levels in fatty tissue: the higher the PUFAs, the stronger was the association, supporting the hypothesis that beta-carotene may play a role in protection against CHD by preventing PUFA oxidation[37]. Two large cohort studies supported the theory that a high carotenoid intake may protect against CHD. The emblematic Health Professionals' Follow-Up Study described an inverse association between dietary beta-carotene and CHD in male smokers[38], and a similar inverse association was reported in elderly Dutch people in the Rotterdam Study[39]. In contrast, the results of randomized trials using supplements were disappointing and did not confirm the benefits of a high intake of beta-carotene or carotenoids[40-42].

At this stage, it is important to see whether we can clarify the discrepancy between the clinical trials testing beta-carotene (with or without retinol) and the observational studies of the effects of beta-carotene intake or the consumption of carotenoid-rich foods. There are many possible explanations for that discrepancy, which are discussed in other chapters of this book. Regarding the dietary aspect of the question, it is important to remember that blood carotenoids are only crude indicators of vegetable and fruit intake[43] and that many factors, for instance aging, sex, smoking and low grade inflammation[44], may contribute to misclassification of the antioxidant vitamin status in observational studies. Also, it seems that the relative significance of each antioxidant compound in relation with the risk of CHD has not been carefully assessed so far. For instance, whereas beta-carotene has been investigated for many years, lycopene (the acyl form of beta-carotene without provitamin A activity, shown to be a more potent antioxidant than beta-carotene) has only recently attracted substantial interest. As a matter of fact, in recent studies, high blood lycopene concentrations were associated with a lower risk of CHD in women[45] and a lower grade of carotid atherosclerosis[46]. Thus, further clinical trials testing different antioxidant strategies are needed before the hypothesis that dietary carotenoids protect against CHD can be definitively rejected.

Vitamin E

The story with vitamin E is very similar to that with vitamin A and carotenoids.

Alpha-tocopherol (AT) is the major and natural form of vitamin E activity, whereas gamma-tocopherol (GT) has the strongest antioxidant capacity and is most prevalent in the diet[47]. Although GT is the main form of vitamin E in many plant seeds (and vegetable oils) and in the Western diet, it has less attracted attention than AT, the predominant form of vitamin E in tissues and the primary form in supplements (*Table 2*).

Table 2: **Total PUFA content, Alpha-tocopherol (AT) content and ratio of AT to PUFAs** (Data from USDA National Nutrient Database for Standard Reference, Release 17)

Food	Vitamin E (mg AT/100g of food)	PUFA (g/100g of food)	Vitamin E/PUFA
Corn oil *	14.3	54.7	0.3
Grapeseed oil	28.8	69.9	0.4
Olive oil	**14.4**	**10.0**	**1.4**
Almond oil	**39.2**	**17.4**	**2.3**
Hazelnut oil	**47.2**	**10.2**	**4.6**
Peanut oil	15.7	32.0	0.6
Canola oil *	17.1	29.6	0.6
Soybean oil	9.2	57.9	0.2
Sunflower oil	41.1	65.7	0.6

* These oils are particularly rich in gamma-tocopherol

In fact, there are four forms of vitamin E (alpha, beta, gamma, and delta) that differ in vitamin E potency, the most active (when using the traditional "rat fetal resorption assay" in which vitamin E activity is not defined in terms of antioxidant activity, but as the ability of supplemented tocopherol to prevent embryo death in vitamin E-depleted mothers) being the AT natural isomer that accounts for about 90% of the vitamin E present in humans. Unlike most other vitamins, synthetic AT is not identical to the naturally occurring form. The main in vivo physiological role of vitamin E seems to be that of an antioxidant. Because it is a potent peroxyl radical scavenger, it protects PUFAs in membranes and lipoproteins against oxidation. The antioxidant synergy between AT and vitamin C is well established. The chain-breaking reaction converts AT into its radical, and the radical is converted back to AT by reacting with vitamin C. In comparison with AT, GT is a less potent antioxidant as regards electron-donating propensity, but is superior in detoxifying electrophiles such as nitrogen oxide species, usually associated with chronic inflammation[47].

The primary dietary sources of vitamin E are vegetable oils and margarines. Secondary sources are eggs, cheese and olives, while nuts are excellent sources of GT. It is generally assumed that the recommended dietary allowance for vitamin E is about eight to ten mg per day of AT, although vitamin E requirements should ideally be defined in terms of PUFA intake. Vitamin E deficiency rarely occurs, because tocopherols are found in virtually all foods. The rare cases of deficiency are usually associated with fat malabsorption syndromes. This point is important because it means that in most vitamin E trials, patients randomized in the experimental group were actually not deficient in vitamin E and were therefore not expected to benefit from correcting a chronic vitamin E deficiency. They were only expecting hypothetic benefits from receiving higher doses of vitamin E than necessary. As compared with the other lipophilic vitamins, vitamin E is relatively nontoxic when taken orally, with doses of up to 1000 mg/day considered entirely safe and without side effects.

Epidemiologic studies have shown negative correlations between vitamin E consumption and the risk of CHD[48,49]. This led to several randomized trials with various protocols and antioxidant regimens[40,50-54]. Among them, only one Cambridge Heart AntiOxidant Study (CHAOS) did provide positive results with a significant reduction (-47%) of the risk of nonfatal myocardial infarction[54]. However, there were some methodological problems in that trial, which partly invalidate the results. It is noteworthy that in the Gruppo Italiano per lo Studio della Sopravivivenza nell'Infarto miocardico Prevenzione (GISSI) trial, despite a lack of significant difference between groups for the primary endpoint -a combination of all-cause death, nonfatal myocardial infarction and stroke—secondary analysis provided another view of the clinical effect of vitamin E in CHD patients, which cannot be easily dismissed[50]. In fact, among the 193 and 155 cardiac deaths that occurred in the control and vitamin E groups, respectively, during the trial (a difference of 38, p<0.05), there were 99 and 65 sudden deaths (a difference of 34, p<0.05), which indicated that the significant decrease in cardiovascular mortality (by 20%) in the vitamin E group was almost entirely due to a decrease in the incidence of sudden death (by 35%). In contrast, nonfatal cardiac events and non-sudden cardiac deaths were not influenced[50]. These data suggest that vitamin E may be useful for the primary prevention of sudden cardiac death in certain patients with established CHD. The patients recruited in GISSI were Italians who were advised (before randomization) to return to their parents' traditional Mediterranean diet, and did so[50]. This means that the diet of the GISSI patients was probably very different from those followed (but never described) by the patients included in other (negative) trials. This is a major potential confounder because the intakes of both PUFAs and vitamin E may have been different in the various trials. For instance, the GISSI patients may have been relatively deficient in vitamin E (as compared with patients of other trials with diet rich in PUFAs and vitamin E), and may therefore have benefited from vitamin E supplementation. The vitamin E data of the GISSI trial do not stand in isolation. In an in vivo dog model of myocardial ischemia[55,] a protective effect of vitamin E on the incidence of ventricular fibrillation (the main mechanism of sudden cardiac death) was reported, with

a 16% rate in the vitamin E group and 44% in the placebo group (p<0.05).
Also in line with the GISSI results, infarct size, the main determinant of
acute heart failure and non-sudden cardiac death, was larger in the
supplemented group (58.5% of the ischemic area) than in the placebo group
(41.9%, p<0.05). Such two-sided effects of vitamin E may at least partly
explain why its effects were neutral or nonsignificant in many studies, with
the negative effects hiding the beneficial ones. Nevertheless, the GISSI trial
showed that cardiovascular mortality and sudden cardiac death were
significantly reduced by vitamin E, and the effect on overall mortality
showed a favorable trend (p=0.07).

   Although much less is known about GT than about AT, a lot of evidence
suggests that GT (the main form of dietary vitamin E) may be important in
the defense against CHD. Several investigations found that plasma GT
concentrations are inversely associated with increased mortality due to
CHD[56,57]. Also, in a seven-year follow-up study of more than 34,000 postmenopausal women, Kushi et al reported that dietary GT, but not
supplemental vitamin E, was inversely associated with the risk of CHD[58].
No trial so far has specifically tested the effect of GT on CHD. In contrast,
in a study of a low-risk population, Hak et al reported a surprising positive
association between plasma GT and the risk of CHD[59]. There are several
explanations to these discrepant data. First, AT (and not GT) is the major
form of vitamin E in supplements, and high doses of AT reduce plasma GT
levels. Second, plasma GT may not reflect dietary vitamin E, due to the
active urinary excretion of GT. Finally, both dietary and plasma GT are
correlated with the intake of trans fatty acids[59], a family of fatty acids
known to be toxic for the heart. Thus, GT could be a marker of trans fatty
acid intake that is strongly and positively associated with CHD. This means
that these different dietary and blood factors are intimately connected and
that in spite of various adjustments, it seems difficult to adequately control
for these many confounders. On the whole, the above mentioned data seem
to warrant further investigations into the role of dietary vitamin E (either AT
or GT) in CHD. At present, however, scientific evidence supports
recommending consumption of a diet high in foods providing antioxidants
and other cardioprotective nutrients, such as fruit, vegetables, whole grains
and nuts, instead of antioxidant supplements, to reduce the risk of CHD, as
recently summarized in an American Heart Association Science Advisory[60].
On the other hand, this does not mean that antioxidant supplements cannot
be useful for purposes other than the secondary prevention of CHD. It is
another question not discussed in the present text.

Vitamin C

Vitamin C (ascorbic acid) also is an essential micronutrient required for normal metabolic functioning of the human body. A lack of vitamin C in the diet causes scurvy, a potentially fatal deficiency disease that can be prevented with as little as ten mg vitamin per day, an amount easily obtained from fresh fruit and vegetables. The current recommended dietary allowance (RDA) is 60 mg/day for healthy adults and is determined by the turnover and depletion rates of an initial body pool of 1500 mg vitamin C and an assumed absorption of 85% of the vitamin at usual intakes. This amount would prevent the development of scurvy for about one month with a diet lacking vitamin C[61]. However, the amount of vitamin C required to prevent scurvy is lower than that necessary to maintain optimal health and prevent chronic diseases such as cancer, cataract and CHD. The antiscorbutic effect of vitamin C is assumed to be based on its action on the biosynthesis of collagen, carnitine and neurotransmitters (catecholamines), whereas the preventive effect of vitamin C against CHD is primarily based on its antioxidant effects. As a matter of fact, vitamin C readily scavenges ROS and nitrogen species in various conditions[61]. On the other hand, the reduction of metal ions such as copper and iron by vitamin C can result in the formation of highly reactive oxygen radicals, a process known as Fenton reaction. There is no convincing evidence that this process occurs in vivo in humans. Finally, vitamin C autoxidation can yield products (ascorbates) that can react with some proteins and result in the formation of carboxymethyllysine (protein carbonyls), which has been identified in human tissues and may contribute to the development of chronic diseases such as CHD and Alzheimer's disease[62,63]. Thus, vitamin C seems to be a quite ambiguous prooxidant-antioxidant compound in humans.

Epidemiological studies investigating the relation between vitamin C intake and CHD have yielded conflicting results. So far, all the evidence from prospective studies suggests that only a minimal intake of vitamin C is required to optimally reduce the risk of CHD, and that there is little or no additional benefit from vitamin C intakes higher than 100 mg/day, probably because of tissue saturation at this level[61]. Several investigators have measured blood vitamin C levels, which is a more accurate and reliable measure of body vitamin C status than the dietary intake as estimated from questionnaires. From these observational studies, it can be proposed that plasma vitamin C concentrations higher than 50 µmol/L (usually achieved with a dietary intake of 100 mg/day) provide an optimal benefit with regard to CHD prevention[61]. It is noteworthy, however, that the inverse association between plasma vitamin C and the risk of CHD was substantially reduced in most studies after adjustment for smoking. This finding is not surprising, given the known effect of smoking on plasma vitamin C. This suggests that the increased risk of CHD for smokers is partly related to reduced vitamin C concentrations. Thus, at least in theory, smokers need more vitamin C than nonsmokers. The elderly also are prone to vitamin C deficiency and also have a higher requirement for vitamin C. In fact, in a recent study, low blood vitamin C levels were strongly predictive of mortality in the older British population[64]. Thus, it seems that the protective effect of vitamin C against CHD seen in population studies essentially results from an effect in smokers and the elderly. The next question is whether data from randomized trials would confirm epidemiological studies regarding the protective effect of vitamin C against CHD. As far as we know, there is no published trial (with an acceptable methodology) testing the effect of vitamin C alone in patients with established CHD or in primary prevention, in particular in smokers and the elderly. Studies combining vitamin C with vitamin E at various doses produce conflicting data, with either encouraging results[65,66] when using a surrogate endpoint (progression of atherosclerosis as evaluated by ultrasonography) or negative results when assessing clinical endpoints[53].

Another major question raised from these quite confusing data is whether a purified nutrient, for instance vitamin C, has the same health benefit as the whole food or mixture of foods in which the nutrient is present. It has been recently shown that the vitamin C in unpeeled fresh apples accounts for only less than 1% of the total antioxidant activity, suggesting that most of the antioxidant activity of fruit and vegetables may come from phenolics and flavonoids[67]. Thus, if such data are confirmed, the obvious conclusion is that we must get our dietary antioxidants by eating fruit and vegetables (and drinking antioxidant-rich beverages such as wine and tea) rather than by taking supplements, even under the form of "antioxidant cocktails".

Polyphenols

Polyphenols are reducing agents that protect body tissues against oxidative stress, together with other dietary reducing agents (see above). They are the most abundant antioxidants in our diets, and epidemiological studies have suggested associations between the consumption of polyphenol-rich foods (fruit and vegetables) or beverages (wine and tea) and the prevention of major chronic diseases such as cancers and CHD. No trial results have been published to date.

Polyphenols are characterized by a considerable diversity of structures, and several thousands of natural polyphenols have been identified in plants and plant foods. In order to understand their impact on human health, we need to know the nature of the main polyphenols ingested with our daily diet and their bioavailability[68]. Another issue is how (by which methods) the effects of exposure to dietary polyphenols should be assessed. Several studies have tried and identified the nature of the polyphenols to which circulating cells and tissues are exposed in vivo. Dietary polyphenols actually undergo extensive modifications during first-pass metabolization, so that the forms entering the blood and tissues are generally not the same as the dietary sources. Thus, great efforts are warranted to define the biological activities of polyphenols in humans, taking into account their specific bioavailability and metabolization[69].

Nature and dietary intake of polyphenols

The main classes of polyphenols are defined according to the nature of their carbon skeleton: simple phenols and phenolic acids(1), flavonoids(2), the less common stilbenes and lignans(3) and other ill-defined phenolic polymers(4). See *Table 3* for a schematic description of polyphenols.

Table 3: **Main polyphenols**

Polyphenols			
Simple phenols and phenolic acids	Flavonoids	Stilbenes and Lignans	Ill-defined phenolic polymers
Tea	See table 4	Red grapes	Wines
Coffee		Wine	Tea
Vanilla		Berries	
Cherry		Peanuts	
Blueberry		Flaxseed	
Citrus fruit		Whole-grain foods	
Plum		Prunes	
Whole-grain foods		Garlic	
		Asparagus	

Phenolic acids

Phenolic acids are quite abundant in foods. The most common one is caffeic acid, often found in the form of esters (chlorogenic acid) that are present in many fruits and in coffee.

Flavonoids

Flavonoids are the most abundant polyphenols in our diet. They can be divided into several classes according to the degree of oxidation of oxygen heterocycles (*Table 4*): flavones, flavonols, flavanols, isoflavones, flavanones, anthocyanins and proanthocyanidins. However, the occurrence of some of these flavonoids is restricted to a few foodstuffs. For instance, the main source of isoflavones is soy, which contains about 1 mg of genistein and daidzein per gram of dry bean and has received considerable attention due to its estrogenic properties (see below). Citrus fruits are the main sources of flavanones, the most commonly consumed form being hesperidin from oranges.

Table 4: **Main flavonoids according to Scalbert et al** (réf 68)

Flavonoids						
Isoflavones	Proantho-cyanidins (polymeric flavanols)	Anthocyanins	Flavonols	Flavones	Flavanols	Flavanones
Soy beans Red clover leaf Barley Brown rice Whole wheat Flaxseed	Fruit (pears, apples, grapes, …) Wine Tea	Berries Wine Grapes Tea	Onion Curly kale Leek Broccoli Blueberry Red wine Green tea Tomatoes	Parsley Red pepper Celery Citrus fruit Onion	Apricot Tea Red wine Grapes Chocolate Apple	Citrus fruit

Other flavonoids are common to various foods. The main flavonol in our diet is quercetin, which is present in many fruits, vegetables and beverages (wine). It is particularly abundant in onions and tea. Flavones are less common and were identified in red pepper and celery. The main flavanols are catechins, which are very abundant in tea. An infusion of green tea contains about 1 g/L catechins, whereas their content in black tea is reduced by about 50% due to fermentation. Other major sources of catechins are red wine and chocolate. Proanthocyanidins are polymeric flavanols present in plants as complex polymer blends. They are responsible for the astringency of foods. They are present in many fruits, including pears, apples and grapes, and in beverages such as wine and tea. Anthocyanins are pigments in red fruits such as berries, cherries, plums and grapes.

Stilbenes

Stilbenes are not common in food plants. One of them, resveratrol, has recently received considerable attention for its potential anticarcinogenic properties and presence in very large amounts in wine. The dietary sources of lignans are essentially flaxseed (linseed) and flaxseed oil. These substances have been recognized as phytoestrogens.

Other dietary polyphenols

Other dietary polyphenols are ill-defined chemical entities, usually resulting from food processing (fermentation, storage, cooking and other processes). These phenolic compounds are the main polyphenols in black tea and wine[68].

For a number of reasons, it is difficult to estimate the average daily intake of polyphenols. Most authors refer to data published more than 25 years ago and reporting a daily intake of one gram of total phenols[70]. Plasma concentrations of the intact parent polyphenols are often low and do not account on their own for the increase in the antioxidant capacity of the plasma[68]. Metabolites also contribute to increase this antioxidant capacity. For instance, polyphenols can be methylated, and about 20% of the catechin present in the plasma one hour only after the ingestion of red wine has been found to be methylated[71]. Microbial metabolites formed in the colon are also important, and equol may be three to four times more abundant in the plasma than the parent isoflavones[72]. The measurement of total plasma antioxidant capacity after consuming polyphenol-rich foods allows comparing the relative contribution of metabolites and parent polyphenols. Scalbert *et al.* have calculated that after drinking 300 ml of red wine containing about 500 mg of polyphenols, the total polyphenol concentration is about ten times higher than the calculated peak concentration of parent polyphenols[68], indicating that the metabolites formed in our tissues or by the microflora in the colon significantly contribute to the acquired antioxidant activity.

Clinical and epidemiological data

Clinical and epidemiological data about the effects of polyphenols on CHD shall now be presented and discussed on the basis of selected polyphenol-rich foods and beverages.

Tea,

Tea, the major source of flavonoids in certain Western populations, seems to reduce the risk of CHD. Several studies in various populations have indeed suggested an inverse association between tea consumption and CHD[73-75], and a meta-analysis confirmed this trend in spite of highly heterogeneous results between studies[76]. Geographic variations may explain this heterogeneity, with a positive association between tea consumption and CHD in the United Kingdom (where people usually add milk to their tea) and negative associations almost everywhere else. Interestingly, the negative associations were found among drinkers of either black tea, as in Saudi Arabia[77], or green tea, as in Japan[78]. Finally, it is noteworthy that tea consumption was associated with beneficial effects on some major risk factors of CHD such as hypertension[79], obesity and body fat distribution[80], as well as on the risk of osteoporosis[81] and cancers[82]. However, data from randomized trials are not available.

Wine

Wine is another polyphenol-rich beverage whose moderate consumption has been associated with a reduced risk of CHD. Contrary to tea, in which there is practically no substance other than water and polyphenols to explain any health effect, wine also contains ethanol which is, by itself, a potent cardioprotective compound especially when taken in moderate amounts[83,84]. One question is whether wine is more protective against CHD than other alcoholic beverages in relation with the presence of high amounts of polyphenols[85-88]. The presence of polyphenols in abundance in wine, but not in beer or spirits, should intuitively lead to think that wine drinking results in better protection. In fact, clinical and epidemiological data do not provide a concluding answer, because no study has been prospectively and specifically designed to compare the effect of the various alcoholic beverages. On the other hand, experimental data suggest that, in addition to an effect on various parameters assumed to be associated with CHD, polyphenols may have a specific protective effect on the ischemic myocardium, a phenomenon called preconditioning[89]. Among polyphenols, resveratrol has been particularly studied in various experimental models, and data suggest that it may act through an effect on nitric oxide (NO) synthase activity and NO generation[90-93]. However, as suggested by other investigators, resveratrol may be cardioprotective through other mechanisms, in particular by interfering with the aryl hydrocarbon receptor involved in dioxin (and cigarette smoke) toxicity[94]. Finally, other polyphenols such as proanthocyanidins may play a role in the cardioprotective (preconditioning) effect of wine drinking[95]. Whether that protection is directly linked to an antioxidant or anti-inflammatory[96] effect remains an open question.

Soy foods

The present renaissance in soy foods is driven largely by documented research on the potential health benefits of soy isoflavones[97]. This is the consequence of the discovery that soybeans and most soy protein products are the richest source of isoflavones, an important class of bioactive phytoestrogens that, once absorbed, exceed estradiol levels by several orders of magnitude[98]. However, it has been discovered that the clinical effectiveness of soy protein in CHD (or bone and menopausal health) may be a function of the ability to biotransform soy isoflavones into equol, a more potent estrogenic isoflavone that is exclusively a product of intestinal bacterial metabolization of daidzein, a dietary isoflavone found in abundance in soybeans and most soy foods[99]. However, equol is not produced in all healthy adults and the highest clinical responses to soy protein diets seem to occur in people who are good "equol producers"[99]. For unclear reasons, about 40-50% of adults are "non-equol producers". It is likely that some specific components of the diet influence bacterial conversion of daidzein to equol, while the use of antibiotic swiping out the intestinal flora can stop the formation of equol. Finally, equol has the greatest in vitro antioxidant activity among all the isoflavones tested[100], and most studies conducted in vivo in humans concluded that soy protein diets significantly reduce lipid peroxidation (in particular F2-isoprostane concentrations) and increase the resistance of lipoproteins to oxidation[101], which theoretically may reduce the risk of CHD.

Whole-grain foods

Whole-grain foods are emerging as dietary constituent that delivers significant health benefits. Several studies have provided strong support for a beneficial role of whole grain intake in reducing the risk of CHD[102]. Whole grains supply complex carbohydrates, resistant starch, dietary fiber, minerals, vitamins, and phytochemicals that can serve as antioxidants. Whole-grain foods are indeed rich in phenolic acids as well as lignans that are formed of two phenylpropane units (a structure not very different from that of resveratrol). The main dietary source of lignans in the Western diet is linseed (flaxseed). Other cereals (wheat), grains, fruit (prunes), and certain vegetables (garlic, asparagus) also contain traces of lignans that are metabolized to enterodiol and enterolactone by the intestinal microflora and found in the blood and urine of animals and humans. However, the low amounts of lignans supplied by our normal diet do not account for the high concentrations of their metabolites measured in blood and urine. Other dietary sources of lignans, the precursors of enterodiol and enterolactone, have yet to be identified[103]. In a recently published prospective study, Finnish investigators found an inverse relation between high serum enterolactone levels (as a marker of a diet high in fiber and vegetables) and the risk of CHD death[104]. They also found an inverse association between F2-isoprostanes, a measure of lipid peroxidation, and serum enterolactone levels, suggesting that lignans may be cardioprotective through an antioxidant effect[105].

Vegetables and fruits

Vegetables and fruits are major sources of the different classes of polyphenols[106]. Their importance in the prevention of CHD has been the subject of many reviews, and a high consumption of vegetables and fruit is

now one of the major lifestyle recommendations of the American Heart
Association, the European Society of Cardiology and various Sciences and
Research Councils[107].

Garlic and onion

Allium vegetables (vegetables containing allylsulfides), including garlic
and onions, are rich in flavonols and organosulfur compounds that have
antioxidant properties. They have been recognized as medicinal plants for
the prevention of CHD and other circulatory disorders. Knowledge of the
therapeutic benefits of garlic goes back thousands of years to the
civilizations of ancient Egypt, Persia and India. Garlic was an important part
of the diets of both Greek and Roman soldiers and was used as food and
medicine in ancient China. While complementary and alternative medicine,
including the consumption of foods believed to have medicinal properties,
has become increasingly popular in Europe and the US over the past two
decades, experiments in animals have shown that garlic may be a strong
antilipidemic, antihypertensive and antiatherogenic food. Human studies,
however, have been conflicting, mainly because of methodological issues in
relation with the difficulty to plan well-controlled, well-sized, blind studies
that subjects can follow for sufficiently long periods. The main reason of
that difficulty is the characteristic aroma of garlic (leading to loss of blinding
and poor compliance) due to the many organosulfur compounds it contains,
as well as the absence of a standardized preparation. However, most recent
studies used *Aged Garlic Extract* (AGE), a standardized preparation
obtained after dehydration and soaking in 15-20% aqueous ethanol solution
at room temperature for at long as 20 months. AGE contains most natural
constituents of fresh garlic, including all the essential amino acids and a
variety of vitamins and minerals, in particular selenium. The
hypocholesterolemic effect of garlic is believed to result from organosulfur
compounds and their inhibitory effect on HMGCoA reductase activity.
Several meta-analyses have been published and, taking into account the
methodological difficulties mentioned above, it can be concluded that AGE
may be an interesting way of reducing serum cholesterol in association (or
not) with classical cholesterol-lowering drugs, with the major advantage that
no significant adverse effects have been reported[108].

Some garlic preparations have been claimed to possess antioxidant
properties, whereas others are said to stimulate oxidation[109]. Dillon et al
showed that AGE was antioxidant (using the peroxidation marker
isoprostane) and more effective in smokers than in nonsmoking men[110].
However, further studies are needed to ascertain the in vivo biological
effects (including the antioxidant effect) of AGE in humans.

Onions are one of the richest sources of polyphenols, especially flavonoids, in the human diet (see the section about polyphenols). Although milder onions are more popular, the bitter and more pungent onions seem to have more flavonoids and could be more healthful. According to recent data, yellow onions are ten times more flavonoids than whites, the onions with fewest flavonoids.

Finally, in addition to organosulfur compounds, onions are extremely rich in polyphenols, especially quercetin (see above the section about polyphenols). Allium vegetables, especially garlic (including AGE), are also rich in steroid saponins that seem to be responsible for the cholesterol-lowering effect of these foods.

Olive oil

The growing enthusiasm about the Mediterranean diet and olive oil is mainly due to the belief that this diet has a positive role in the prevention of CHD. The prevailing theory to explain that protection relates, at least partly, to the antioxidant properties of this diet. Lipoprotein oxidation (actually peroxidation of the PUFAs present in lipoproteins) is currently thought to cause accelerated atherogenesis[111]. Elevated plasma levels of oxidized LDL have indeed been associated with CHD, and the plasma level of malondialdehyde-modified LDL is higher in patients with unstable CHD syndromes (usually associated with plaque rupture) than in patients with clinically stable CHD[112]. In addition, ROS influence thrombus formation[113]. Diets high in PUFAs increase the polyunsaturated fatty acid content of lipoproteins and render them more susceptible to oxidation[114]. In the secondary prevention of CHD, such diets failed to improve the prognosis of the patients[115]. In this context, the traditional Mediterranean diet with its high contents in oleic acid was shown to increase the resistance of lipoproteins to oxidation, whatever the antioxidant contents[116,117], and also to cause leukocyte inhibition[118]. This means that oleic acid by itself protects lipoproteins from oxidation. Apart from oleic acids, other constituents of olive oil may also inhibit LDL oxidation[119], including possibly vitamin E— mainly as alpha-tocopherol (AT)—, squalene, carotenoids, and polyphenols[120]. The tocopherol content of olive oil is highly variable and is mainly accounted for by AT[120]. The adequacy of AT in any oil is evaluated by the ratio of vitamin E to PUFAs, which should be higher than 0.6[121]. This ratio is approximately two in most extra-virgin olive oils[120], indicating that olive oils, essentially because their content in PUFAs is low, are major sources of antioxidant activity as compared with other vegetable oils.

Squalene, a highly unsaturated aliphatic hydrocarbon with antioxidant properties[122], is though to play an active role in the healthy effect of olive oil[120]. It probably regenerates AT by reducing tocopherol radicals.

However, there are a few clinical or biological data to support a role for squalene in the cardioprotective effect of the Mediterranean diet.

The main carotenoids present in olive oil are beta-carotene and lutein. As discussed above, while studies have indicated an inverse relation between carotenoid intake and CHD, it is still not clear whether carotenoids have an effect on lipoprotein oxidation and whether the health effect of a high consumption of fruit and vegetables is mediated through an effect of carotenoids. Finally, it is not known whether the concentrations of carotenoids in olive oil could result in a significant antioxidant effect in vivo in humans.

Olive oil contains polyphenolic substances that affect its stability and flavor. When their content exceeds 300 mg/kg, the oil may have a bitter taste. In addition to tyrosol and hydroxytyrosol, other compounds that often appear in the tables of olive oil polyphenol composition are caffeic acid, cinnamic acid, elenolic acid, gallic acid, oleuropein and vanillic acid[120]. Among the olive oil polyphenols tested for their contribution to the antioxidant effect, hydroxytyrosol and caffeic acid were found to be the most potent[123]. Oleuropein (in large amounts in olive tree leaves) is claimed to have many biological (including antioxidant) properties. However, its amount in olive oil is very small, whereas it is found in very high amounts in olives[120]. Finally, the color of olive oil is mainly due to the presence of chlorophylls that have weak antioxidant properties in the absence of light[120].

The antiatherogenic properties of olive oil and oleic acid have been assessed in vitro by testing the direct effect of oleate on the stimulated adhesion of a monocytoid cell line on human umbilical vein endothelial cells[124]. Preincubation of endothelial cells with oleate for 48 hours significantly inhibited the adhesion of monocytoid cells and consistently inhibited the endothelial expression of VCAM-1, which plays a pivotal role in cell recruitment. Under similar experimental conditions, the effects of oleuropein and hydroxytyrosol were also tested and both cell adhesion and VCAM-1 expression were inhibited, suggesting that olive oil polyphenols may favorably affect early stages of CHD by interfering with oxidant-antioxidant mechanisms[124].

Ginseng

In the Chinese culture, traditional medicine is often used to maintain good health rather than to cure illness once it has developed, much in the same way that vitamin or mineral supplements or herbal preparations are used in Western countries. One of the ways in which many traditional (including Chinese) medicines are thought to act is an antioxidant effect.

Ginseng has been extensively used in Chinese traditional medicine and has become increasingly popular in the Western world for its various (but ill-defined) health effects, and in particular for its possible beneficial effect in CHD. Although there are extensive biological and animal data in the literature dealing with the myriad of effects of ginseng, the underlying mechanisms are not elucidated and the information regarding the clinical effects of ginseng in CHD is even more scattered.

There are two major species of ginseng, *Panax ginseng* from Asia and *Panax quinquefolius* from North America. Both contain flavonoids, vitamins and ginsenosides, a diverse group of steroid saponins producing an array of pharmacologic responses[125] and thought to be the main constituents of ginseng. Among many possible effects on CHD (including effects on platelets, lipid metabolism, and glucose metabolism), ginseng was shown to be protective against free-radical damage in various experimental models[126-129]. However, the authors of a systematic review of randomized clinical trials (published in 1999) concluded that the efficacy of ginseng root extract was not established beyond reasonable doubt for several indications which, however, excluded CHD[130]. The variability in the effectiveness of ginsenosides observed in certain studies[131] further complicates the prediction of the clinical outcome. Thus, despite the widespread use of ginseng as an herbal remedy, more clinical rigorous investigations are needed to assess its actual efficacy and safety. In addition, future investigations of the effectiveness of ginseng must focus on the use of standard methods of preparation.

Ginkgo biloba, aromatic herbs and honey

Antioxidant mechanisms have been proposed to underlie the beneficial pharmacological effects of *Ginkgo biloba* extract for treating some forms of circulatory diseases. However, the antioxidant activity of these products is very variable, probably because of differences in the manufacturing processes between suppliers[132]. Among the biologically active secondary metabolites from *Ginkgo biloba* identified as having an antioxidant activity, the main ones (quercetin, kampferol) are polyphenols[133] described in the above section.

Antioxidant activities and polyphenol composition of various *aromatic and culinary herbs* have been examined using the oxygen radical absorbance capacity (ORAC) technique[134,135] or other techniques[136]. Both a remarkably high phenolic content and radical scavenging activities were found in various herb extracts (especially those from the Mediterranean area) with a linear relationship between ORAC values and total phenolic content. One of the major polyphenol components was rosmarinic acid, whereas the presence

216 M. de Lorgeril and P. Salen

of the flavones luteolin and apigenin and the flavonol quercetin was confirmed in most of the extracts.

Little is known about the components of *honey* that are responsible for its antioxidant activity. In fact, most honeys have similar but quantitatively different polyphenol profiles. Again, a linear correlation between polyphenol content and ORAC activity was demonstrated[137]. Dark-colored honeys, such as buckwheat honey, had the highest ORAC values in one study[138]. These data show that honey may be used as a healthy alternative to sugar in many products and thereby serve as a source of dietary antioxidants.

Supplements

Many antioxidant supplements (with various compositions, various preparations and for various purposes) are currently used by many patients or healthy people all over the world. In the specific context of the treatment and prevention of CHD, where a narrow range of antioxidant nutrients (essentially vitamin E and beta-carotene) has been tested in randomized trials, there is no reason to systematically prescribe antioxidant supplements. However, knowing the apparent benefits observed in epidemiological studies with antioxidant-rich foods, there is no reason to systematically reject the use of antioxidant supplements, in particular by people who are unable to adapt their dietary habits and prefer taking supplements. At this time, scientific evidence actually supports recommending a diet high in sources of antioxidants nutrients, such as fruit, vegetables, whole grains, soy foods, tea, olive oil and wine, allium vegetables (garlic and onions), and aromatic herbs to reduce the risk of CHD and cancers. Such a diet is often called Mediterranean or Mediterranean-like diet and has been unambiguously associated with a striking cardioprotective effect[139-144]. The exact role of the various antioxidant nutrients and foods found with that type of diet remains to be defined.

References

1. Berger A. What does zinc do? BMJ 2002;325:1062-3.
2. Bray TM, Bettger WJ. The physiological role of zinc as antioxidant. Free Rad Biol Med 1990;8:281-91.
3. Rayman MP. Dietary selenium: time to act. BMJ 1997;314:387-8.
4. Goyer RA. Toxic and essential metal interactions. Ann Rev Nutr 1997;17:35-50.
5. de Lorgeril M, Salen P, Accominotti M, et al. Dietary and blood antioxidants in patients with chronic heart failure. Insights into the potential importance of selenium in heart failure. Eur J Heart Failure 2001;3:661-9.
6. Cowie MR, Mostred A, Wood DA, et al. The epidemiology of heart failure. Eur Heart J 1997;18:208-25.
7. Gheorghiade M, Bonow RO. Chronic heart failure in the United States. Circulation 1998;97282-9.
8. Keith M, Geranmayegan A, Sole MJ, et al. Increased oxidative stress in patients with congestive heart failure. J Am Coll Cardiol 1998;31:1352-6.
9. Mallat Z, Philip I, Lebret M, Chatel D, Maclouf J, Tedgui A. Elevated levels of 8-iso-prostaglandin F2 alpha in pericardial fluid of patients with heart failure. A potential role for in vivo oxidant stress in ventricular dilatation and progression to heart failure. Circulation 1998;97:1536-9.
10. Dhalla AK, Hill M, Singal PK. Role of oxidative stress in transition of hypertrophy to heart failure. J Am Coll Cardiol 1996;28:506-14.
11. Bauersachs J, Bouloumié A, Fraccarollo D, Hu K, Busse R, Ertl G. Endothelial dysfunction in chronic myocardial infarction despite increased vascular endothelial nitric oxide synthase and soluble guanylate cyclase expression: role of enhanced vascular superoxide production. Circulation 1999;100:292-8.
12. Ge K, Yang G. The epidemiology of selenium deficiency in the etiological study of endemic diseases in China. Am J Clin Nutr (Suppl) 1993;57:259S-263S.
13. Chariot P, Perchet H, Monnet I. Dilated cardiomyopathy in HIV-infected patients. N Engl J Med 1999;340:732.
14. Ferrari R. Origin of heart failure: cardiac or generalized myopathy? Eur Heart J 1999;20:1613-4.
15. Coats AJS. Exercise training for heart failure. Coming of age. Circulation 1999;99:1138-40.
16. Inoko M, Konishi T, Matsusue S, Kobashi Y. Midmural fibrosis of left ventricle due to selenium deficiency. Circulation 1998;98:2638-9.
17. Xu GL, Wang SC, Gu BQ, et al. Further investigation on the role of selenium deficiency in the etiology and pathogenesis of Keshan disease. Biomed Environ Sci 1997;10:316-26.
18. Recommended Dietary Allowances, 1989. Food and Nutrition Board, National Research council, 10ed. National Acad Press.

19. Yang GQ, Xia YM. Studies on human dietary requirements and safe range of dietary intakes of selenium in China and their application in the prevention of related endemic diseases. Biomed Environ Sci 1995;8:187-201.

20. Coats AJ. Origins of symptoms in heart failure. Cardiovasc Drugs Ther 1997;11(suppl 1):265-72.

21. Takahashi K, Newburger PE, Cohen HJ. Glutathione peroxidase protein. Absence in selenium deficiency states and correlation with enzymatic activity. J Clin Invest 1986;77:1402-4.

22. Burk RF, Hill KE. Selenoprotein P. A selenium-rich extracellular glycoprotein. J Nutr 1994;124:1891-7.

23. May JM, Mendiratta S, Hill KE, Burk RF. Reduction of dehydroascorbate to ascorbate by the selenoenzyme thioredoxin reductase. J Biol Chem 1997;272:22607-10.

24. Zelis R, Flaim SF. Alterations in vasomotor tone in chronic heart failure. Prog Cardiovasc Dis 1982;24:437-59.

25. Okita K, Yonezawa K, Nishijima H, et al. Skeletal muscle metabolism limits exercise capacity in patients with chronic heart failure. Circulation 1998;98:1886-91.

26. Drexler H. Endothelium as a therapeutic target in heart failure. Circulation 1998;98:2652-5.

27. Hambrecht R, Fiehn E, Weigl C, et al. Regular physical exercise corrects endothelial dysfunction and improves exercise capacity in patients with chronic heart failure. Circulation 1998;98:2709-15.

28. Frei B, England L, Ames BN. Ascorbate is an outstanding antioxidant in human blood plasma. Proc Natl Acad Sci U S A 1989;86:6377-81.

29. Meister A. Glutathione-ascorbic acid antioxidant system in animals. J Biol Chem 1994;269:9397-400.

30. Tanguy S, Morel S, Berthonneche C et al. Preischemic selenium status as a major determinant of myocardial infarct size in vivo in rats. Antioxid Redox Signal 2004;6:792-6.

31. Tanguy S, Toufektsian MC, Besse S, et al. Dietary selenium intake affects cardiac susceptibility to ischemia/reperfusion in male senescent rats. Age Ageing 2003;32:273-8.

32. Boucher F, Coudray C, Tirard V, et al. Oral selenium supplementation in rats reduces cardiac toxicity of adriamycin during ischemia and reperfusion. Nutrition 1995;11:708-11.

33. Lopes C, Casal S, Oliveira B, et al. Retinol, beta-carotene and alpha-tocopherol in heart disease, in *Nutrition and Heart Disease, Causation and Prevention,* edited by Watson RR and Preedy VR, CRC Press, Boca Raton, Florida, 2004, chap 8.

34. Ness AR, Powles JW. Fruits and vegetables and cardiovascular diseases: a review. Int J Epidemiol 1997;26:1-12.

35. Asplund K. Antioxidant vitamins in the prevention of cardiovascular disease: a systematic review. J Intern Med 2002;251:372-7.

36. Kardinaal AF, Kok FJ, Ringstad J, et al. Antioxidants in adipose tissue and risk of myocardial infarction. The EURAMIC Study. Lancet 1993,342:1379-84.

37. Kardinaal AF, Aro A, Kark JD, et al. Association between beta-carotene and acute myocardial infarction depends on polyunsaturated fatty acid status. The EURAMIC Study on antioxidants. Arterioscl Thromb Vasc Biol 1995;15:726-32.

38. Rimm EB, Stampfer MJ, Ascherio A, et al. Vitamin E consumption and the risk of coronary heart disease in men. N Engl J Med 1993;328:1450-6.

39. Klipstein-Grobusch K, Geleijnse JM, Breeijen JH. Dietary antioxidants and the risk of myocardial infarction in the elderly. The Rotterdam Study. Am J Clin Nutr 1999;69:261-7.

40. Alpha-Tocopherol-Beta-Carotene Cancer Prevention Study Group. The effect of vitamin E and beta-carotene on the incidence of lung cancer and other cancers in male smokers. N Engl J Med 1994;330:1029-34.

41. Omenn GS, Goodman E, Thornquist MD, et al. Effect of a combination of beta-carotene and vitamin A on lung cancer and cardiovascular disease. N Engl J Med 1996;334:1150-5

42. Hennekens CH, Buring JE, Manson JE, et al. Lack of effect of long term supplementation with beta-carotene on the incidence of malignant neoplasm and cardiovascular disease. N Engl J Med 1996;334:1145-51.

43. Jansen MC, Van Kappel AL, Ocke MC, et al. "Plasma carotenoid levels in Dutch men and women, and in relation with vegetable and fruit consumption. Eur J Clin Nutr 2004;58:1386-95.

44. Stephensen CB, Gildengorin G. Serum retinol, the acute phase response, and the apparent misclassification of vitamin A status in the third National Health and Nutrition Examination Survey. Am J Clin Nutr 2000;72:1170-8.

45. Sesso HD, Buring JE, Norkus EP, Gaziano JM. Plasma lycopene, other carotenoids, and retinol and the risk of cardiovascular disease in women. Am J Clin Nutr 2004;79:47-53.

46. Rissanan TH, Voutilainen S, Nyyssönen K, et al. Serum lycopene concentrations and carotid atherosclerosis: The Kuopio Ischaemic Heart Disease Risk Factor Study. Am J Clin Nutr 2003;77:133-8.

47. Jiang Q, Christen S, Shigenaga MK, Ames BN. Gamma-tocopherol, the major form of vitamin E in the US diet, deserves more attention. Am J Clin Nutr 2001;74:714-22.

48. Rimm EB, Stampfer MJ, Ascherio A, et al. Vitamin E consumption and the risk of coronary heart disease in men. N Engl J Med 1993;328:1450-6.

49. Stampfer MJ, Hennekens CH, Manson JE, et al. Vitamin E consumption and the risk of coronary heart disease in women. N Engl J Med 1993;328:1444-9.

50. GISSI-Prevenzione Investigators. Dietary supplementation with n-3 polyunsaturated fatty acids and vitamin E after myocardial infarction: results of the GISSI-Prevenzione trial. Lancet 1999;354:447-55.

51. The Heart Outcome Prevention Evaluation (HOPE) Study Investigators. Vitamin E supplementation and cardiovascular events in high-risk patients. N Engl J Med 2000;342:154-60.

52. Rapola JM, Virtamo J, Ripatti S et al. Randomised trial of alpha-tocopherol and beta-carotene supplements on incidence of major coronary events in men with previous myocardial infarction. Lancet 1997;349:1715-20.

53. MRC/BHF Heart Protection Study of antioxidant vitamin supplementation in 20,536 high-risk individuals: a randomised placebo-controlled trial. Lancet 2002;360:23-33.

54. Stephens NG, Parsons A, Schofield PM et al. Randomised controlled trial of vitamin E in patients with coronary heart disease. The Cambridge Heart Antioxidant Study (CHAOS). Lancet 1996;347:781-6.

55. Sebbag L, Forrat R, Canet E, et al. Effect of dietary supplementation with alpha-tocopherol on myocardial infarct size and ventricular arrhythmias in a dog model of ischemia and reperfusion. J Am Coll Cardiol 1994;24:1580-5.

56. Ohrvall M, Sundlof G, Vessby B. Gamma, but not alpha, tocopherol levels in serum are reduced in coronary heart disease patients. J Intern Med 1996;239:111-7.

57. Kontush A, Spranger T, Reich A, et al. Lipophilic antioxidants in blood plasma as markers of atherosclerosis: the role of alpha-carotene and gamma-tocopherol. Atherosclerosis 1999;144:117-22.

58. Kushi LH, Folsom AR, Prineas RJ, et al. Dietary antioxidant vitamins and death from coronary heart disease in postmenopausal women. N Engl J Med 1996;334:1156-62.

59. Hak AE, Stampfer MJ, Campos H, et al. Plasma carotenoids and tocopherols and risk of myocardial infarction in a low risk population of US male physicians. Circulation 2003;108:802-7.

60. Kris-Etherton P, Lichtenstein AH, Howard BV, et al. Antioxidant vitamins supplements and cardiovascular disease. AHA Science Advisory. Circulation 2004;110:637-41.

61. Carr AC, Frei B. Toward a new recommended dietary allowance for vitamin C based on antioxidant and health effects in humans. Am J Clin Nutr 1999;69:1086-107.

62. Miyata T, Inagi R, Asahi K, et al. Generation of protein carbonyls by glycoxidation and lipoxidation reactions with autoxidation products of ascorbic acid and polyunsaturated fatty acids. FEBS Lett 1998;437:24-8.

63. Picklo MJ, Montine TJ, Amarnath V, Neely MD. Carbonyl toxicology and Alzheimer disease. Toxicol Appl Pharmacol 2002;184:187-97.

64. Fletcher AE, Breeze E, Shetty PS. Antioxidant vitamins and mortality in older persons: findings from the nutrition add-on study to the Medical Research Council Trial of Assessment and Management of Older People in the Community. Am J Clin Nutr 2003;78:999-1010.

65. Fang JC, Kinlay S, Beltrame J, et al. Effects of vitamins C and E on progression of transplant-associated arteriosclerosis: a randomised trial. Lancet 2002;359:1108-13.

66. Salonen RM, Nyyssonen K, Kaikkonen J, et al. Six-year effect of combined vitamin C and E supplementation on atherosclerotic progression: the Antioxidant Supplementation in Atherosclerosis Prevention (ASDAP) Study. Circulation 2003;107:947-53.

67. Liu RH. Health benefits of fruit and vegetables are from additive and synergistic combination of phytochemicals. Am J Clin Nutr 2003;78(suppl):517S-20S.

68. Scalbert A, Williamson G. Dietary intake and bioavailability of polyphenols. J Nutr 2000;130:2073S-85S.

69. Kroon PA, Clifford MN, Crozier A, et al. How should we assess the effects of exposure to dietary polyphenols in vitro? Am J Clin Nutr 2004;80:15-21.

70. Kühnau J. The flavonoids: a class of semi-essential food components: their role in human nutrition. World RevNutr Diet 1976;24:117-91.

71. Donovan JL, Bell JR, Kasin-Karakas S, et al. Catechin is present as metabolites in human plasma after consumption of red wine. J Nutr 1999;129:1662-8.

72. Cassidy A, Bingham S, Setchell KD. Biological effects of a diet of soy protein rich in isoflavones on the menstrual cycle of premenopausal women. Am J Clin Nutr 1994;60:333-40.

73. Geleijnse JM, Launer JL, van der Kuip DAM, et al. Inverse association of tea and flavonoid intakes with incident myocardial infarction: the Rotterdam Study. Am J Clin Nutr 2002;75:880-6.

74. Arts ICW, Hollman PCH, Feskens EJM, et al. Catechin intake might explain the inverse association between tea consumption and ischemic heart disease: the Zutphen Elderly Study. Am J Clin Nutr 2001;74:227-32.

75. Mukamal KJ, Maclure M, Muller JE, et al. Tea consumption and mortality after acute myocardial infarction. Circulation 2002;105:2474-9.

76. Peters U, Poole C, Arab L. Does tea affect cardiovascular disease? A meta-analysis. Am J Epidemiol 2001;154:495-503.

77. Hakim IA, Alsaif MA, Alduwaihy M, et al. Tea consumption and the prevalence of coronary heart disease in Saudi adults: results from a Saudi national Study. Prev Med 2003;36:64-70.

78. Sasazuki S, Kodama H, Yoshimasu K, et al. Relation between green tea consumption and the severity of coronary atherosclerosis among Japanese men and women. Ann Epidemiol 2000;10:401-8.

79. Yang YC, Lu FH, Wu JS, Chang CJ. The protective effect of habitual tea consumption on hypertension. Arch Intern Med 2004;164:1534-40.

80. Wu CH, Lu FH, Chang CS, et al. Relationship among habitual tea consumption, percent body fat, and body fat distribution. Obes Res 2003;11:1088-95.

81. Wu CH, Yang YC, Yao WJ, et al. Epidemiological evidence of increased bone mineral density in habitual tea drinkers. Arch Intern Med 2002;162:1001-6.

82. Wu AH, Yu MC, Tseng CC, et al. Green tea and risk of breast cancer in Asian Americans. Int J Cancer 2003;106:574-9.

83. Rimm EB, Giovannucci EL, Willett WC, et al. Prospective study of alcohol consumption and risk of coronary disease in men. Lancet 1991;338:464-8.

84. Thun MJ, Peto R, Lopez AD, et al. Alcohol consumption and mortality among middle-aged and elderly US adults. N Engl J Med 1997;337:1705-14.

85. Gronbaek M, Deis A, Sorensen T, et al. Mortality associated with moderate intakes of wine, beer, or spirits. BMJ 1995;310:1165-9.

86. Di Castelnuovo A, Rotondo S, Iacoviello L, Donati MB, de Gaetano G. Meta-analysis of wine and beer consumption in relation to vascular risk. Circulation 2002;105:2836-44.

87. Renaud S, de Lorgeril M. Wine, alcohol, platelet aggregation and the French Paradox for coronary heart disease. Lancet 1992;339:1523-6.

88. de Lorgeril M, Salen P, Martin JL, et al. Wine drinking and risks of cardiovascular complications after recent acute myocardial infarction. Circulation 2002;106:1465-9.

89. de Lorgeril M, Salen P, Guiraud A, Boucher F, de Leiris J. Resveratrol and non-ethanolic components of wine in experimental cardiology. Nutr Metab Cardiovasc Dis 2003;13:100-3.

90. Hattori R, Otani H, Maulik N, Das DK. Pharmacological preconditioning with resveratrol: role of nitric oxide. Am J Physiol Heart Circ Physiol 2002;282:H1988-95.

91. Imamura G, Bertelli AA, Bertelli A, et al. Pharmacological preconditioning with resveratrol: an insight with iNOS knockout mice. Am J Physiol Heart Circ Physiol 2002;282:H1996-2003.

92. Wallerath T, Deckert G, Ternes T, et al. Resveratrol, a polyphenolic phytoalexin present in red wine, enhances expression and activity of endothelial NO synthase. Circulation 2002;106:1652-8.

93. Leikert JF, Rathel TR, Wohlfart P, Cheynier V, Vollmar AM, Dirsch VM. Red wine polyphenols enhance endothelial NO synthase expression and subsequent NO release from endothelial cells. Circulation 2002;106:1614-7.

94. Savouret JF, Berdeaux A, Casper RF. The aryl hydrocarbon receptor and its xenobiotic ligands: a fundamental trigger for cardiovascular diseases. Nutr Metab Cardiovasc Dis 2003;13:104-13.

95. Pataki T, Bak I, Kovacs P, Bagchi D, Das DK, Tosaki A. Grape seed proanthocyanidins improved cardiac recovery during reperfusion after ischemia in isolated hearts. Am J Clin Nutr 2002;75:894-9.

96. de Lorgeril M, Salen P. Is alcohol anti-inflammatory in the context of coronary heart disease? Heart 2004;90:355-7.

97. Setchell KDR. Phytoestrogens: the biochemistry, physiology, and implications for human health of soy isoflavones. Am J Clin Nutr 1998;68(suppl):1333S-46S.

98. Setchell KDR, Boriello SP, Hulme P, et al. Nonsteroidal estrogens of dietary origin: possible roles in hormone-dependent diseases. Am J Clin Nutr 1984;40:569-78.

99. Setchell KDR, Brown NM, Lydeking-Olsen E. The clinical importance of the metabolite equol: a clue to the effectiveness of soy and its isoflavones. J Nutr 2002;132:3577-84.

100. Mitchell JH, Gardner PT, McPhail DB, et al. Antioxidant efficacy of phytoestrogens in chemical and biological model systems. Arch Biochem Biophys 1998;360:142-8.

101. Wiseman H, O'Reilly JD, Adlercreutz H, et al. Isoflavone phytoestrogens consumed in soy decrease F2-isoprostane concentrations and increase resistance of low-density lipoproteins to oxidation in humans. Am J Clin Nutr 2000;72:395-400.

102. Anderson JW, Hanna TJ. Whole grains and protection against coronary heart disease: what are the active components and mechanisms? Am J Clin Nutr 1999;70:307-8.

103. Heinonen S, Nurmi T, Liukkonen K, et al. In vitro metabolism of plant lignans: new precursors of mammalian lignans enterolactone and enterodiol. J Agric Food Chem 2001;49:3178-86.

104. Vanharanta M, Voutilainen S, Rissanen TH, et al. Risk of cardiovascular disease-related and all-cause death according to serum concentrations of enterolactone: Kuopio Ischaemic Heart Disease Risk Factor Study. Arch Intern Med 2003;163:1099-104.

105. Vanharanta M, Voutilainen S, Nurmi T, et al. Association between low serum enterolactone and increased plasma F2-isoprostanes, a measure of lipid peroxidation. Atherosclerosis 2002;160:465-9.

106. Manach C, Scalbert A, Morand C, et al. Polyphenols: food sources and bioavailability. Am J Clin Nutr 2004;79:727-47.

107. National Academy of Sciences, Committee on Diet and Health, National Research Council. Diet and health: implications for reducing chronic disease risk. Washington DC: National Academy Press, 1989.

108. Stevinson C, Pittler MH, Ernst E. Garlic for treating hypercholesterolemia. A meta-analysis of randomized clinical trials. Ann Intern Med 2001;133:420-9.

109. Amagase H, Petesch BL, Matsuura H, et al. Intake of garlic and its bioactive components. J Nutr 2001,131:955S-62S.

110. Dillon SA, Lowe GM, Billington D, Rahman K. Dietary supplementation with aged garlic extract reduces plasma and urine concentrations of 8-iso-prostaglandine F(2 alpha) in smoking and non-smoking men and women. J Nutr 2002;132:168-71.

111. Steinberg D, Parthasarathy S, Carew TE, Khoo JC, Witztum JL. Beyond cholesterol: modifications of low-density lipoproteins that increase its atherogenicity. N Engl J Med 1989;320:915-24.

112. Holvoet P, Vanhaecke J, Janssens S, et al. Oxidized LDL and malondialdehyde-modified LDL in patients with acute coronary syndromes and stable coronary artery disease. Circulation 1998;98:1487-94.

113. Ambrosio G, Tritto I, Golino P. Reactive oxygen metabolites and arterial thrombosis. Cardiovasc Res 1997;34:445-52.

114. Louheranta AM, Porkkala-Sarataho EK, Nyyssönen MK, et al. Linoleic acid intake and susceptibility of very-low-density and low-density lipoproteins to oxidation in men. Am J Clin Nutr 1996;63:698-703.

115. de Lorgeril M, Salen P, Monjaud I, et al. The diet heart hypothesis in secondary prevention of coronary heart disease. Eur Heart J 1997;18:14-18.

116. Bonamone A, Pagnan A, Biffanti S et al. Effect of dietary monounsaturated and polyunsaturated fatty acids on the susceptibility of plasma low density lipoproteins to oxidative modification. Arterioscl Thromb 1992;12:529-33.

117. Tsimikas S, Reaven PD. The role of dietary fatty acids in lipoprotein oxidation and atherosclerosis. Curr Opin Lipidol 1998;9:301-7.

118. Mata P, Alonso R, Lopez-Farre A et al. Effect of dietary fat saturation on LDL and monocyte adhesion to human endothelial cells in vitro. Arterioscler Thromb Vasc Biol 1996;16:1347-55.

119. Visioli F, Bellomo G, Montedoro G et al. Low density lipoprotein oxidation is inhibited in vitro by olive oil constituents. Atherosclerosis 1995;117:25-32.

120. Boskou D. Olive oil. World Rev Nutr Diet 2000;87:56-77.

121. Harris PL, Embee ND. Quantitative consideration of the effect of polyunsaturated fatty acid content of the diet upon the requirement for vitamin E. Am J Clin Nutr 1963;13:385-92.

122. Kohno Y, Egawa Y, Itoh S, et al. Kinetic studies of quenching reaction of singlet oxygen and scavenging reaction of free radical by squalene in n-butanol. Biochem Biophys Acta 1995;1256:52-6.

123. Papadopoulos G, Boskou D. Antioxidant effects of natural phenols in olive oil. J Am Oil Chem Soc 1991;68:669-71.

124. Massaro M, Carluccio MA, Ancora MA, Scoditti E, De Caterina R. Vasculoprotective effect of olive oil: epidemiological background and direct vascular antiatherogenic properties. In *"Nutrition and Heart Diseases. Causation and prevention"* edited by Watson RR and Preedy VR, CRC Press 2004;chap 12:193-213.

125. Attele AS, Wu JA, Yuan CS. Multiple pharmacological effects of ginseng. Biochem Pharmacol 1999;58:1685-93.

126. Zhou W, Chai H, Lin PH, et al. Molecular mechanisms and clinical applications of ginseng root for cardiovascular disease. Med Sci Monit 2004;10:187-92.

127. Fu Y, Ji LL. Chronic ginseng consumption attenuates age-associated oxidative stress in rats. J Nutr 2003;133:3603-9.

128. Liu ZQ, Luo XY, Liu GZ, et al. In vitro study of the relationship between the structure of ginsenosides and its antioxidative or prooxidative activity in free radical-induced hemolysis of human erythrocyte. J Agric Food Chem 2003;51:2555-8.

129. Shao ZH, Xie JT, Vanden Hoek TL, et al. Antioxidant effect of American ginseng berry extract in cardiomyocyte exposed to acute oxidant stress. Biochim Biophys Acta 2004;1670:165-71.

130. Vogler BK, Pittler MH, Ernst E. The efficacy of ginseng. A systematic review of randomised clinical trials. Eur J Clin Pharmacol 1999;55:567-75.

131. Yuan C, Wu JA, Osinski J. Ginsenoside variability in American ginseng samples. J Nutr 2002;75:600-1.

132. Mantle D, Wilkins RM, Gok MA. Comparison of antioxidant activity in commercial Ginkgo biloba preparations. J Altern Complement Med 2003;9:625-9.

133. Bedir E, Tatli II, Khan RA, et al. Biologically active secondary metabolites from Ginkgo biloba. J Agric Food Chem 2002;50:3150-5.

134. Zheng W, Wang SY. Antioxidant activity and phenolic compounds in selected herbs. J Agric Food Chem 2001;49:5165-70.

135. Exarchou V, Nenadis N, Tsimidou M, et al. Antioxidant activities and phenolic composition of extracts from Greek oregano, Greek sage, and summer savory. J Agric Food Chem 2002;50:5294-9.

136. Parejo I, Viladomat F, Bastida J, et al. Comparison between the radical scavenging activity and antioxidant activity of six distilled and nondistilled Mediterranean herbs and aromatic plants. J Agric Food Chem 2002;50:6882-90.

137. Gheldof N, Wang XH, Engeseth NJ. Identification and quantification of antioxidant components of honeys from various floral sources. J Agric Food Chem 2002;50:5870-7.

138. Gheldof N, Engeseth NJ. Antioxidant capacity of honeys from various floral sources based on the determination of oxygen radical absorbance capacity and inhibition of in vitro lipoprotein oxidation in human serum samples. J Agric Food Chem 2002;50:3050-5.

139. de Lorgeril M, Salen P. Modified Mediterranean diet in the prevention of coronary heart disease and cancer. World Rev Nutr Diet 2000;87:1-23.

140. de Lorgeril M, Renaud S, Mamelle N, et al. Mediterranean alpha-linolenic acid-rich diet in secondary prevention of coronary heart disease. Lancet 1994;343:1454-9.

141. de Lorgeril M, Salen P, Martin JL, et al. Effect of a Mediterranean-type of diet on the rate of cardiovascular complications in coronary patients. Insights into the cardioprotective effect of certain nutriments. J Am Coll Cardiol 1996;28:1103-8.

142. de Lorgeril M, Salen P, Caillat-Vallet E, et al. Control of bias in dietary trial to prevent coronary recurrences. The Lyon Diet Heart Study. Eur J Clin Nutr 1997;51:116-22.

143. de Lorgeril M, Salen P, Martin JL et al. Mediterranean diet, traditional risk factors and the rate of cardiovascular complications after myocardial infarction. Final report of the Lyon Diet Heart Study. Circulation 1999;99:779-85.

144. Singh RB, Dubnov G, Niaz M, et al. Effect of an Indo-Mediterranean diet on progression of coronary artery disease in high-risk patients (Indo-Mediterranean Diet Heart Study): a randomised single-blind trial. Lancet 2002;360:1455-61.

Chapter 9

ANTIOXIDANTS AND CHRONIC VASCULAR DISEASE: ANIMAL STUDIES

Tillman Cyprus[1] and Domenico Pratico[2]

[1]Washington University, Saint Louis, MO; [2]University of Pennsylvania, Philadelphia, PA

Introduction

In the late 1980s experimental and clinical evidence showing an increased risk for atherosclerosis in the setting of high circulating levels of cholesterol led to the formulation of two major hypotheses.

The first is the cholesterol or lipid hypothesis, originally based on observational studies in the 1950s, which has now gained support from primary and secondary prevention trials showing that reducing levels of cholesterol resulted in fewer complications of atherosclerosis[1-3]. However, this hypothesis did not address the mechanisms by which high levels of low-density lipoprotein (LDL) cholesterol influence atherogenesis.

Searching to delineate these mechanisms led to the formulation of the second hypothesis, the oxidative modification hypothesis of atherosclerosis[4]. Although it was recognized that fatty streaks, predominantly consisting of cholesterol-loaded macrophages, were one of the earliest signs of atherosclerosis, macrophages incubated with LDL failed to accumulate cholesterol and form foam-cells. The discovery of scavenger receptors recognizing chemically altered LDL such as due to acetylation[5,6] led to further research showing that oxidation of LDL rendered it susceptible to uptake by these receptors[7,8]. Further, basic research accumulated evidence indicating that oxidative modification of LDL increases its atherogenicity[9-11]. So far, several pathways for oxidative modification of LDL in the human artery wall have been proposed (reviewed in[12]), yet, the mechanisms of LDL oxidation in humans in vivo are still not completely known. The oxidative modification hypothesis gained popularity in the 1990s and consequently antioxidants were studied to determine if they could prevent LDL from becoming atherogenic.

Since then, we have seen a wealth of publications with many animal studies lending support, yet the larger human studies failing to show beneficial effects. These discordant findings have generated significant controversy, and many questions still need to be answered and hypotheses have been formulated. For this topic we refer to some excellent recent review articles[13-15]. The aim of this chapter is to critically review the published literature on several distinct antioxidants in animal models of chronic vascular disease, i.e. atherosclerosis.

First, we will present a brief summary of the most common oxidants and relative metabolic pathways, which have been frequently involved in this disease; in the second part we will describe the studies where different exogenous compounds, with putative anti-oxidant ability, were used.

Oxidants and atherogenesis

Metal ions

An extensively studied pathway for LDL oxidation involves metal ions, among them iron and copper have been the most investigated. Animal studies in hypercholesterolemic rabbits came to conflicting conclusions. In this setting, iron deficiency or overload were induced based on the hypothesis that oxidation of LDL may be modulated as iron is a major oxidant in vivo. One study used New Zealand White rabbits on a diet containing 1% (wt/wt) cholesterol fed for six weeks. Interestingly the rabbits with induced iron overload had decreased plasma levels of cholesterol compared with control and iron deficient animals both before and after cholesterol feeding[16]. Neither iron overload nor iron deficiency had a significant effect on the levels of antioxidants and lipid peroxidation products in plasma and aortic tissue or on the susceptibility of LDL to ex-vivo oxidation, yet iron overload significantly decreased aortic arch lesion formation by 56% compared with controls, and iron deficiency resulted in no significant effect. These findings suggest that the effects were due to the lowering of cholesterol and not related to iron's effect on oxidation. Another study used the same animals but on a diet containing 0.5% (wt/wt) cholesterol. Lipoperoxides in liver and spleen homogenates of iron-overloaded rabbits and iron deposits in the arterial walls were increased[17]. Interestingly, aortic lesion involvement was significantly enhanced in the iron overload group in the setting of hypercholesterolemia, but not in the iron overload only group. However, the iron overload plus hypercholesterolemia group had greater lesional involvement than the hypercholesterolemia only group. Statistical significance was reached only in the distal aorta, whereas trends were observed in the arch and proximal aorta. In another study, an iron-deficient diet reduced atherosclerotic lesion formation in apoE-/- mice, and this was associated with a reduction in autoantibody against oxidized LDL[18], and an increase in plaque stability[19].

In summary, animal studies offer no conclusive support for the notion that iron contributes to atherosclerotic vascular disease. This is especially interesting since iron overload in hereditary hemochromatosis (HHC) is causing myocardial injury resulting in cardiomyopathy. The exact mechanisms are not completely understood. However, a recent study in the *HFE* gene knockout mouse model that replicates HHC implicated a direct effect of iron on myocardial injury mediated by generation of free radicals[20]. *HFE* was discovered as the gene for HHC[21], and it has been found to be mutated in a large proportion of HHC patients[22].

Another metal that has been implicated in atherosclerosis is copper. Elevated serum copper concentrations were associated with cardiovascular disease but a causal relationship remains to be determined[23]. The presence of metal ions such as iron or copper has been examined in atherosclerotic plaques, but not conclusive results have been obtained[24-27]. Importantly, copper treatment of macrophages increased the expression of several genes whose products are involved in cholesterol uptake and metabolism[28]. In animal models it has been shown that dietary copper supplementation modulates the formation of atherosclerotic lesions. Surprisingly, dietary copper supplementation was associated with significantly smaller intimal lesions in the cholesterol-fed New Zealand White rabbits[29]. The composition of lesions containing increased amounts of copper was changed towards less smooth muscle cells and a reduction in intimal collagen staining[30]. The areas staining for macrophages did not change. In another study it has been shown that there is a biphasic modulation of atherosclerosis by copper, with dietary copper deficiency or excess being associated with an increased susceptibility to aortic atherosclerosis[31]. While further studies may be conducted to investigate these mechanisms in more detail and resolve discrepancies between human and animal studies, it appears that copper metabolism in humans is tightly regulated and offers little target for intervention in the absence of deficiency or excess, i.e. Wilson's disease.

Reactive oxygen species (ROS)

As members of an aerobic life, we utilize oxygen to transform a large pool of biomolecules in order to obtain chemical energy. This means that when we oxidize these substrates, oxygen itself can become reduced and originate intermediates which we generally call reactive oxygen species (ROS). This is a collective name that includes not only oxygen centered (O_2) and hydroxyl radicals (OH'), but also some non-radical species of oxygen such as hydrogen peroxide (H_2O_2). Nowadays, it is well accepted that ROS are continuously produced in vivo, some accidentally (e.g., by auto-oxidation reactions), some deliberately (e.g., for phagocyte killing mechanisms and intra- and extra-cellular signaling)[32]. Many ROS are involved in vascular physiology and pathophysiology.

The role of macrophage derived ROS in chronic vascular disease has been investigated in animals deficient in a receptor for oxidatively modified LDL (CD36) or 12/15-lipoxygenase (an enzyme that is involved in lipid peroxidation) as discussed below. CD36 functions as a scavenger receptor on phagocytotic cells, recognizing and internalizing oxidatively modified lipids[33,34]. Atherosclerosis was significantly decreased in apolipoprotein E deficient (apoE$^{-/-}$) mice also lacking the class B scavenger receptor CD36[33]. This finding was concomitant with ex vivo inhibition of oxidation of LDL suggesting that blockade of CD36 may be anti-atherogenic[35]. Deletion of the scavenger receptor class B type 1 (SR-B1) was also shown to be pro-atherogenic in animal models using low-density lipoprotein receptor deficient (LDLR$^{-/-}$) mice[36,37] and apoE$^{-/-}$ mice[38] suggesting that upregulation of this receptor may be atheroprotective. More recently, specific macrophage expression of the SR-B1 receptor via bone marrow transplant was compared to mice completely deficient in SR-B1[39]. Inactivation of macrophage SR-B1 promoted the development of atherosclerosis in apoE$^{-/-}$ mice in the absence of changes in plasma lipids.

Superoxide anion

There are several oxidases and other enzymes that produce superoxide anion in the vascular wall, and superoxide dismutase (SOD) is the major enzymatic defense against this anion. Extracellular superoxide dismutase (EC-SOD) is increased in the intima of atherosclerotic arteries, colocalizes with epitopes for oxidized LDL[40] and reduces LDL oxidation by endothelial cells in vitro[41]. With the creation of EC-SOD knockout mice (EC-SOD$^{-/-}$) an animal model was generated where antioxidant action in relation to atherogenesis could be tested. Surprisingly, EC-SOD$^{-/-}$ mice, which had been crossbred with apoE$^{-/-}$ mice, did not have more atherosclerosis than control mice after three months of high-fat diet or eight months on normal chow. Initially, after one month of the high-fat diet the double-knockout mice had even smaller lesions than the apoE$^{-/-}$ mice[42]. The urinary excretion of lipid peroxidation markers correlated with the extent of atherosclerosis, but was not influenced by the EC-SOD genotype. Interestingly, despite initially smaller and later equal lesion areas in the EC-SOD$^{-/-}$ mice, their cholesterol levels were mildly, albeit not significantly, higher. Two more studies with apoE$^{-/-}$ mice as background reported no significant effect of disruption of components of the neutrophil-type superoxide radical producing NADPH oxidases. One used mice deficient in the qp91*phox* subunit of the NADPH oxidase (gp91*phox*$^{-/-}$) to explore the role of superoxide in atherosclerotic disease[43]. The other study investigated effects of homozygous disruption of the cytosolic oxidase p47*phox*[44]. The p47*phox*$^{-/-}$ mice had a reduction in vascular superoxide production. However, neither study showed a difference in the extent of atherosclerotic plaque. More recently however decreased lesion development was reported in ApoE$^{-/-}$/p47*phox*$^{-/-}$ mice regardless of whether they were fed a chow or high-fat diet[45]. These apparent contradictory findings appear to be due to the analysis of more distal parts of the aortic tree in the current study. Indeed, proximal atherosclerosis was unchanged as was previously reported. The suppressed atherogenesis in the distal aorta may be due to a time-delay. Recently, a new animal model of oxidant stress was created overexpressing p22*phox* (Tg^{p22vsmc}) in C57BL/6 mice. Increased atherogenesis in the setting of elevated hydrogen peroxide and vascular endothelial growth factor levels was observed[46]. Interestingly, lesions in Tg^{p22vsmc} mice showed extensive neointimal angiogenesis. Another line of evidence supporting the importance of superoxide anion comes from animal models of restenosis after balloon injury. NAD(P)H oxidoreductase activity is upregulated after balloon injury[47]. In a rat model p22*phox* and gp91*phox* and 2 homologues of gp91*phox*, the novel NAD(P)H oxidases nox1 and nox4 were upregulated at different time points after balloon injury[48]. This was accompanied by an increase in superoxide production and a decrease in glutathione levels immediately after balloon injury[47], which could be prevented by administration of antioxidants in a model using New Zealand White rabbits[49].

In summary, ROS appear to have influence on atherogenesis in different animal models. However, the multitude and complexity of individual ROS-generating or scavenging enzyme systems, and synergistic and counterregulatory mechanisms make it very difficult to assess specific antioxidant therapies.

Reactive nitrogen species (RNS)

Nitric oxide (NO) is a gaseous free radical synthesized in mammalian cells by a family of NO synthases (NOs). It has a relative low chemical reactivity and does not significantly oxidize or nitrate biological molecules directly. However, in the presence of other ROS it can form potent reactive nitrogen species (RNS)[50]. The initial evidence that NO is associated with chronic vascular diseases derives from the finding that metabolites of NO are elevated in hypercholesterolemia, a condition where also the normal smooth-muscle cell relaxation in response to NO is inhibited[51,52]. However, reports suggesting an anti- or pro-atherogenic effect for NO have also been described[53,54]. One possible explanation is that NO alone is anti-oxidant and anti-inflammatory, but in the presence of ROS potent pro-atherogenic RNS are formed[50]. Among them peroxynitrate (ONOO-), the product of the reaction between NO and superoxide anion, is considered the major player in the early vascular lesion development[55]. The pro-atherogenic role of peroxynitrate is supported by data showing the presence of NO mediated oxidative damage in the form of 3-nitrotyrosine in atherosclerotic lesions[56]. Furthermore, LDL isolated from atherosclerotic vascular lesions have also clear signatures of nitration[57].

Myeloperoxidase

Myeloperoxidase (MPO) is a heme protein of 150kDa, which is very abundant in neutrophils and monocytes, where it is stored in their azurophilic granules and secreted in the extracellular or the lysosome compartment following phagocytic activation[58]. In general, this secretion is accompanied by an oxidative burst where ROS are formed, and MPO can amplify their oxidizing potential by generating several reactive oxidants and radicals[59]. MPO can oxidatively modify its targets via several pathways. One pathway involves the conversation of L-tyrosine to the tyrosyl radical and subsequently forming *o,o'*-dityrosine[60-62], and another involves the generation of hypochlorous acid which converts L-tyrosine to 3-chlorotyrosine and chlorinates cholesterol[63-66]. Recently, evidence has been accumulating suggesting that these pathways contribute to protein and lipid oxidation during the development of chronic vascular diseases. Thus, several distinct MPO products are present in atherosclerotic lesions and LDL recovered from vascular atheroma[67-70].

Lipoxygenase

Lipoxygenases form a family of non-heme iron dioxygenase enzymes with a size range of 75-80kDa, which insert oxygen into molecules of poly-unsaturated fatty acids and thereby synthesize inflammatory eicosanoids or lipid oxidation products[71]. Among them, 5-lipoxygenase and 15-lipoxygenase are probably the most investigated. The observation that purified soybean lipoxygenase in the presence of phospholipase A_2 caused LDL oxidation in vitro[72] and the detection of 15-lipoxygenase mRNA and protein with epitopes of oxidized LDL in atherosclerotic lesions[73] ignited interest in delineating this potential pathway for LDL oxidation in animal models. Significant next findings were that 15-lipoxygenase was expressed in atherosclerotic lesions in rabbit aortas fed a cholesterol-rich diet[74] and that transient over-expression of 15-lipoxygenase protein in rabbit iliac arteries resulted in the appearance of oxidation-specific lipid-protein adducts characteristic of oxidized LDL[75]. Also, over-expression of 15-lipoxygenase in vascular endothelium of LDLR$^{-/-}$ mice was found to accelerate early atherosclerosis[76]. LDL from these mice was more susceptible to copper-induced oxidation ex vivo, yet no difference in levels of serum anti-oxidized

LDL antibodies was observed compared to the control group. In contrast, in a model using Watanabe heritable hyperlipidemic rabbits, over-expression of 15-lipoxygenase in a macrophage-specific manner resulted in smaller lesion areas than in the controls[77]. More recent pharmacological and genetic animal studies and their impact on our understanding of lipoxygenase involvement in atherosclerosis will be discussed below.

Antioxidants and atherogenesis

Probucol

Probucol [4,4'-isopropylidenedithio(2,6-di-*t*-butyl-phenol)] is a lipid-lowering agent with powerful antioxidant properties. A great number of studies have been conducted eliciting the effects of probucol on atherogenesis in different animal models. Probucol was originally developed as an antioxidant but has a unique pharmacodynamic and clinical profile and is most effective in lowering total cholesterol and LDL cholesterol[78]. However, it has also been shown to lower HDL cholesterol. Because of the associated HDL lowering and its side effects including QT-prolongation, it is not widely used in clinical practice. Probucol has been shown to prevent oxidative modification of LDL in vitro[79]. It also reduces autoantibody titers to MDA-LDL, a measure of in vivo oxidation status, in hypercholesterolemic rabbits[80]. Numerous studies have shown that probucol treatment results in decreased atherosclerotic lesion development. Such atheroprotective effects were reported in animal models such as Watanabe heritable hyperlipidemic (WHHL) rabbits[81-88], New Zealand White rabbits[89-94], rats[95], JCR:LA-corpulent strain of rats[96], apoE$^{-/-}$ mice[94], high-density lipoprotein receptor SR-B1/apoE$^{-/-}$ double-knockout mice[97], pigs[98], and monkeys[99,100].

Despite this long list of "positive" studies, no effects[101,102] or even pro-atherogenic effects were also found in studies with WHHL rabbits[101,103], Syrian hamsters[104], apoE$^{-/-}$ mice[102,105], apoE$^{+/-}$ mice[105], and LDLR$^{-/-}$ mice[106,107]. One confounder in many of these studies is that probucol lowers cholesterol levels. In order to account for that effect, some study designs used different chows to result in unchanged lipid levels compared to non-probucol treated animals, or the studies matched animals for plasma cholesterol levels and still observed reduced atherosclerotic lesion development[82,83,86,87,90,93,95,96]. While these studies negate some of the above concerns, it needs to be kept in mind that several of those studies showing no effect or pro-atherogenic effects of probucol did so even while the animals had lower cholesterol[101-103,105,106] and triglyceride[104,106,107] levels. Interestingly, some had significant decreases in the HDL fraction[102,105,107]. Some of the varying effects of probucol on atherosclerotic lesion development appear to be dependent on the animal model used and the section of arterial vessel examined. A major confounder in many animal models is the effect of probucol on lipid and lipoprotein levels. Although, some of these effects are adjusted for in several studies, it seems likely that probucol reduces atherogenesis by mechanisms not shared by all antioxidants. One potentially anti-atherogenic pathway may be the increased selective cholesteryl ester uptake in vivo by modifying HDL by probucol, which has been documented in C57BL/6 mice[108] and humans[109].

It appears that different and complex cellular events are involved in the effect of probucol. For instance immunohistologic examination of lesions often find the atherosclerotic lesions in probucol treated animals to be changed in favor of smooth muscle cells and less macrophages than untreated animal lesions. Thus, as atherosclerosis has an immune and inflammatory component, the effects of this drug on growth factors and immunologic factors such as cytokines involved in monocyte adhesion may also be important.

Butylated hydroxytoluene

Butylated hydroxytoluene (BHT) [3,5-di-*tert*-butyl-4-hydroxytoluene] is a fat-soluble molecule that can prevent oxidative reactions and thus has been studied for its antioxidant effects. It was patented in 1947 and received FDA approval for use as a food additive and preservative in 1954. One study showed significantly reduced surface areas of atherosclerosis in rabbit aortas despite BHT raising total cholesterol, LDL, VLDL, and triglycerides in plasma[110]. Serum levels of cholesterol auto-oxidation products (7-ketocholesterol and cholesterol 5 alpha,6 alpha-epoxide) were lower in the group of rabbits treated with BHT, and serum levels of vitamin E were slightly higher in the BHT group. Another study using New Zealand White rabbits also showed anti-atherogenic effects of BHT, this time in the absence of differences in serum lipid levels[111].

DPPD

DPPD [*N,N'*-diphenyl-1,4-phenylenediamine] is another potent, orally active antioxidant molecule, which is mostly used as a preservative. Feeding New Zealand White rabbits 1% (wt/wt) DPPD resulted in increased levels of triglycerides (73%) and HDL cholesterol (26%) with total cholesterol not being different between the DPPD and control groups[112]. After 10 weeks, the DPPD fed rabbits had less severe thoracic aortic atherosclerosis and decreased aortic cholesterol content. DPPD also decreased atherogenesis in apoE$^{-/-}$ mice in the absence of changes of plasma total cholesterol levels[113].

In summary, despite lipoproteins from DPPD-fed animals being more resistant to oxidation ex vivo, other effects such as the rise of HDL cannot be ruled out as at least partially responsible for the anti-atherogenic effect of DPPD.

Of note, DPPD is an orally active antioxidant, which cannot be given to humans because it is mutagenic.

Lipoxygenase inhibition

The first conclusive evidence for an involvement of lipoxygenase in atherosclerosis came with a study on 12/15-lipoxygenase gene knockout mice (12/15-LO$^{-/-}$)[114]. These mice crossed with apoE$^{-/-}$ to generate 12/15-LO$^{-/-}$/apoE$^{-/-}$ mice, had significantly reduced lesion development in the absence of differences in cholesterol and lipoprotein levels when compared to apoE$^{-/-}$ mice. Autoantibodies to oxidized LDL epitopes were diminished. These findings were further extended in a different mouse model crossing 12/15-LO$^{-/-}$ with LDLR$^{-/-}$ mice[115]. Atherosclerotic lesions were reduced in this double-knockout compared with the LDLR$^{-/-}$ mice in the aortic root as well as throughout the aorta at 3,9,12, and 18 weeks on a high-fat diet. The cellular composition of the plaques, however, did not differ between the animal groups with respect to macrophage and T-lymphocyte content.

Using another mouse model, the apolipoprotein B mRNA editing catalytic polypeptide-1/LDLR$^{-/-}$ double-knockout mice were crossbred with 12/15-LO$^{-/-}$ mice[116]. These animals had an approximate 50% decrease in aortic lesions on a chow diet in the absence of cholesterol differences. Lack of 12/15-lipoxygenase was also shown to result in diminished growth factor-induced migration of vascular smooth muscle cells and reduced superoxide production[117]. Data on long-term effects of 12/15-lipoxygenase deficiency were subsequently published[118]. 12/15-LO$^{-/-}$/apoE$^{-/-}$ mice had significantly decreased atherosclerotic lesion areas at all time points from 10 weeks to 15 months of age when compared to apoE$^{-/-}$ mice. Indices of lipid peroxidation: urinary and plasma levels of the specific isoprostane 8,12-*iso*-iPF$_{2\alpha}$-VI and IgG autoantibodies against malondialdehyde-LDL (an epitope of LDL formed as a result of oxidative modification) were significantly reduced in the double-knockout mice in parallel with decreased atherosclerosis at all time points.

Recently, 5-lipoxygenase, which is the rate-limiting enzyme in leukotriene synthesis, has also been implicated as contributing to atherosclerosis[119]. The exact mechanisms and effects of blocking this enzyme on atherosclerosis remain to be determined. These data suggest that lipoxygenases could be potential targets for drug development in atherosclerosis. If this will result in antioxidant effect is not conclusively proven. The available data support indirectly a role for 12/15-lipoxygenase in the oxidative modification of LDL and suggest a proatherogenic role for 12/15-lipoxygenase in several mouse models[114-116,118]. One specific 15-

lipoxygenase inhibitor (PD146176) has been shown to limit the progression of macrophage enrichment of atherosclerotic lesions in New Zealand White rabbits[120,121]. This drug is a specific inhibitor of the enzyme in vitro and lacks significant non-specific antioxidant properties.

Lipoxygenases can contribute to the pathophysiology of atherosclerosis not only via LDL oxidation, but also via biosynthesis of pro-inflammatory eicosanoids. And indeed, data from a mouse model link the 12/15-lipoxygenase pathway to a known immunomodulatory Th1 cytokine in atherogenesis[116]. Another mechanism by which 12/15-lipoxygenase may be involved in atherogenesis may be by the involvement of peroxisome proliferator-activated receptor-γ (PPAR-γ)[122]. Finally, lack of 12/15-lipoxygenase has been linked with diminished vascular smooth muscle cell migration which would be another "non"-antioxidant mechanism[117].

Antioxidant vitamins

Much of the data on antioxidants and chronic vascular diseases in animal models has been accumulated using different antioxidant vitamins. However, α-tocopherol, the chemically and biologically most active form of vitamin E[123], is the most intensively studied in animal models.

Vitamin E

Vitamin E is the most important lipid soluble chain-breaking antioxidant in mammalian cells, and α-tocopherol is its major component and most active form[124]. Therefore the term vitamin E is often identified with α-tocopherol and vice versa. In this chapter, we will use the term vitamin E to indicate α-tocopherol. In the last 50 years a large number of studies have conclusively demonstrated that its principal function in vivo is to defend tissues against oxidative damage. However, in recent years it has become evident that vitamin E also regulates different cellular events all implicated in atherogenesis, by mechanisms only in part related to its antioxidant functions[125]. Numerous animal studies have found atheroprotective effects of vitamin E supplementation. Even if one critically confers less significance to those studies that found these effects with concomitantly observed hypolipidemic effects of treatment[126-128], an impressive number of studies show atheroprotective effects of vitamin E in the absence of changes in lipid profiles. These are seen in animal models using rabbits[126,129-131], hamsters[132,133], guinea pigs[134], apoE[-/-] mice[135], and LDLR[-/-] mice[136,137]. However, other studies have shown no effect of vitamin E treatment on atherosclerotic lesion development in the absence of changes in lipid profiles in animal models of New Zealand White rabbits[91,93,138], WHHL rabbits[88,101,139,140], hamsters[132], and monkeys[141]. Furthermore, studies in rabbits[142-144], chicken[145,] hamsters[104], and C57BL/6 mice[146] found lack of anti-atherogenic effects even in the setting of concomitant hypolipidemic effects.

In summary, a large body of evidence points toward effectiveness of vitamin E in atheroprotection in different animal models. Most of the studies failing to show an effect of vitamin E used low doses and/or could not suppress markers of oxidant stress[147]. In contrast, using the same apoE[-/-] animal model and dosages of vitamin E sufficient to significantly suppress markers of oxidative stress, atherosclerosis was reduced by about 50%[135]. Of note, the dosages effective in this animal model would exceed those given in clinical trials.

Combinations of natural antioxidants inhibit both LDL oxidation and atherogenesis in hyperlipidemic animals but often no strong correlation between measured LDL oxidation and atherogenesis exists among individual animals[137,148]. Hence, inhibition of LDL oxidation alone may not prevent atherogenesis and other anti-oxidative defense mechanisms or anti-inflammatory actions may be important. Thus, combination of antioxidant vitamins (E and C) attenuates myocardial neovasculararization in hypercholesterolemia by preventing up-regulation of VEGF, HIF-1α and protecting SOD expression and activity[149].

One effect of α-tocopherol may be the inhibition of cytokine or oxidized LDL-induced expression of adhesion molecules such as, ICAM-1, VCAM-1, or E-selectin, on endothelial cells. This effect has been observed in cell culture studies[150-152], but could not initially be confirmed in animal studies[153,154]. Another key regulator of inflammation is the nuclear factor-kappa beta (NF-κB). NF-κB activation in macrophages is implicated in atherogenesis and indeed in LDLR[-/-] mice with a macrophage-restricted deletion of IkappaB kinase 2 (IKK2) atherosclerosis is augmented[155].

Not surprisingly, in pigs vitamin E given with vitamin C resulted in interruption of hypercholesterolemia induced NF-κB activation and led to normalized NO activity indicating a role for increased oxidative stress and NF-κB activation in early atherosclerosis[156,157]. Another potential atheroprotective mechanism of α-tocopherol could be the prevention of endothelial dysfunction due to oxidized LDL by inhibiting protein kinase C. This effect has been observed in New Zealand White rabbits[158]. Recently, improved endothelial function, reduced superoxide production and NAD(P)H oxidase activity, and increased eNOS activity and NO generation have been observed in rat aortas in response to treatment with vitamin E and/or vitamin C[159]. Moreover, α-tocopherol is implicated to have effects on several genes at the transcriptional level resulting in effects on CD36, α-tropomyosin, and collagenase, which are involved in smooth muscle cell proliferation, monocyte adhesion and platelet aggregation.

Lastly, under certain conditions, α-tocopherol has pro-oxidant activity, which can be abrogated by co-antioxidants such as vitamin C[160].

Vitamin C

Vitamin C, or ascorbic acid, represents an important water-soluble dietary anti-oxidant in biological fluids[161]. It scavenges ROS and RNS, and effectively protects other substrates from oxidative damage. Thus, vitamin C is a primary antioxidant in plasma, within the cytosol, and also interacts with the plasma membrane. It donates electrons to the α-tocopheroxyl radical and thus recycles oxidized vitamin E[160]. Fed in combination with α-tocopherol ascorbic acid has been shown to reduce atherosclerosis in New Zealand White rabbits[93] and LDLR$^{-/-}$ mice[148]. In the absence of other antioxidants such as α-tocopherol vitamin C does not appear to influence atherosclerosis[93]. However, it is important to note that differently from humans, mice can endogenously synthesize ascorbic acid[162]. Thus, unless mice are in a situation of oxidative stress where vitamin C is used at a high rate and they become relatively depleted, all the studies using this vitamin are inconclusive[163].

Polyphenols

More than 8000 polyphenols in more than a dozen chemical subclasses have been identified. They have a similar basic structural chemistry including an aromatic or phenol ring structure. Present in foods and beverages such as tea, grape juice, wine, and even beer polyphenols have antioxidant properties in vitro. Administration of these compounds resulted in a reduced susceptibility of LDL to oxidation ex vivo and decreased atherosclerotic lesion formation in some animal models: i.e., hamsters[164], New Zealand White rabbits[165,166], and apoE$^{-/-}$ mice[167,168]. However, polyphenols also inhibited atherogenesis in the absence of changes in markers of oxidant stress[169], or lipoprotein oxidation in the artery wall[168]. Interestingly, red wine polyphenols have also been found to inhibit endothelial activation. VCAM-1 expression and monocyte adhesion were reduced as well as NF-κB activation[170]. The implication that polyphenols can transcriptionally inhibit endothelial adhesion molecule expression would be one explanation of their atheroprotective action and constitute a mechanism independent of their antioxidant properties.

Newer antioxidants

In recent years, several synthetic new molecules, all with putative anti-oxidant properties, have been developed and used in different animal models.

TMG

TMG [2-(alpha-D-glucopyranosyl)methyl-2,5,7,8-tetramethylchroman-6-ol] is a novel water-soluble vitamin E derivative, which does not decrease LDL, VLDL, or HDL. It has been shown to reduce the serum concentration of thiobarbituric acid-reactive substances (TBARS; an index of lipid peroxidation) in cholesterol-fed New Zealand rabbits but not WHHL rabbits[171]. Nevertheless, it inhibits aortic atherosclerosis as effectively as probucol in both animal models.

BO-653

BO-653 [2,3-dihydro-5-hydroxy-2,2-dipentyl-4,6-di-*tert*-butylbenzofuran] was designed to exhibit antioxidative potency comparable to that of α-tocopherol, but with a degree of lipophilicity comparable to that of probucol[172,173]. Initial animal studies showed decreased atherogenesis in WHHL rabbits, C57BL/6J mice, and LDLR mice[173]. BO-653 in these models also decreased VLDL and LDL levels. Similar results were observed in another study of diet-induced atherosclerosis in C57BL/6J mice[174].

BO-653,1f

BO-653,1f [4,6-di-tert-butyl-2,3-dihydro-2,2-dipentyl-5-benzofuranol] is another newly developed antioxidant and a member of the benzofuranol group. This compound shows the highest concentration in plasma in WHHL rabbits[175]. LDL from rabbits treated with this compound are highly resistant to oxidation ex vivo. Data on prevention of atherosclerosis in animal studies has not yet been published, but this drug has recently been taken into clinical trials.

KY-455

KY-455 [N-(4,6-dimethyl-1-pentylindolin-7-yl)-2,2-dimethylpropanamide] is a novel acyl-CoA:cholesterol acyltransferase (ACAT) inhibitor. Investigations in hyperlipidemic rabbits and normolipidemic hamsters showed inhibition of LDL oxidation and ACAT activity[176]. In addition, it lowers serum esterified and free LDL-cholesterol.

AGI-1067

AGI-1067 [mono[4-[[1-[[3,5-bis(1,1-dimethylethyl)-4-hydroxyphenyl] thio]-1-methylethyl]thio]-2,6-bis(1,1-dimethylethyl)phenyl] ester] (butanedioc acid) is a novel antioxidant, which has additional anti-inflammatory and lipid lowering properties[177]. It is a derivative of probucol that was designed to retain the LDL-lowering but omit the HDL-lowering potency of probucol and improve the side effect profile. This novel compound has been studied regarding its impact on atherogenesis and shown to inhibit atherosclerosis in

LDLR$^{-/-}$ mice and apoE$^{-/-}$ mice even in the absence of a lipid-lowering effect[178]. Human trials have begun, and recently favorable effects were reported in a trial on prevention of restenosis after coronary angioplasty[179].

Conclusions

Many animal studies show that antioxidant therapies do generally inhibit atherosclerosis, yet some compounds do not provide protection, and most importantly, some of the results cannot be directly translated to the human condition. One of the benefits of animal studies is that they offer more controlled settings and confounders can be more easily controlled. Thus, animal models often allow to delineate pathways and mechanisms of action, that are difficult or impossible to evaluate in primates or humans. This advantage however has pitfalls as the more complex organisms get, the more confounders, alternate pathways and counterregulatory mechanisms may be encountered. An abundance of studies has delineated the mechanisms of oxidative injury in vitro, in animal models, and often confirmed either directly or indirectly in humans. The seemingly logical conclusion that known antioxidants such as several vitamins will efficiently hinder oxidative processes involved in atherogenesis in humans has proven premature, though. Atherosclerotic processes in humans are complex and occur over decades with periods of progression and regression and dramatic events occurring within seconds. Here we performed a review of animal studies involving antioxidants and analyze them for clues as to why inhibition of LDL peroxidation by antioxidants may not account for all of their effects on chronic vascular disease. Many studies seem to support the hypothesis that oxidation of LDL plays an important role in the atherosclerosis of different animal models. Yet, if this role is causative and if antioxidants ameliorate atherogenesis by means of inhibiting oxidative modification of LDL alone remains elusive. Oxidized LDL and lipoproteins are found in atherosclerotic lesions, yet we still have to identify how LDL and lipoproteins in general become oxidized in vivo.

Supplementation with antioxidants has effects on atherosclerosis and markers of oxidative stress in many animal models. However, other actions such as anti-inflammatory mechanisms may be of equal or even predominant significance. As seen with the inhibition of lipoxygenase, the effects that are more predominant for the inhibition of atherogenesis may be anti-inflammatory. Thus, agents with a pure antioxidant function may be of limited benefit in the modification of atherogenesis.

References

1. Blan Kenhorn DH, Nessim SA, Johnson RL, Sanmarco ME, Azen SP, Cashin-Hemphill L. Beneficial effects of combined colestipol-niacin therapy on coronary atherosclerosis and coronary venous bypass grafts. JAMA 1987;257:3233-40.

2. Brown BG, Albers JJ, Fisher LD, et al. Regression of coronary artery disease as a result of intensive lipid-lowering therapy in men with high levels of apolipoprotein B. N Engl J Med 1990;323:1289-98.

3. Maher VMG, Brown BG, Marcovina SM, et al. Effects of lowering elevated LDL cholesterol on the cardiovascular risk of lipoprotein(a). JAMA 1995;274:1771-4.

4. Steinberg D, Parthasarathy S, Carew TE, Khoo JC, Witztum JL. Beyond cholesterol: modifications of low-density lipoprotein that increase its atherogenicity. N Engl J Med 1989;320:915-24.

5. Goldstein JL, Ho YK, Basu SK, Brown MS. Binding site on macrophages that mediates uptake and degradation of acetylated low density lipoprotein, producing massive cholesterol deposition. Proc Nat Acad Sci U S A 1979;76:333-7.

6. Fogelman AM, Shechter I, Seager J, Hokom M, Child JS, Edwards PA. Malondialdehyde alteration of low density lipoproteins leads to cholesteryl ester accumulation in human monocyte-macrophages. Proc Nat Acad Sci U S A 1980;77:2214-8.

7. Henriksen T, Mahoney EM, Steinberg D. Enhanced macrophage degradation of low density lipoprotein previously incubated with cultured endothelial cells: recognition by receptors for acetylated low density lipoproteins. Proc Nat Acad Sci U S A 1981;78:6499-503.

8. Steinbrecher UP, Parthasarathy S, Leake DS, Witztum JL, Steinberg D. Modification of low density lipoprotein by endothelial cells involves lipid peroxidation and degradation of low density lipoprotein phospholipids. Proc Nat Acad Sci U S A 1984;81:3883-7.

9. Daugherty A, Zweifel BS, Sobel BE, Schonfeld G. Isolation of low density lipoprotein from atherosclerotic vascular tissue of Watanabe heritable hyperlipidemic rabbits. Arteriosclerosis 1988;8:768-77.

10. Haberland ME, Fong D, Cheng L. Malondialdehyde-altered protein occurs in atheroma of Watanabe heritable hyperlipidemic rabbits. Science 1988;241:215-8.

11. Ylä-Herttuala S, Palinski W, Rosenfeld ME, et al. Evidence for the presence of oxidatively modified low density lipoprotein in atherosclerotic lesions of rabbit and man. J Clin Invest 1989;84:1086-95.

12. Heinecke JW. Oxidants and antioxidants in the pathogenesis of atherosclerosis: implications for the oxidized low density lipoprotein hypothesis. Atherosclerosis 1998;141:1-15.

13. Gotto AM. Antioxidants, statins, and atherosclerosis. J Am Coll Cardiol 2003;41:1205-10.

14. Griendling KK, FitzGerald GA. Oxidative stress and cardiovascular injury: Part II: animal and human studies. Circulation 2003;108:2034-40.

15. Keaney JF, Vita JA. Vascular oxidative stress and antioxidant protection in atherosclerosis: what do the clinical trials say? J Cardiopulm Rehab 2002;22:225-33.

16. Dabbagh AJ, Shwaery GT, Keaney JF, Frei B. Effect of iron overload and iron deficiency on atherosclerosis in the hypercholesterolemic rabbit. Arterioscler Thromb Vasc Biol 1997;17:2638-45.

17. Araujo JA, Romano EL, Brito BE, et al. Iron overload augments the development of atherosclerotic lesions in rabbits. Arterioscler Thromb Vasc Biol 1995;15:1172-80.

18. Lee TS, Shiao MS, Pan CC, Chau LY. Iron-deficient diet reduces atherosclerotic lesions in apoE-deficient mice. Circulation 1999;99:1222-9.

19. Lee HT, Chiu LL, Lee TS, Tsai HL, Chau LY. Dietary iron restriction increases plaque stability in apolipoprotein-E-deficient mice. J Biomed Sci 2003;10:510-7.

20. Turoczi T, Jun L, Cordis G, et al. HFE mutation and dietary iron content interact to increase ischemia/reperfusion injury of the heart in mice. Circ Res 2003;92:1240-6.

21. Feder JN, Gnirke A, Thomas W, et al. A novel MHC class I-like gene is mutated in patients with hereditary haemochromatosis. Nature Genetics 1996;13:399-408.

22. Hanson EH, Imperatore G, Burke W. HFE Gene and hereditary hemochromatosis: A HuGE review. Am J Epidemiol 2001;154:193-206.

23. Ford ES. Serum copper concentration and coronary heart disease among US adults. Am J Epidemiol 2000;151:1182-8.

24. Smith C, Mitchinson MJ, Aruoma OI, Halliwell B. Stimulation of lipid peroxidation and hydroxyl-radical generation by the contents of human atherosclerotic lesions. Biochem J 1992;286:901-5.

25. Swain J, Gutteridge JMC. Prooxidant iron and copper, with ferroxidase and xanthine oxidase activities in human atherosclerotic material. FEBS Letters 1995;368:513-5.

26. Yuan XM, Li W, Olsson AG, Brunk U, T. Iron in human atheroma and LDL oxidation by macrophages following erythrophagocytosis. Atherosclerosis 1996;124:61-73.

27. Stadler N, Lindner RA, Davies MJ. Direct detection and quantification of transition metal ions in human atherosclerotic plaques: evidence for the presence of elevated levels of iron and copper. Arterioscler Thromb Vasc Biol 2004;24:949-54.

28. Svensson P-A, Englund MCO, Markström E, et al. Copper induces the expression of cholesterogenic genes in human macrophages. Atherosclerosis 2003;169:71-6.

29. Lamb DJ, Reeves GL, Taylor A, Ferns GAA. Dietary copper supplementation reduces atherosclerosis in the cholesterol-fed rabbit. Atherosclerosis 1999;146:33-43.

30. Lamb DJ, Avades TY, Allen MD, Anwar K, Kass GEN, Ferns GAA. Effect of dietary copper supplementation on cell composition and apoptosis in atherosclerotic lesions of cholesterol-fed rabbits. Atherosclerosis 2002;164:229-36.

31. Lamb DJ, Avades TY, Ferns GAA. Biphasic modulation of atherosclerosis induced by graded dietary copper supplementation in the cholesterol-fed rabbit. Int J Exp Path 2001;82:287-94.

32. Praticò D. In vivo measurement of the redox state. Lipids 2001;36:S45-7.

33. Endemann G, Stanton LW, Madden KS, Bryant CM, White RT, Protter AA. CD36 is a receptor for oxidized low density lipoprotein. J Biol Chem 1993;268:11811-6.

34. Podrez EA, Poliakov E, Shen Z, et al. A novel family of atherogenic oxidized phospholipids promotes macrophage foam cell formation via the scavenger receptor receptor CD36 and is enriched in atherosclerotic lesions. J Biol Chem 2002;277:38517-23.

35. Febbraio M, Podrez EA, Smith JD, et al. Targeted disruption of the class B scavenger receptor CD36 protects against atherosclerotic lesion development in mice. J Clin Invest 2000;105:1049-56.

36. Covey SD, Krieger M, Wang W, Penman M, Trigatti BL. Scavenger receptor class B type 1-mediated protection against atherosclerosis in LDL receptor-negative mice involves its expression in bone marrow-derived cells. Arterioscler Thromb Vasc Biol 2003;23:1589-94.

37. Huszar D, Varban ML, Rinninger F, et al. Increased LDL cholesterol and atherosclerosis in LDL receptor-deficient mice with attenuated expression of scavenger receptor B1. Arterioscler Thromb Vasc Biol 2000;20:1068-73.

38. Braun A, Trigatti BL, Post MJ, et al. Loss of SR-B1 expression leads to the early onset of occlusive atherosclerotic coronary artery disease, spontaneous myocardial infarctions, severe cardiac dysfunction, and premature death in apolipoprotein E-deficient mice. Circ Res 2002;90:270-6.

39. Zhang W, Yancey PG, Su YR, et al. Inactivation of macrophage scavenger receptor class B type I promotes atherosclerotic lesion development in apolipoprotein E-deficient mice. Circulation 2003;108:2258-63.

40. Luoma J, Stralin P, Marklund S, Hiltunen S, Sarkioja T, Yla-Herttuala S. Expression of extracellular SOD and iNOS in macrophages and smooth muscle cells in human and rabbit atherosclerotic lesions: colocalization with epitopes characteristic of oxidized LDL and peroxynitrite-modified proteins. Arterioscler Thromb Vasc Biol 1998;18:157-67.

41. Laukkanen MO, Letholainen P, Turunen P, et al. Rabbit extracellular superoxide dismutase: expression and effect on LDL oxidation. Gene 2000;254:173-9.

42. Sentman M-L, Brannstrom T, Westerlund S, et al. Extracellular superoxide dismutase deficiency and atherosclerosis in mice. Arterioscler Thromb Vasc Biol 2001;21:1477-82.

43. Kirk EA, Dinauer MC, Rosen H, Chait A, Heinecke JW, LeBoeuf RC. Impaired superoxide production due to a deficiency in phagocyte NADPH oxidase fails to inhibit atherosclerosis in mice. Arterioscler Thromb Vasc Biol 2000;20:1529-35.

44. Hsich E, Brahm SH, Pagano PJ, et al. Vascular effects following homozygous disruption of p47-phox. An essential component of NADPH oxidase. Circulation 2000;101:1234-6.

45. Barry-Lane PA, Patterson C, van der Merwe M, et al. p47phox is required for atherosclerotic lesion progression in ApoE$^{-/-}$ mice. J Clin Invest 2001;108:1513-22.

46. Khatri JJ, Johnson C, Magid R, et al. Vascular oxidant stress enhances progression and angiogenesis of experimental atheroma. Circulation 2004;109:520-5.

47. Souza HP, Souza LC, Anastacio VM, et al. Vascular oxidant stress early after balloon injury: evidence for increased NAD(P)H oxidoreductase activity. Free Radic Biol Med 2000;28:1232-42.

48. Szöcs K, Lassègue B, Sorescu D, et al. Upregulation of nox-based NAD(P)H oxidases in restenosis after carotid injury. Arterioscler Thromb Vasc Biol 2002;22:21-7.

49. Pollman MJ, Hall JL, Gibbons GH. Determinants of vascular smooth muscle cell apoptosis after balloon angioplasty injury: influence of redox state and cell phenotype. Circ Res 1999;84:113-21.

50. Patel RP, Moellering D, Murphy-Ullrich J, Jo H, Beckman JS, Darley-Usmar VM. Cell signaling by reactive nitrogen and oxygen species in atherosclerosis. Free Radic Biol Med 2000;28:1780-94.

51. Minor RLJ, Myers PR, Guerra RJ, Bates JN, Harrison DG. Diet-induced atherosclerosis increases the release of nitrogen oxides from rabbit aorta. J Clin Invest 1990;86:2109-16.

52. White CR, Brock TA, Chang L-Y, et al. Superoxide and peroxynitrite in atherosclerosis. Proc Nat Acad Sci U S A 1994;91:1044-8.

53. Naruse K, Shimizu K, Muramatsu M, et al. Long-term inhibition of NO synthesis promotes atherosclerosis in the hypercholesterolemic rabbit thoracic aorta. PGH2 does not contribute to impaired endothelium-dependent relaxation. Arterioscler Thromb Vasc Biol 1994;14:746-52.

54. Cooke JP, Singer AH, Tsao P, Zera P, Rowan RA, Billingham ME. Antiatherogenic effects of L-arginine in the hypercholesterolemic rabbit. J Clin Invest 1992;90:1168-72.

55. Beckman JS, Beckman TW, Chen J, Marshall PA, Freeman BA. Apparent hydroxyl radical production by peroxynitrite: Implications for endothelial injury from nitric oxide and superoxide. Proc Nat Acad Sci U S A 1990;87:1620-4.

56. Beckmann JS, Ye YZ, Anderson PG, et al. Extensive nitration of protein tyrosines in human atherosclerosis detected by immunohistochemistry. Biol Chem Hoppe-Seyler 1994;375:81-8.

57. Leeuwenburgh C, Hardy MM, Hazen SL, et al. Reactive nitrogen intermediates promote low density lipoprotein oxidation in human atherosclerotic intima. J Biol Chem 1997;272:1433-6.

58. Hurst JK. Myeloperoxidase-active site structure and catalytic mechanisms. In: Everse J, Everse KE, Grisham MB, eds. Peroxidases in Chemistry and Biology. Boca Raton, Florida: CRC Press; 1991.

59. Hazen SL, Zhang R, Shen Z, et al. Formation of nitric oxide-derived oxidants by myeloperoxidase in monocytes: pathways for monocyte-mediated protein nitration and lipid peroxidation in vivo. Circ Res 1999;85:950-8.

60. Heinecke J, Li W, Daehnke H, 3d, Goldstein J. Dityrosine, a specific marker of oxidation, is synthesized by the myeloperoxidase-hydrogen peroxide system of human neutrophils and macrophages. J Biol Chem 1993;268:4069-77.

61. Heinecke JW, Li W, Francis GA, Goldstein JA. Tyrosyl radical generated by myeloperoxidase catalyzes the oxidative cross-linking of proteins. J Clin Invest 1993;91:2866-72.

62. Francis GA, Mendez AJ, Bierman EL, Heinecke JW. Oxidative tyrosylation of high density lipoprotein by peroxidase enhances cholesterol removal from cultured fibroblasts and macrophage foam cells. Proc Nat Acad Sci U S A 1993;90:6631-5.

63. Hazen SL, Hsu FF, Mueller DM, Crowley JR, Heinecke JW. Human neutrophils employ chlorine gas as an oxidant during phagocytosis. J Clin Invest 1996;98:1283-9.

64. Heinecke JW, Li W, Mueller DM, Bohrer A, Turk J. Cholesterol chlorohydrin synthesis by the myeloperoxidase-hydrogen peroxide-chloride system: potential markers for lipoproteins oxidatively damaged by phagocytes. Biochemistry 1994;33:10127-36.

65. Hazen SL, Hsu FF, Duffin K, Heinecke JW. Molecular chlorine generated by the myeloperoxidase-hydrogen peroxide-chloride system of pPhagocytes converts low density lipoprotein cholesterol into a family of chlorinated sterols. J Biol Chem 1996;271:23080-8.

66. Hazen SL, Heinecke JW. 3-chlorotyrosine, a specific marker of myeloperoxidase-catalyzed oxidation, is markedly elevated in low density lipoprotein isolated from human atherosclerotic intima. J Clin Invest 1997;99:2075-81.

67. Podrez EA, Abu-Soud HM, Hazen SL. Mycloperoxidase-generated oxidants and atherosclerosis. Free Radic Biol Med 2000;28:1717-25.

68. Daugherty A, Dunn JL, Rateri DL, Heinecke JW Myeloperoxidase, a catalyst for lipoprotein oxidation, is expressed in human atherosclerotic lesions. J Clin Invest 1994;94:437-44.

69. Hazell LJ, Arnold L, Flowers D, Waeg G, Malle E, Stocker R. Presence of hypochlorite-modified proteins in human atherosclerotic lesions. J Clin Invest 1996;97:1535-44.

70. Leeuwenburgh C, Rasmussen JE, Hsu FF, Mueller DM, Pennathur S, Heinecke JW. Mass spectrometric quantification of markers for protein oxidation by tyrosyl radical, copper, and hydroxyl radical in low density lipoprotein isolated from human atherosclerotic plaques. J Biol Chem 1997;272:3520-6.

71. Funk CD, Cyrus T. 12/15-lipoxygenase, oxidative modification of LDL and atherogenesis. Trends Cardiovasc Med 2001;11:116-124.

72. Sparrow CP, Parthasarathy S, Steinberg D. Enzymatic modification of low density lipoprotein by purified lipoxygenase plus phospholipase A2 mimics cell-mediated oxidative modification. J Lipid Res 1988;29:745-53.

73. Ylä-Herttuala S, Rosenfeld ME, Parthasarathy S, et al. Colocalization of 15-lipoxygenase mRNA and protein with epitopes of oxidized low density lipoprotein in macrophage-rich areas of atherosclerotic lesions. Proc Nat Acad Sci U S A 1990;87:6959-63.

74. Kühn H, Belkner J, Zaiss S, Fahrenklemper T, Wohlfeil S. Involvement of 15-lipoxygenase in early stages of atherogenesis. J Exp Med 1994;179:1903-11.

75. Ylä-Herttuala S, Luoma J, Viita H, Hiltunen T, Sisto T, Nikkari T. Transfer of 15-lipoxygenase gene into rabbit iliac arteries results in the appearance of oxidation-specific lipid-protein adducts characteristic of oxidized low density lipoprotein. J Clin Invest 1995;95:2692-8.

76. Harats D, Shaish A, George J, et al. Overexpression of 15-lipoxygenase in vascular endothelium accelerates early atherosclerosis in LDL receptor-deficient mice. Arterioscl Thromb Vasc Biol 2000;20:2100-5.

77. Shen J, Herderick E, Cornhill FJ, et al. Macrophage-mediated 15-lipoxygenase expression protects against atherosclerosis development. J Clin Invest 1996;98:2201-8.

78. Buckley MM, Goa KL, Price AH, Brogden RN. Probucol. A reappraisal of its pharmacological properties and therapeutic use in hypercholesterolemia. Drugs 1989;37:761-800.

79. Parthasarathy S, Young SG, Witztum JL, Pittman RC, Steinberg D. Probucol inhibits oxidative modification of low density lipoprotein. J Clin Invest 1986;77:641-4.

80. Schwenke DC, Behr SR. Alpha-tocopherol and probucol reduce autoantibody titer to MDA-LDL in hypercholesterolemic rabbits. Free Radic Biol Med 2001;31:778-89.

81. Kita T, Nagano Y, Yokode M, et al. Probucol prevents the progression of atherosclerosis in Watanabe heritable hyperlipidemic rabbit, an animal model for familial hypercholesterolemia. Proc Nat Acad Sci U S A 1987;84:5928-31.

82. Carew TE, Schwenke DC, Steinberg D. Antiatherogenic effect of probucol unrelated to its hypocholesterolemic effect: evidence that antioxidants in vivo can selectively inhibit low density lipoprotein degradation in macrophage-rich fatty streaks and slow the progression of atherosclerosis in Watanabe heritable hyperlipidemic rabbit. Proc Nat Acad Sci U S A 1987;84:7725-9.

83. Steinberg D, Parthasarathy S, Carew TE. In vivo inhibition of foam cell development by probucol in Watanabe rabbits. Am J Card 1988;62:6B-12B.

84. O'Brien K, Nagano Y, Gown A, Kita T, Chait A. Probucol treatment affects the cellular composition but not anti-oxidized low density lipoprotein immunoreactivity of plaques from Watanabe heritable hyperlipidemic rabbits. Arterioscler Thromb 1991;11:751-9.

85. Nagano Y, Nakamura T, Matsuzawa Y, Cho M, Ueda Y, Kita T. Probucol and atherosclerosis in the Watanabe heritable hyperlipidemic rabbit - long term antiatherogenic effect and effects on established plaques. Atherosclerosis 1992;92:131-40.

86. Fruebis J, Bird DA, Pattison J, Palinski W. Extent of antioxidant protection of plasma LDL is not a predictor of the antiatherogenic effects of antioxidants. J Lipid Res 1997;38:2455-64.

87. Oshima R, Ikeda T, Watanabe K, Itakura H, Sugiyama N. Probucol treatment attenuates the aortic atherosclerosis in Watanabe heritable hyperlipidemic rabbits. Atherosclerosis 1998;137:13-22.

88. Brasen JH, Koenig K, Bach H, et al. Comparison of the effects of alpha-tocopherol, ubiquinone-10 and probucol at therapeutic doses on atherosclerosis in WHHL rabbits. Atherosclerosis 2002;163:249-59.

89. Ferns G, Forster L, Stewart-Lee A, Konneh M, Nourooz-Zadeh J, Anggard E. Probucol inhibits neointimal thickening and macrophage accumulation after balloon injury in the cholesterol-fed rabbit. Proc Nat Acad Sci U S A 1992;89:11312-6.

90. Daugherty A, Zweifel BS, Schonfeld G. Probucol attenuates the development of atherosclerosis in cholesterol-fed rabbits. Brit J Pharmacol 1989;98:612-8.

91. Shaish A, Daugherty A, O'Sullivan F, Schonfeld G, Heinecke JW. Beta-carotene inhibits atherosclerosis in hypercholesterolemic rabbits. J Clin Invest 1995;96:2075-82.

92. Sharma RC, Hodis HN, Mack WJ, Sevanian A, Kramsch DM. Probucol suppresses oxidant stress in hypertensive arteries. Immunohistochemical evidence. Am J Hypert 1996;9:577-90.

93. Schwenke DC, Behr SR. Vitamin E combined with selenium inhibits atherosclerosis in hypercholesterolemic rabbits independently of effects on plasma cholesterol concentrations. Circ Res 1998;83:366-77.

94. Lau AK, Witting PK, Chaufour X, Celermajer DS, Pettersson K, Stocker R. Protective effects of probucol in two animal models of atherosclerosis. Redox Report 2000;5:116-8.

95. Shankar R, Sallis JD, Stanton H, Thomson R. Influence of probucol on early experimental atherogenesis in hypercholesterolemic rats. Atherosclerosis 1989;78:91-7.

96. Russell JC, Graham SE, Amy RM, Dolphin PJ. Cardioprotective effect of probucol in the atherosclerosis-prone JCR:LA-cp rat. Eur J Pharmacol 1998;350:203-10.

97. Braun A, Zhang S, Miettinen HE, et al. Probucol prevents early coronary heart disease and death in the high-density lipoprotein receptor SR-B1/apolipoprotein E double knockout mouse. Proc Nat Acad Sci U S A 2003;100:7283-8.

98. Schneider JE, Berk BC, Gravanis MB, et al. Probucol decreases neointimal formation in a swine model of coronary artery balloon injury. A possible role for antioxidants in restenosis. Circulation 1993;88:628-37.

99. Wissler RW, Vesselinovitch D. Combined effects of cholestyramine and probucol on regression of atherosclerosis in rhesus monkey aortas. Applied Pathology 1983;1:89-96.

100. Sasahara M, Raines EW, Chait A, et al. Inhibition of hypercholesterolemia-induced atherosclerosis in the nonhuman primate by probucol. I. Is the extent of atherosclerosis related to resistance of LDL to oxidation? J Clin Invest 1994;94:155-64.

101. Kleinveld HA, Demacker PNM, Stalenhoef AFH. Comparative study on the effect of low-dose vitamin E and probucol on the susceptibility of LDL to oxidation and the progression of atherosclerosis in Watanabe heritable hyperlipidemic rabbits. Arterioscler Thromb Vasc Biol 1994;14:1386-91.

102. Yoshikawa T, Shimano H, Chen Z, Ishibashi S, Yamada N. Effects of probucol on atherosclerosis of apoE-deficient or LDL receptor-deficient mice. Horm Metab Res 2001;33:472-9.

103. Daugherty A, Zweifel BS, Schonfeld G. The effects of probucol on the progression of atherosclerosis in mature Watanabe heritable rabbits. Brit J Pharmacol 1991;103:1013-8.

104. El-Swefy S, Schaefer EJ, Seman LJ, et al. The effect of vitamin E, probucol, and lovastatin on oxidative status and aortic fatty lesions in hyperlipidemic-diabetic hamsters. Atherosclerosis 2000;149:277-86.

105. Zhang SH, Reddick RL, Avdievich E, et al. Paradoxical enhancement of atherosclerosis by probucol treatment in apolipoprotein E-deficient Mice. J Clin Invest 1997;99:2858-66.

106. Benson GM, Schiffelers R, Nicols C, et al. Effect of probucol on serum lipids, atherosclerosis and toxicology in fat-fed LDL receptor deficient mice. Atherosclerosis 1998;141:237-47.

107. Bird DA, Tangirala RK, Fruebis J, Steinberg D, Witztum JL, Palinski W. Effect of probucol on LDL oxidation and atherosclerosis in LDL receptor-deficient mice. J Lipid Res 1998;39:1079-90.

108. Rinninger F, Wang N, Ramakrishnan R, Jiang XC, Tall AR. Probucol enhances selective uptake of HDL-associated cholesteryl esters in vitro by a scavenger receptor B-1-dependent mechanism. Arterioscler Thromb and Vasc Biol 1999;19:1325-32.

109. Ishigami M, Yamashita S, Sakai N, et al. High-density lipoproteins from probucol-treated patients have increased capacity to promote cholesterol efflux from mouse peritoneal macrophages loaded with acetylated low-density lipoproteins. Eur J Clin Invest 1997;27:285-92.

110. Bjorkhem I, Henriksson-Freyschuss A, Breuer O, Diczfalusy U, Berglund L, Henriksson P. The antioxidant butylated hydroxytoluene protects against atherosclerosis. Arterioscler Thromb 1991;11:15-22.

111. Freyschuss A, Stiko-Rahm A, Swedenborg J, et al. Antioxidant treatment inhibits the development of intimal thickening after balloon injury of the aorta in hypercholesterolemic rabbits. J Clin Invest 1993;91:1282-8.

112. Sparrow CP, Deobber TW, Olszewski J, et al. Low density lipoprotein is protected from oxidation and the progression of atherosclerosis is slowed in cholesterol-fed rabbits by the antioxidant N,N'-diphenyl-phenylenediamine. J Clin Invest 1992;1992:1885-93.

113. Tangirala RK, Casanada F, Miller E, Witztum JL, Steinberg D, Palinski W. Effect of the antioxidant N,N'-diphenyl 1,4-phenylenediamine (DPPD) on atherosclerosis in apoE-deficient mice. Arterioscler Thromb Vasc Biol 1995;15:1625-30.

114. Cyrus T, Witztum JL, Rader DJ, et al. Disruption of the 12/15-lipoxygenase gene diminishes atherosclerosis in apo E-deficient mice. J Clin Invest 1999;103:1597-1604.

115. George J, Afek A, Shaish A, et al. 12/15-Lipoxygenase gene disruption attenuates atherogenesis in LDL receptor-deficient mice. Circulation 2001;104:1646-50.

116. Zhao L, Cuff CA, Moss E, et al. Selective interleukin-12 synthesis defect in 12/15-lipoxygenase deficient macrophages associated with reduced atherosclerosis in a mouse model of familial hypercholesterolemia. J Biol Chem 2002;277:35350-6.

117. Reddy MA, Kim Y-S, Lanting L, Natrajan R. Reduced growth factor responses in vascular smooth muscle cells derived from 12/15-lipoxygenase-deficient mice. Hypertension 2003;41:1294-300.

118. Cyrus T, Praticò D, Zhao L, et al. Absence of 12/15-lipoxygenase expression decreases lipid peroxidation and atherogenesis in apolipoprotein E-deficient mice. Circulation 2001;103:2277-82.

119. Mehrabian M, Allayee H, Wong J, et al. Identification of 5-lipoxygenase as a major gene contributing to atherosclerosis susceptibility in mice. Circ Res 2002;91:120-6.

120. Sendobry SM, Cornicelli JA, Welch K, et al. Attenuation of diet-induced atherosclerosis in rabbits with a highly selective 15-lipoxygenase inhibitor lacking significant antioxidant properties. Brit J Pharmacol 1997;120:1199-206.

121. Bocan TM, Rosebury WS, Mueller SB, et al. A specific 15-lipoxygenase inhibitor limits the progression and monocyte-macrophage enrichment of hypercholesterolemia-induced atherosclerosis in the rabbit. Atherosclerosis 1998;136:203-16.

122. Huang JT, Welch JS, Ricote M, et al. Interleukin-4-dependent production of PPAR-γ ligands in macrophages by 12/15-lipoxygenase. Nature 1999;400:378-82.

123. Brigelius-Flohe R, Traber MG. Vitamin E: function and metabolism. FASEB J 1999;13:1145-55.

124. Azzi A, Ricciarelli R, Zingg JM. Non-antioxidant molecular functions of α-tocopherol (vitamin E). FEBS Lett 2002;519:8-19.

125. Praticò D. Vitamin E: murine studies versus clinical trials. Ital Heart J 2001;2:878-81.

126. Wilson RB, Middleton CC, Sun GY. Vitamin E, antioxidants and lipid peroxidation in experimental atherosclerosis of rabbits. J Nutr 1978;108:1858-67.

127. Williams RJ, Motteram JM, Sharp CH, Gallagher PJ. Dietary vitamin E and the attenuation of early lesion development in modified Watanabe rabbits. Atherosclerosis 1992;94:153-9.

128. Özer NK, Sirikçi Ö, Taha S, San T, Moser U, Azzi A. Effect of vitamin E and probucol on dietary cholesterol -induced atherosclerosis in rabbits. Free Radic Biol Med 1998;24:226-33.

129. Prasad K, Kalra J. Oxygen free radicals and hypercholesterolemic atherosclerosis: Effect of vitamin E. Am Heart J 1993;125:958-73.

130. Sun J, Giraud DW, Moxley RA, Driskell JA. beta-carotene and alpha-tocopherol inhibit the development of atherosclerotic lesions in hypercholesterolemic rabbits. Int. J Vit Nutr Res 1997;67:155-63.

131. Böger RH, Bode-Böger SM, Phivthong-Ngam L, et al. Dietary L-arginine and alpha-tocopherol reduce vascular oxidative stress and preserve endothelial function in hypercholesterolemic rabbits via different mechanisms. Atherosclerosis 1998;141:31-43.

132. Parker RA, Sabrah T, Cap M, Gill BT. Relation of vascular oxidative stress, α-tocopherol, and hypercholesterolemia to early atherosclerosis in hamsters. Arterioscler Thromb Vasc Biol 1995;15:349-58.

133. Xu R, Yokoyama WH, Irving D, Rein D, Walzem RL, German JB. Effect of dietary catechin and vitamin E on aortic fatty streak accumulation in hypercholesterolemic hamsters. Atherosclerosis 1998;137:29-36.

134. Qiao Y, Yokoyama M, Kameyama K, Asano G. Effect of vitamin E on vascular integrity in cholesterol-fed guinea pigs. Arterioscler Thromb 1993;13:1885-92.

135. Praticò D, Tangirala RK, Rader DJ, Rokach J, FitzGerald GA. Vitamin E suppresses isoprostane generation in vivo and reduces atherosclerosis in ApoE-deficient mice. Nature Medicine 1998;4:1189-92.

136. Cyrus T, Tang LX, Rokach J, FitzGerald GA, Praticò D. Lipid peroxidation and platelet activation in murine atherosclerosis. Circulation 2001;104:1940-5.

137. Cyrus T, Yuemang Y, Rokach J, Tang LX, Praticò D. Vitamin E reduces progression of atherosclerosis in low-density lipoprotein receptor-deficient mice with established vascular lesions. Circulation 2003;107:521-3.

138. Godfried SL, Combs GFJ, Saroka JM, Dillingham LA. Potentiation of atherosclerotic lesions in rabbits by a high dietary level of vitamin E. Brit J Nutr 1989;61:607-17.

139. Fruebis J, Carew TE, Palinski W. Effect of vitamin E on atherogenesis in LDL receptor-deficient rabbits. Atherosclerosis 1995;117:217-24.

140. Kleinveld HA, Hak-Lemmers HL, Hectors MP, de Fouw NJ, Demacker PN, Stalenhoef AF. Vitamin E and fatty acid intervention does not attenuate the progression of atherosclerosis in Watanabe heritable hyperlipidemic rabbits. Arterioscler Thromb Vasc Biol 1995;15:290-7.

141. Verlangieri AJ, Bush MJ. Effects of d-alpha-tocopherol supplementation on experimentally induced primate atherosclerosis. J Am Coll Nutr 1992;11:131-8.

142. Wojcicki J, Rozewicka L, Barcew-Wiszniewska B, et al. Effect of selenium and vitamin E on the development of experimental atherosclerosis in rabbits. Atherosclerosis 1991;87:9-16.

143. Willingham AK, Bolanos C, Bohannan E, Cenedella RJ. The effects of high levels of vitamin E on the progression of atherosclerosis in the Watanabe heritable hyperlipidemic rabbit. J Nutr Biochem 1993;4:651-4.

144. Keaney JFJ, Gaziano JM, Xu A, et al. Low dose α-tocopherol improves and high-dose α-tocopherol worsens endothelial vasodilator function in cholesterol-fed rabbits. J Clin Invest 1994;93:844-51.

145. Smith TL, Kummerow FA. Effect of dietary vitamin E on plasma lipids and atherogenesis in restricted ovulator chickens. Atherosclerosis 1989;75:105-9.

146. Munday JS, Thompson KG, James KA, Manktelow BW. Dietary antioxidants do not reduce fatty streak formation in the C57BL/6 mouse atherosclerosis model. Arterioscler Thromb Vasc Biol 1998;18:114-9.

147. Shaish A, George J, Gilburd B, Keren P, Levkovitz H, Harats D. Dietary β-carotene and α-tocopherol combination does not inhibit atherogenesis in an apoE-deficient mouse model. Arterioscler Thromb Vasc Biol 1999;19:1470-5.

148. Crawford RS, Kirk EA, Rosenfeld ME, LeBoeuf RC, Chait A. Dietary antioxidants inhibit development of fatty streak lesions in the LDL receptor-deficient mouse. Arterioscler Thromb Vasc Biol 1998;18:1506-13.

149. Zhu XY, Rodriguez-Porcel M, Bentley MD, et al. Antioxidant intervention attenuates myocardial neovascularization in hypercholesterolemia. Circulation 2004;109:2109-15.

150. Faruqi R, de la Motte C, DiCorleto PE. α-tocopherol inhibits agonist-induced monocytic cell adhesion to cultured human endothelial cells. J Clin Invest 1994;94:592-600.

151. Cominacini L, Garbin U, Pasini AF, et al. Antioxidants inhibit the expression of intercellular cell adhesion molecule-1 and vascular cell adhesion molecule-1 induced by oxidized LDL on human umbilical vein endothelial cells. Free Radic Biol Med 1997;22:117-27.

152. Martin A, Foxall T, Blumberg JB, Meydani M. Vitamin E inhibits low-density lipoprotein-induced adhesion of monocytes to human aortic endothelial cells in vitro. Arterioscler Thromb Vasc Biol 1997;17:429-36.

153. Lehr HA, Frei B, Arfors KE. Vitamin C prevents cigarette smoke-induced leukocyte aggregation and adhesion to endothelium in vivo. Proc Nat Acad Sci U S A 1994;91:7688-92.

154. Lehr HA, Frei B, Olofsson AM, Carew TE, Arfors KE. Protection from oxidized LDL-induced leukocyte adhesion to microvascular and macrovascular endothelium in vivo by vitamin C but not by vitamin E. Circulation 1995;91:1525-32.

155. Kanters E, Pasparakis M, Gijbels MJ, et al. Inhibition of NF-kappaB activation in macrophages increases atherosclerosis in LDL receptor-deficient mice. J Clin Invest 2003;112:1176-85.

156. Rodriguez-Porcel M, Lerman LO, Holmes DRJ, Richardson D, Napoli C, Lerman A. Chronic antioxidant supplementation attenuates nuclear factor-κB activation and preserves endothelial function in hypercholesterolemic pigs. Cardiovasc Res 2002;53:1010-8.

157. Rodriguez-Porcel M, Herman J, Chade AR, et al. Long-term antioxidant intervention improves myocardial microvascular function in experimental hypertension. Hypertension 2004;43:493-8.

158. Keaney JF, Guo Y, Cunningham D, Shwaery GT, Xu A, Vita JA. Vascular incorporation of α-tocopherol prevents endothelial dysfunction due to oxidized LDL by inhibiting protein kinase C stimulation. J Clin Invest 1996;98:386-94.

159. Ulker S, McKeown PP, Bayraktutan U. Vitamins reverse endothelial dysfunction through regulation of eNOS and NAD(P)H oxidase activities. Hypertension 2003;41:534-9.

160. Scarpa M, Rigo A, Maiorino M, Ursini F, Gregolin C. Formation of α-tocopherol radical and recycling of α-tocopherol by ascorbate during peroxidation of phosphatidylcholine liposomes. An electron paramagnetic resonance study. Biochem Biophys Acta 1984;801:215-9.

161. Carr AC, Frei B. Toward a new recommended dietary allowance for vitamin C based on antioxidant and health effects in humans. Am J Clin Nutr 1999;69:1086-107.

162. Nakata Y, Maeda N. Vulnerable atherosclerotic plaque morphology in apolipoprotein E-deficient mice unable to make ascorbic acid. Circulation 2002;105:1485-90.

163. d'Uscio LV, Milstien S, Richardson D, Smith L, Katusic ZS. Long-term vitamin C treatment increases vascular tetrahydrobiopterin levels and nitric oxide synthase activity. Circ Res 2003;92:88-95.

164. Vinson JA, Mandarano M, Hirst M, Trevithick JR, Bose P. Phenol antioxidant quantity and quality in foods: beers and the effect of two types of beer on an animal model of atherosclerosis. J Agric Food Chem 2003;51:5528-33.

165. Wu Y-J, Hong C-Y, Lin S-J, Wu P, Shiao M-S. Increase of vitamin E content in LDL and reduction of atherosclerosis in cholesterol-fed rabbits by a water-soluble antioxidant-rich fraction of salvia miltiorrhiza. Arterioscler Thromb Vasc Biol 1998;18:481-6.

166. Yamakoshi J, Kataoka S, Koga T, Ariga T. Proanthocyanidin-rich extract from grape seeds attenuates the development of aortic atherosclerosis in cholesterol-fed rabbits. Atherosclerosis 1999;142:139-49.

167. Hayek T, Fuhrman B, Vaya J, et al. Reduced progression of atherosclerosis in apolipoprotein E-deficient mice following consumption of red wine, or its polyphenols Quercetin or catechin, is associated with reduced susceptibility of LDL to oxidation and aggregation. Arterioscler Thromb Vasc Biol 1997;17:2744-752.

168. Stocker R, O'Halloran RA. Dealcoholized red wine decreases atherosclerosis in apolipoprotein E gene-deficient mice independently of inhibition of lipid peroxidation in the artery wall. Am J Clin Nutr 2004;79:123-30.

169. Waddington E, Puddley IB, Croft KD. Red wine polyphenolic compounds inhibit atherosclerosis in apolipoprotein E-deficient mice independently of effects on lipid peroxidation. Am J Clin Nutr 2004;79:54-61.

170. Carluccio MA, Siculella L, Ancora MA, et al. Olive oil and red wine antioxidant polyphenols inhibit endothelial activation: antiatherogenic properties of Mediterranean diet phytochemicals. Arterioscler Thromb Vasc Biol 2003;23:622-9.

171. Yoshida N, Murase H, Kunieda T, et al. Inhibitory effect of a novel water-soluble vitamin E derivative on atherosclerosis in rabbits. Atherosclerosis 2002;162:111-7.

172. Noguchi N, Iwaki Y, Takahashi M, et al. 2,3-Dihydro-5-hydroxy-2,2-dipentyl-4,6-di-tert-butylbenzofuran: design and evaluation as a novel radical-scavenging antioxidant against lipid peroxidation. Arch Biochem Biophys 1997;342:236-43.

173. Cynshi O, Kawabe Y, Suzuki T, et al. Antiatherogenic effects of the antioxidant BO-653 in three different animal models. Proc Nat Acad Sci U S A 1998;95:10123-8.

174. Kamada N, Kodama T, Suzuki H. Macrophage scavenger receptor (SR-A I/II) deficiency reduced diet-induced atherosclerosis in C57BL/6J mice. J Atheroscler Thromb 2001;8:1-6.

175. Tamura K, Kato Y, Ishikawa A, et al. Design and synthesis of 4,6-di-tert-butyl-2,3-dihydro-5-benzofuranols as a novel series of antiatherogenic antioxidants. J Med Chem 2003;46:3083-93.

176. Nakamura S, Kamiya S, Shirahase H, et al. Hypolipidemic and antioxidant activity of the novel acyl-CoA:cholesterol acyltransferase (ACAT) inhibitor KY-455 in rabbits and hamsters. Arzneimittel-Forschung 2004;54:102-8.

177. Meng CQ, Somers PK, Rachita CL, et al. Novel phenolic antioxidants as multifunctional inhibitors of inducible VCAM-1 expression for use in atherosclerosis. Bioorg Med Chem Lett 2002;12:2545-8.

178. Sundell CL, Somers PK, Meng CQ, et al. AGI-1067: A multifunctional phenolic antioxidant, lipid modulator, anti-inflammatory and antiatherosclerotic agent. J Pharmacol Exp Ther 2003;305:1116-23.

179. Tardif J-C, Gregoire J, Schwartz L, et al. for the Canadian Antioxidant Restenosis Trial (CART-1) Investigators. Effects of AGI-1067 and probucol after percutaneous coronary interventions. Circulation 2003;107:552-8.

Chapter   10

SYNTHETIC ANTIOXIDANTS AND ATHEROSCLEROSIS: HUMAN STUDIES

Martial G. Bourassa and Jean-Claude Tardif
Montreal Heart Institute, Montreal, Quebec, Canada

Introduction

Atherosclerosis is the leading cause of death worldwide[1]. Coronary atherosclerosis accounted for 7.2 million deaths worldwide in 1996, representing one-third of all deaths in industrialized countries; during the same year, cerebrovascular atherosclerosis accounted for an additional 4.6 million deaths. Moreover, a 28% increase in cardiovascular deaths is predicted over the next five years in developing countries. Based on global trends, the World Health Organization projects that, by 2020, approximately half of all deaths in developed countries and one-third in developing countries will be related to cardiovascular disease. Moreover, coronary artery disease (CAD) creates a substantial economic burden: aggregate costs of CAD in the U.S. exceeded 100 billion dollars in 2000[2].

In spite of significant advances in the management of risk factors such as dyslipidemia and hypertension, many patients still remain at risk for major cardiovascular events which include death, myocardial infarction (MI), stroke, worsening angina, and need for revascularization procedures. It is now understood that atherosclerosis is a chronic inflammatory disease characterized by an excess accumulation of macrophages within the arterial wall[3]. Compelling evidence points to oxidative stress as an important trigger in the complex chain of events leading to vascular inflammation and atherosclerosis[4-10]. Both inflammation and oxidative stress may be responsible for high rates of cardiovascular events in spite of currently available therapies.

Several clinical trials using natural antioxidants in patients with or without documented cardiovascular disease have yielded disappointing results[11-16]. On the other hand, therapeutic agents with known antioxidant properties such as angiotensin converting enzyme (ACE) inhibitors[17-25], 3-hydroxy-3-methylglutaryl coenzyme A reductase inhibitors (statins)[26-30], beta-blockers[31-37], and calcium channel blockers[38-42] have been shown to improve cardiovascular morbidity and mortality in clinical trials of patients with known or suspected vascular atherosclerosis. Probucol, a synthetic compound with potent direct antioxidant activity, which has been shown to prevent atherosclerosis and restenosis after PCI in clinical studies, is no longer in clinical use because of its major side effects[43-48]. More recently, an analog of probucol, AGI-1067, has demonstrated clinical benefits and is under active investigation[49-52]. This chapter briefly reviews the mechanisms of action and the effects of antioxidants, with a special emphasis on synthetic antioxidants, in the prevention of vascular astherosclerosis in humans.

Oxidative stress and atherosclerosis

Oxidative stress plays a central role in the chain of events that lead to and promote atherosclerosis[3-10] (*Figure 1*). Atherosclerosis initially results from endothelial cell injury, leading to impaired endothelial function, macrophage infiltration and smooth muscle cell (SMC) dysfunction[3]. Oxidation of low-density lipoproteins (LDL) and its interaction with the endothelium constitute the first step leading to formation of fatty streaks and to atherogenesis. All vascular cells produce reactive oxygen species (ROS) and ROS mediate diverse physiological functions in these cells.

Current models of atherogenesis link abnormalities in the oxidative state of the vascular wall to interactions with the immune system and to a cycle of localized inflammatory and growth responses that result in mature atherosclerotic lesions[4]. The oxidative modification of LDL may be an important mediator of this process, although the extent of its contribution to atherogenesis has not been directly assessed[5]. Oxidative stress plays a major role in the expression of a subset of genes, which are regulated by oxidation-mediated signals[5]. Monocyte chemotactic protein-1 (MCP-1) and vascular cell adhesion molecule-1 (VCAM-1) are both regulated through a redox sensitive pathway[53,54]. Animal studies show that antioxidants modulate the expression of certain endothelial inflammatory response genes such as VCAM-1[55]. Oxidative modification of lipids, mainly oxidized LDL-cholesterol, is thought to be an important step in the pathogenesis of atherosclerosis[7,8,56]. Observational studies have shown an association between oxidized LDL and presence of atherosclerotic lesions[57] as well as progression of carotid atherosclerosis[56]. Increased oxidative stress has been reported in association with several cardiovascular risk factors such as diabetes mellitus, hypertension, hypercholesterolemia and smoking.

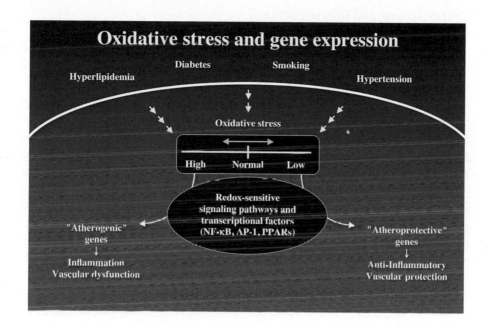

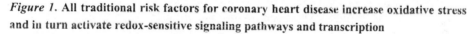

Figure 1. All traditional risk factors for coronary heart disease increase oxidative stress and in turn activate redox-sensitive signaling pathways and transcription

The expression of chemotactic factors such as MCP-1 is enhanced by oxidative stress and oxidized LDL[57]. Endothelial expression of VCAM-1 promotes the adhesion of monocytes to the endothelium. The release of macrophage colony-stimulating factor (M-CSF) is also enhanced by modified LDL[58]. The expression of these factors results in the attraction and adhesion of monocytes to the arterial wall and promotion of their differentiation into tissue macrophages. Exposure of the superoxide ion activates the nuclear factor kappa-B (NF kappa-B) regulatory complex and triggers the transcription of several atherosclerosis-related genes (VCAM-1, MCP-1, tumour necrosis factor (TNF), matrix metalloproteinase (MMP)-9 and procoagulant tissue factor[59]. This series of events leads to accumulation of macrophages in the arterial wall, which then avidly incorporate oxidized LDL to form foam cells. Oxidized LDL, in turn, stimulates the release of interleukin-1 from macrophages[60]. The activity of MMPs is also regulated by oxidative stress and appears to be closely linked to SMC activation and migration[61]. MMPs have also been implicated in the pathophysiology of plaque rupture. Furthermore, ROS can lead to platelet activation and thrombus formation[62]. Therefore, oxidative stress appears to be important not only in the early, but also in the late, stages of the atherosclerotic process.

Atherosclerosis and inflammation

Atherosclerosis is a chronic inflammatory disease, which is characterized by focal accumulation of leucocytes, lipid-laden macrophages, SMCs and extracellular matrix[3,4]. One of the earliest events in this inflammatory process is adherence, migration and accumulation of lipid-laden macrophages and T lymphocytes at the site of atherosclerotic lesions and this event is regulated in part by VCAM-1[63]. Atherosclerosis may be accelerated or enhanced by factors that cannot be influenced such as age and male gender, as well as factors that are responsive to interventions such as cigarette smoking, diabetes mellitus, or hypercholesterolemia. Many existing therapies target these acquired secondary factors without treating the underlying chronic inflammatory process. The nature of the inflammatory signals and molecular mechanisms that activate these inflammatory genes in endothelial cells in the early atherogenic lesion is not fully understood. However, endothelial cells are thought to play a major role in defining the types of leucocytes recruited to the site of vascular inflammation by expressing adhesion molecules such as VCAM-1, intercellular adhesion molecule-1 (ICAM-1), E-selectin, and chemotactic factors such as MCP-1[64]. MCP-1 is highly expressed in human atherosclerotic lesions and is postulated to play a central role in monocyte recruitment into the arterial wall and in the development of atherosclerotic lesions[65]. Factors commonly found in the inflammatory atherosclerotic lesion, such as the cytokines TNF-alpha, and interleukin-1 beta (IL-1 beta), have also been shown to induce the expression of inflammatory response genes including VCAM-1, ICAM-1, E-selectin, and MCP-1[66].

There is strong evidence supporting a major role of VCAM-1 in the pathogenesis of atherosclerosis[67-73]. Animal studies suggest a dominant role for VCAM-1, but not ICAM-1, in the initiation of atherosclerosis[67]. VCAM-1 has been shown to contribute to the predominance of macrophages over lymphocytes in atherosclerotic lesions[68]. Focal increases in the expression of endothelial VCAM-1 has been observed in coronary and carotid artery specimens from patients with documented atherosclerosis[69,70]. Several investigators have also shown a correlation between soluble vascular cell adhesion molecule-1 (sVCAM-1) and degree of atherosclerotic burden[70-73]. Elevated levels of sVCAM-1 have also been shown to be independent risk factors for future fatal cardiovascular events in patients with CAD[74].

Markers of oxidative stress and inflammation

Measurement of ROS in vivo represents a complex challenge. Recent attention has focused on the identification of indirect in vivo biomarkers of oxidative stress such as chemically stable, free radical-catalyzed products of lipid peroxidation (isoprostanes), modified proteins (nitrated fibrinogen) and indices of free radical catalyzed modification of DNA (8-oxo-deoxyguanosine). Autoantibodies directed against oxidation-dependent epitomes in LDL have also been found to be useful in the quantification of lipid peroxidation in humans[9,10].

Although these different assays strongly support the role of oxidative stress in atherosclerosis, it is perhaps the mediators of inflammation and endothelial cell activation that have been most useful recently in assessing the risk for cardiovascular events as well as providing new therapeutic targets[75,76]. The acute-phase reactant C-reactive protein (CRP) is one of the strongest independent predictors of cardiovascular death in patients with CAD[77]. Moreover, recent observations suggest that CRP can also directly promote endothelial cell inflammation and atherosclerosis[75]. The CD40/CD40L system has been implicated in the pathophysiology of severe chronic inflammatory diseases, including atherosclerosis. The CD40/CD40L signaling dyad is present within both early and advanced human atherosclerotic plaques and its role in plaque development and evolution has been demonstrated in LDL receptor-deficient mice that are fed a high-cholesterol diet. In patients with acute coronary syndromes, elevated soluble CD40L levels indicate an increased risk of death and nonfatal MI, which is reduced by abciximab[78]. Indeed, the proinflammatory dyad CD40/CD40L has been shown to induce not only proatherogenic but also prothrombotic conditions. Interleukin-18 (IL-18), a member of the IL-1 cytokine family is highly expressed in atherosclerotic plaques and is localized in plaque macrophages. Significantly higher levels of IL-18 mRNA are found in unstable plaques, and serum levels of IL-18 are increased in patients having suffered an MI or experienced unstable angina[79,80]. Serum IL-18 is a strong independent predictor of cardiovascular death in patients with CAD[80]. Finally, several emerging markers of inflammation and endothelial cell activation are currently under investigation and at least some of them may yield new targets to predict, prevent and treat cardiovascular disease[76]. They include lectin-like oxidized LDL receptor-1, protein-activated receptors, lipoprotein-associated phospholipase A2 and secretory phospholipase A2, MPP-9, and endothelial progenitor cells.

Lack of efficacy of vitamin supplementation

As discussed in chapter 13, the results of large, prospective epidemiological studies have supported a protective role for antioxidant vitamins in cardiovascular diseases. In spite of sophisticated statistical approaches, such observational studies are inherently limited in their ability to control for the effects of unknown or unmeasured confounders. Indeed, persons with greater intake of antioxidant vitamins through food sources or supplements are likely to differ from others in important ways that may alter the risk of cardiovascular diseases, such as lifestyle factors or other dietary habits. In contrast to the epidemiological studies, results of randomized clinical trials with antioxidant vitamins have been disappointing[11-16].

An excess risk of cancer and cardiovascular mortality was observed with beta-carotene in the large Alpha-Tocopherol/Beta Carotene (ATBC) and Carotene and Retinol Efficacy Trial (CARET) studies[11,12]. For vitamin E, the results of the Cambridge Heart Antioxidant Study (CHAOS) were initially encouraging in secondary prevention, showing a 47% reduced risk of the combined primary endpoint of cardiovascular death and nonfatal MI in subjects with angiographically-proven CAD[13]. This risk reduction was due to a significant benefit for nonfatal MI, and there was a nonsignificant 18% excess of cardiovascular deaths in the vitamin E group.

Recent results from three other major secondary prevention trials with vitamin E, in which more than 40,000 patients were randomized, were not supportive[14-16]. The Gruppo Italiano per lo Studio della Sopravivenza nell'Infarcto miocardico (GISSI) prevention trial assessed dietary supplements of vitamin E and n-3 polyunsaturated fatty acids in 11,324 patients with a recent MI[14]. The Heart Outcome Protection Evaluation (HOPE) study of over 9000 high-risk vascular patients tested both an ACE inhibitor and vitamin E, in a factorial design, for the prevention of cardiovascular morbidity and mortality[15]. The Heart Protection Study (HPS) randomized over 20,000 patients at high risk of atherosclerosis-related events to receive, in a 2 by 2 factorial design, simvastatin alone, antioxidant vitamins (vitamin E, vitamin C and beta-carotene), the combination of simvastatin and vitamins, or placebo[16]. Vitamin E did not offer vascular protection in either the GISSI, HOPE or HPS trials[14-16].

Major problems associated with the use of vitamins, such as their potential prooxidant effects, have been offered as explanations for the neutral clinical results[81,82]. Alpha-tocopherol itself becomes a radical when it scavenges a free electron. Because the tocopherol radical is relatively unstable, it can become a donor of free radicals or act as a prooxidant. Bowry et al.[81] showed that, with high concentrations of vitamin E, lipid peroxidation is actually faster in the presence of alpha-tocopherol and it is propagated within LDL particles by reaction with the tocopherol radical. This may explain why high-dose alpha-tocopherol worsens endothelial-dependent vasodilatation, whereas a low dose improves it in cholesterol-fed rabbits[82]. Moreover, the negative interaction of vitamins with lipid-lowering agents and with other antioxidants that have been reported in the HDL Atherosclerotic Treatment Study (HATS) and in the MultiVitamins and Probucol (MVP) trial may be related to their prooxidant activity or to other mechanisms[46,83].

Potential anti-proliferative and anti-inflammatory effects of indirect antioxidant compounds

ACE inhibitors

Antioxidative properties

There is accumulating evidence that angiotensin II (AII) increases vascular oxidative stress as well as vasoconstriction[84-86]. Activation of the renin-angiotensin system enhances the production of ROS, in part through activation of membrane-bound NADH and NADPH oxidases. These enzymes are present in endothelial cells, vascular SMCs, fibroblasts and phagocytic monocytes. ROS production is enhanced through several pathways including activation of xanthine oxidase, auto-oxidation of NADPH, and inactivation of superoxide dismutase. Enhanced ROS production inactivates nitric oxide, impairing endothelium-dependent vasodilation, and generates peroxynitrite, a potent oxidant that further contributes to vasoconstriction and vascular injury. In addition, as a potent proinflammatory agent, AII upregulates the expression of many redox-sensitive cytokines, chemokines, and growth factors that have been implicated in the pathogenesis of atherosclerosis. Thus, it can be postulated that the beneficial effects of blockade of the renin-angiotensin system by ACE inhibitors (and presumably also by AII receptor antagonists) on progression of atherosclerosis and on the risk of associated cardiovascular complications may be related at least in part to decreased ROS production in the vascular wall.

Beneficial effects

Recognition that the majority of patients benefiting from the use of ACE inhibitors in heart failure studies also suffered from CAD led to the suspicion that this class of agents might prevent cardiovascular events in coronary subjects even in the absence of heart failure[17]. Indeed, ACE inhibition has proven to be beneficial in a variety of subjects with CAD, especially in post-MI patients[18-21], and in those at high risk for cardiovascular events[22]. In large mixed populations of patients with suspected MI, but undetermined left ventricular function, GISSI-3 and the fourth International Study of Infarct Survival (ISIS-4) showed significant reductions in short term overall mortality[18,19]. As shown in the Survival And Ventricular Enlargement (SAVE) and the TRAndolapril Cardiac Evaluation (TRACE) studies, mortality reduction in post-MI patients was even greater when ejection fraction was less than 40% and 35%, respectively[20,21]. The HOPE trial opened a new era for ACE inhibition in the treatment of CAD[22]. The trial targeted patients at high risk for cardiovascular events: either with a history of CAD, stroke, or peripheral vascular disease, or a combination of diabetes plus at least one other cardiovascular risk factor. The primary composite endpoint of MI, stroke, or death from cardiovascular causes was reduced by 22% at five years in the ramipril group as compared to placebo (p<0.001). The MICRO-HOPE study confirmed benefits in the subgroup of HOPE patients with diabetes mellitus[23]. More recently, the EUropean trial on Reduction Of cardiac events with Perindopril in stable coronary Artery disease (EUROPA) assessed the ACE inhibitor, perindopril, in patients with stable CAD but no clinical heart failure. After a mean follow-up of 4.2 years, patients receiving perindopril experienced a 20% relative risk reduction in the composite primary endpoint of cardiovascular death, nonfatal MI, or cardiac arrest with successful resuscitation as compared to placebo-treated patients (p=0.0003)[24]. On the other hand, in the Prevention of Events with Angiotensin-Converting Enzyme inhibition (PEACE) trial, the combined incidence of cardiovascular death, MI, and coronary revascularization was not improved by the ACE inhibitor, trandolapril, over a median follow-up period of 4.8 years, in patients with CAD and preserved LV function [25]. These patients were receiving intensive cardiac therapy (for example, 72% had previously undergone coronary revascularization and 70% were taking lipid-lowering drugs). The authors concluded that, in patients with stable CAD and preserved LV function who are receiving "current standard" therapy and in whom the rate of cardiovascular events is lower than in previous trials of ACE inhibitors in patients with vascular disease, there is no evidence that the addition of an ACE inhibitor provides further benefit in terms of death from cardiovascular causes, MI, and coronary revascularization. Finally, the beneficial effects of ACE inhibitors, in patients with CAD with or without LV dysfunction, are probably related to several mechanisms which are discussed elsewhere in this book, one of them being reduced oxidative stress.

Statins

Antioxidative properties

The discrepancy of a relatively large clinical benefit in the presence of only minimal regression of atherosclerotic lesions, when serum cholesterol was lowered by 3-hydroxy-3-methylglutaryl coenzyme A reductase inhibitors (statins) in patients with CAD, has led to the hypothesis of a pleiotropic action of statins on the arterial wall[87-89]. Endothelial dysfunction occurs early in the atherosclerotic process, often preceding the formation of the atherosclerotic plaque. Statins improve endothelial function through several mechanisms, including plaque stabilization, decreased oxidative stress, and reduced vascular inflammation. In particular, they increase nitric oxide production, enhance fibrinolytic activity, and reduce monocyte recruitment as well as expression of adhesion molecules and biomarkers of inflammation such as CRP and lipoprotein-associated phospholipase A2[88,89].

Beneficial effects

In 2002, the HPS showed an overall 25% reduction in the incidence of coronary events by simvastatin as compared to placebo and this was associated with a 40 mg/dl (1.03 mmol/L) reduction in LDL cholesterol levels[26]. However, patients with normal baseline LDL cholesterol levels (<100 mg/dl or 2.59 mmol/L) received just as much benefit as those with high LDL cholesterol levels. This finding raised the question of whether the benefits of statins are related only to their lipid-lowering properties. The Reversal of Atherosclerosis with Aggressive Lipid Lowering (REVERSAL) trial compared intensive lipid-lowering therapy with 80 mg of atorvastatin daily to moderate lipid-lowering therapy with 40 mg of pravastatin daily on progression of coronary atherosclerosis[27]. LDL cholesterol levels were lowered more with atorvastatin and intensive lipid-lowering therapy was also superior in limiting atherosclerotic progression. However, intensive lipid-lowering therapy also lowered CRP levels significantly as compared to the moderate regimen, suggesting that LDL-cholesterol lowering alone perhaps did not explain all the differences in efficacy. The PRavastatin Or atorVastatin Evaluation and Infection Therapy (PROVE-IT) trial compared, in patients with acute coronary syndromes that were followed for a mean of 24 months, the effects on a composite of major cardiovascular events of the same daily doses of atorvastatin and pravastatin as in REVERSAL[28]. Compared to the standard regimen, the intensive lipid-lowering statin regimen provided substantially lower levels of LDL cholesterol (median of 62 mg/dl versus 95 mg/dl) as well as a significant reduction in death or major cardiovascular events. The precise mechanism of action responsible for atorvastatin superiority is still uncertain.[29]. Although much of the benefit may be attributable to the difference in the degree of LDL-cholesterol lowering, one cannot exclude the possibility that the difference in clinical outcomes may be due in part to non-lipid-related pleiotropic effects, which may differ between these two statins[30]. Lowering LDL-cholesterol also results in other anti-inflammatory effects, such as reductions in the levels of high-sensitivity CRP and soluble CD40 ligand. Interestingly, however, no correlation seems to exist between LDL-cholesterol reduction and the levels of these inflammatory markers.

Beta-blockers

Antioxidative properties

Unlike second generation beta-blockers, beta-adrenergic receptor antagonists of the third generation such as carvedilol and nebivolol have been shown to possess important antioxidant and antiproliferative properties[90-93]. Carvedilol is a nonselective beta-blocker that blocks all three adrenergic receptors (beta-1, alpha-1, and beta-2) that mediate a positive inotropic response in human cardiac myocytes. Thus, unlike selective beta-1 compounds such as metroprolol and bisoprolol, carvedilol also blocks beta-2 adrenergic receptors, and because of its alpha-1 blocking properties, carvedilol is a moderate vasodilator[32,33]. Nebivolol is a beta-1 selective adrenergic receptor antagonist with nitric oxide-mediated vasodilating properties in humans[94,95]. In the rat aorta, nebivolol alleviates ROS-induced impairment of endothelium-dependent vasorelaxation. This protective effect is very likely the result of a direct ROS-scavenging action by the nebivolol molecule itself[96]. Both drugs inhibit endothelin-1 secretion and SMC and endothelial cell proliferation in human coronary arteries[92] These additional actions may enhance their ability to attenuate the adverse effects of the sympathetic nervous system on the heart and circulation[33].

Beneficial effects

Adrenergic activation may become excessive and may have deleterious effects on cardiovascular function, especially in post-MI patients and in patients with chronic congestive heart failure. Several trials have examined the secondary prevention effect of beta-blockers on survival after MI and pooled data from these trials show a significant reduction in total mortality and in the occurrence of sudden death[31]. Large, randomized, placebo-controlled trials involving long-term treatment with carvedilol[32,33], metroprolol [34] and bisoprolol[35] have shown marked reductions in overall mortality and in the need for hospitalizations in patients with chronic heart failure. In a recent meta-analysis of over 10,000 patients with heart failure, the odds ratio was 0.65 for deaths and 0.64 for hospitalizations for heart failure[36]. In the Carvedilol Or Metoprolol European Trial (COMET), both total and cardiovascular mortality were significantly lower in patients with chronic heart failure receiving carvedilol than in those receiving metroprolol[37]. Further studies are needed to determine whether their antioxidant properties confer to carvedilol and nebivolol additional cardioprotective effects and whether they can protect against progression of coronary atherosclerosis as well as atherosclerosis in other vascular territories.

Calcium channel blockers

Antioxidative properties

Several dihydropyridine calcium channel blockers, especially highly lipophilic compounds such as amlodipine, lacidipine lercanidipine and nisoldipine, are known to possess important antioxidant properties[97-100]. Lipophilic calcium antagonists inhibit lipid peroxidation in cellular membranes and this effect is independent of calcium channel inhibition. Amlodipine possesses potent antioxidant activity as a result of distinct biophysical interactions with the membrane lipid bilayer[97]. Amlodipine improves endothelial function via enhanced formation and prolonged half-life of nitric oxide through antioxidatve properties[98]. As a result of its antiproliferative properties, amlodipine inhibits SMC proliferation and migration, prevents cytokine-induced endothelial apoptosis, and modulates vascular gene expression and extracellular matrix formation[97]. Finally, amlodipine, lacidipine and lercanidipine decrease the expression of the adhesion molecules ICAM-1, VCAM-1, and E-selectin and this effect is determined both by their lipophilicity and by their intrinsic antioxidant activity[99]. Other dihydropyridine-like calcium antagonists have anti-atherosclerotic effects which may or may not be related to an antioxidant activity. For example, both nifedipine and nicardipine have been shown, using quantitative coronary angiographic analysis, to interfere with new atherosclerotic lesion formation without affecting the size of existing lesions[101,102]. Moreover, the recent Evaluation of Nifedipine and Cerivastatin On Recovery of Endothelial function (ENCORE 1) has shown that long-acting nifedipine significantly improves coronary endothelial function, as compared to placebo, in patients with CAD[103].

Beneficial effects

In the Prospective Randomized Evaluation of the Vascular Effects of Norvasc (amlodipine) Trial (PREVENT), amlodipine significantly reduced intimal/medial thickness in the carotid arteries and decreased hospitalizations for unstable angina and revascularization procedures[38]. Although atheroclerotic progression in the coronary arteries was not reduced, a post hoc analysis of the angiographic data suggested that amlodipine had a favourable effect on regression of coronary lesions with >70% diameter stenosis at baseline[39]. In the Coronary Angioplasty Amlodipine Restenosis Study (CAPARES), angiographic luminal loss did not decrease after the percutaneous coronary intervention, but the incidence of repeated procedures was significantly reduced by amlodipine. The composite incidence of major adverse clinical events was significantly reduced in the patients treated with amlodipine, but the difference was mainly due to a reduction in the number of repeat angioplasties[40]. The Comparison of AMlodipine versus Enalapril to Limit Occurrences of Thrombosis (CAMELOT) study compared the effects of amlodipine or enalapril versus placebo on cardiovascular events in 1,991 patients with CAD and normal blood pressure at baseline[41]. Compared to placebo, amlodipine reduced adverse cardiovascular events by 31% (p=0.003). Directionally similar, but smaller and nonsignificant treatment effects were observed with enalapril. CAMELOT included a substudy of 274 patients entitled Norvasc for Regression of Manifest Atherosclerotic Lesions by Intravascular Sonographic Evaluation (NORMALISE) in which atherosclerosis progression was measured by IVUS. Compared with baseline, IVUS showed progression in the placebo group (p=0.001), a trend toward progression in the enalapril group (p=0.08), and no progression in the amlodipine group (p=0.31).

Whether the antioxidant activity of amlodipine contributed, in addition to its hemodynamic effects, to prevention of carotid atherosclerosis and of clinical events in PREVENT, and of cardiovascular events and coronary atherosclerosis prevention in CAMELOT, remains to be established. In A Coronary disease Trial Investigating Outcome with Nifedipine GITS (gastro-intestinal therapeutic system) (ACTION), addition of long-acting nifedipine to conventional treatment of angina had no effect on major cardiovascular event-free survival, but reduced the need for coronary angiography and coronary artery bypass surgery[42].

Direct synthetic antioxidants

Probucol

Mechanisms of action

Animal studies have shown a beneficial effect of probucol on the development of atherosclerotic lesions[104,105]. In Watanabe Heritable Hyperlipemic (WHHL) rabbits, the ability of probucol to inhibit atherosclerosis was independent of its lipid-lowering effects[104]. The antioxidant activity of probucol has also been directly linked to its ability to reduce atherosclerosis in cholesterol-fed monkeys[105].

Clinical effects

It has been hypothesized that the lack of beneficial effects of probucol on progression of femoral atherosclerosis in the Probucol Quantitative Regression Swedish Trial (PQRST) was due to the prolonged 40% reduction in HDL-cholesterol levels[43,44]. However, the design of the study raised several important issues[43]. The primary endpoint in PQRST was lumen volume of femoral arteries using three-dimensional reconstruction of angiograms, an approach rarely used in other clinical trials. The choice of the femoral location for assessment is also questionable, in light of the preferential effect of probucol on younger lesions in the proximal thoracic aorta compared to the more advanced iliac lesions in experimental atherosclerosis in non-human primates[104]. In addition, probucol was given to all patients (including those in the placebo group) for two months during the pre-randomization phase, which represents another problematic design feature considering that probucol accumulates in tissues for prolonged periods. In contrast, the recently published Fukuoka AtheroSclerosis Trial (FAST) showed that probucol reduced progression of carotid atherosclerosis despite significant HDL lowering[45]. Atherosclerosis-related clinical events were also significantly reduced by probucol in FAST. We have also shown in the MultiVitamins and Probucol (MVP) trial that probucol reduces coronary restenosis after balloon angioplasty[46-48]. However, despite the beneficial effects of probucol, prolongation of the QT interval and lowering of HDL-cholesterol with probucol remain long-term safety concerns.

AGI-1067

Mechanisms of action

AGI-1067 is part of a new therapeutic class of agents, which combines antioxidant properties with unique anti-atherosclerotic activity: intracellular redox-signaling blockade and VCAM-1 inhibition[106,107]. In CART-1, we observed both an inhibition of negative remodeling and a reduction of plaque burden. These favourable results are supported by demonstration of atherosclerosis prevention by AGI-1067 in all tested animal models[106,107], including the apo-E knockout and LDL-receptor deficient mice. Recently, AGI-1067 almost entirely inhibited the development of atherosclerosis in the non-human primate, to a much greater extent than probucol[106,107]. However, in light of its potential negative effect on HDL cholesterol, demonstration of a neutral or beneficial effect on atherosclerosis must be directly proven in a clinical trial before AGI-1067 can be used for prolonged periods.

Clinical effects

Canadian Antioxidant Restenosis Trial (CART-1)
Volumetric (3-D) changes of non-intervened coronary reference segments, away from the PCI site, were also evaluated with intravascular ultrasound (IVUS) in CART-1[49]. The mean changes in lumen volume (follow-up minus baseline) in the reference segments were: -5.3 mm2 in the placebo group; -0.2 mm2 for probucol; -2.4 mm2 with AGI-1067 70 mg; +3.5 mm2 with AGI-1067 140-mg dose; +1.8 mm2 with AGI-1067 280-mg group (p=0.05 for AGI-1067 140 mg versus placebo; p=0.077 for dose-response relationship; *Figure 2*). This improvement in non-PCI site coronary artery lumen may represent the first clinical evidence of vascular protection with AGI-1067. Therefore, a key objective of CART-2 is to assess the effect of AGI-1067 on changes in coronary atherosclerosis[50].

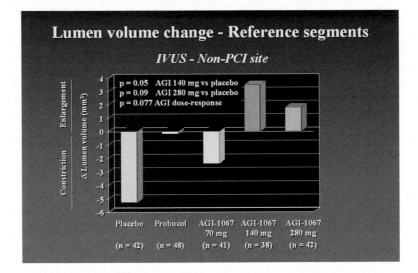

Figure 2. **Changes in reference segments, away from the PCI site, at six months of follow-up.** Patients had stopped receiving study medication for five months at the time of follow-up IVUS examination. [49]

The Canadian Atherosclerosis Restenosis Trial (CART-2)
Patients in the CART-2 study were randomized to placebo plus standard of care, or to one of three active treatment groups. Starting 14 days prior to a scheduled angioplasty (PCI) procedure, the first treatment group received AGI-1067 for the full 14 days, the second group received placebo for the first 11 days and AGI-1067 for the last three days, and the third group received placebo for the full 14 days. Following the angioplasty, all three active treatment groups continued receiving AGI-1067 for 12 consecutive

months. The dose of AGI-1067 used for all patients in the treatment groups was 280 mg, dosed orally once per day, plus standard of care. The trial was originally designed as a restenosis study, primarily assessing the minimal lumen diameter at the site of PCI, measured by Quantitative Coronary Angiogram (QCA), on the 12-month follow-up angiogram. During the course of the trial, but before the results were known to the investigators or to the sponsor (AtheroGenics, Inc.), it was decided to modify the protocol of the study and to make this a secondary endpoint, the new primary endpoint being a change in plaque volume at follow-up in a 30-mm segment of a non-PCI coronary artery on 3-D IVUS.

The Aggressive Reduction of Inflammation Stops Events (ARISE) Trial

Despite improvements in imaging modalities, visualization of morphological details indicative of plaque stability is not yet possible with IVUS[51]. The predictive value of anatomical changes for future clinical events is not yet known. The greatest impact AGI-1067 may have clinically is in the prevention of plaque rupture and subsequent cardiovascular morbidity and mortality. Modifications resulting from the administration of AGI-1067, which stabilize the plaque but do not result in overall plaque volume changes are only evaluable with a properly conducted clinical events trial. Therefore, the ARISE trial was designed to evaluate the potential utility of AGI-1067. The primary objective of ARISE is to determine whether long-term treatment with AGI-1067 will prevent major cardiovascular events in modernly-managed patients with CAD. Since the beneficial effects of AGI-1067 would likely be related to its potent antioxidant and anti-inflammatory propertics, another key objective is to determine the effects of AGI-1067 on markers of inflammation and oxidation. ARISE represents a unique opportunity to test, in a definitive fashion, that antioxidant/anti-inflammatory hypothesis[52].

ARISE is a multicenter, double blind, randomized, placebo-controlled trial of two parallel groups involving approximately 250 study sites (*Figure 4*). Approximately 6,000 patients with a recent diagnosis of CAD (unstable angina or MI) and one additional risk factor have been enrolled in the U.S., Canada, Europe, and South Africa. Patients have been randomized to AGI-1067 or placebo in 1: 1 ratio. The primary study endpoint is the combined incidence of cardiovascular mortality, resuscitated cardiac arrest, non-fatal MI, non-fatal stroke, need for coronary revascularization, and urgent hospitalization for angina pectoris with objective evidence of ischemia. The study will be complete when at least 980 patients have experienced a primary event or when all patients have been treated for at least 12 months, whichever occurs first.

As of July 2005, the original patient enrolment target of 6,000 patients has been reached for ARISE.

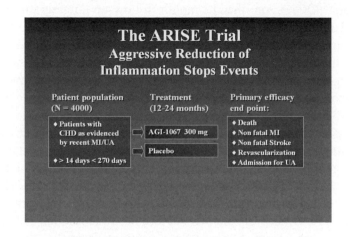

Figure 3. **The ARISE trial (Aggressive Reduction of Inflammation Stops Events)** [52]

Conclusions

Medical advances over the past decade have resulted in a greater ability to detect and treat atherosclerotic cardiovascular disease. Nevertheless, atherosclerotic disease inflicts a large burden in terms of life expectancy, quality of life, and societal costs. Since aging of the population and recent trends in environmental and lifestyle factors contribute to an increasing risk of atherosclerosis in our societies, it is anticipated that this burden will not dissipate soon. There is, therefore, a need for a novel pharmacological intervention that would provide further cardiovascular protection in patients with atherosclerosis, over and above the protection afforded by other available medications, such as aspirin, statins and ACE inhibitors. In view of its promising effects, two important and large clinical trials are ongoing with AGI-1067. CART-2 and ARISE are respectively evaluating its value on atherosclerosis progression and clinical outcomes.

References

1. Aboderin I, Kalache A, Ben-Shlomo Y, et al. Life course perspectives on coronary heart disease, stroke and diabetes: key issues and implications for policy and research. Geneva, World Health Organization, 2002.
2. American Heart Association. Heart and Stroke Statistical Update. Dallas, Texas: American Heart Association, 2000.
3. Ross R. Atherosclerosis - An inflammatory disease. N Engl J Med 1999;340:115-26.
4. Libby P. Changing concepts of atherogenesis. J Intern Med 2000;247:349-58.
5. Offerman MK, Medford RM. Antioxidants and atherosclerosis: a molecular perspective, Heart Dis Stroke 1994;3:52-7.
6. Kunsch C, Medford RM. Oxidative stress as a regulator of gene expression in the vasculature. Circ Res 1999;85:753-66.
7. Steinberg D, Parthasarathy S, Carew TE, Khoo JC, Witztum JL. Beyond cholesterol. Modifications of low-density lipoprotein that increase its atherogenecity. N Engl J Med 1989;320:915-24.
8. Witztum JL. The oxidative hypothesis of atherosclerosis. Lancet 1994;344:793-5.
9. Griendling KK, FitzGerald GA. Oxidative stress and cardiovascular injury. Part I: Basic mechanisms and in vivo monitoring of ROS. Circulation 2003;108:1912-6.
10. Griendling KK, FitzGerald GA. Oxidative stress and cardiovascular injury. Part II: Animal and human studies. Circulation 2003;108:2034-40.
11. The Alpha-Tocopherol, Beta-Carotene Cancer Prevention Study Group. The effect of vitamin E and beta carotene on the incidence of lung cancer and other cancers in male smokers. N Engl J Med 1994;330:1029-35.
12. Omenn GS, Goodman GE, Thornquist MD, et al. Effects of a combination of beta carotene and vitamin A on lung cancer and cardiovascular disease. N Engl J Med 1996;334:1150-5.
13. Stephens NG, Parsons A, Schofield PM, et al. Randomized controlled trial of vitamin E in patients with coronary disease: Cambridge Heart Antioxidant Study (CHAOS). Lancet 1996;347:781-6.
14. Gruppo Italiano per lo Studio della Sopravivenza nell'Infarcto miocardico. Dietary supplementation with n-3 polyunsaturated fatty acids and vitamin E after myocardial infarction: results of the GISSI-Prevenzione trial. Lancet 1999;354:447-55.
15. The HOPE study investigators. Vitamin E supplementation and cardiovascular events in high-risk patients. N Engl J Med 2000;342:154-60.
16. MRC/BHF Heart Protection Study Collaborative Group. MRC/BHF heart protection study of cholesterol-lowering therapy and of antioxidant vitamin supplementation in a wide range of patients at increased risk of coronary heart disease death: early safety and efficacy experience Eur Heart J 1999;20:725-41.
17. Larose E, Tardif JC, Bourassa MG. Use of ACE inhibitors for secondary prevention. Current Treatment Opinions in Cardiovasc Med 2003;5:51-61.

18. GISSI-3 Collaborators. GISSI-3: Effects of lisinopril and transdermal glyceryl trinitrate singly and together on 6-week mortality and ventricular function after acute myocardial infarction. Lancet 1994;343:1115-22.

19. ISIS-4 Collaborative Group. ISIS-4: A randomized factorial trial assessing early oral captopril, oral mononitrate, and intravenous magnesium sulphate in 58050 patients with suspected acute myocardial infarction. Lancet 1995;345:669-85.

20. Pfeffer MA, Braunwald E, Moye LA, et al. Effect of captopril on mortality and morbidity in patients with left ventricular dysfunction after myocardial infarction. Results of the survival and left ventricular enlargement trial. N Engl J Med 1992;327:669-77.

21. Kober L, Torp-Pedersen C, Carlsen JE, et al. A clinical trial of the angiotensin-converting-enzyme inhibitor trandolapril in patients with left ventricular dysfunction after myocardial infarction. N Engl J Med 1995;333:1670-6.

22. The Heart Outcome Prevention Evaluation Study Investigators. Effects of an ACEI, ramipril, on cardiovascular events in high risk patients. N Engl J Med 2000;342:145-53.

23. HOPE Investigators. Effects of ramipril on CV and microvascular outcomes in people with DM: results of the HOPE study and MICRO-HOPE substudy. Lancet 2000;355:253-8.

24. EURopean trial On reduction of cardiac events with Perindopril in stable coronary Artery disease investigators. Efficacy of perindopril in reduction of cardiovascular events among patients with stable coronary artery disease: randomized, double-blind, placebo-controlled, multicentre trial (the EUROPA study). Lancet 2003;362:782-8.

25. The PEACE Investigators. Angiotensin-converting-enzyme inhibition in stable coronary artery disease. N Engl J Med 2004;351:2058-68.

26. Heart Protection Study Collaboration Group. MRC/BHF Heart Protection Study of cholesterol lowering with simvastatin in 20 536 high-risk individuals: a randomized placebo-controlled trial. Lancet 2002;360:7-22.

27. Nissen SE, Tuzcu EM, Schoenhagen P, et al. Effect of intensive compared with moderate lipid-lowering therapy on progression of coronary atherosclerosis: a randomized controlled trial. JAMA 2004;291:1071-80.

28. Cannon CP, Braunwald E, McCabe CH, et al. Comparison of intensive and moderate lipid lowering with statins after acute coronary syndromes. N Engl J Med 2004;350:1495-504.

29. Topol EJ. Intensive statin therapy – A sea change in cardiovascular prevention. N Engl J Med 2004;350:1562-4.

30. Bonetti PO, Lerman LO, Napoli C, Lerman A. Statin effects beyond lipid lowering - are they clinically relevant? Eur Heart J 2003;24:225-48.

31. Yusuf S, Peto R, Lewis J, Collins R, Sleight P. Beta blockade during and after myocardial infarction: an overview of the randomized trials. Prog Cardiovasc Dis 1985;27:335-71.

32. Packer M, Bristow MR, Cohn JN, et al. The effect of carvedilol on morbidity and mortality in chronic heart failure. N Engl J Med 1996;334:1349-55.

33. Packer M, Coats AJS, Fowler M, et al. Effect of carvedilol on survival in severe chronic heart failure. N Engl J Med 2001;344:1668-75.

34. MERIT-HF Study Group. Effect of metoprolol CR/XL in chronic heart failure: Metoprolol CR/XL Randomized Intervention Trial in Congestive Heart Failure (MERIT-HF). Lancet 1999;353:2001-7.

35. CIBIS-II Investigators and Committees. The Cardiac Insufficiency Bisoprolol Study II (CIBIS II): a randomized trial. Lancet 1999;353:9-13.

36. Brophy JM, Joseph L, Rouleau JL. β-blockers in congestive heart failure: a Bayesian meta-analysis. Ann Intern Med 2001;134:550-60.

37. Poole-Wilson PA, Swedberg K, Cleland JGF, et al. Comparison of carvedilol and metoprolol on clinical outcomes in patients with chronic heart failure in the Carvedilol Or Metoprolol European Trial (COMET): randomized, controlled trial. Lancet 2003; 362:7-13.

38. Pitt B, Byington RP, Furberg CD, et al. Effect of amlodipine on the progression of atherosclerosis and the occurrence of clinical events. Circulation 2000;102:1503-10.

39. Mancini GB, Miller ME, Evans GW, et al. Post hoc analysis of coronary findings from the Prospective Randomized Evaluation of the Vascular Effects of the Norvasc Trial (PREVENT). Am J Cardiol 2002;89:1414-6.

40. Jorgensen B, Simonsen S, Endresen K, et al. Restenosis and clinical outcome in patients treated with amlodipine after angioplasty: results from the Coronary Angioplasty Amlodipine Restenosis Study (CAPARES). J Am Coll Cardiol 2000;35:592-9.

41. Nissen SE, Tuzcu EM, Libby P, et al. Effects of antihypertensive agents on cardiovascular events in patients with coronary disease and normal blood pressure. The CAMELOT Study: a randomized controlled trial. JAMA 2004;292:2217-26.

42. Poole-Wilson PA, Lubsen J, Kirwan BA, et al. Effect of long-acting nifedipine on mortality and cardiovascular morbidity in patients with stable angina requiring treatment (ACTION trial) : randomized controlled trial. Lancet 2004;364:849-57.

43. Waldius G, Erikson U, Olsson AG, et al. The effect of probucol on femoral atherosclerosis: the Probucol Quantitative Regression Swedish Trial (PQRST). Am J Cardiol 1994;74:875-83.

44. Johansson J, Olsson AG, Bergstrand L, et al. Lowering of HDL2b by probucol partly explains the failure of the drug to affect femoral atherosclerosis in subjects with hypercholesterolemia. A Probucol Quantitative Regression Swedish Trial (PQRST) Report. Arterioscler Thromb Vasc Biol 1995;15:1049-56.

45. Sawayama Y, Shinizu C, Maeda N, et al. Effects of probucol and pravastatin on common carotid atherosclerosis in patients with asymptomatic hypercholesterolemia. J Am Coll Cardiol 2002;39:610-6.

46. Tardif JC, Coté G, Lespérance J, et al. Probucol and multivitamins in the prevention of restenosis after coronary angioplasty. N Engl J Med 1997;337:365-72.

47. Rodes J, Tardif JC, Lespérance J, et al. Prevention of restenosis after angioplasty in small coronary arteries with probucol. Circulation 1998;97:429-36.

48. Coté G, Tardif JC, Lespérance J, et al. Effects of probucol on vascular remodeling after coronary angioplasty. Circulation 1999;99:30-5.

49. Tardif JC, Grégoire J, Schwartz L, et al. Effects of AGI-1067 and probucol after percutaneous coronary interventions. Circulation 2003;107:552-8.

50. Tardif JC. Clinical results with AGI-1067: a novel antioxidant vascular protectant. Am J Cardiol 2003;91 (suppl.):41A-49A.

51. Tardif JC. The future of intravascular ultrasound in the detection and management of coronary artery disease. Can J Cardiol 2000;16 (Suppl.D):12D-15D.

52. Tardif JC. Insights into oxidative stress and atherosclerosis. Can J Cardiol 2000;16 (Suppl.D):2D-4D.

53. De Keulenaer GW, Ushio-Fukai M, Yin Q, et al. Convergence of redox-sensitive and mitogen-activated protein kinase signaling pathways in tumour necrosis factor-alpha-mediated monocyte chemoattractant protein-1 induction in vascular smooth muscle cells. Arterioscler Thromb Vasc Biol 2000;20:385-91.

54. Marui N, Offerman MK, Swerlick R, et al. Vascular cell adhesion molecule (VCAM-1) gene transcription and expression are regulated through an antioxidant-sensitive mechanism in human vascular endothelial cells. J Clin Invest 1993;92:1866-74.

55. Fruebis J, Gonzales V, Silvestre M, Palinski W. Effect of probucol treatment on gene expression of VCAM-1, MCP-1, and M-CSF in the aortic wall of LDL-receptor-deficient rabbits during early atherosclerosis. Arterioscler Thromb Vasc Biol. 1997;17:1289-302.

56. Salonen JT, Yla-Herttuala S, Yamamoto R, et al. Autoantibody against oxidized LDL and progression of carotid atherosclerosis. Lancet 1992;339:883-7.

57. Cushing SD, Berliner JA, Valente AJ, et al. Minimally modified low density lipoprotein induces monocyte chemotactic protein 1 in human endothelial cells and smooth muscle cells. Proc Natl Acad Sci USA 1990;87:5134-38.

58. Rajavashisth TB, Andalibi A, Territo, et al. Induction of endothelial cell expression of granulocyte and macrophage colony-stimulating factors by modified low density lipoproteins. Nature 1990;344:254-7.

59. Bourcier T, Sukhova G, Libby P. The nuclear factor kappa-B signaling pathway participates in dysregulation of vascular smooth muscle cells in vitro and in human atherosclerosis. J Biol Chem 1997;272:15817-24.

60. Thomas CE, Jackson RL, Ohlweiler DF, et al. Multiple lipid oxidation products in low density lipoproteins induce interleukin-1 beta release from human blood mononuclear cells. J Lipid Res 1994;35:417-27.

61. Rajapopalan S, Meng XP, Ramasamy S, et al. Reactive oxygen species produced by macrophage-derived foam cells regulate the activity of vascular matrix metalloproteinases in vitro. J Clin Invest 1996;98:2572-9.

62. Ikeda H, Koga Y, Oda T, et al. Free oxygen radicals contribute to platelet aggregation and cyclic flow variations in stenosed and endothelium-injured canine coronary arteries. J Am Coll Cardiol 1994;24:1749-56.

63. Li H, Cybulsky MI, Gimbrone MA, Jr., Libby P. An atherogenic diet rapidly induces VCAM-1, a cytokine-regulated mononuclear leucocyte adhesion molecule, in rabbit aortic endothelium. Arterioscler Thromb 1993;13:197-204.

64. Harrington JR. The role of MCP-1 in atherosclerosis. Stem Cells 2000;18:65-6.

65. Reape TJ, Groot PH. Chemokines and atherosclerosis. Atherosclerosis 1999;147:213-25.

66. Gerszten RE, Mach F, Sauty A, Rosenzweig A, Luster Ad. Chemokines, leucocytes, and atherosclerosis. J Lab Clin Med 2000;136:87-92.

67. Cybulsky MI, Iiyama K, Li H, et al. A major role for VCAM-1, but not ICAM-1, in early atherosclerosis. J Clin Invest 2001;107:1255-62.

68. Davies MJ, Gordon JL, Gearing AJ, et al. The expression of the adhesion molecules ICAM-1, VCAM-1, PECAM, and E-selectin in human atherosclerosis. J Pathol 1993;171:223-9.

69. Gerszten RE, Lim YC, Ding HT, et al. Adhesion of monocytes to vascular cell adhesion molecule-1-transduced human endothelial cells: implications for atherogenesis. Circ Res 1998;82:871-8.

70. Rohde LE, Lee RT, Rivero J, et al. Circulating cell adhesion molecules are correlated with ultrasound-based assessment of carotid atherosclerosis. Arterioscler Thromb Vasc Biol 1998;18:1765-70.

71. De Caterina R, Basta G, Lazzerini G, et al. Soluble vascular cell adhesion molecule-1 as a biohumoral correlate of atherosclerosis. Arterioscler Thromb Vasc Biol 1997;17:2646-54

72. Peter K, Weirich U, Nordt TK, Ruef J, Bode C. Soluble vascular cell adhesion molecule-1 (VCAM-1) as potential marker of atherosclerosis. Thromb Haemost 1999;82(Suppl.1):38-43.

73. Peter K, Nawroth P, Conradt C, et al. Circulating vascular cell adhesion molecule-1 correlates with the extent of human atherosclerosis in contrast to circulating intercellular adhesion molecule-1, E-selectin, P-selectin, and thrombomodulin. Arterioscler Thromb Vasc Biol 1997;17:505-12.

74. Blankenberg S, Rupprecht HJ, Bickel C, et al. Circulating cell adhesion molecules and death in patients with coronary artery disease. Circulation 2001;104:1336-42.

75. Szmitko PE, Wang CH, Weisel RD, de Almeida JR, Anderson TJ, Verma S. New markers of inflammation and endothelial cell activation. Part I. Circulation 2003;108:1917-23.

76. Szmitko PE, Wang CH, Weisel RD, Jeffries GA, Anderson TJ, Verma S. Biomarkers of vascular disease linking inflammation to endothelial activation. Part II. Circulation 2003;108:2041-8.

77. Ridker PM, Rifai N, Rose I, et al. Comparison of C-reactive protein and low-density lipoprotein cholesterol levels in the prediction of first cardiovascular events. N Engl J Med 2002;347:1557-65.

78. Heeschen C, Dimmeler S, Hamm CW, et al. Soluble CD40 ligand in acute coronary syndromes. N Engl J Med 2003;348:1104-11.

79. Mallat Z, Corbaz A, Scoazec A, et al. Expression of interleukin-18 in human atherosclerotic plaques and relation to plaque stability. Circulation 2001;104:1598-603.

80. Blankenberg S, Tiret L, Bickel C, et al. Interleukin-18 is a strong predictor of cardiovascular death in stable and unstable angina. Circulation 2002;106:24-30.

81. Bowry VW, Ingold KU, Stocker R. Vitamin E in human low-density lipoprotein: when and how this antioxidant becomes a pro-oxidant. Biochem J 1992;288:341-4.

82. Keaney JF Jr., Gaziano JM, Xu A, et al. Low-dose alpha-tocopherol improves and high-dose alpha-tocopherol worsens endothelial vasodilator function in cholesterol-fed rabbits. J Clin Invest 1994;93:844-51.

83. Brown BG, Zhao XQ, Chait A, et al. Simvastatin and niacin, antioxidant vitamins, or the combination for the prevention of coronary disease. N Engl J Med 2001;345:1583-92.

84. Griendling KK, Minieri CA, Ollerenshaw JD, et al. Angiotensin II stimulates NADH and NADPH oxidase activity in cultured vascular smooth muscle cells. Circ Res 1994;74:1141-8.

85. Dzau VJ. Theodore Cooper Lecture: tissue angiotensin and pathobiology of vascular disease: a unifying hypothesis. Hypertension 2001;37:1047-52.

86. Weiss D, Sorescu D, Taylor WR. Angiotensin II and atherosclerosis. Am J Cardiol 2001;87(suppl.):25C-32C.

87. Brown BG, Zhao XQ, Sacco DE, Albers JJ. Lipid lowering and plaque regression. New insights into prevention of plaque disruption and clinical events in coronary disease. Circulation 1993;87:1781-91.

88. Langer A, Constance C, Fodor JG, et al. Statin therapy and the management of acute coronary syndromes. Can J Cardiol 2003;19:921-7.

89. Saini HK, Arneja AS, Dhalla NS. Role of cholesterol in cardiovascular dysfunction. Can J Cardiol 2004;20:333-46.

90. Yue TL, Cheng HY, Lysko PG, et al. Carvedilol, a new vasodilator and beta adrenoreceptor antagonist, is an antioxidant and free radical scavenger. J Pharmacol Exp Ther 1992;263:92-8.

91. Ohlstein EH, Douglas SA, Sung CP, et al. Carvedilol, a cardiovascular drug, prevents vascular smooth muscle cell proliferation, migration, and neointimal formation following vascular injury. Proc Natl Acad Sci USA 1993;90:6189-93.

92. Brehm BR, Bertsch D, von Fallois J, Wolf SC. Beta-blockers of the third generation inhibit endothelin-1 liberation, mRNA production and proliferation of human coronary smooth muscle and endothelial cells. J Cardiovasc Pharmacol 2000;36 (suppl. 1):S401-3.

93. Yasunari K, Maeda K, Nakamura M, Watanabe T, Yoshikawa J, Asada A. Effects of carvedilol on oxidative stress in polymorphonuclear and mononuclear cells in patients with essential hypertension. Am J Med 2004;116:460-5.

94. Broeders MA, Doevendans PA, Bekkers BC, et al. Nebivolol, a third-generation beta-blocker that augments vascular nitric oxide release: endothelial beta (2)-adrenergic receptor-mediated nitric oxide production. Circulation 2000;102:677-84.

95. Cominacini L, Fratta Pasini A, Garbin U, et al. Nebivolol and its 4-keto derivative increase nitric oxide in endothelial cells by reducing its oxidative inactivation. J Am Coll Cardiol 2003;42:1838-44.

96. de Groot AA, Mathy MJ, van Zwieten PA, Peters SL. Antioxidant activity of nebivolol in the rat aorta. J Cardiovasc Pharmacol 2004;43:148-53.

97. Mason RP, Mak IT, Trumbore MW, Mason PE. Antioxidant properties of calcium antagonists related to membrane biophysical interactions. Am J Cardiol 1999;84:16L-22L.

98. Berkels R, Taubert D, Bartels H, Breitenbach T, Klaus W, Roesen R. Amlodipine increases endothelial nitric oxide by dual mechanisms. Pharmacology 2004;70:39-45.

99. Cominacini L, Pasini AF, Pastorino AM, et al. Comparative effects of different dihydropyridines on the expression of adhesion molecules induced by TNF-alpha on endothelial cells. J Hypertens 1999;17:1837-41.

100. Cominacini L, Garbin U, Fratta Pacini A, et al. Lacidipine inhibits the activation of the transcription factor NF-kappaB and the expression of adhesion molecules induced by pro-oxidant signals on endothelial cells. J Hypertens 1997;15:1633-40.

101. Lichtlen PR, Hugenholtz PG, Rafflenbeul W, Hecker H, Jost S, Deckers JW, Retardation of angiographic progression of coronary artery disease by nifedipine. Results of the International Nifedipine Trial on Antiatherosclerotic Therapy (INTACT). INTACT Group Investigators. Lancet 1990;335:1109-13.

102. Waters DD, Lesperance J. Interventions that beneficially influence the evolution of coronary atherosclerosis. The case for calcium channel blockers. Circulation 1992;86 (Suppl) III:111-6.

103. ENCORE Investigators. Effect of nifedipine and cerivastatin on coronary endothelial function in patients with coronary artery disease: the ENCORE 1 study (Evaluation of Nifedipine and Cerivastatin On Recovery of coronary Endothelial function). Circulation 2003;107:422-8.

104. Carew TE, Schwenke DC, Steinberg D. Antiatherogenic effect of probucol unrelated to its hypocholesterolemic effect: evidence that antioxidants in vivo can selectively inhibit low density lipoprotein degradation in macrophage-rich fatty streaks and slow the progression of atherosclerosis in the Watanabe heritable hyperlipidemic rabbit. Proc Natl Acad Sci USA 1987;84:7725-9.

105. Sasahara M, Raines EW, Chait A, et al. Inhibition of hypercholesterolemia-induced atherosclerosis in the non-human primate by probucol. Is the extent of atherosclerosis related to resistance of LDL to oxidation? J Clin Invest 1994;94:155-64.

106. Wasserman MA, Sundell CL, Kunsch C, et al. Chemistry and pharmacology of vascular protectants. A novel approach to the treatment of atherosclerosis and coronary artery disease. Am J Cardiol 2003;91(suppl.):34A-40A.

107. Meng CQ, Somers PK, Rachita CL, et al. Novel phenolic antioxidants as multifunctional inhibitors of inducible VCAM-1 expression for use in atherosclerosis. Bioorg Med Chem Lett 2002;12:2545-8.

Chapter 11

ANTIOXIDANTS AND ENDOTHELIAL FUNCTION: HUMAN STUDIES

Christian Bingelli, Isabella Sudano, Bernd van der Loo, Francesco Cosentino, Georg Noll, and Thomas F. Lüscher
University Hospital and Cardiovascular Research, Institute of Physiology, University of Zürich, Switzerland

Introduction

Endothelial dysfunction is an early manifestation of atherosclerosis. Abnormal responses to endothelium-dependent vasodilators in the absence of structural changes have been described for various cardiovascular risk states including hypertension, hyperlipidemia, smoking, diabetes, hyperhomocysteinemia and aging. The discovery of oxidatively modified Low Density Lipoprotein (LDL) particles being involved in foam cell generation and the pivotal role of nitric oxide (NO), its antiatherogenic properties and interactions with superoxide and other radicals, have led to the concept that oxidative stress is a hallmark of vascular disease and atherosclerosis, and have suggested a protective role of exogenous antioxidative substances.

Methods to assess endothelial function in vivo

Venous occlusion plethysmography

Venous occlusion plethysmography measures total forearm blood flow, of which, under resting conditions, the main proportion occurs through skeletal muscle. The principle of venous occlusion plethysmography is simple: when venous return from the arm is obstructed by a cuff, inflated above venous pressure, the arm volume gradually increases due to unobstructed arterial inflow (*Figure 1*). The hands are normally excluded, although it seems that this does not substantially influence the measurements[1]. The arm swells proportional to the rate of arterial inflow[1].

Excluding the hand is achieved by inflation of a wrist cuff above systemic arterial pressure. Arrest of venous return is achieved by inflation of a cuff placed around the upper arm. The cuff is usually inflated to 40 mmHg for about five to eight seconds, triggered in some installations by the electrocardiogram. It is important to achieve complete emptying of the forearm veins before subsequent measurements. Therefore, the forearm is placed above the level of the right atrium. Complete emptying is normally achieved by five to eight seconds of cuff deflation; however at high flow rates, it may be necessary to decrease the time of cuff inflation and to increase the period of venous return to avoid high venous pressure.

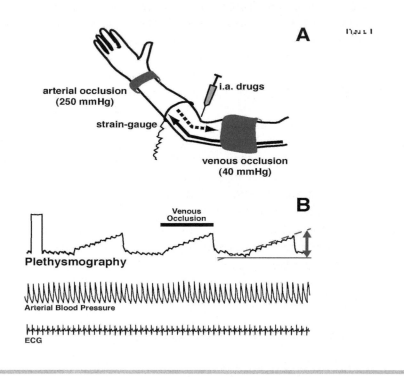

Figure 1. **Venous occlusion plethysmography:**
A: Venous return is obstructed by inflating a cuff to 40 mmHg. The arm-volume gradually increases, measured by strain gauges. Drugs are applied through an arterial catheter. The hand is normally excluded by inflating a cuff to supra-systolic pressure.
B: The volume increase is proportional to the blood flow to the arm. The recording of arterial blood pressure and or the ECG allows pulse-triggered, computer assisted evaluation of the plethysmographic recording.

Combining this method with cannulation of the brachial artery, it is possible to test endothelium-dependent vasodilation with agonists like acetylcholine, methacholine, serotonin, substance-P, bradykinin, as well as endothelium-independent vasodilators like sodium-nitroprusside, and vasoconstrictors like phenylephrine, norepinephrine, angiotensin II or endothelin.

Echo Doppler flow measurements

This method allows a non-invasive assessment of endothelial function. With a Doppler flow probe placed over the brachial or the radial artery, the velocity and diameter of large sized vessels can be measured (*Figure 2*). This technique allows simultaneous study of large conduit vessels, assessed by the diameter of the brachial artery, and of small vessels, and by measurement of total flow[2]. However, small errors in measuring the diameter result in large errors in calculating flow, and the difference in diameter between systole and diastole presents a problem of the technique, although sophisticated models have largely overcome this problem. The method is particularly suitable for measuring flow increase and flow-mediated vasodilatation (FMD) after ischemia of the arm. FMD is partly NO-dependent and can thus serve as a marker of endothelial function[3].

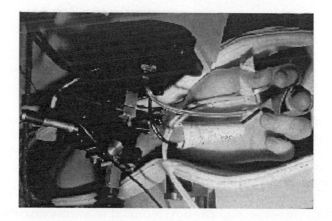

Figure 2. **Flow mediated dilatation of the radial artery:** The arm is fixed and the transducer is held in place by a stereotaxic arm. The diameter of the radial artery and flow velocity are continuously measured.

Quantitative coronary angiography flow measurements

Functional studies can also be conducted in coronary arteries using the same vasoactive drugs. To quantify the vascular response the vessel diameters can be quantified using mono- or biplane angiography and computer-assisted calculation of the vessel diameter[4] (*Figure 3*). The flow-velocity in coronary arteries can be measured using a flow-wire. Applied together, these techniques provide measurements of coronary flow and vasomotion.

Quantitative Coronary Angiography

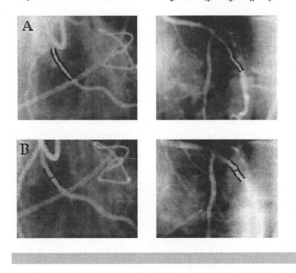

Figure 3. **Quantitative coronary angiography:** Corresponding vessel segments (biplane) are selected by an operator. Border detection is performed by an edge detection algorithm. Changes of vessel diameter can be studied at rest (A) and during various provoked changes such as exercise or intracoronary infusion of vasoactive substances. The intracoronary infusion of papaverine led to endothelium-dependent vasodilation (B).

Endothelial dysfunction and the development of cardiovascular disease

The principal changes that take place in the arterial wall during the development of atherosclerosis occur largely within the intima of medium-size and large arteries, although functional changes also occur in the microcirculation in the presence of risk factors[5]. Thus the entry of substances and cells from the blood into the artery wall as well as from the artery wall into the blood depends upon alterations in the function of endothelial cells (*Figure 4*). The endothelium is a living organ and has, besides its barrier function, important regulatory properties, being capable of producing substances influencing vascular tone, hemostasis, adhesion of leucocytes, migration and proliferation of smooth muscle cells.

NO plays a pivotal role in the endothelium. NO has inhibitory effects on smooth muscle cell proliferation, platelet function and on chemotaxis, adhesion and internalization of monocytes. NO can be inactivated by oxygen-derived free radicals, the production of which is augmented in various cardiovascular risk states. This leads to reduced bioavailability of NO and to a loss of its inhibitory functions (*Figure 4*).

When endothelial cells are presented with LDL, they will bind, internalize, and modify the lipoprotein and can oxidize it, making it available for macrophage uptake via the scavenger receptor on the surface of the macrophage. OxLDL has profound effects on endothelial function, in particular it reduces NO production and enhances the expression and release of ET-1 (*Figure 4*).

The response to injury hypothesis of atherosclerosis suggests that some form of injury to the endothelial lining of the artery wall results in a sequence of events that lead to endothelial dysfunction, and the development of the lesions of atherosclerosis. The injury may be subtle and may result in functional impairment but no observable alteration. Those forms of injury that do not lead to phenotypic alterations in the endothelium may lead to increased endothelial turnover. Morphological observation of the vessel surface may provide no evidence for such an increased turnover. Nevertheless this may be enough to stimulate the expression of genes for chemotactic factors (MCP-1, etc.), monocytes, and growth factors within the endothelium. Expression of selectins and adhesion molecules allow monocytes to attach to the endothelium and to migrate into the subendothelial space where they can become activated macrophages. They are then capable of expressing genes for numerous mediators, including PDGF-A and B chains, TGF-α, TGF-β, CSF-1 PGE, ET-1, and γ-IFN (*Figure 4*). Macrophages in the subendothelial space lead to the formation of fatty streaks. In a further step, endothelial cells and macrophages are capable of forming growth factors that can attract smooth muscle cells from the media into the intima, causing intimal smooth muscle cell migration, proliferation and accumulation. Furthermore, when vascular wall integrity is lost (i.e. endothelial denudation, plaque rupture) and platelets come into contact with subendothelial structures, causing platelet-vessel wall interactions, platelets are also important sources of vasoconstrictors, coagulation factors and growth factors. Thus, the varying forms of injury, such as hypercholesterolemia, hypertension, toxins, viruses, bacteria, substances from cigarette smoke or homocysteine, are the primary agents leading to these early changes in the endothelium and the vessel wall that ultimately result in advanced atherosclerosis.

Endothelium dysfunction and oxidative stress

Endothelial injury and dysfunction have been proposed as initiating events of atherosclerosis. They are associated with a decrease in the bioavailability of NO, and often an increased production of constricting factors (i.e. ET, PGH_2, TXA_2). The nature of the endothelial dysfunction resulting in an attenuation of endothelium-mediated responses to endothelium-dependent agonists is not completely understood (*Figure 5*), but may include: 1) decreased substrate availability (e.g. L-arginine), 2) reduced NO-synthase (NOS) activity (e.g. reduced levels of cofactors such as tetrahydrobiopterin, BH_4) 3) decreased expression of NOS, 4) imbalance between the production of endothelium-derived constricting and relaxing factors, 5) production of an endogenous NOS inhibitor, and 6) overproduction of oxygen-derived free radicals with inactivation of NO. While experimental evidence has been provided to support almost all of these possibilities (and in fact several may be important at different stages of the disease process), increased production of superoxide anions (O_2-) within the vascular wall is currently favored as an explanation for the observed changes in vascular responsiveness and the characteristic loss of the anti-adhesive properties of the endothelium in the presence of cardiovascular risk factors. There are three major endothelial sources of O_2^-: NAD(P)H-oxidases, eNOS and mitochondria (*Figure 6*). In the presence of low intracellular levels of the essential cofactor tetrahydrobiopterin (BH_4), eNOS is a source of O_2-. It is likely that the formation of BH_4 through GTP-cyclohydrolase is reduced in hypercholesterolemia, early hypertension, and other risk factors[6,7] NAD(P)H-oxidases are activated by angiotensin II[8,9]. O_2- as a free radical is very reactive. It oxidizes LDL, reacts with NO to form peroxynitrite (ONOO-), and activates NF-κB which leads to the expression of adhesion molecules.

Endothelium dysfunction and oxidative stress

Endothelial injury and dysfunction have been proposed as initiating events of atherosclerosis. They are associated with a decrease in the bioavailability of NO, and often an increased production of constricting factors (i.e. ET, PGH_2, TXA_2). The nature of the endothelial dysfunction resulting in an attenuation of endothelium-mediated responses to endothelium-dependent agonists is not completely understood (*Figure 5*), but may include: 1) decreased substrate availability (e.g. L-arginine), 2) reduced NO-synthase (NOS) activity (e.g. reduced levels of cofactors such as tetrahydrobiopterin, BH_4) 3) decreased expression of NOS, 4) imbalance between the production of endothelium-derived constricting and relaxing factors, 5) production of an endogenous NOS inhibitor, and 6) overproduction of oxygen-derived free radicals with inactivation of NO. While experimental evidence has been provided to support almost all of these possibilities (and in fact several may be important at different stages of the disease process), increased production of superoxide anions (O_2-) within the vascular wall is currently favored as an explanation for the observed changes in vascular responsiveness and the characteristic loss of the anti-adhesive properties of the endothelium in the presence of cardiovascular risk factors. There are three major endothelial sources of O_2^-: NAD(P)H-oxidases, eNOS and mitochondria (*Figure 6*). In the presence of low intracellular levels of the essential cofactor tetrahydrobiopterin (BH_4), eNOS is a source of O_2-. It is likely that the formation of BH_4 through GTP-cyclohydrolase is reduced in hypercholesterolemia, early hypertension, and other risk factors[6,7] NAD(P)H oxidases are activated by angiotensin II[8,9]. O_2- as a free radical is very reactive. It oxidizes LDL, reacts with NO to form peroxynitrite (ONOO-), and activates NF-κB which leads to the expression of adhesion molecules.

Oxidized LDL and endothelial function

Oxidative modification of LDL has been recognized as a key factor in the formation of foam cells. Normally, LDL in the circulation is well protected against oxidation by highly effective antioxidant defense mechanisms of human plasma. Native LDL is taken up by the classic Goldstein/Brown LDL receptor. As cholesterol rises in the cell, the expression of the LDL receptor is down-regulated. In this way, there is no cholesterol accumulation even when cells are exposed in vitro to very high concentrations of native cholesterol. However, in patients with cardiovascular risk factors, oxidative modification of LDL can occur. Oxidized LDL (oxLDL) is taken up into macrophages by specific oxLDL (scavenger) receptors that are not down-regulated and metabolic effects as well as lipid accumulation can occur (*Figure 5*). Recently, a novel lectin-like receptor for ox-LDL (LOX-1) has been identified, primarily in the endothelial cells. It allows uptake of ox-LDL into endothelial cells[10]. This receptor is transcriptionally upregulated by tumor necrosis factor-alpha, angiotensin II, shear stress and ox-LDL itself. This receptor is highly expressed in the blood vessels of animals and humans with hypertension, diabetes mellitus and atherosclerosis[11]. OxLDL has many properties. It is chemotactic for monocytes and for T-cells and is cytotoxic for endothelial cells. It interferes with G_i-protein mediated signal transduction for eNOS activation by serotonin[12] and NO as well as ET production[13]. It can also stimulate the expression of adhesion molecules (ICAM-1, VCAM-1, selectins) and chemoattractant proteins like MCP-1. Oxygen-derived radicals and oxLDL, among other factors, stimulate NF-κB, inducing increased expression of ICAM-1 (*Figure 5*).

Hypercholesterolemia is most commonly associated with an elevation of plasma LDL, and LDL is the ultimate source of the cholesterol that accumulates in developing foam cells. Yet, paradoxically, the uptake of LDL into macrophages and into smooth muscle cells almost certainly does not occur by way of the classic Goldstein/Brown LDL receptor. Foam cells develop in patients and in animals that totally lack LDL receptors, and their foam cells resemble the ones developing in atherosclerotic lesions of patients with hypercholesterolemia and normal LDL receptors. Incubation of either macrophages[14] or smooth muscle cells[15] with even very high concentrations of LDL does not increase the cell content of cholesterol. This reflects in part the fact that the native LDL receptor of macrophages, smooth muscle cells, and other cells, downregulates when the cell cholesterol content builds up. These experiments made it necessary to postulate that LDL in the circulation must somehow be altered before it could be a source of foam cell cholesterol. Goldstein et al[14] showed that pretreating LDL in vitro with acetic anhydride caused a markedly increased uptake of acetyl LDL by macrophages, by way of a new receptor distinct from the LDL receptor. Most importantly, this acetyl LDL receptor, unlike the LDL receptor, did not downregulate and macrophages became engorged with stored cholesterol esters. However, there is little evidence that this process is of much significance in vivo. Therefore, the search for other modifications of LDL that do occur in vivo continued. In the early 1980s, Henriksen et al[16-18] showed that endothelial cells and smooth muscle cells are able to modify LDL in vitro, in such a way as to enhance its uptake by macrophages. Later studies by Steinbrecher et al[19] and Morel et al[20] showed that the cells actually simply oxidize LDL. The effects could be mimicked by incubating LDL with copper ions as catalyst. Thus, the oxidative modification hypothesis originally rested on the finding that cell-modified (oxidized) LDL had the potential to cause foam cell formation. Oxidation of LDL is a very complex process. Both the protein and the lipid part can be oxidatively modified, and each of the lipid classes can be attacked, including sterols, fatty acids in phospholipids, cholesterol esters, and triglycerides and in fact almost all components, including the many antioxidants in LDL. The extent of the changes in the LDL particle induced by oxidation depends on the prooxidant conditions used, and the length of time the particle is exposed to those prooxidant conditions. Therefore, there is no unique LDL particle corresponding to "oxidized LDL". OxLDL molecules can differ not only structurally but also functionally. It was shown that LDL, only exposed to minimal oxidative stress, does not change its interaction with the LDL receptor[21]. Yet it can acquire important functions such as the ability to stimulate the release of cytokines from endothelial cells[22,23]. The ability of oxLDL to induce cholesterol accumulation in macrophages was the first proatherogenic property of oxLDL to be described[18], and was the basis of the hypothesis that oxidation of LDL might be a crucial step in the atherogenic process.

There is strong evidence that LDL oxidation does occur in vivo under certain conditions. First, cholesterol extracted from plaques is in part oxidatively modified[24]. Second, atherosclerotic lesions contain material reactive with antibodies against oxLDL[25-27]. Third, there are circulating antibodies against oxLDL[26], indicating the presence of oxLDL or of a very similar antigen.

Thus the oxidative modification hypothesis says that LDL is somehow altered and taken up into cells by specific oxLDL-receptors that do not downregulate as cholesterol builds up in the cell, and is able to induce cholesterol accumulation. The necessary modifications do occur in vivo, especially in the endothelium. Macrophages and smooth muscle cells are protected against accumulation of non-modified cholesterol by compensatory downregulation of the classic Goldstein/Brown receptor as intracellular cholesterol content rises.

Antioxidants in the treatment of atherosclerosis

Oxidative stress is a common feature induced by aging and cardiovascular risk factors in the endothelium and the vascular wall (*Figure 6*), leading to oxidative modification of LDL, NO inactivation, formation of ONOO- and nitrotyrosine residues, and in turn inactivation of important enzymes. Thus, it seems very reasonable to try to inhibit or scavenge reactive oxygen species (ROS). This approach, which also prevents activation of NF-κB and expression of adhesion molecules and oxidative modification of LDL, may finally slow down the progression of atherosclerosis.

Whereas there is good evidence from animal models that the process of atherosclerosis can be slowed by different antioxidants (*Table 1*)[28-40], in humans, there are conflicting data. The Cambridge Heart Antioxidant Study (CHAOS), a double-blind, randomized trial involving 2002 patients with proven CAD, showed a 47% reduced risk of combined cardiovascular death and non-fatal myocardial infarction in patients treated with vitamin E 400 to 800 IU/d, compared to placebo[41]. But there was no difference in cardiovascular death and all-cause mortality (*Table 2*)[41-46]. The Finnish α-tocopherol and β-carotene cancer prevention study involved about 27,000 Finnish male smokers aged between 50 and 70 years. Patients either received small dosages of these antioxidants or placebo, in a primary preventive setting. There were no significant differences among the groups concerning cardiovascular risk[47] as well as in the vitamin E arm of the Heart Outcome Prevention Evaluation (HOPE) [45] or in the Heart Protection Study (HPS)[46]. The slow development of atherosclerosis in humans and the relatively short observation period (two to six years) might be a problem of such trials. Therefore, for a better understanding of the pathophysiology, the assessment of endothelial function in vivo has been proposed[48] as a surrogate endpoint. However, long-term oral vitamins C and E did not affect biomarkers of oxidative stress and gave inconsistent results in adults with CAD[49,50]. The concept that endothelial dysfunction can predict clinical outcome has recently been supported by forearm studies with a mean observation time of 2.5 and 4.5 years[51,52] and by studies in the coronary circulation[53].

Hyperlipidemia:

Hypercholesterolemia is associated with endothelial dysfunction in the forearm[54-56] and in the coronary circulation[57,58]. The mechanisms by which hypercholesterolemia impairs endothelial function are not yet fully understood. OxLDL and/or total LDL, as outlined above, seem to play a key role in the reduction of NO bioavailabilty and induction of adhesive properties of the endothelium, allowing monocytes to adhere to endothelial cells[59,60]. Reduction of LDL by a single LDL apheresis improves endothelial-dependent vasodilation to acetylcholine[61], indicating a role of LDL as well. An increase of extracellular NO breakdown does not seem to occur because the administration of superoxide-dismutase – a scavenger of superoxide anion – did not improve endothelial function in hypercholesterolemic patients[56]. This could be explained by: 1) the relatively slow reaction of superoxide with superoxide-dismutase and the much faster reaction of NO with the radical, and 2) the fact that superoxide-dismutase does not penetrate into endothelial cells.

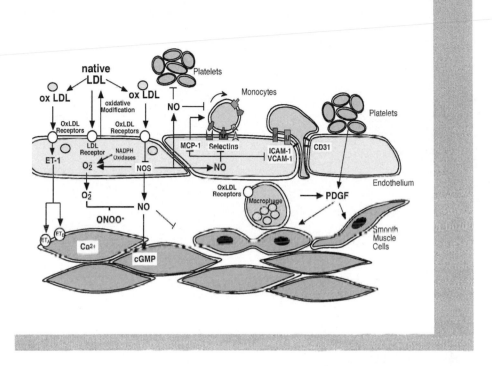

Figure 4. **Endothelial dysfunction in hypcrlipidemia and atheriosclerosis.** The major componcnts are oxLDL which impair the activity of the L-arginine NO pathway. The expression of MCP-1, selectins and adhesion molecules (ICAM-1, VCAM-1) is normally inhibited by NO; however, in states of increased production of O2-, NO-bioavailabilty is reduced. Peroxynitrite leads to nitrotyrosine residues and in turn inactivation of important enzymes. The expression of adhesion molecules allows monocytes to attach to the endothelium. In the subendothelial space, they become macrophages with scavenger receptors, taking up oxLDL and forming foam cells. OxLDL activate endothelin gene expression and production.

OxLDL: oxidized low density lipoprotein; NO: nitric oxide; O2-: Superoxide-anion; ET-1: Endothelin-1; NOS: nitric oxide synthase; ONNO-: Peroxynitrite; PDGF: Platelet derived growth factor; ICAM-1: intercellular adhesion molecule-1; VCAM-1: vascular cell adhesion molecule-1; MCP-1: monocyte chemoattractant protein 1

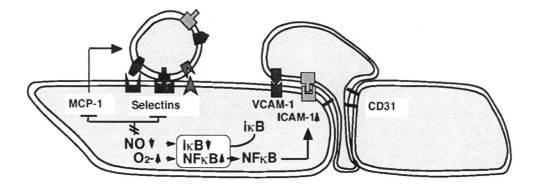

Figure 5. **In atherosclerosis, NO availability is reduced, leading to decreased ikB.** Oxygen-derived radicals, oxLDL and other stimuli lead to increased production of NF-kB that in turn stimulates the expression of ICAM-1. NF-kB in its inactive form is bound to iκB.

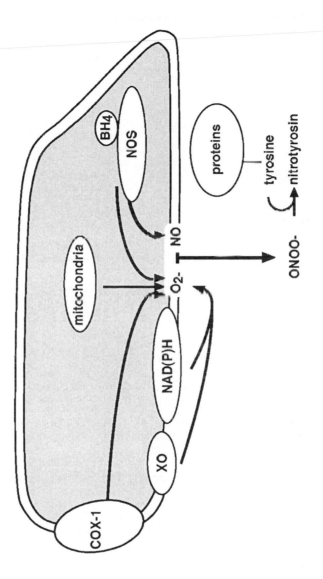

Figure 6. **Sources of superoxide:** Superoxide (O2-) is produced by NAD(P)H oxidases, mitochondria, and by nitric oxide synthase (NOS). BH4 (tetrahydrobiopterin) is a cofactor for NOS. ONOO- (peroxynitrite) is formed by the fast reaction of O2- and NO. Peroxynitrite can structurally and functionally modify proteins, forming nitrotyrosines.

Table 1: **Antioxidants in animal models of atherosclerosis**

Type of Study	Authorship and Date	Reference
Probucol in LDL-R deficient rabbits	Carew et al, 1987	28
	Kita et al, 1987	29
	Daugherty et al, 1991	30
	Mao et al, 1991	31
	Fruebis et al, 1994	32
	Morel et al, 1994	33
Probucol in cholesterol-fed rabbits	Stein et al, 1989	34
	Daugherty et al, 1989	35
Vitamin E in rabbits	Prasad et al, 1993	36
	Morel et al, 1994	33
	Kleinveld et al, 1995	37
	Fruebis et al, 1995	38
Vitamin E in hamsters	Parker et al, 1995	39
Vitamin E in primates	Verlangieri et al, 1992	40

Table 2: **Human trials with antioxidants**

Study	Authorship and Date	Reference	Result	
Vitamin E, beta-carotene	The ABC Cancer Prevention Study Group, 1994	42	cardiovascular:	0
			all-cause mortality:	0
Beta-carotene	Hennekens et al, 1996	43	cardiovascular:	0
			all-cause mortality:	0
Beta-carotene and retinol	Omenn et al, 1996	44	all-cause mortality:	-
Cambridge Heart Antioxidant Study (CHAOS)	Stephens et al, 1996	41	myocardial infarction: all-cause mortality:	+ 0
HOPE vitamin E	Yusuf et al. 2000	45	Cardiovascular	0
HPS vitamin E, beta-carotene	MRC/BHF Heart Protection Study	46	major coronary event	0

0 = no significant effect; **+** = positive effect (significant reduction of risk); **-** = negative effect.

Endothelial function, as assessed by FMD, appears already reduced early in childhood in patients with familial hypercholesterolemia and familial combined hyperlipidemia, and endothelial dysfunction can be restored by oral vitamin E and vitamin C[62,63]. In hypercholesterolemic patients, endothelial dysfunction can acutely be improved by vitamin C[64]. Stroes et al demonstrated a restoration of endothelial function in the same setting after supplementation with tetrahydrobiopterin, an antioxidant and co-factor of NO synthases (*Figure 6*)[6]. Similarly, BH$_4$ infusion in the coronary circulation improves endothelial function under acute conditions[65]. These studies suggest that reduced BH$_4$ levels in hypercholesterolemia may cause eNOS dysfunction and oxidative stress (increased O$_2$- production) (*Figure 6*). Long term vitamin E supplementation in patients with hypercholesterolemia was not effective[66]. Thus, various antioxidants are able to improve endothelial function acutely, whereas the results for long term supplementation are still conflicting.

Remnant hyperlipidemia is also characterized by impaired endothelial function. The mechanisms are not well understood. A double blind study recently showed that treatment with vitamin E, but not with placebo, significantly increased flow-mediated dilation in patients with high remnants levels. This indicates a role of oxidative damage in patients with remnant hyperlipidemia[67]. Statins are able to improve endothelial-dependent vasodilation in the forearm and coronary circulation in hypercholesterolemic patients[68,69]. Similar experiments have shown an improvement of FMD in the brachial artery of patients with hypercholesterolemia after a vitamin E and simvastatin combination therapy[70]. In the coronary circulation lovastatin and probucol for one year significantly improved vasomotion compared to an American Heart Association step 1 diet[71]. How exactly statins improve endothelial function is not clear. It might not be lipid lowering alone, since it has been demonstrated that atorvastatin restored endothelium-dependent vasodilation in normocholesterolemic cigarette smokers, independent of changes in lipids[72]. Several statins have recently been shown to induce endothelial NO synthase expression[73], or improved the oxidative state[74].

Smoking

Cigarette smoking is associated with endothelial dysfunction[75-77] that is further aggravated in the presence of hypercholesterolemia[78]. Smokers show impaired endothelium- dependent vasodilation in the brachial artery. Acute smoking causes a further impairment of FMD. FMD is improved after 200 mg of vitamin C[79] or consumption of 250ml of red wine[80].

Long-term cigarette smoking is also associated with impaired endothelium-dependent coronary vasodilation, regardless of the presence or absence of coronary atherosclerotic lesions[81]. Long-term vitamin E supplementation[66], as well as the acute administration of tetrahydrobiopterin[82], improve endothelium- dependent relaxation in forearm resistance vessels, whereas long term vitamin C was ineffective[83].

Hypertension

In human hypertension, available data clearly indicate the presence of reduced basal production of NO[84], and impaired vasodilation to endothelium-dependent agonists[48,85-90]. Using the local infusion of the NO synthase inhibitor N[G]-monomethyl-L-arginine (L-NMMA), the basal production of NO was found to be reduced in the forearm circulation[48,90] and in the coronary macro- and micro-circulation of hypertensive patients[85,91]. Vasodilation to endothelium-dependent agonists is impaired in the forearm[89,90], coronary[91] and renal circulation[92] of essential hypertensive patients.

Several mechanisms seem to be involved in the endothelial dysfunction found in essential hypertension. The alteration of the L-arginine-NO pathway is associated with an increased production of endothelium-derived contracting factors (EDCF) such as vasoconstrictor prostanoids (tromboxane A_2 and prostaglandin H_2) and oxygen free radicals that can inactivate NO, reducing its bioavailability[93,94].

In epicardial coronary arteries of essential hypertensive patients, the local infusion of vitamin C is able to improve the response to acetylcholine and the FMD in response to papaverine[71,95]. In the forearm circulation, impaired endothelial vasodilation can be improved by oral administration[96], or by intrabrachial infusion, of vitamin C[97]. The effect obtained by intrabrachial infusion of vitamin C can be reversed by L-NMMA[97], a finding supporting the hypothesis that NO inactivation by oxygen free radicals contributes to endothelial dysfunction in essential hypertension.

The positive effect of vitamin C is not observed in the presence of indomethacin; for this reason, it is conceivable that the major source of the oxidative stress that causes NO breakdown is endothelial cyclooxygenase[97]. This possibility is consistent with the finding that intrabrachial superoxide dismutase[98], a scavenger that does not penetrate into endothelial cells, and oxypurinol[99], a specific inhibitor of xantine oxidase, a major source of oxygen derived free radicals in experimental hypertension, do not improve vasodilation to acetylcholine in essential hypertensive patients.

Hyperhomocysteinemia

In healthy subjects, the elevation of the plasma concentration of homocysteine, after oral L-methionine, is associated with an acute impairment of vascular endothelial function[100,101] that can be prevented by pretreatment with vitamin C[102-104]. These results support the hypothesis that the adverse effects of homocysteine on vascular endothelial cells are mediated by oxidative stress mechanisms. Long term supplementation with folic acid in healthy subjects with hyperhomocysteinemia yielded conflicting results[105,106].

Diabetes mellitus

NO-mediated vasodilation is impaired in insulin-dependent[107] and non-insulin-dependent diabetes mellitus[108,109]. Also, acute normoinsulinemic hyperglycemia impairs endothelium-dependent vasodilation in healthy humans in vivo[110]. Inactivation of endothelium-derived NO by oxygen-derived free radicals contributes to abnormal vascular reactivity in experimental models of diabetes[7]. Ting et al have shown that vitamin C improved the endothelium-dependent vasodilation elicited by methacholine in non-insulin dependent patients, whereas the vasodilatatory answer was the same as in the control group[111]. These findings support the hypothesis that NO inactivation by oxygen derived free radicals contributes to abnormal vascular reactivity in diabetes.

Aging

Aging is associated with diminished vasodilator response to reactive hyperemia[114] by acetylcholine in the forearm[112,113], and the coronary circulation[57]. Although NOS is upregulated in older rats, increased generation of O_2- results in a net diminished availability of NO[115]. Medium-term supplementation with vitamin E has no major impact on arterial endothelial function when age-related dysfunction is already present[116]. In a small study, a 'Mediterranean-type' diet-rich in vitamin C improved vascular function, but neither acute intra-arterial nor sustained administration of one gram of oral vitamin C improved vascular function in healthy older subjects[117]. Regular physical activity can at least in part prevent the age-induced endothelial dysfunction, probably by preventing the production of oxidative stress, since vitamin C restored the response to acetylcholine in elderly sedentary subjects, while it was unaltered by vitamin C in elderly athletes[118].

Conclusions

Thus, the current review of the available literature suggests that oxidative stress is a major feature of vascular disease and atherosclerosis. O_2- is produced mainly in the endothelium and derived from NAD(P)H oxidases, eNOS (in the presence of low BH_4 levels), cyclooxygenase, and mitochondrial enzymes. O_2- leads to NO inactivation, formation of ONOO- and in turn, nitrotyrosine residues of vascular enzymes. In addition O_2- activates NF-κB, leads to expression of adhesion molecules and oxidizes

LDL. Oxidized LDL in turn has important properties. It is cytotoxic for endothelial cells, chemotactic, and stimulates the expression of adhesion molecules, allowing monocytes to adhere to the vascular wall. Antioxidants include probucol, vitamin E, folic acid, vitamin C, and polyphenols. Large human studies with antioxidants, and primary or secondary cardiovascular endpoints, showed mainly negative results. However, there is evidence that endothelial dysfunction, as an early manifestation of developing atherosclerosis, can acutely be improved with different antioxidants. Long term supplementation with vitamin antioxidants was ineffective in the majority of studies.

Acknowledgements

Clinical research work of the authors has been supported by grants of the Swiss National Research Foundation 32-51069.97 and 32–45878.95) and the Swiss Heart Foundation.

References

1. Whitney RJ. The measurement of volume changes in human limbs. J Physiol (Lond). 1953;121:1-27.

2. Celermajer DS, Sorensen KE, Gooch VM et al. Non-invasive detection of endothelial dysfunction in children and adults at risk of atherosclerosis. Lancet 1992;340:1111-5.

3. Joannides R, Haefeli WE, Linder L et al. Nitric oxide is responsible for flow-dependent dilation of human peripheral conduit arteries in vivo. Circulation 1995;91:1314-9.

4. Egashira K, Inou T, Hirooka Y, Yamada A, Urabe Y, Takeshita A. Evidence of impaired endothelium-dependent coronary vasodilatation in patients with angina pectoris and normal coronary angiograms. N Engl J Med 1993;328:1659-64.

5. Binggeli C, Spieker LE, Corti R et al. Statins enhance postischemic hyperemia in the skin circulation of hypercholesterolemic patients: a monitoring test of endothelial dysfunction for clinical practice? J Am Coll Cardiol 2003;42:71-7.

6. Stroes E, Kastelein J, Cosentino F et al. Tetrahydrobiopterin restores endothelial function in hypercholesterolemia. J Clin Invest 1997;99:41-6.

7. Cosentino F, Hishikawa K, Katusic ZS, Luscher TF. High glucose increases nitric oxide synthase expression and superoxide anion generation in human aortic endothelial cells. Circulation 1997;96:25-8.

8. Griendling KK, Minieri CA, Ollerenshaw JD, Alexander RW. Angiotensin II stimulates NADH and NADPH oxidase activity in cultured vascular smooth muscle cells. Circ Res 1994;74:1141-8.

9. Fukai T, Siegfried MR, Ushio-Fukai M, Griendling KK, Harrison DG. Modulation of extracellular superoxide dismutase expression by angiotensin II and hypertension. Circ Res 1999;85:23-8.

10. Sawamura T, Kume N, Aoyama T et al. An endothelial receptor for oxidized low-density lipoprotein. Nature 1997;386:73-7.

11. Mehta JL, Li D. Identification, regulation and function of a novel lectin-like oxidized low-density lipoprotein receptor. J Am Coll Cardiol 2002;39:1429-35.

12. Shimokawa H, Vanhoutte PM. Impaired endothelium-dependent relaxation to aggregating platelets and related vasoactive substances in porcine coronary arteries in hypercholesterolemia and atherosclerosis. Circ Res 1989;64:900-14.

13. Boulanger CM, Tanner FC, Bea ML, Hahn AW, Werner A, Luscher TF. Oxidized low density lipoproteins induce mRNA expression and release of endothelin from human and porcine endothelium. Circ Res 1992;70:1191-7.

14. Goldstein JL, Ho YK, Basu SK, Brown MS. Binding site on macrophages that mediates uptake and degradation of acetylated low density lipoprotein, producing massive cholesterol deposition. Proc Natl Acad Sci U S A 1979;76:333-7.

15. Weinstein DB, Carew TE, Steinberg D. Uptake and degradation of low density lipoprotein by swine arterial smooth muscle cells with inhibition of cholesterol biosynthesis. Biochim Biophys Acta 1976;424:404-21.

16. Henriksen T, Mahoney EM, Steinberg D. Enhanced macrophage degradation of biologically modified low density lipoprotein. Arteriosclerosis 1983;3:149-59.

17. Henriksen T, Mahoney EM, Steinberg D. Interactions of plasma lipoproteins with endothelial cells. Ann N Y Acad Sci 1982;401:102-16.

18. Henriksen T, Mahoney EM, Steinberg D. Enhanced macrophage degradation of low density lipoprotein previously incubated with cultured endothelial cells: recognition by receptors for acetylated low density lipoproteins. Proc Natl Acad Sci U S A 1981;78:6499-503.

19. Steinbrecher UP, Parthasarathy S, Leake DS, Witztum JL, Steinberg D. Modification of low density lipoprotein by endothelial cells involves lipid peroxidation and degradation of low density lipoprotein phospholipids. Proc Natl Acad Sci U S A 1984;81:3883-7.

20. Morel DW, DiCorleto PE, Chisolm GM. Endothelial and smooth muscle cells alter low density lipoprotein in vitro by free radical oxidation. Arteriosclerosis 1984;4:357-64.

21. Berliner JA, Navab M, Fogelman AM et al. Atherosclerosis: basic mechanisms. Oxidation, inflammation, and genetics. Circulation 1995;91:2488-96.

22. Rajavashisth TB, Andalibi A, Territo MC et al. Induction of endothelial cell expression of granulocyte and macrophage colony-stimulating factors by modified low-density lipoproteins. Nature 1990;344:254-7.

23. Cushing SD, Berliner JA, Valente AJ et al. Minimally modified low density lipoprotein induces monocyte chemotactic protein 1 in human endothelial cells and smooth muscle cells. Proc Natl Acad Sci U S A 1990;87:5134-8.

24. Yla-Herttuala S, Palinski W, Rosenfeld ME et al. Evidence for the presence of oxidatively modified low density lipoprotein in atherosclerotic lesions of rabbit and man. J Clin Invest 1989;84:1086-95.

25. Haberland ME, Fong D, Cheng L. Malondialdehyde-altered protein occurs in atheroma of Watanabe heritable hyperlipidemic rabbits. Science 1988;241:215-8.

26. Palinski W, Rosenfeld ME, Yla-Herttuala S et al. Low density lipoprotein undergoes oxidative modification in vivo. Proc Natl Acad Sci U S A 1989;86:1372-6.

27. Rosenfeld ME, Palinski W, Yla-Herttuala S, Butler S, Witztum JL. Distribution of oxidation specific lipid-protein adducts and apolipoprotein B in atherosclerotic lesions of varying severity from WHHL rabbits. Arteriosclerosis 1990;10:336-49.

28. Carew TE, Schwenke DC, Steinberg D. Antiatherogenic effect of probucol unrelated to its hypocholesterolemic effect: evidence that antioxidants in vivo can selectively inhibit low density lipoprotein degradation in macrophage-rich fatty streaks and slow the progression of atherosclerosis in the Watanabe heritable hyperlipidemic rabbit. Proc Natl Acad Sci U S A 1987;84:7725-9.

29. Kita T, Nagano Y, Yokode M et al. Probucol prevents the progression of atherosclerosis in Watanabe heritable hyperlipidemic rabbit, an animal model for familial hypercholesterolemia. Proc Natl Acad Sci U S A 1987;84:5928-31.

30. Daugherty A, Zweifel BS, Schonfeld G. The effects of probucol on the progression of atherosclerosis in mature Watanabe heritable hyperlipidaemic rabbits. Br J Pharmacol 1991;103:1013-8.

31. Mao SJ, Yates MT, Rechtin AE, Jackson RL, Van Sickle WA. Antioxidant activity of probucol and its analogues in hypercholesterolemic Watanabe rabbits. J Med Chem 1991;34:298-302.

32. Fruebis J, Steinberg D, Dresel HA, Carew TE. A comparison of the antiatherogenic effects of probucol and of a structural analogue of probucol in low density lipoprotein receptor-deficient rabbits. J Clin Invest 1994;94:392-8.

33. Morel DW, de la Llera-Moya M, Friday KE. Treatment of cholesterol-fed rabbits with dietary vitamins E and C inhibits lipoprotein oxidation but not development of atherosclerosis. J Nutr 1994;124:2123-30.

34. Stein Y, Stein O, Delplanque B, Fesmire JD, Lee DM, Alaupovic P. Lack of effect of probucol on atheroma formation in cholesterol-fed rabbits kept at comparable plasma cholesterol levels. Atherosclerosis 1989;75:145-55.

35. Daugherty A, Zweifel BS, Schonfeld G. Probucol attenuates the development of aortic atherosclerosis in cholesterol-fed rabbits. Br J Pharmacol 1989;98:612-8.

36. Prasad K, Kalra J. Oxygen free radicals and hypercholesterolemic atherosclerosis: effect of vitamin E. Am Heart J 1993;125:958-73.

37. Kleinveld HA, Hak-Lemmers HL, Hectors MP, de Fouw NJ, Demacker PN, Stalenhoef AF. Vitamin E and fatty acid intervention does not attenuate the progression of atherosclerosis in Watanabe heritable hyperlipidemic rabbits. Arterioscler Thromb Vasc Biol 1995;15:290-7.

38. Fruebis J, Carew TE, Palinski W. Effect of vitamin E on atherogenesis in LDL receptor-deficient rabbits. Atherosclerosis 1995;117:217-24.

39. Parker RA, Sabrah T, Cap M, Gill BT. Relation of vascular oxidative stress, alpha-tocopherol, and hypercholesterolemia to early atherosclerosis in hamsters. Arterioscler Thromb Vasc Biol 1995;15:349-58.

40. Verlangieri AJ, Bush MJ. Effects of d-alpha-tocopherol supplementation on experimentally induced primate atherosclerosis. J Am Coll Nutr 1992;11:131-8.

41. Stephens NG, Parsons A, Schofield PM, Kelly F, Cheeseman K, Mitchinson MJ. Randomised controlled trial of vitamin E in patients with coronary disease: Cambridge Heart Antioxidant Study (CHAOS). Lancet 1996;347:781-6.

42. The effect of vitamin E and beta carotene on the incidence of lung cancer and other cancers in male smokers. The Alpha-Tocopherol, Beta Carotene Cancer Prevention Study Group. N Engl J Med 1994;330:1029-35.

43. Hennekens CH, Buring JE, Manson JE et al. Lack of effect of long-term supplementation with beta carotene on the incidence of malignant neoplasms and cardiovascular disease. N Engl J Med 1996;334:1145-9.

44. Omenn GS, Goodman GE, Thornquist MD et al. Effects of a combination of beta carotene and vitamin A on lung cancer and cardiovascular disease. N Engl J Med 1996;334:1150-5.

45. Yusuf S, Dagenais G, Pogue J, Bosch J, Sleight P. Vitamin E supplementation and cardiovascular events in high-risk patients. The Heart Outcomes Prevention Evaluation Study Investigators. N Engl J Med 2000;34:154-60.

46. MRC/BHF Heart Protection Study of antioxidant vitamin supplementation in 20,536 high-risk individuals: a randomised placebo-controlled trial. Lancet 2002;360:23-33.

47. Virtamo J, Rapola JM, Ripatti S, et al. Effect of vitamin E and beta carotene on the incidence of primary nonfatal myocardial infarction and fatal coronary heart disease. Arch Intern Med 1998;158:668-75.

48. Luscher TF, Noll G. Endothelial function as an end-point in interventional trials: concepts, methods and current data. J Hypertens Suppl 1996;14:S119-21.

49. Kinlay S, Behrendt D, Fang JC et al. Long-term effect of combined vitamins E and C on coronary and peripheral endothelial function. J Am Coll Cardiol 2004;43:629-34.

50. Gokce N, Keaney JF, Jr., Frei B et al. Long-term ascorbic acid administration reverses endothelial vasomotor dysfunction in patients with coronary artery disease. Circulation 1999;99:3234-40.

51. Heitzer T, Schlinzig T, Krohn K, Meinertz T, Munzel T. Endothelial dysfunction, oxidative stress, and risk of cardiovascular events in patients with coronary artery disease. Circulation 2001;104:2673-8.

52. Perticone F, Ceravolo R, Pujia A et al. Prognostic significance of endothelial dysfunction in hypertensive patients. Circulation 2001;104:191-6.

53. Schachinger V, Britten MB, Zeiher AM. Prognostic impact of coronary vasodilator dysfunction on adverse long-term outcome of coronary heart disease. Circulation 2000;101:1899-906.

54. Creager MA, Cooke JP, Mendelsohn ME et al. Impaired vasodilation of forearm resistance vessels in hypercholesterolemic humans. J Clin Invest 1990;86:228-34.

55. Gilligan DM, Guetta V, Panza JA, Garcia CE, Quyyumi AA, Cannon RO, 3rd. Selective loss of microvascular endothelial function in human hypercholesterolemia. Circulation 1994;90:35-41.

56. Garcia CE, Kilcoyne CM, Cardillo C, Cannon RO, 3rd, Quyyumi AA, Panza JA. Evidence that endothelial dysfunction in patients with hypercholesterolemia is not due to increased extracellular nitric oxide breakdown by superoxide anions. Am J Cardiol 1995;76:1157-61.

57. Vita JA, Treasure CB, Nabel EG et al. Coronary vasomotor response to acetylcholine relates to risk factors for coronary artery disease. Circulation 1990;81:491-7.

58. Drexler H, Zeiher AM, Meinzer K, Just H. Correction of endothelial dysfunction in coronary microcirculation of hypercholesterolaemic patients by L-arginine. Lancet 1991;338:1546-50.

59. Quinn MT, Parthasarathy S, Fong LG, Steinberg D. Oxidatively modified low density lipoproteins: a potential role in recruitment and retention of monocyte/macrophages during atherogenesis. Proc Natl Acad Sci U S A 1987;84:2995-8.

60. Frostegard J, Nilsson J, Haegerstrand A, Hamsten A, Wigzell H, Gidlund M. Oxidized low density lipoprotein induces differentiation and adhesion of human monocytes and the monocytic cell line U937. Proc Natl Acad Sci U S A 1990;87:904-8.

61. Tamai O, Matsuoka H, Itabe H, Wada Y, Kohno K, Imaizumi T. Single LDL apheresis improves endothelium-dependent vasodilatation in hypercholesterolemic humans. Circulation 1997;95:76-82.

62. Mietus-Snyder M, Malloy MJ. Endothelial dysfunction occurs in children with two genetic hyperlipidemias: improvement with antioxidant vitamin therapy. J Pediatr 1998;133:35-40.

63. Engler MM, Engler MB, Malloy MJ et al. Antioxidant vitamins C and E improve endothelial function in children with hyperlipidemia: Endothelial Assessment of Risk from Lipids in Youth (EARLY) Trial. Circulation 2003;108:1059-63.

64. Ting HH, Timimi FK, Haley EA, Roddy MA, Ganz P, Creager MA. Vitamin C improves endothelium-dependent vasodilation in forearm resistance vessels of humans with hypercholesterolemia. Circulation 1997;95:2617-22.

65. Fukuda Y, Teragawa H, Matsuda K, Yamagata T, Matsuura H, Chayama K. Tetrahydrobiopterin restores endothelial function of coronary arteries in patients with hypercholesterolaemia. Heart 2002;87:264-9.

66. Heitzer T, Yla Herttuala S, Wild E, Luoma J, Drexler H. Effect of vitamin E on endothelial vasodilator function in patients with hypercholesterolemia, chronic smoking or both. J Am Coll Cardiol 1999;33:499-505.

67. Kugiyama K, Motoyama T, Doi H et al. Improvement of endothelial vasomotor dysfunction by treatment with alpha-tocopherol in patients with high remnant lipoproteins levels. J Am Coll Cardiol 1999;33:1512-8.

68. O'Driscoll G, Green D, Taylor RR. Simvastatin, an HMG-coenzyme A reductase inhibitor, improves endothelial function within 1 month. Circulation 1997;95:1126-31.

69. Stroes E, de Bruin T, de Valk H et al. NO activity in familial combined hyperlipidemia: potential role of cholesterol remnants. Cardiovasc Res 1997;36:445-52.

70. Neunteufl T, Kostner K, Katzenschlager R, Zehetgruber M, Maurer G, Weidinger F. Additional benefit of vitamin E supplementation to simvastatin therapy on vasoreactivity of the brachial artery of hypercholesterolemic men. J Am Coll Cardiol 1998;32:711-6.

71. Anderson TJ, Meredith IT, Yeung AC, Frei B, Selwyn AP, Ganz P. The effect of cholesterol-lowering and antioxidant therapy on endothelium-dependent coronary vasomotion. N Engl J Med 1995;332:488-93.

72. Beckman JA, Liao JK, Hurley S et al. Atorvastatin restores endothelial function in normocholesterolemic smokers independent of changes in low-density lipoprotein. Circ Res 2004;95:217-23.

73. Laufs U, La Fata V, Plutzky J, Liao JK. Upregulation of endothelial nitric oxide synthase by HMG CoA reductase inhibitors. Circulation 1998;97:1129-35.

74. Yilmaz MI, Baykal Y, Kilic M et al. Effects of statins on oxidative stress. Biol Trace Elem Res 2004;98:119-27.

75. Celermajer DS, Sorensen KE, Georgakopoulos D et al. Cigarette smoking is associated with dose-related and potentially reversible impairment of endothelium-dependent dilation in healthy young adults. Circulation 1993;88:2149-55.

76. Heitzer T, Just H, Munzel T. Antioxidant vitamin C improves endothelial dysfunction in chronic smokers. Circulation 1996;94:6-9.

77. McVeigh GE, Lemay L, Morgan D, Cohn JN. Effects of long-term cigarette smoking on endothelium-dependent responses in humans. Am J Cardiol 1996;78:668-72.

78. Heitzer T, Yla Herttuala S, Luoma J et al. Cigarette smoking potentiates endothelial dysfunction of forearm resistance vessels in patients with hypercholesterolemia. Role of oxidized LDL. Circulation 1996;93:1346-53.

79. Motoyama T, Kawano H, Kugiyama K et al. Endothelium-dependent vasodilation in the brachial artery is impaired in smokers: effect of vitamin C. Am J Physiol 1997;273:H1644-50.

80. Papamichael C, Karatzis E, Karatzi K et al. Red wine's antioxidants counteract acute endothelial dysfunction caused by cigarette smoking in healthy nonsmokers. Am Heart J 2004;147:E5.

81. Zeiher AM, Schachinger V, Minners J. Long-term cigarette smoking impairs endothelium-dependent coronary arterial vasodilator function. Circulation 1995;92:1094-100.

82. Heitzer T, Brockhoff C, Mayer B et al. Tetrahydrobiopterin improves endothelium-dependent vasodilation in chronic smokers: evidence for a dysfunctional nitric oxide synthase. Circ Res 2000;86:E36-41.

83. Raitakari OT, Adams MR, McCredie RJ, Griffiths KA, Stocker R, Celermajer DS. Oral vitamin C and endothelial function in smokers: short-term improvement, but no sustained beneficial effect. J Am Coll Cardiol 2000;35:1616-21.

84. Forte P, Copland M, Smith LM, Milne E, Sutherland J, Benjamin N. Basal nitric oxide synthesis in essential hypertension. Lancet 1997;349:837-42.

85. Drexler H, Hornig B. Endothelial dysfunction in human disease. J Mol Cell Cardiol 1999;31:51-60.

86. Boulanger CM. Secondary endothelial dysfunction: hypertension and heart failure. J Mol Cell Cardiol 1999;31:39-49.

87. Noll G, Tschudi M, Nava E, Luscher TF. Endothelium and high blood pressure. Int J Microcirc Clin Exp 1997;17:273-9.

88. Panza JA. Endothelial dysfunction in essential hypertension. Clin Cardiol 1997;20(Suppl 2):II-26-33.

89. Taddei S, Virdis A, Mattei P, Salvetti A. Vasodilation to acetylcholine in primary and secondary forms of human hypertension. Hypertension 1993;21:929-33.

90. Taddei S, Virdis A, Mattei P et al. Hypertension causes premature aging of endothelial function in humans. Hypertension 1997;29:736-43.

91. Quyyumi AA, Mulcahy D, Andrews NP, Husain S, Panza JA, Cannon RO, 3rd. Coronary vascular nitric oxide activity in hypertension and hypercholesterolemia. Comparison of acetylcholine and substance P. Circulation 1997;95:104-10.

92. Mimran A, Ribstein J, DuCailar G. Contrasting effect of antihypertensive treatment on the renal response to L-arginine. Hypertension 1995;26:937-41.

93. Tschudi MR, Mesaros S, Luscher TF, Malinski T. Direct in situ measurement of nitric oxide in mesenteric resistance arteries. Increased decomposition by superoxide in hypertension. Hypertension 1996;27:32-5.

94. Munzel T, Heitzer T, Harrison DG. The physiology and pathophysiology of the nitric oxide/superoxide system. Herz 1997;22:158-72.

95. Solzbach U, Hornig B, Jeserich M, Just H. Vitamin C improves endothelial dysfunction of epicardial coronary arteries in hypertensive patients. Circulation 1997;96:1513-9.

96. Levine GN, Frei B, Koulouris SN, Gerhard MD, Keaney JF, Jr., Vita JA. Ascorbic acid reverses endothelial vasomotor dysfunction in patients with coronary artery disease. Circulation 1996;93:1107-13.

97. Taddei S, Virdis A, Ghiadoni L, Magagna A, Salvetti A. Vitamin C improves endothelium-dependent vasodilation by restoring nitric oxide activity in essential hypertension. Circulation 1998;97:2222-9.

98. Garcia CE, Kilcoyne CM, Cardillo C, Cannon RO, 3rd, Quyyumi AA, Panza JA. Effect of copper-zinc superoxide dismutase on endothelium-dependent vasodilation in patients with essential hypertension. Hypertension 1995;26:863-8.

99. Cardillo C, Kilcoyne CM, Cannon RO, 3rd, Quyyumi AA, Panza JA. Xanthine oxidase inhibition with oxypurinol improves endothelial vasodilator function in hypercholesterolemic but not in hypertensive patients. Hypertension 1997;30:57-63.

100. Bellamy MF, McDowell IF, Ramsey MW et al. Hyperhomocysteinemia after an oral methionine load acutely impairs endothelial function in healthy adults. Circulation 1998;98:1848-52.

101. Tawakol A, Omland T, Gerhard M, Wu JT, Creager MA. Hyperhomocyst(e)inemia is associated with impaired endothelium- dependent vasodilation in humans. Circulation 1997;95:1119-21.

102. Chambers JC, McGregor A, Jean-Marie J, Obeid OA, Kooner JS. Demonstration of rapid onset vascular endothelial dysfunction after hyperhomocysteinemia: an effect reversible with vitamin C therapy. Circulation 1999;99:1156-60.

103. Nappo F, De Rosa N, Marfella R et al. Impairment of endothelial functions by acute hyperhomocysteinemia and reversal by antioxidant vitamins. JAMA 1999;281:2113-8.

104. Virdis A, Ghiadoni L, Cardinal H et al. Mechanisms responsible for endothelial dysfunction induced by fasting hyperhomocystinemia in normotensive subjects and patients with essential hypertension. J Am Coll Cardiol 2001;38:1106-15.

105. Woodman RJ, Celermajer DE, Thompson PL, Hung J. Folic acid does not improve endothelial function in healthy hyperhomocysteinaemic subjects. Clin Sci (Lond) 2004;106:353-8.

106. Woo KS, Chook P, Chan LL et al. Long-term improvement in homocysteine levels and arterial endothelial function after 1-year folic acid supplementation. Am J Med 2002;112:535-9.

107. Johnstone MT, Creager SJ, Scales KM, Cusco JA, Lee BK, Creager MA. Impaired endothelium-dependent vasodilation in patients with insulin- dependent diabetes mellitus. Circulation 1993;88:2510-6.

108. McVeigh GE, Brennan GM, Johnston GD et al. Impaired endothelium-dependent and independent vasodilation in patients with type 2 (non-insulin-dependent) diabetes mellitus. Diabetologia 1992;35:771-6.

109. Williams SB, Cusco JA, Roddy MA, Johnstone MT, Creager MA. Impaired nitric oxide-mediated vasodilation in patients with non-insulin-dependent diabetes mellitus. J Am Coll Cardiol 1996;27:567-74.

110. Williams SB, Goldfine AB, Timimi FK et al. Acute hyperglycemia attenuates endothelium-dependent vasodilation in humans in vivo. Circulation 1998;97:1695-701.

111. Ting HH, Timimi FK, Boles KS, Creager SJ, Ganz P, Creager MA. Vitamin C improves endothelium-dependent vasodilation in patients with non-insulin-dependent diabetes mellitus. J Clin Invest 1996;97:22-8.

112. Corretti MC, Plotnick GD, Vogel RA. The effects of age and gender on brachial artery endothelium-dependent vasoactivity are stimulus-dependent. Clin Cardiol 1995;18:471-6.

113. Taddei S, Virdis A, Mattei P et al. Aging and endothelial function in normotensive subjects and patients with essential hypertension. Circulation 1995;91:1981-7.

114. Celermajer DS, Sorensen KE, Bull C, Robinson J, Deanfield JE. Endothelium-dependent dilation in the systemic arteries of asymptomatic subjects relates to coronary risk factors and their interaction. J Am Coll Cardiol 1994;24:1468-74.

115. van der Loo B, Labugger R, Skepper JN et al. Enhanced peroxynitrite formation is associated with vascular aging. J Exp Med 2000;192:1731-44.

116. Simons LA, von Konigsmark M, Simons J, Stocker R, Celermajer DS. Vitamin E ingestion does not improve arterial endothelial dysfunction in older adults. Atherosclerosis 1999;143:193-9.

117. Singh N, Graves J, Taylor PD, MacAllister RJ, Singer DR. Effects of a 'healthy' diet and of acute and long-term vitamin C on vascular function in healthy older subjects. Cardiovasc Res 2002;56:118-25.

118. Taddei S, Galetta F, Virdis A et al. Physical activity prevents age-related impairment in nitric oxide availability in elderly athletes. Circulation 2000;101:2896-901.

Chapter 12

ANTIOXIDANT VITAMINS AND CARDIOVASCULAR DISEASE:
RANDOMIZED TRIALS FAIL TO FULFILL THE PROMISES OF OBSERVATIONAL EPIDEMIOLOGY

Danielle Hollar[1] and Charles H. Hennekens[2]
[1]Agatston Research Institute (ARI) Miami Beach FL; [2]University of Miami School of Medicine, Miami, FL

Introduction

Advances in medical knowledge proceed on several fronts, optimally simultaneously, based on contributions of different types of evidence. Basic researchers describe biological mechanisms and answer the crucial question of why an agent or intervention reduces premature death. Clinicians, through their daily practice, are providing enormous benefits to their patients by their applications of advances in diagnosis and treatment. They also formulate hypotheses based on their clinical experiences, specifically their case reports and case series. Clinical investigators test the relevance of basic research findings to affected patients and healthy individuals. Epidemiologists and statisticians, optimally collaborating with researchers in other disciplines, formulate hypotheses from descriptive studies and test them in analytic studies, both case-control and cohort as well as, where necessary, randomized trials. This strategy addresses the equally crucial and complementary question of whether an agent or intervention reduces premature death. Thus, each discipline and indeed every strategy within a discipline provide importantly relevant and complementary information to a totality of evidence on which rational clinical decisions for individuals, and policy decisions for the health of the general public, can be safely based[1].

For many exposure-disease hypotheses, randomized trials are neither necessary nor desirable. When the postulated effect sizes are small to moderate (i.e. 10-50%), however, as is the case with antioxidant vitamins and cardiovascular disease (CVD), the amount of uncontrolled and uncontrollable confounding inherent in all observational epidemiological study designs may be as big as the effect size. Randomized trials of sufficient size will tend to evenly distribute all known and unknown confounders between the treatment groups. Thus, for small to moderate effects, randomized trials represent the most reliable design strategy[2].

Basic research provides plausible biologic mechanisms to explain why antioxidant vitamins reduce risk of CVD events, and some but not all, observational epidemiologic studies indicate that individuals who self-select for antioxidant vitamins have decreased risks of CVD. Several large-scale randomized trials of sufficient size, dose, and duration, as well as their meta-analyses, demonstrate no significant benefit of antioxidant vitamins in the treatment or prevention of CVD.

In this chapter, we review the available data from prospective cohort studies as well as randomized trials and their meta-analyses. Specifically, we review the observational epidemiologic studies of both dietary-based and supplement-based antioxidant vitamins in the treatment and prevention of CVD. Then we review the blood-based observational epidemiologic studies. Finally, we review completed and ongoing randomized trials, and their meta-analyses, according to type of trial (secondary prevention or primary prevention), and by type of antioxidant intervention (single agent/vitamin or combined agent/multivitamin).

Observational epidemiologic studies

Prospective cohort studies

In a large prospective cohort study of 87,245 healthy female nurses followed for an average of eight years, a total of 552 new cases of major coronary disease (437 non-fatal myocardial infarctions (MIs) and 115 deaths due to cardiac causes) were documented[3]. Women in the highest quintile of vitamin E intake, including both dietary and supplement sources, had a 34% reduced risk of coronary heart disease (CHD) (relative risk [RR], 0.66, 95% confidence interval [95% CI], 0.50-0.87) compared to those in the lowest quintile of intake, after adjustment for age and smoking. The findings persisted after adjustment for a large number of potential confounders. When women taking vitamin E from supplements were excluded, there was no longer a significant result, suggesting that only women who consumed vitamin E as supplements experienced a CVD benefit. Vitamin C or multivitamins had no independent beneficial effect on major coronary events.

Another large prospective cohort study, the Health Professionals Follow-Up Study (HPFS), was composed of 39,910 U.S. male health professionals free of CHD, diabetes, and hypercholesterolemia[4]. A total of 667 cases of CHD (360 coronary surgical procedures, 201 nonfatal MIs, and 106 death due to cardiac causes) were documented during four years of follow-up. Men in the highest quintile of vitamin E intake, including both dietary and supplement sources, had a 40% lower risk of CHD (RR, 0.60; 95% CI, 0.44-0.81) compared to those in the lowest quintile after controlling for other risk factors and the intake of other antioxidants. Further analysis indicated only men who consumed vitamin E from supplements had a significant CVD benefit. A significant benefit was also observed among men with high intake of carotene (comparing the highest and lowest quintiles; RR, 0.71; 95% CI, 0.53-0.86), but not for those taking vitamin C, after adjustment for confounding factors as well as the use of other antioxidants.

In a prospective cohort study of 34,486 postmenopausal women, 242 CHD deaths were documented during seven years of follow-up[5]. Women who consumed high amounts of vitamin E had significantly lower risk of coronary death. The apparently beneficial effects of vitamin E were not observed among women who took supplements. Women in the highest quintile of vitamin E intake from diet had a multivariate RR of death from CHD of 0.38 (95% CI, 0.18-0.80) when compared to those in the lowest quintile. Additionally, women consuming high amounts of vitamins A or C had lower a risk of coronary death.

In another large prospective cohort study of 83,639 male U.S. physicians with no history of CVD or cancer, data for vitamin E, ascorbic acid, and multivitamin supplements were collected via self-administered questionnaires. During a mean follow-up period of 5.5 years, 1,037 CVD deaths occurred, including 608 CHD deaths. This study showed no significant association among physicians using antioxidant vitamin supplements and risk of total CVD mortality or CHD mortality either crudely or after controlling for confounding risk factors. Relative risks for vitamin E were 0.92 for total CVD mortality (95% CI, 0.70-1.21, p=.52) and 0.88 for CHD mortality (95% CI, 0.61-1.27, p=.47); for vitamin C, relative risks were 0.88 for total CVD mortality (95% CI, 0.70-1.12, p=.29) and 0.86 for CHD mortality (95% CI, 0.63-1.18, p=.34); and for multivitamins, relative risks were 1.07 for total CVD mortality (95% CI, 0.91-1.25, p=.46) and 1.02 for CHD mortality (95% CI, 0.83-1.25, p=.88)[6].

Blood-based studies

Serum antioxidant levels in 2,974 middle-aged men in the Basel Prospective Study were measured at baseline[7]. During 12 years of follow-up, there were 163 cardiovascular deaths, including 132 due to ischemic heart disease. Men in the lowest quartile of serum carotene concentrations had a 53% higher risk of death from ischemic heart disease (RR, 1.53; 95%

CI, 1.07-2.20) compared to those in the other quartiles after adjustment for age, smoking, total plasma cholesterol, and blood pressure. For vitamin C, men in the lowest quartile had a statistically nonsignificant 25% increased risk for ischemic heart disease mortality. There was no association between vitamin E concentrations and ischemic heart disease mortality, although the baseline vitamin E levels in this population were unusually high with relatively little variation.

Baseline serum cartenoid levels were assessed in 1,899 hyperlipidemic men aged 40 to 59 who were assigned to the placebo arm of the Lipid Research Clinics Coronary Primary Prevention Trial[8]. A total of 282 CHD events (non-fatal MIs and CHD deaths) were documented during 13 years of follow-up. Men in the highest quartile of serum beta-carotene had a 36% lower risk of a CHD event (RR, 0.64; 95% CI, 0.44-0.92) as compared to those in the lowest quartile after adjustment for a number of CHD risk factors. This association appeared to be stronger among men who never smoked.

In a prospective nested case-control study, serum antioxidant levels for 123 cases of first MI, identified from a population of approximately 25,000 residents of Washington County, Maryland, were compared to levels for a combined group of 123 hospital-based and 123 community-based controls matched to the cases on sex and age (within two years) at diagnosis of MI[9]. Blood specimens were collected 7 to 14 years before the onset of MI. Overall, persons in the highest quintile of beta-carotene concentration had a 55% reduced risk of MI (RR, 0.45; 95% CI, 0.22-0.90) compared to those in the lowest quintile. Further analysis showed that the apparent protective effect was restricted to current smokers. Alpha-tocopherol levels appeared to be associated with the risk of MI, only among post-hoc subgroups with elevated cholesterol.

Completed randomized trials

Since the postulated benefits of antioxidants in the treatment and prevention of CVD are small to moderate in size (i.e., 10-50%), those with greater intake of antioxidant vitamins may share other dietary or nondietary lifestyle practices that account for some or all of any observed associations[10]. Thus, randomized trials of sufficient size and duration of treatment and follow-up are necessary. As shown below, recent results of several large-scale randomized trials of antioxidants in the treatment and prevention of CVD have not supported the previously described promising but unproven results from epidemiologic studies. Of the 13 completed randomized trials reviewed below, one was conducted in a poorly nourished population in China, while the other 12 were conducted among well-nourished populations in Canada, France, Finland, Israel, Italy, the United Kingdom, and the United States. Six trials focused on secondary prevention of CVD, of which three examined the benefits of single agents/vitamins and three examined combined agents/multivitamins. Seven trials evaluated antioxidant vitamins in primary prevention, of which five examined the effectiveness of single agents/vitamins and two examined combined agents/multivitamins. (*Table 1*).

Completed secondary prevention (treatment) trials of single agents/vitamins for CVD

Cambridge Heart Antioxidant Study (CHAOS)

The Cambridge Heart Antioxidant Study (CHAOS) was a randomized double-blind, placebo-controlled, trial of 2,002 patients with angiographically proven coronary atherosclerosis[11]. After median treatment and follow-up of 1.4 years, patients assigned to vitamin E (800 IU daily for 546 patients and 400 IU daily for 489 patients) had a 47% reduced risk of a combined endpoint of cardiovascular death and nonfatal MI (RR, 0.53; 95% CI, 0.34-0.83) compared to those assigned to placebo. This reduced risk was due to a significant benefit of vitamin E on nonfatal MI (RR, 0.23; 95% CI, 0.11-0.47). For cardiovascular death, those assigned to vitamin E had a possible but nonsignificant 18% increased risk associated with vitamin E (RR, 1.18; 95% CI, 0.62-2.27).

Gruppo Italiano Per lo Studio della Sopravvivenza nell'Infarto (GISSI) Prevention study

The Gruppo Italiano Per lo Studio della Sopravvivenza nell'Infarto (GISSI) prevention trial was a randomized, 2x2 factorial trial using an open design that investigated the effects of vitamin E and an n-3 polyunsaturated fatty acid (n-3 PUFA) in 11,324 patients surviving a recent MI (≤ 3 months). Patients received vitamin E (300 mg daily), n-3 PUFA (1 g daily), both supplements, or neither. Results of four-way analyses indicated no significant benefit of vitamin E on subsequent cardiovascular outcomes[12].

Secondary Prevention with Antioxidants of Cardiovascular Disease in Endstage Renal Disease (SPACE)

Secondary Prevention with Antioxidants of Cardiovascular Disease in Endstage Renal Disease (SPACE) randomized 196 haemodialysis patients with preexisting CVD to receive 800 IU/day vitamin E or matching placebo. Vitamin E supplementation was found to significantly reduce the number of composite CVD endpoints as well as acute MI.

Table 1. Completed randomized trials of antioxidants in the treatment and prevention of CVD

Type of Trial	Single Agent/Vitamin	Combined Agents/Multivitamins
Secondary Prevention	Cambridge Heart Antioxidant Study (CHAOS) Gruppo Italiano Per lo Studio della Sopravvivenza nell'Infarto (GISSI) Prevention Study Secondary Prevention with Antioxidants of Cardiovascular Disease in Endstage Renal Disease (SPACE)	Heart Protection Study (HPS) HDL-Atherosclerosis Treatment Study (HATS) Women's Angiographic Vitamin and Estrogen (WAVE) Trial
Primary Prevention	Finnish Alpha-tocopherol, Beta-carotene (ATBC) Cancer Prevention Trial Heart Outcomes Prevention Evaluation Study (HOPE) Physicians' Health Study I (PHS I) Primary Prevention Project (PPP) Vitamin E Atherosclerosis Prevention Study (VEAPS)	Beta-Carotene and Retinol Efficacy Trial (CARET) Chinese Cancer Prevention Trial

Specifically, a 54% (p=0.014) reduction in primary endpoint risk (a composite of fatal and nonfatal MI, ischaemic stroke, peripheral vascular disease [with the exception of arteriovenous fistula], and unstable angina) was associated with intake of vitamin E. Seventy percent (p=0.016) fewer MIs occurred during follow up in the vitamin E treatment group as compared to placebo.

If all sudden deaths were added to fatal MI, those assigned to vitamin E had a 55% lower risk of marginal significance because the 95% confidence intervals were wide due to the small number of endpoints. (RR, 0.45; 95% CI, 0.2-0.99, p=0.04)[13]. Vitamin E did not seem to protect against the secondary outcome, CVD mortality.

Completed secondary prevention (treatment) trials of combined agents/multivitamins for CVD

Heart Protection Study (HPS)

The Heart Protection Study (HPS) tested a daily antioxidant vitamin mixture including vitamin E (600mg), beta-carotene (20mg), and vitamin C (250mg) in a randomized, 2x2 factorial design with a cholesterol-lowering medication (40 mg simvastatin daily). The study population in the United Kingdom included 20,536 adults (15,454 men; 5,082 women) with CHD, other occlusive arterial disease, or diabetes during a five year treatment period. Results showed that the antioxidant mixture was safe, but added no significant cardiovascular benefits. With respect to mortality, there was a possible small but non-significant association between intake of study vitamins and all-cause mortality (RR, 1.04; 95% CI 0.97-1.12). There were slight, but non-significant, adverse trends in mortality due to CHD (RR, 1.06; 95%CI 0.95-1.18), other vascular causes (RR, 1.02; 95% CI 0.84-1.24), and non-vascular causes (RR, 1.04; 95% CI 0.92-1.17) among those taking vitamins. With respect to major vascular events (defined as major coronary events, strokes of any type, and coronary or non-coronary revascularizations), study vitamins did not reduce the risk of major vascular events when compared to placebo (RR, 1.0; 95% CI 0.94-1.06). No significant differences were found between treatment groups for non-fatal MI or coronary death (RR, 1.02; 95% CI 0.93-1.11), coronary or non-coronary revascularization (RR, 0.98; 95% CI 0.9-1.06), non-fatal or fatal stroke, (RR, 0.99; 95% CI 0.87-1.12), or strokes of any type of severity[14].

HDL-Atherosclerosis Treatment Study (HATS)

The HDL-Atherosclerosis Treatment Study (HATS) was a randomized 2x2 factorial trial including 160 patients assigned to one of four treatments: (1) simvastatin plus niacin with antioxidant vitamin placebo, (2) simvastatin-niacin plus antioxidant vitamins (vitamins C and E, beta-carotene, and selenium), (3) antioxidant vitamins (vitamins C and E, beta-carotene, and selenium) and placebos for simvastatin and niacin, or (4) all placebos. No significant benefits of antioxidant treatment were found, despite increased presence of vitamins in participants' plasma. In fact, combining antioxidants with simvastatin and niacin tended to reduce the proven benefits achieved with the simvastatin-niacin combination alone. Specifically, the adverse interaction between antioxidants and the simvastatin-niacin combination was significant (p=0.02) with respect to angiographic end points, but not significant (p=0.13) with respect to the clinical end points (death from coronary causes, confirmed MI or stroke, or revascularization for worsening ischemic symptoms). Antioxidants had no effect on stenoses of 0 to 29% of the luminal diameter, and with the exception of a 15% reduction in HDL2 for those who received only antioxidants (p=0.05 when compared to placebo treatment group), lipid levels overall were not affected by intake of antioxidants[15].

A plasma substudy was conducted using samples from 123 HATS patients, with clinical CHD and with three or more stenoses of at least 30% of the luminal diameter or one stenosis of at least 50%, collected at two points in time: on treatment (at 24 months) and off treatment (at 38 months). With respect to the group that received only antioxidant vitamins, lipid and lipoprotein levels, as well as markers of cholesterol synthesis and absorption, remained unchanged between on and off treatment[16]. Specifically, none of the measured plasma parameters changed significantly, but there was a nonsignificant trend for antioxidants to increase levels of cholesterol synthesis markers including concentrations of very-low-density-lipoprotein cholesterol (VLDL-C), remnant-like particle cholesterol (RLP-C), and plasma triglycerides (TG)[17]. The combination of simvastatin-niacin plus antioxidant vitamins reduced desmosterol and lathosterol, and elevated campesterol and beta-sisterol levels, but the changes were not significant. As mentioned previously, for reasons that are not entirely clear, antioxidants appeared to mitigate the efficacy of statin treatment on regression of coronary disease. Among-treatment group analyses showed no significant differences between the placebo and antioxidant groups with respect to percent change in cholesterol synthesis and absorption markers[16].

Women's Angiographic Vitamin and Estrogen (WAVE) trial

The Women's Angiographic Vitamin and Estrogen (WAVE) trial was a 2x2 factorial trial that randomized 423 postmenopausal women, with at least one 15% to 75% coronary stenosis at baseline coronary angiography, to receive either 0.625 mg/d of conjugated equine estrogen (plus 2.5 mg/d of medroxyprogesterone acetate for women who had not had a hysterectomy), or matching placebo, and 400 IU of vitamin E daily plus 500 mg of vitamin C twice daily, or placebo. Mean duration of follow-up was 2.8 years. Neither hormone replacement therapy (HRT) nor vitamin supplementation were found to reduce coronary progression, and in fact, there was the suggestion of harm associated with both treatments. The composite end point of death and nonfatal MI was more prevalent in women receiving HRT treatment as compared to women receiving HRT placebo, but the association did not reach statistical significance. With respect to the vitamin supplementation arm, all-cause mortality was significantly higher in women assigned to active treatment versus placebo (HR, 2.8; 95% CI, 1.1-7.2, p=0.47). A nonsignificant trend towards increased risk for cardiovascular death also was found for those taking vitamins versus placebo (p=.17)[18].

Completed primary prevention trials of single agents/vitamins for CVD

Finnish Alpha-Tocopherol, Beta-Carotene (ATBC) cancer prevention trial

The Finnish Alpha-tocopherol, Beta-carotene (ATBC) Cancer Prevention Trial (ATBC) was the first large-scale randomized trial to test antioxidant vitamins in a well-nourished population[19]. A total of 29,133 Finish male smokers, 50 to 69 years of age, were randomly assigned to alpha-tocopherol (50 mg daily) and/or beta-carotene (20 mg daily), both treatments, or placebos. Treatment and follow-up continued for more than six years, during which time there were 1,239 deaths due to ischemic heart disease and 233 fatal strokes (100 hemorrhagic strokes and 123 ischemic strokes). There was no apparent CVD benefit from either alpha tocopherol or beta-carotene, and in fact, alpha tocopherol and beta-carotene were shown to increase the risk of fatal CHD[20]. Specifically, persons assigned to beta-carotene had a significant 12% increase in ischemic heart disease mortality (RR, 1.12; 95% CI, 1.00-1.25), while those assigned to alpha tocopherol experienced a significant 50% increase in mortality from cerebral hemorrhage (RR, 1.50; 95% CI, 1.02-2.20)[19]. Additionally, all persons assigned to either antioxidant vitamin regimen, or both, were more at risk of fatal MI, with greatest risk among those taking beta-carotene (RR, 3.44; 95% CI 1.70-6.94)[20]. In regard to other end points, assignment to beta-carotene was associated with statistically significant increases of 18% in lung cancer and 8% in total mortality [ATBC Study Group, 1994]. These findings for CVD and cancer were unexpected and had not been specified in advance.

An ATBC substudy examined the effectiveness of antioxidant supplementation on the prevention of angina pectoris. Similar to the findings regarding trial end points, neither alpha tocopherol nor beta-carotene had preventive effects on angina, although a trend towards decreased incidence was seen for those taking alpha tocopherol as compared to placebo (95% CI, 0.85-1.10, p=0.63). Those taking beta-carotene had a borderline significant 13% increase in incidence of angina (RR, 1.13; 95% CI, 1.0-2.7, p=0.06)[21].

Heart Outcomes Prevention Evaluation study (HOPE)

The Heart Outcomes Prevention Evaluation Study (HOPE) was a large, simple randomized trial that used a 2x2 factorial design to test an angiotensin-converting enzyme inhibitor (ramipril) and vitamin E (400 IU daily from natural sources) in the prevention of MI, stroke, or cardiovascular death[22]. The study population included 2,545 women and 6,996 men aged 55 years and older who were at high risk for cardiovascular events such as MI and stroke. Results showed that taking vitamin E for an average of 4.5 years had no effect on cardiovascular outcomes. Specifically, there were no differences between the vitamin E and placebo groups with respect to the primary cardiovascular outcomes including deaths from CVD (RR, 1.05; 95% CI 0.90-1.22), MI (RR, 1.02; 95% CI 0.90-1.15), or stroke (RR, 1.17; 95% CI 0.95-1.42). Neither were there differences between groups for the secondary cardiovascular and combined outcomes including number of hospitalizations for unstable angina (RR, 1.04; 95% CI 0.93-1.17), hospitalizations for heart failure (RR, 1.12; 95% CI 0.90-1.41), revascularizations or limb amputations (RR, 1.09; 95% CI 0.99-1.20), number of patients with angina of new onset (RR, 1.15; 95% CI 0.97-1.37), or microvascular complications of diabetes (RR, 1.06; 95% CI 0.91-1.23)[23].

Physicians' Health Study I (PHS I)

In the Physicians' Health Study I (PHS I), 22,071 male U.S. physicians, aged 42-84 years, were randomized in a 2x2 factorial design to receive beta-carotene (50 mg on alternate days), aspirin (325 mg on alternate days), or placebo[24]. At baseline in 1982, 11% of the men were current smokers and 39% were past smokers. During more than 12 years of treatment and follow-up, there were 957 MIs, 749 strokes, and 651 deaths from cardiovascular causes. There was no significant evidence of benefit or harm of beta-carotene on total MI (RR, 0.96; 95% CI, 0.84-1.09), total stroke (RR, 0.96; 95% CI, 0.83-1.11), cardiovascular death (RR, 1.09; 95% CI, 0.93-1.27), or the combined end point of nonfatal MI, nonfatal stroke, and total cardiovascular death (RR, 1.00; 95% CI, 0.91-1.08). Subgroup analysis of current smokers also indicated no significant evidence of benefit or harm, but the confidence limits were wide. In a preliminary subgroup analysis using five-year data at the time the aspirin component of the PHS I was terminated early, beta-carotene supplementation among 333 men with prior angina or revascularization procedures decreased the risk of subsequent important vascular events by 54%[25].

Primary Prevention Project (PPP)

In the Primary Prevention Project (PPP), 4,495 people were randomized in an open 2x2 factorial trial to test low-dose aspirin (100mg/day) and vitamin E (300 mg/day) for the prevention of cardiovascular events. Although this trial was stopped early due to findings from other trials regarding the efficacy of aspirin therapy, mean follow-up was three to six years. With respect to the effectiveness of vitamin E for the prevention of cardiovascular events, the results showed no effect on any prespecified end point, including the main combined end point of cardiovascular death, non-fatal MI, and non-fatal stroke [RR, 1.07; 95% CI 0.74-1.56], except for the end point of peripheral artery disease [RR, 0.54; 95% CI 0.30-0.99], for those taking vitamin E[26].

Vitamin E Atherosclerosis Prevention Study (VEAPS)

The Vitamin E Atherosclerosis Prevention Study (VEAPS) randomized 353 patients with LDL $\geq$ 3.37 mmol/L and no clinical signs or symptoms of CVD to DL alpha tocopherol 400 IU per day or placebo. Although alpha tocopherol treatment significantly increased plasma vitamin E levels (p<0.0001), reduced circulating oxidized LDL (p=0.03), and reduced LDL oxidative susceptibility (p<0.01), the rate of change in the intima-media thickness (IMT) of the common carotid artery far-wall, the primary trial end point, was not reduced over a three year period as compared to placebo treatment[27].

Completed primary prevention trials of combined agents/multivitamins for CVD

Beta-Carotene and Retinol Efficacy Trial (CARET)

The Beta-Carotene and Retinol Efficacy Trial (CARET) evaluated combined treatment with beta-carotene (30 mg daily) and retinyl palmitate (25,000 IU daily) among 18,314 men and women, aged 40 to 74 years, at high risk of lung cancer due to cigarette smoking and/or occupational exposure to asbestos. The trial was terminated early, after an average duration of treatment of four years, primarily because interim analyses suggested that no evidence of benefit could be demonstrated with longer treatment, but also because of concern that the interim findings regarding cancer end points and combined treatment with beta-carotene and retinyl palmitate appeared to be compatible with the ATBC results for beta-carotene alone. Specifically, for lung cancer, the primary trial end point, there was a statistically significant 28% increase (p=0.02) among the combined treatment group. Regarding CVD, the combined treatment group had a nonsignificant 26% increased risk (p=0.06) of cardiovascular mortality at the time of the study's early termination. Of note, neither end point reached the prespecified stopping boundary for early termination (P<0.007), and the finding for cardiovascular mortality did not even reach the level of conventional statistical significance (p<0.05)[28].

Chinese Cancer Prevention Trial

The Chinese Cancer Prevention Trial evaluated antioxidant vitamin and other micronutrient supplements among 29,584 poorly nourished residents of Linxian, China. Various combinations of nine different agents (retinol, zinc, riboflavin, niacin, vitamin C, molybdenum, beta-carotene, vitamin E, and selenium) were tested. After nearly six years of treatment and follow-up, a total of 2,127 deaths were documented, including 523 (25%) due to cerebrovascular disease (CHD is rare in this population and could not be evaluated). Persons assigned to combined daily treatment of beta-carotene (15mg), vitamin E (30mg), and selenium (50 mg) had a nonsignificant 10% decrease in cerebrovascular mortality compared with those assigned to placebo (RR, 0.90; 95% CI, 0.76-1.07)[29]. It is doubtful whether these findings are generalizable to well-nourished populations, and because three agents were tested in combination, the specific benefit of beta-carotene, vitamin E, or selenium cannot be determined.

Ongoing Randomized Trials of Antioxidants for CVD

Currently, four trials of antioxidants for CVD are in process. One trial focuses on secondary prevention of both single agents/vitamins and combined agents/multivitamins. Three trials are evaluating antioxidants in primary prevention, of which one focuses on a single agent/vitamin, a second focuses on combined agents/multivitamins, and a third on both single agents/vitamins and combined agents/multivitamins (*Table 2*).

Ongoing secondary prevention (treatment) trials of single agents/vitamins and combined agents/multivitamins for CVD in factorial designs

Women's Antioxidant Cardiovascular Disease Study (WACS)

The Women's Antioxidant Cardiovascular Disease Study (WACS) is a randomized, double-blind, placebo-controlled secondary prevention trial using a 2x2x2x2 factorial design to test beta-carotene (50 mg on alternate days), vitamin E (600 IU on alternate days), vitamin C (500 mg daily), and a combination of folate (2.5 mg daily), vitamin B_6 (50 mg daily), and vitamin B_{12} (1 mg daily)[30]. The study population includes 8,171 female health professionals, aged 40 years or older, who are at high risk for cardiovascular disease because of a prior event or because they have three or more risk factors.

Ongoing primary prevention trials of single agents/vitamins for CVD

Women's Health Study (WHS)

The Women's Health Study (WHS) is a randomized, double-blind, placebo-controlled trial utilizing a 2x2 factorial design to test vitamin E (600 IU on alternate days) and low-dose aspirin (100 mg on alternate days) in the prevention of CVD and cancer[31,32]. The study population is 39,876 apparently healthy U.S. female health professionals, aged 45 years and older.

Ongoing primary prevention trials of combined agents/multivitamins for CVD in factorial designs

SUpplementation en VItamines et Mineraux AntiXydants (SU.VI.M.AX) study

The SUpplementation en VItamines et Mineraux AntiXydants (SU.VI.M.AX) Study is a randomized, double-blind, placebo-controlled, primary prevention trial that is testing the efficacy of daily supplementation at nutritional doses with antioxidant vitamins (vitamin C, 120 mg; vitamin E, 30 mg; and beta-carotene, 6 mg) and minerals (selenium, 100 mg; and zinc, 20 mg) in reducing risk of CVD and cancer[33]. The study began in 1994 and is comprised of 12,735 French men (aged 45-60) and women (aged 35-60).

Ongoing primary prevention trials of single agents/vitamins and combined agents/multivitamins for CVD in factorial designs

Physicians' Health Study II (PHS II)

PHS II is a randomized, double-blind, placebo-controlled trial of beta-carotene (50 mg on alternate days), vitamin E (400 IU on alternate days), vitamin C (500 mg daily), and a multivitamin (Centrum Silver daily) in the prevention of total and prostate cancer, CVD, and the age-related eye diseases, cataract and macular degeneration[34]. The trial uses a 2x2x2x2 factorial design with participant recruitment and randomization occurring in two phases. In Phase I, approximately 7,600 PHS I participants who were willing and eligible to participate in PHS II retained their randomized beta-carotene assignment from PHS I and have been newly randomized to vitamin E, vitamin C, a multivitamin, or placebos. In Phase II, new physician participants are randomly assigned to the same interventions.

Summary of results from completed randomized trials and contributions of ongoing trials

Large-scale randomized trials of sufficient size, dose, and duration, as well as their meta-analyses, demonstrate no significant benefit of antioxidant vitamins in the treatment or prevention of CVD. With respect to beta-carotene supplementation for durations up to 12 years, there was no overall benefit on the incidence of CVD in well-nourished populations at usual risk. The present review also shows no benefit of vitamin E for the treatment or prevention of CVD, a finding that was supported by a recent meta-analysis of seven vitamin E trials with a combined total of 106,625 randomized participants in secondary and primary prevention who experienced a total of 9,727 CVD end points[35]. Further evidence will emerge from the recently completed Women's Health Study (WHS)[32,33]. Finally, none of the five trials of multivitamins resulted in beneficial effects on cardiovascular morbidity or mortality. SU.V.I.MAX should provide additional data on combined use of antioxidant vitamins.

Table 2. Ongoing randomized trials of antioxidants in the treatment and prevention of CVD

Type of Trial	Single Agent/Vitamin	Combined Agents/Multivitamins
Secondary Prevention	Women's Antioxidant Cardiovascular Disease Study (WACS)*	Women's Antioxidant Cardiovascular Disease Study (WACS)*
Primary Prevention	Physicians Health Study II (PHS II)*	Physicians Health Study II (PHS II)*
	Women's Health Study (WHS)	SUpplementation en VItamines et Mineraux AntiXydants (SU.VI.M.AX) Study

*PHS II and WACS include both single agent/vitamin and combined agents/multivitamins in a factorial design.

In addition to the finding of no benefit of antioxidants in the treatment and prevention of CVD, some results of trials suggest the possibility of adverse effects. In populations with excess risk for some cardiovascular (and cancer) end points, as shown in the ATBC study and in CARET – two trials conducted among smokers – unexpected findings of harm were observed among those taking beta-carotene as a single agent/vitamin (ATBC) and among those taking beta-carotene and retinyl (CARET). In HATS, antioxidant supplements containing beta-carotene mitigated the effectiveness of proven statin therapy (simvastatin and niacin). In HPS, there was a slight, nonsignificant trend in cardiovascular mortality among those taking a multivitamin containing vitamins E, C, and beta-carotene. Finally, a suggestion of harm was found in WAVE in the vitamin E plus C arm.

However, these findings may be due to the play of chance – the hypothesis of adverse effects in the ATBC trial was not pre-specified, hence the data should be viewed as hypothesis formulating. In CARET, which was terminated early, the results for neither the primary end point, lung cancer, nor for cardiovascular mortality, reached the prespecified stopping boundary for early termination ($P<0.007$). Moreover, the results of ATBC, CARET, HATS, and the HPS should be viewed in the context of the findings from PHS I which are particularly reliable because the trial lasted more than twice as long as any other beta-carotene trial and because the narrow confidence intervals in PHS I exclude even small amounts of harm among non-smokers with a high degree of assurance. Finally, the PHS I subgroup findings for men with prior angina or revascularization procedures raise the possibility that beta-carotene may exert a beneficial effect among those with atherosclerosis, an unexpected finding being tested in ongoing trials of men[34] and women[30].

Conclusions

With respect to antioxidant vitamins and CVD, the randomized trials have failed to fulfill the promises of observational epidemiologic studies which are also supported by a body of evidence from basic research that supports plausible biological mechanisms. Interestingly this situation also occurred with the use of post-menopausal hormones[36]. For antioxidant vitamins, at present, we believe the most plausible interpretation of the totality of evidence to be that there is no significant evidence of benefit or harm in the treatment or prevention of CVD. These considerations should be viewed in light of the preponderance of evidence that suggests that diets high in fruits and vegetables may have beneficial effects on CVD, cancer, as well as other chronic conditions[37]. It remains plausible that either antioxidant vitamin supplements in combination with other components of fruits and vegetables or even these other components alone contribute to the lower risks of CVD, cancer, and other chronic conditions consistently observed among people who consume diets rich in fruits and vegetables.

Nonetheless, antioxidant vitamins as supplements are consumed by large numbers of U.S. adults, perhaps over one-third of the population[38]. Unfortunately, use of agents of proven lack of benefit on CVD which are more readily available over the counter such as antioxidant vitamins may well be contributing to the underutilization of agents of proven benefit in CVD such as aspirin[39], statins[40], beta-blockers and angiotensin converting inhibitors[41]. Finally, many individuals in the U.S. prefer prescription of pills, even of proven lack of benefit, to avoiding harmful lifestyles[37,42]. All of these considerations underscore the importance of avoiding harmful lifestyles, adopting healthy lifestyles that include diet and exercise, as well as the prescription of drugs of proven benefit as adjuncts not alternatives, and finally, the avoidance of agents of lack of proven benefit.

Acknowledgements

We are indebted to Theodore Lucas Hollar for advice and help.

References

1. Hennekens CH and Buring JE. Epidemiology in Medicine (MA: Little, Brown, & Co., Boston, 1987).

2. Hennekens CH and Buring JE. In: Clinical Trials in Cardiovascular Disease: A Companion to Braunwald's Heart Disease, edited by CH Hennekens, JE Buring, PM Ridker, and JE Manson, WB Saunders Co., Philadelphia, 1998: pp. 3-7.

3. Stampfer MJ, Hennekens CH, Manson JE, Colditz GA, Rosner B, Willett WC. Vitamin E consumption and the risk of coronary disease in women. N Engl J Med 1993;328:1444-9.

4. Rimm EB, Stampfer MJ, Ascherio A, Giovannucci F, Colditz GA, Willett WC. Vitamin E consumption and the risk of coronary disease in men. N Engl J Med 1993;329:1450-6.

5. Kushi LH, Folsom AR, Prineas RJ, Mink PJ, Wu Y, Bostick RM. Dietary antioxidant vitamins and death from coronary heart disease in postmenopausal women. N Engl J Med 1996;334:1156-62.

6. Muntwyler J, Hennekens CH, Manson JE, Buring JE, Gaziano JM. Vitamin supplement use in a low-risk population of US male physicians and subsequent cardiovascular mortality. Arch Intern Med 2002;162:1472-6.

7. Gey KF, Moser UK, Jordan P, Stahein HB, Eichholzer, Ludin E. Increased risk of cardiovascular disease at suboptimal plasma concentrations of essential antioxidants: an epidemiologic update with special attention to carotene and vitamin E. Am J Clin Nutr 1993;57(suppl):S787-97.

8. Morris DL, Kritchevsky SB, Davis CE. Serum carotenoids and coronary heart disease: The Lipid Research Clinics Coronary Primary Prevention Trial and Follow-up Study. JAMA 1994;272:1439-41.

9. Street DA, Comstock GW, Salkeld RM, Schuep W, Klag MA. Serum antioxidants and myocardial infarction: are low levels of carotenoids and alpha-tocopherol risk factors for myocardial infarction? Circulation 1994;90:1154-61.

10. Hennekens CH. Increasing burden of cardiovascular disease; current knowledge and future directions for research on risk factors (Special Report). Circulation 1998;97:1095-102.

11. Stephens NG, Parsons A, Schofield PM et al. Randomized controlled trial of vitamin E in patients with coronary disease: Cambridge Heart Antioxidant Study (CHAOS)., Lancet 1996;347:781-6.

12. GISSI-Prevenzione Investigators. Dietary supplementation with n-3 polyunsaturated fatty acids and vitamin E after myocardial infarction: results of the GISSI-Prevenzione trial. Lancet 1999;354:447-55.

13. Boaz M, Smetana S, Weinstein T, et al. Secondary prevention with antioxidants of cardiovascular disease in endstage renal disease (SPACE): randomized placebo-controlled trial. Lancet 2000;356:1213-8.

14. Heart Protection Study Collaborative Group. MRC/BHF Heart Protection Study of antioxidant vitamin supplementation in 20,536 high-risk individuals: a randomized placebo-controlled trial. Lancet 2002;360:23-33.

15. Brown BG, Zhao XQ, Chai, A, et al., Simvastatin and niacin, antioxidant vitamins, or the combination for the prevention of coronary disease. N Engl J Med 2001;345:1583-92.

16. Matthan NR, Giovanni A, Schaefer EJ, Brown BG, Lichtenstein AH. Impact of simvastatin, niacin, and/or antioxidants on cholesterol metabolism in CAD patients with low HDL. J Lipid Res 2003; 44:800-6.

17. Asztalos F, Bela B, Marcelo H, et al. Change in alpha$_1$ HDL concentration predicts progression in coronary artery stenosis. Arterioscler Thromb Vasc Biol 2003;23:847-52.

18. Waters DD, Alderman EL, Hsia J, et al. Effects of hormone replacement therapy and antioxidant vitamin supplements on coronary atherosclerosis in postmenopausal women. JAMA 2002;288:2432-40.

19. The Alpha-Tocopherol, Beta Carotene Cancer Prevention Study Group. The effect of vitamin E and beta carotene on the incidence of lung cancer and other cancers in male smokers. N Engl J Med 1994;330:1029-35.

20. Rapola JM, Virtamo J, Ripatti S et al. Randomised trial of alpha-tocopherol and beta-carotene supplements on incidence of major coronary events in men with previous myocardial infarction. Lancet 1997;349:1715-20.

21. Rapola MJ, Virtamo J, Haukika KJ et al. Effect of vitamin E and beta carotene on the incidence of angina pectoris: A randomized, double-blind, controlled trial. JAMA 1996;275:693-8.

22. The HOPE Study Investigators. The HOPE (Heart Outcomes Prevention Evaluation) Study. The design of a large, simple randomized trial of an angiotensin-converting enzyme inhibitor (ramipril) and vitamin E in patients at high risk of cardiovascular events. Can J Cardiol 1996;12:127-37.

23. Heart Outcomes Prevention Evaluation Study Investigators. Vitamin E supplementation and cardiovascular events in high-risk patients. N Engl J Med 2000;42:154-60.

24. Hennekens CH, Buring JE, Manson JE et al. Lack of effect of long-term supplementation with beta carotene on the incidence of malignant neoplasms and cardiovascular disease. N Engl J Med 1996;334:1145-9.

25. Gaziano JM, Manson JE, Ridker PM, Buring JE, Hennekens CH. Beta carotene therapy for chronic stable angina. Circulation 1990; 82(suppl):202.

26. Collaborative Group of the Primary Prevention Project. Low-dose aspirin and vitamin E in people at cardiovascular risk: a randomized trial in general practice. Lancet 2001;357:89-95.

27. Hodis HN, Mack WJ, LaBree L et al. Alpha-tocopherol supplementation in healthy individuals reduces low-density lipoprotein oxidation but not atherosclerosis: The Vitamin E Atherosclerosis Prevention Study (VEPS). Circulation 2002;106:1453-9.

28.   Omenn GS, Goodman GE, Thornquist MD et al. Effects of a combination of beta carotene and vitamin A on lung cancer and cardiovascular disease. N Engl J Med 1996;334:1150-5.

29.   Blot WJ, Li JY, Taylor RP et al. Nutrition intervention trials in Linxian, China: supplementation with specific vitamin/mineral combinations, cancer incidence, and disease-specific mortality in the general population. J Natl Cancer Inst 1993;85:1483-92.

30.   Manson JE, Gaziano JM, Spelsberg A et al for the WACS Research Group. A secondary prevention trial of antioxidant vitamins and cardiovascular disease in women; rationale, design, and methods. Ann Epidemiol 1995;5:261-9.

31.   Buring JE, Hennekens CH for the Women's Health Study Research Group. The Women's Health Study: Summary of the study design. J Myocardial Ischemia 1992;4:27-9.

32.   Buring JE, Hennekens CH. For the Women's Health Study Research Group. The Women's Health Study: Rationale and background. J Myocardial Ischemia 1992;4:30-40.

33.   Hercberg S, Preziosi P, Briancon S et al. A primary prevention trial using nutritional doses of antioxidant vitamins and minerals in cardiovascular disease and cancers in a general population: The SU.VI.MAX Study – design, methods, and participant characteristics. Controlled Clin Trials 1998;19:336-51.

34.   Christen WG, Gaziano JM, Hennekens CH. For the Steering Committee of Physician's Health Study II, Design of Physician's Health Study II: A randomized trial of beta-carotene, vitamins E and C, and multivitamins in prevention of cancer, cardiovascular disease, and eye disease – and review of results of completed trials. Ann Epidemiol 2000;10:125-134.

35.   Eidelman RS, Hebert PR, Hollar D, Lamas GA, Hennekens CH. Randomized trials of vitamin E in the treatment and prevention of cardiovascular disease. Arch Int Med 2004;164:1552-6.

36.   Women's Health Initiative Steering Committee. Effects of conjugated equine estrogen in postmenopausal women with hysterectomy: The Women's Health Initiative Randomized Controlled Trial. JAMA 2004;291:1701-12.

37.   Panel on Dietary Antioxidants and Related Compounds. Dietary Reference Intakes for Vitamin C, Vitamin E, Selenium, and Carotenoids. A report for the Panel on Dietary Antioxidants and Related Compounds. Subcommittees on Upper Reference Levels of Nutrients and Interpretation and Uses of DRIs. Standing Committee on the Scientific Evaluation of Dietary Reference Intakes, Food and Nutrition Board, Institute of Medicine. National Academy Press, Washington, D.C., 2000.

38.   Hensrud DD, Engle DD, Scheitel SM. Underreporting the use of the dietary supplements and nonprescription medications among patients undergoing a periodic health examination. Mayo Clin Proc 1999;74:443-77.

39.   Cook NR, Chae C, Mueller FB, Landis S, Saks AM, Hennekens CH. Mis-medication and under-utilization of aspirin in the prevention and treatment of cardiovascular

disease. (accessed on January 22, 2003); Medscape General Medicine, 1999, www.medscape.com/viewarticle/408025_1.

40. Eidelman RS, G. Lamas A, Hennekens CH. The new National Cholesterol Education Program guidelines: Clinical challenges for more widespread therapy of lipids to treat and prevent coronary heart disease. Arch Intern Med 2003;162:2033-6.

41. Stafford RS, Radley DC. The underutilization of cardiac medications of proven benefit, 1990-2002. J Am Coll Cardiol 2003;41:56-61.

42. Hennekens CH, Buring JE. eds, Introduction: Thematic Review Series IV: Antioxidant vitamins—The search for definitive answers. Proc Assoc Amer Phys 1999;111:1-21.

Chapter 13

ANTIOXIDANTS AND RESTENOSIS AFTER PERCUTANEOUS CORONARY INTERVENTION: ANIMAL STUDIES

Eric Durand, Ayman Al Haj Zen, Camille Brasselet, Antoine Lafont
European Georges Pompidou Hospital and INSERM E00-16, Faculté de Médecine Necker-Enfants Malades, Paris, France

Introduction

Restenosis remains the principal limitation of percutaneous coronary intervention (PCI). We have learned from animal studies that constrictive remodeling is the principal mechanism of restenosis after balloon angioplasty[1-6]. In contrast, in-stent restenosis is related to neointimal hyperplasia[7]. These data were confirmed in humans by intravascular ultrasound (IVUS)[8,9]. After balloon arterial injury, oxidative stress is increased and contributes to endothelial dysfunction, macrophage activation, and release of cytokines and growth factors[10]. In the past decade, several antioxidants have been evaluated in various animal models after balloon angioplasty. Probucol and vitamins (E with or without C) effectively reduced restenosis by promoting favorable remodeling (i.e., enlargement remodeling). Moreover, these treatments decreased neointimal hyperplasia which is the target for in-stent restenosis. In an era of nearly 100% stent implantation, it is now time to evaluate their efficacy in animal models of in-stent restenosis after either systemic administration or local delivery.

Mechanisms of restenosis after balloon or stent angioplasty

In the 1980s, neointimal hyperplasia was considered the principal mechanism of restenosis. We have learned from animal models in the 1990s that neointimal hyperplasia is not the principal target of restenosis (i.e., lumen loss at the site of angioplasty) after balloon angioplasty. Indeed, there was no correlation between restenosis and severity of neointimal hyperplasia[1-6]. In contrast, restenosis was closely correlated with arterial remodeling in rabbit, pig, and non-human primate models[1-6]. Schematically, constrictive remodeling is observed in the presence of restenosis, and enlargement remodeling in its absence. Interestingly, these findings were confirmed by IVUS in humans[8]. During the same period, we learned from two clinical trials that stents reduce the incidence of restenosis by about 30% as compared to balloon angioplasty[11,12]. In animal models and in humans, it has been clearly demonstrated that neointimal hyperplasia is the principal mechanism of in-stent restenosis after PCI[7,9]. Indeed, the severity of in-stent restenosis is closely correlated with the extent of neointimal hyperplasia[9]. Neointimal hyperplasia is related to the severity of injury, smooth muscle cell proliferation, collagen synthesis and inflammation[13,14].

Antioxidants and restenosis after balloon angioplasty

The methodology and results of these experimental studies are summarized in *tables 1 and 2*. First, it is surprising to note that none of these studies evaluated the amount of reactive oxygen species (ROS) produced after angioplasty as well as the effect of antioxidants on ROS production. However, in 1997, Nunes *et al* showed that ROS production increased after balloon injury, and decreased with antioxidants[10]. The principal source of ROS was recently attributed to NAD(P)H oxidases after vascular injury[15,16].

In the 1990s, a large number of studies evaluated the effect of probucol after arterial injury in rat, pig, and rabbit models (*Table 1, 17-23*). Probucol was administrated before angioplasty (from two hours to two weeks) and was continued during two or four weeks[17-23]. In these studies, neointimal hyperplasia was significantly reduced as compared to control animals[17-23]. However, these authors neither evaluated restenosis nor arterial remodeling[17-23].

Similarly, the effect of vitamin E with or without vitamin C was evaluated in cholesterol fed rabbit, rat and swine models (*Table 2, 24-27*). With a pretreatment (from one to nine weeks) and a treatment duration of one to three weeks after balloon angioplasty, all studies (except Nunes *et al*[10]) observed that neointimal hyperplasia was reduced as compared to control animals[24-27]. Only two studies evaluated the effect on restenosis and one the effect on remodeling[24,27]. Vitamin E or the combination of vitamins C and E reduced restenosis by promoting favorable remodeling[24].

Table 1. Probucol animal studies

	Ferns et al (17)	Shinomiya et al (18)	Schneider et al (19)	Ihizaka et al (20)	Miyauchi et al (21)	Tanaka et al (22)	Jackson et al (23)	Yokoyama et al (41)
Model	Rabbit	Rabbit	Swine	Rat	Rabbit	Rabbit	Rat	Porcine
Artery	Carotid	Carotid	Coronary	Carotid	Carotid	Carotid	Carotid	Coronary
Animal number	30	18	26	50	32	10	24	9
Pretreatment	1 week	2 weeks	2 days	2 days	2 weeks	No	No	1 week
Treatment duration	4 weeks	2 weeks	2 weeks	2 weeks	2-4 weeks	2 weeks	2 weeks	4 weeks
Double injury	No	No	No	No	No	No	No	No
Type of injury	Fogarty denudation	Fogarty denudation	Balloon angioplasty	Fogarty denudation	Fogarty denudation	Fogarty denudation	Fogarty denudation	Stent
Angiography	ND	ND	Yes	ND	ND	ND	ND	ND (IVUS)
Restenosis	ND	ND	ND	ND	ND	ND	ND	NS
Morphometry	Yes	Yes	Yes	Yes	Yes	Yes	Yes	Yes
Lumen area	ND	ND	+15% (p=0.02)	ND	ND	ND	ND	4.2 vs 3.8 mm², p=0.6
Intimal hyperplasia	↓	↓	↓	↓	↓	↓	↓	3.7 vs 4.0 mm², p=0.7
Arterial remodeling	ND	ND	↑(p=NS)	ND	ND	ND	ND	ND

ND: Not done, NS: non significant

Table 2. Vitamins C and E in animal studies

	Lafont et al (25)	Nunes et al (24)	Konneh et al (26)	Chen et al (27)
Model	Rabbit	Swine	Rat	Rabbit
Artery	Femoral	Coronary	Carotid	Aorta
Animal number	29	44	?	96
Pretreatment	3 weeks (vitamin E)	1 week (vitamins E+C)	9 weeks (vitamin E)	2 weeks (vitamin E)
Treatment duration	3 weeks	2 weeks	1 week	3 weeks
Double injury	Yes	No	No	No
Type of injury	Air desiccation+ balloon injury	Balloon angioplasty	Fogarty denudation	Fogarty denudation
Angiography	Yes	ND	ND	ND
Restenosis	↓	↓	ND	ND
Morphometry	Yes	Yes	Yes	Yes
Lumen area	↑	↑	ND	ND
Intimal hyperplasia	↓	NS	↓	↓
Arterial remodeling	ND	↑	ND	ND

ND: not done, NS: not significant

Interestingly, similar results were reported in humans. The MultiVitamin Probucol (MVP) trial evaluated by angiography and IVUS the effect of vitamins C and E or probucol on restenosis after balloon angioplasty[28,29]. In summary, they confirmed that probucol, but not vitamins C and E, reduced restenosis[28]. This beneficial effect was attributed to a favorable effect on arterial remodeling[29].

The effect of adenovirus-mediated gene transfer of superoxide dismutase (SOD) with or without catalase was evaluated after balloon injury in the rabbit model[30, 31]. ROS production was decreased as compared to control animals. After adenovirus-mediated gene transfer of SOD and catalase, neointimal hyperplasia and constrictive remodeling were significantly reduced and resulted in less restenosis[30,31].

In conclusion, antioxidants reduced both neointimal hyperplasia and constrictive remodeling resulting in less restenosis after balloon injury. The beneficial effect on restenosis is limited to the remodeling process since the extent of neointimal hyperplasia is not related to restenosis[1-6].

The next step is to understand how it works (i.e., how antioxidants promote favorable remodeling after balloon injury). Vessel remodeling after arterial injury is a complex healing process. Endothelial dysfunction, collagen accumulation, and inflammation are probably the three principal mechanisms of constrictive remodeling after balloon angioplasty[32,33]. After angioplasty, some endothelium is removed, and preserved adjacent endothelial cells migrate and proliferate to reline the vascular wall. Arteries with regenerated endothelium may exhibit impaired endothelium-dependent relaxation via reduction of nitric oxide (NO) production[32,34]. Interestingly, the severity of endothelial dysfunction is correlated with restenosis and with constrictive remodeling[32]. The mechanisms controlling re-endothelialization after angioplasty are not well established. Re-endothelialization does not seem to be mediated by NO since L-arginine and L-NAME have no effects on the re-endothelialization process after arterial balloon injury[35]. Recently, Lau *et al* elegantly demonstrated that probucol accelerates re-endothelialization and improves endothelium-dependent relaxation after balloon injury[36]. Interestingly, we also observed that adenovirus-mediated gene transfer of SOD and catalase accelerates re-endothelialization and improves endothelium-dependent response to acetylcholine[31]. The more effective re-endothelialization may be explained in part by the fact that antioxidants are known to inhibit endothelial cell apoptosis after angioplasty[37,38]. In turn, improved re-endothelialization might contribute to the reduction of neointimal medial growth observed in probucol-treated animals. Therefore, the beneficial effect of antioxidants on remodeling after balloon injury may be mediated via an acceleration of functional re-endothelialization.

Collagen accumulation is the second determinant of constrictive remodeling after balloon angioplasty. Indeed, we and others showed that collagen increases after angioplasty, and that this increase correlates with severity of restenosis and constrictive remodeling[32]. The interaction between antioxidant therapies and collagen content has recently been evaluated after balloon injury. Antioxidants decrease collagen content after arterial injury but it is not known whether they interact with collagen synthesis or degradation[31]. However, it has been shown in other experimental models that oxidative stress increases collagen synthesis and decreases metalloproteinase activity[39,40].

Finally, inflammatory cell infiltration is the third determinant of arterial remodeling via production of cytokines and growth factors. It has been shown that antioxidant therapies reduce monocyte-macrophage infiltration after balloon injury[30,31]. Therefore the beneficial effect of antioxidant therapies on remodeling after balloon injury may be mediated by an improvement of functional re-endothelialization, and a reduction of collagen content and inflammation.

Antioxidants and in-stent restenosis

As described above, the principal mechanism of in-stent restenosis is neointimal hyperplasia. It is logical to hypothesize that antioxidants are capable of preventing in-stent restenosis since it has been demonstrated that probucol and vitamins reduce neointimal hyperplasia after balloon injury[17-27]. However, to our knowledge, antioxidants have been poorly evaluated in animal models of in-stent restenosis. Surprisingly, only one negative study has been published concerning the effect of probucol on restenosis after stent angioplasty in animal models[41]. Probucol was administrated one week before stent implantation in porcine coronary arteries[41]. The authors did not find any positive effect by IVUS. Indeed, restenosis and neointimal hyperplasia were similar in the probucol and control group[41]. In humans, the effect of probucol after stent angioplasty were evaluated in the Canadian Antioxidant Restenosis Trial (CART-1) pilot study[42]. Patients were treated for two weeks before and four weeks after PCI. As compared to placebo, probucol significantly reduced in-stent restenosis. This study was also designed to evaluate the best dose of AGI-1067, a metabolically stable modification of probucol, for a larger trial, the Canadian Atherosclerosis and Restenosis Trial (CART-2). This trial was mandatory since it is known that probucol induces a prolongation of the QT interval which remains a long-term safety concern. This new metabolite does not increase the QT interval. To our knowledge, AGI-1067 has never been tested in animal models of in-stent restenosis. In human, AGI-1067 with a pretreatment period of two weeks, and a treatment duration of four weeks, reduced in-stent restenosis through a favorable effect on neointimal hyperplasia. A randomized multicenter study is therefore conducted (CART-2) to evaluate the effect of AGI-1067 with a treatment duration of six weeks in a larger population. One can regret that preclinical studies were not published or performed prior to this study.

Conclusions

Antioxidants therapies reduce constrictive remodeling and restenosis after experimental balloon injury. These favorable results led to the MVP trial which clearly demonstrated that probucol reduces restenosis after balloon angioplasty in humans. In contrast, antioxidants have been poorly evalued in the setting of in-stent restenosis in animal models. However, promising premilinary results have been obtained in humans with AGI-1067, a metabolically stable modification of probucol. However, we must keep in mind that systemic antioxidant therapies need a pre-treatment period of at least two weeks before angioplasty, which is not available in the setting of PCI during acute coronary syndromes.

References

1. Post MJ, Borst C, Kuntz RE. The relative importance of arterial remodeling compared with intimal hyperplasia in lumen renarrowing after balloon angioplasty. A study in the normal rabbit and the hypercholesterolemic Yucatan micropig. Circulation 1994;89:2816-21.

2. Lafont A, Guzman LA, Whitlow PL, Goormastic M, Cornhill JF, Chisolm GM. Restenosis after experimental angioplasty. Intimal, medial, and adventitial changes associated with constrictive remodeling. Circ Res 1995;76:996-1002.

3. Guzman LA, Mick MJ, Arnold AM, Forudi F, Whitlow PL. Role of intimal hyperplasia and arterial remodeling after balloon angioplasty: an experimental study in the atherosclerotic rabbit model. Arterioscler Thromb Vasc Biol 1996;16:479-87.

4. Mondy JS, Williams JK, Adams MR, Dean RH, Geary RL. Structural determinants of lumen narrowing after angioplasty in atherosclerotic nonhuman primates. J Vasc Surg 1997;26:875-83.

5. Kakuta T, Usui M, Coats WD Jr, Currier JW, Numano F, Faxon DP. Arterial remodeling at the reference site after angioplasty in the atherosclerotic rabbit model. Arterioscler Thromb Vasc Biol 1998;18:47-51.

6. de Smet BJ, Pasterkamp G, van der Helm YJ, Borst C, Post MJ. The relation between de novo atherosclerosis remodeling and angioplasty-induced remodeling in an atherosclerotic Yucatan micropig model. Arterioscler Thromb Vasc Biol 1998;18:702-7.

7. Karas SP, Gravanis MB, Santoian EC, Robinson KA, Anderberg KA, King SB 3rd. Coronary intimal proliferation after balloon injury and stenting in swine: an animal model of restenosis. J Am Coll Cardiol 1992;20:467-74.

8. Mintz GS, Popma JJ, Pichard AD, et al. Arterial remodeling after coronary angioplasty: a serial intravascular ultrasound study. Circulation 1996;94:35-43.

9. Hoffmann R, Mintz GS, Dussaillant GR et al. Patterns and mechanisms of in-stent restenosis. A serial intravascular ultrasound study. Circulation 1996;94:1247-54.

10. Nunes GL, Robinson K, Kalynych A, King SB 3rd, Sgoutas DS, Berk BC. Vitamins C and E inhibit O2- production in the pig coronary artery. Circulation 1997;96:3593-601.

11. Serruys PW, de Jaegere P, Kiemeneij F, et al. A comparison of balloon-expandable-stent implantation with balloon angioplasty in patients with coronary artery disease. Benestent Study Group. N Engl J Med 1994;331:489-95.

12. Fischman DL, Leon MB, Baim DS, et al. A randomized comparison of coronary-stent placement and balloon angioplasty in the treatment of coronary artery disease. Stent Restenosis Study Investigators. N Engl J Med 1994;331:496-501.

13. Kornowski R, Hong MK, Tio FO, Bramwell O, Wu H, Leon MB. In-stent restenosis: contributions of inflammatory responses and arterial injury to neointimal hyperplasia. J Am Coll Cardiol 1998;31:224-30.

14. Li C, Cantor WJ, Nili N, Robinson R, et al. Arterial repair after stenting and the effects of GM6001, a matrix metalloproteinase inhibitor. J Am Coll Cardiol 2002;39:1852-8.

15. Szöcs K, Lassègue B, Sorescu D, et al. Upregulation of Nox-based NAD(P)H oxidases in restenosis after carotid injury Arterioscler Thromb Vasc Biol 2002;22:21-7.

16. Jacobson GM, Dourron HM, Liu J, et al. Novel NAD(P)H oxidase inhibitor suppresses angioplasty-induced superoxide and neointimal hyperplasia of rat carotid artery. Circ Res 2003;92:637-43.

17. Ferns GA, Forster L, Stewart-Lee A, Konneh M, Nourooz-Zadeh J, Anggard EE. Probucol inhibits neointimal thickening and macrophage accumulation after balloon injury in the cholesterol-fed rabbit. Proc Natl Acad Sci U S A 1992;89:11312-6.

18. Shinomiya M, Shirai K, Saito Y, Yoshida S. Inhibition of intimal thickening of the carotid artery of rabbits of outgrowth of explants of aorta by probucol. Atherosclerosis 1992;97:143-8.

19. Schneider JE, Berk BC, Gravanis MB, et al. Probucol decreases neointimal formation in a swine model of coronary artery balloon injury. A possible role for antioxidants in restenosis. Circulation 1993;88:628-37.

20. Ishizaka N, Kurokawa K, Taguchi J, Miki K, Ohno M. Inhibitory effect of a single local probucol administration on neointimal formation in balloon-injured rat carotid artery. Atherosclerosis 1995;118:53-6.

21. Miyauchi K, Aikawa M, Tani T, et al. Effect of probucol on smooth muscle cell proliferation and dedifferentiation after vascular injury in rabbits: possible role of PDGF. Cardiovasc Drugs Ther 1998;12:251-60.

22. Tanaka K, Hayashi K, Shingu T, et al. Probucol inhibits neointimal formation in carotid arteries of normocholesterolemic rabbits and the proliferation of cultured rabbit vascular smooth muscle cells. Cardiovasc Drugs Ther 1998;12:19-28.

23. Jackson CL, Petterson KS. Effects of probucol on rat carotid artery responses to balloon catheter injury. Atherosclerosis 2001;154:407-14.

24. Nunes GL, Sgoutas DS, Redden RA, et al. Combination of vitamins C and E alters the response to coronary balloon injury in the pig. Arterioscler Thromb Vasc Biol 1995;15:156-65.

25. Lafont A, Whitlow P, Cornhill JF, Chisolm G. Effect of alpha-tocopherol on restenosis after angioplasty in a model of experimental atherosclerosis. J Clin Invest 1995;95:1018-25.

26. Konneh MK, Rutherford C, Li SR, Anggard EE, Ferns GA. Vitamin E inhibits the intimal response to balloon catheter injury in the carotid artery of the cholesterol- fed rat. Atherosclerosis 1995;113:29-39.

27. Chen MF, Hsu HC, Liau CS, Lee YT. Vitamin E supplementation attenuates myointimal proliferation of the abdominal aorta after balloon injury in diet-induced hypercholesterolemic rabbits. Prostaglandins Other Lipid Mediat 1998;56:219-38.

28. Tardif JC, Cote G, Lesperance J, et al. Probucol and multivitamins in the prevention of restenosis after coronary angioplasty. Multivitamins and Probucol Study Group. N Engl J Med 1997;337:365-72.

29. Cote G, Tardif JC, Lesperance J, et al. J. Effects of probucol on vascular remodeling after coronary angioplasty. Multivitamins and Protocol Study Group. Circulation 1999;99:30-5.

30. Laukkanen MO, Kivela A, Rissanen T, et al. Adenovirus-mediated extracellular superoxide dismutase gene therapy reduces neointima formation in balloon-denuded rabbit aorta. Circulation 2002;106:1999-2003.

31. Addad F, Vinchon f, Durand E, et al. Superexpression of superoxyde dismutase and catalase by adenovirus-mediated gene transfert improves endothelial function and experimental balloon angioplasty. XII Congress of the European Society of Cardiology. Amsterdam. August 2000.

32. Lafont A, Durand E, Samuel JL, et al. Endothelial dysfunction and collagen accumulation: two independent factors for restenosis and constrictive remodeling after experimental angioplasty. Circulation 1999;100:1109-15.

33. Breuss JM, Cejna M, Bergmeister H, et al. Activation of nuclear factor-kappa B significantly contributes to lumen loss in a rabbit iliac artery balloon angioplasty model. Circulation 2002;105:633-8.

34. Shimokawa H, Aarhus LL, Vanhoutte PM. Porcine coronary arteries with regenerated endothelium have a reduced endothelium-dependent responsiveness to aggregating platelets and serotonin. Circ Res 1987;61:256-70.

35. Six I, Van Belle E, Bordet R, et al. L-Arginine and L-NAME have no effects on the reendothelialization process after arterial balloon injury. Cardiovasc Res 1999;43:731-8.

36. Lau AK, Leichtweis SB, Hume P, et al. Probucol promotes functional reendothelialization in balloon-injured rabbit aortas. Circulation 2003;107:2031-6.

37. Durand E, Mallat Z, Addad F, et al. Time courses of apoptosis and cell proliferation and their relationship to arterial remodeling and restenosis after angioplasty in an atherosclerotic rabbit model. J Am Coll Cardiol 2002;39:1680-5.

38. Rossig L, Hoffmann J, Hugel B, et al. Vitamin C inhibits endothelial cell apoptosis in congestive heart failure. Circulation 2001;104:2182-7.

39. Nieto N, Friedman SL, Greenwel P, Cederbaum AI. CYP2E1-mediated oxidative stress induces collagen type 1 expression in rat hepatic cells. Hepatology 1999;30:987-96.

40. Mattana J, Margiloff L, Chaplia L. Oxidation of extracellular matrix modulates susceptibility to degradation by the mesangial matrix metalloproteinase-2. Free Radic Biol Med 1999;27:315-21.

41. Yokoyama T, Miyauchi K, Kurata T, Sato H, Daida H. Effect of probucol on neointimal thickening in a stent porcine restenosis model. Jpn Heart J 2004;45:305-13.

42. Tardif JC, Gregoire J, Schwartz L, et al. Canadian Antioxidant Restenosis Trial (CART-1) Investigators. Effects of AGI-1067 and probucol after percutaneous coronary interventions. Circulation 2003;107:552-8.

Chapter 14

ANTIOXIDANTS AND RESTENOSIS AFTER PERCUTANEOUS CORONARY INTERVENTION: HUMAN STUDIES

Martial G. Bourassa and Jean-Claude Tardif
Montreal Heart Institute, Montreal, Quebec, Canada

Introduction

Since its inception in 1977, the use of percutaneous coronary intervention (PCI) has increased to over one million cases per year worldwide[1]. This explosive growth reflects the improvement in initial success rates, an acceptable safety profile, and the acceptance of PCI as an alternative or adjunctive therapy to medical treatment and bypass surgery in patients with coronary artery disease[2,3]. Rapid advances in guide wires and balloon catheters, the introduction of intracoronary stents, including drug-eluting stents (DES), and other interventional devices as well as the accumulation of operator experience allow PCI to be used in more complex lesions, smaller coronary vessels, and in patients with multi-vessel disease, with greater procedural and long-term success.

Restenosis after PCI

Incidence

Restenosis occurs in approximately one-third of patients within the first six to nine months after PCI[4-6] and it remains a vexing problem with major clinical and socio-economic implications. Both the clinical benefits and costs of PCI in relation to surgery and medical therapy rest on occurrence rates. Restenosis usually occurs within the first nine months and most restenotic lesions appear between one and four months after PCI[4]. It occurs more often when PCI is performed in smaller coronary arteries, saphenous vein grafts, total occlusions, and bifurcation and ostial lesions[5,6]. It also occurs more often in diabetic patients, smokers, and patients with unstable coronary syndromes. Within six months of PCI, approximately 20% to 30% of patients undergo repeat PCI, and 5% to 8% receive coronary bypass surgery for symptomatic restenosis. The cost of restenosis is estimated at over two billion dollars annually in the U.S. alone.

Compared to balloon angioplasty, however, the widespread use of bare-metal stents since the mid 1990s has reduced the rate of restenosis after PCI and the need for repeat PCI by about 50%[7]. More recently, as shown in several prospective randomized trials, DES have further reduced its incidence, in low-risk cases, to practically one-digit figure[8-11]. As a rule, both sirolimus-[8,9] and paclitaxel-[10,11] eluting stents have yielded similar results.

Incidence and methods of assessment

Restenosis after PCI is often asymptomatic[12,13] and the predictive values of non-invasive tests, such as exercise stress testing with or without radionuclide scintigraphy and stress echocardiography, are not accurate enough for reliable use in clinical studies[14]. Therefore, coronary angiography has emerged early on as the preferred method of assessing restenosis after PCI. Several angiographic definitions of binary restenosis have been used[5]. Among the best known are a $\geq 50\%$ loss of luminal gain at PCI, a $\geq 30\%$ increase in stenosis after PCI, and a stenosis going from < 50% diameter narrowing at PCI to > 50% at follow-up angiography. A luminal narrowing > 50% at follow-up is generally well accepted for its simplicity and practicality. This definition should include, in addition, a meaningful difference (10% to 15%) from early to follow-up post-PCI measurement.

In addition, late lumen loss often represents the primary angiographic endpoint of restenosis after PCI in clinical studies. This angiographic assessment requires quantitative computer-assisted analysis (QCA)[15,16]. Likewise, intravascular ultrasound (IVUS) allows quantitative assessment of changes in lumen and wall dimensions, such as changes in minimal lumen diameter and lumen area, as well as changes in plaque volume, and is particularly well suited to assess restenosis late after PCI.

Finally, because of the importance of clinical outcome later after PCI, target lesion and target vessel revascularization (TLR and TVR) have been assessed, in the absence of angiographic of IVUS data, as secondary or even as primary endpoints after PCI in recent clinical studies.

Pathophysiology

The pathophysiology of restenosis after PCI is not entirely defined[17]. Restenosis is the result of a complex vascular healing response to injury

(*Figure 1*). The inflammatory and thrombotic responses that occur after injury to blood vessels produce numerous growth factors that stimulate smooth muscle cell (SMC) activation, migration and proliferation. Combined with cellular proliferation, the heightened production and accumulation of extracellular matrix results in neointimal hyperplasia[18]. The same events that lead to neointima formation after PCI, i.e. matrix formation and SMC proliferation, are believed to be involved in the process of vascular remodeling (chronic changes in total vessel size). SMC contraction, along with cross-linking of collagen fibers, may limit compensatory vessel enlargement in response to neointima formation and may even result in vascular constriction[19,20]. In addition, chronic flow-dependent changes in vessel size may be limited by endothelial dysfunction[21]. As described below, vascular remodeling contributes to the presence or absence and severity of luminal encroachment after PCI[19,20].

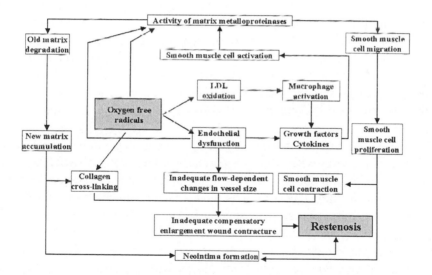

Figure 1. Pathophysiology of restenosis after PCI involving the oxidation hypothesis.

Role of stents and brachytherapy

Bare-metal stents

As a result of the success and growth of stent implantation[22], in-stent restenosis has now become a major clinical problem. Indeed, in-stent restenosis occurs in 20%-25% of patients treated with bare-metal stents[23]. The mechanism of in-stent restenosis has been shown to be neointima formation, which reflects an inflammatory pathogenesis[23]. Diabetics, patients with unstable coronary syndromes, with small coronary arteries and long lesions, and those undergoing multiple stent implantations have been shown to be at high risk for in-stent restenosis[24,25]. Although restenosis may be related to mechanical problems or suboptimal results at the time of stent implantation, there appears to be a biological subset of lesions and patients in whom in-stent restenosis is a chronic recurrent problem, independent of procedural results.

Drug-eluting stents

At least two types of anti-proliferative substances, sirolimus and paclitaxel, have been tested in recent clinical trials in an attempt to prevent or reduce the occurrence of in-stent restenosis after PCI[8-11]. Sirolimus (rapamycin) is a cytostatic macrocyclic lactone with both anti-inflammatory and anti-proliferative properties which can be delivered from a polymer-encapsulated stent. Paclitaxel is a lipophilic molecule derived from the Pacific yew tree *Taxus breviola*, which is capable of inhibiting cellular division, motility, activation, secretory processes and signal transduction. Like sirolimus, paclitaxel can be delivered through a slow- or moderate-release polymer-matrix formulation. Both molecules have been shown, in pivotal clinical trials, to be safe and highly effective in reducing rates of coronary restenosis after PCI[8-11]. However, only patients with single, previously untreated lesions in native coronary artery were enrolled in these trials.

In the SIRolImUS-coated Bx Velocity balloon-expandable stent in the treatment of patients with de novo coronary artery lesions (SIRIUS) trial, which enrolled 1,058 patients in whom the target lesions averaged 14.4 mm in length and the target vessels averaged 2.80 mm in diameter, sirolimus-eluting stents were compared to standard stents. After a follow-up of 270 days, the primary endpoint, i.e. the rate of failure of the target vessel (a composite of cardiac death, myocardial infarction, and repeat PCI or surgical revascularization), was reduced from 21.0% with a standard stent to 8.6% with a sirolimus-eluting stent (p<0.001)[9]. Stent thrombosis was infrequent, and the rate was similar in the two treatment groups (0.4% vs. 0.8%)[9]. In the TAXUS-IV trial, 1,314 patients were randomized to receive either a bare-metal stent or a slow-release, polymer-based, paclitaxel-eluting stent to revascularize a single coronary lesion (lesion length, 10 to 28 mm; vessel diameter, 2.5 to 3.75 mm). The rate of ischemia-driven target-vessel revascularization at nine months (the primary endpoint of the trial) was reduced from 12.0% with the implantation of a bare-metal stent to 4.7% with the implantation of a paclitaxel-eluting stent (p<0.001)[11]. In this study, the rate of angiographic restenosis was reduced from 26.6% to 7.9% with the paclitaxel-eluting stent (p<0.001). Again, stent thrombosis was infrequent (0.6% vs. 0.8%) and similar in both groups[11]. Although the short-term safety of these devices compares favourably with that of bare-metal stents, their long-term safety remains to be documented.

Subgroup analyses of the SIRIUS and TAXUS-IV trials suggest that DES are perhaps most useful in lesions and patients at higher risk for stent restenosis, such as small-diameter lesions, long lesions and patients with diabetes mellitus[9,11]. In several other situations, involving more complex coronary lesions such as chronic total occlusion, bifurcation/ostial lesions, unprotected left main disease, lesions in bypass grafts, multivessel disease and in-stent restenosis, additional data are needed to establish the safety and efficacy of DES, as compared to bare-metal stents. DES may be cost prohibitive in patients with multiple lesions and some vessels may be too small or tortuous to accommodate a DES. In these situations and in others where DES are known to be associated with higher rates of stent restenosis, oral medications with anti-inflammatory properties, such as long-term use of antioxidants, may be of great benefit.

Brachytherapy

In-stent restenosis is due to intimal hyperplasia within the stent and endovascular radiation therapy has emerged as a treatment of choice for its prevention[26]. In 1997, Terstein et al. reported favourable results using gamma-radiation after coronary stenting in patients with previous restenosis[27]. In the Canadian arm of the Beta-Energy Restenosis Trial (BERT), intracoronary beta-radiation has been shown to inhibit neointima formation with no reduction of external elastic membrane area at six-month follow-up[28]. Again, oral antioxidants may prove useful as adjunct anti-inflammatory therapy in these patients.

Oxidative stress and restenosis after PCI

The positive results obtained with the synthetic antioxidant probucol in restenosis trials suggest that the restenosis process is associated with oxidative stress[19,25,29-36]. There is evidence that oxidative stress occurs early after PCI[37,38]. Damaged endothelium and activated platelets and neutrophils at the PCI site can generate reactive intermediates (*Figure 1*). These oxidizing metabolites can induce chain reactions that result in endothelial dysfunction, macrophage activation, SMC migration and proliferation, and matrix remodeling[39,40]. Activated macrophages and dysfunctional endothelium can release cytokines and growth factors that stimulate matrix remodeling and SMC proliferation. Metalloproteinases are involved in matrix remodeling and their activity is modulated by reactive oxygen species

(ROS)[41]. Matrix degradation by metalloproteinases precedes or accompanies early formation of new extracellular matrix after PCI and also is a crucial step before SMC migration and proliferation[42]. In addition, oxidation processes are involved in the nonenzymatic cross-linking of collagen fibers[43] and this could result in chronic vascular constriction.

The accumulation of new extracellular matrix and SMCs results in neointimal formation responsible for lumen narrowing after stent deployment and balloon angioplasty.

Randomized trials of synthetic antioxidants after PCI

Small clinical studies

As discussed in chapter 14, animal studies have shown a beneficial effect of antioxidants on both neointima formation and arterial remodeling after PCI. In addition, small clinical studies have suggested that probucol, a synthetic antioxidant, started before angioplasty may prevent restenosis[31,34]. In a study involving 111 patients, Lee et al. reported a restenosis rate of 8% when probucol therapy was initiated 30 days before balloon coronary angioplasty (p<0.05 vs. all other treatment groups), compared to more than 33% when either probucol was started three days before angioplasty or when pravastatin was used[31]. Probucol and dipyridamole were compared in 67 patients in whom therapy was initiated at least seven days before balloon coronary angioplasty[32]. Rates of restenosis were 19.4% in the probucol group vs. 41.7% in the dipyridamole group in that study (p<0.05). QCA methods were not used in these two studies.

Watanabe et al. randomized 118 patients to probucol therapy (given for at least seven days before and for three months after PCI) or to a control group[33]. The rates of restenosis in that study were 19.7% for probucol and 39.7% for the control group (p<0.05). Finally, the effects of probucol administered for ≥ 30 days or for < 14 days prior to PCI were compared to those of pravastatin in another study[34]. Rates of restenosis per lesion were 14% when probucol was administered for ≥ 30 days prior to PCI (p<0.05 compared to the other treatment groups), 51.8% when probucol was given for < 14 days before PCI, and 40.4% and 34%, respectively, when pravastatin was given for 30 days vs. < 14 days before PCI. These clinical studies were, however, not double-blinded.

The Probucol Angioplasty Restenosis Trial (PART)

The Probucol Angioplasty Restenosis Trial[35] was designed to investigate the preventive effect of probucol on restenosis after balloon coronary angioplasty in a prospective randomized fashion. One hundred and one patients were randomly assigned to receive 1000 mg/day of probucol or control (no lipid-lowering) therapy four weeks before angioplasty. After four weeks of pretreatment, both groups underwent balloon angioplasty. Probucol was continued until follow-up angiography 24 weeks after the procedure. Results were analyzed by QCA. At follow-up angiography, restenosis occurred in 23% of patients in the probucol group and in 58% in the control group (p=0.001). Minimal lumen diameter was significantly greater at follow-up angiography in the probucol than in the control group. The loss/gain ratio tended to be lower and net gain was greater in the probucol than in the control group. The higher than expected restenosis rate in the control group was attributed to a high proportion of type B lesions in their population.

The beneficial effect of probucol on the prevention of restenosis in small coronary arteries was evaluated in a subgroup of 78 patients. In that study, the effectiveness of probucol was restricted to arteries ≤ 2.7 mm, with a resultant restenosis rate of 24% in the probucol group compared with 75% in the control group[36]. Again, these data strongly suggest that oxidative stress plays an important role in the restenosis process.

The Multivitamins and Probucol (MVP) study

The MVP study[19,25,29,30] was a double-blind, placebo-controlled randomized trial using a 2 by 2 factorial design. The objective of the trial was to evaluate whether drugs with antioxidant properties decrease the incidence and severity of restenosis as assessed by QCA within the first six months after successful balloon coronary angioplasty. Patients referred for elective angiography were evaluated at least 30 days prior to their scheduled procedure. Patients were eligible if they were scheduled to undergo standard balloon angioplasty on at least one native coronary artery and had at least one target lesion with ≥ 50% stenosis of the luminal diameter as measured by caliper on the angiogram.

Beginning 30 days before the scheduled angioplasty, patients were randomly assigned to receive one of four treatments: probucol alone, multivitamins alone, the combination of probucol and multivitamins, or placebo. Two tablets of the multivitamin complex, each of which contained 15,000 IU of beta-carotene, 250 mg of vitamin C, and 350 IU of vitamin E (*dl*-alpha-tocopherol) or the matched placebo were administered twice daily. All patients received an extra dose of 2000 IU of vitamin E, 1000 mg of probucol, both the vitamin E and probucol, or placebo 12 hours before angioplasty, according to their random treatment assignment. All patients in whom angioplasty was successful and who did not have procedure-related cardiac complications continued to receive the assigned study treatment until follow-up angiography was performed.

Data from the MVP study provide strong evidence that probucol therapy initiated 30 days before and given for six months after angioplasty prevents angiographic restenosis[29] (*Figures 2 and 3*). Luminal loss was 0.38 mm in the placebo group, 0.33 mm in the multivitamin group, 0.22 mm in the combined-treatment group, and 0.12 mm in the probucol group (p=0.006 for probucol vs. no probucol). Restenosis occurred in 38.9% of the dilated segments in the placebo group, 40.3% in the multivitamin group, 28.9% in the combined-treatment group, and 20.7% in the probucol group (p=0.003 for probucol vs. no probucol). Compared to the placebo, probucol given alone resulted in reduction of 68% in late lumen loss, 47% in restenosis rate per segment and 58% in the need for repeat intervention. The importance of pre-angioplasty therapy with probucol appears critical, considering the negative results from the Angioplasty Plus Probucol/Lovastatin Evaluation (APPLE) study in which probucol was started between 48 hours before and 24 hours after angioplasty[44]. Data suggesting that probucol accumulates slowly in tissue probably explain these results[45].

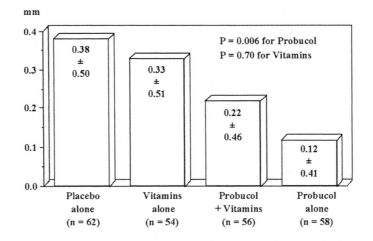

Figure 2. Angiographic late luminal loss after PCI for the four groups of treatment of the per-protocol population in the MVP study[29]

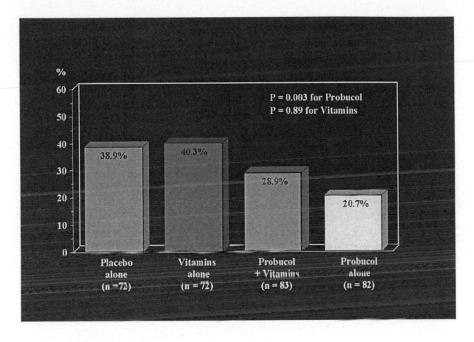

Figure 3. Restenosis rates per dilated segment for the four study groups in the MVP trial[29]

The MVP results were obtained without imposing any restriction relative to vessel size at entry into the trial. Interestingly, the benefit of probucol therapy was maintained in the subgroup of 189 patients who underwent successful balloon angioplasty of at least one coronary segment with a reference diameter <3.0 mm[25,46]. Mean reference diameter in this study population was 2.5 mm. Lumen loss was 0.12 mm for probucol vs. 0.38 mm for placebo (p=0.005) and restenosis rates per segment were 20% vs. 37%, respectively (p=0.006) (*Figure 4*). This represents a 68% reduction in late lumen loss and a 46% reduction in restenosis rate per segment. In this subgroup as in the whole MVP study, there was a tendency for probucol to have better results when given alone than when it was combined with vitamins. The possible prooxidant effect of the very high doses of vitamins used in the MVP study may explain this observation[47].

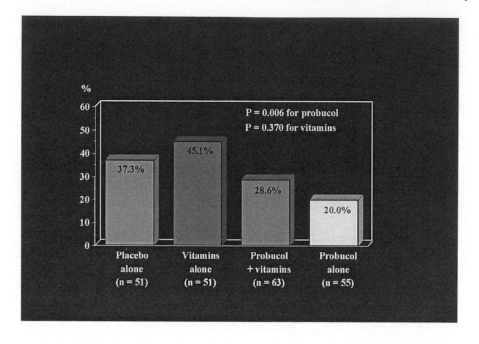

Figure 4. **Rates of restenosis for segments with a reference diameter of less than 3.0mm in the MVP study**[25]**.**

The Canadian Antioxidant Restenosis Trial (CART-1)

The Canadian Antioxidant Restenosis Trial (CART-1)[48] was a double-blind, double-dummy, multicenter trial in which 305 patients scheduled to undergo elective PCI with or without stent placement (85% received stents) were randomly assigned to placebo, probucol 500 mg twice daily (as a positive control) AGI-1067 70 mg, 140 mg or 280 mg once daily. Patients were treated for two weeks prior to and four weeks after PCI in this phase 2 trial. The primary endpoint in CART-1, the minimal lumen area at the site of PCI on follow-up intravascular ultrasound (IVUS), was on average: 2.66 mm2 in the placebo group; 3.69 mm2 with probucol; 2.75 mm2 for AGI-1067 70 mg; 3.17 mm2 in the AGI-1067 140-mg group; and 3.36 mm2 with AGI-1067 280 mg (p<0.05 for larger lumen with AGI-1067 280 mg and probucol versus placebo). There was a significant dose-response relationship of AGI-1067 (p=0.02) (*Figure 5*).

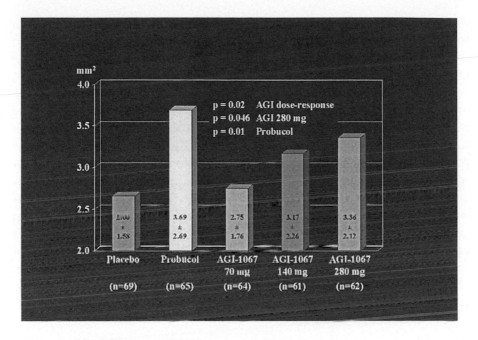

Figure 5. **Minimal lumen area at the site of PCI on follow-up intravascular ultrasound in the CART-1 study**[48].

The volumetric assessment with IVUS supported these results[48]. The early benefits of AGI-1067 and probucol after PCI raise the possibilities that countering oxidative stress may rapidly improve endothelial function[49] and/or that these agents may produce changes in plaque content[50] that contributed to an improved response to PCI.

In CART-1, AGI-1067 did not prolong QT interval like probucol. Therefore, this compound has now entered the next phase of testing of the antioxidant/anti-inflammatory hypothesis.

The Canadian Atherosclerosis and Restenosis Trial (CART-2)

CART-2 was a 12-month, double blind, randomized, placebo-controlled trial of AGI-1067 280 mg QD versus placebo. In order to yield 425 patients who underwent PCI and were eligible for the trial, approximately 1500 patients were randomized to one of four treatment regimens starting 14 days prior to their scheduled diagnostic angiogram. Two groups received placebo for 14 days, one group received AGI-1067 (280 mg/day) for three days, and one group received AGI-1067 (280 mg/day) for 14 days. These 425 patients were continued on study medication for 12 months according to the randomized treatment arm assigned initially. Although change in plaque volume at follow-up in a 30-mm segment of a non-PCI coronary artery on 3-D IVUS[51] was the primary endpoint of the trial, the minimal lumen diameter (MLD) at the site of PCI, measured by QCA, on the 12-month follow-up angiogram, was a major secondary endpoint of CART-2. To confirm and extend the results on reduction of coronary restenosis after PCI in CART-1, two major hypotheses are being tested in CART-2. First, considering that oxidative stress and inflammation may persist for a prolonged period after stenting[52], treatment with AGI-1067 for the entire period of risk after PCI (instead of only four weeks in CART-1) may result in enhanced protection against luminal renarrowing[53]. Second, restenosis reduction with AGI-1067 started two weeks before PCI was the initial proof of concept in CART-1. However, this strategy cannot be applied to patients undergoing non-elective PCI or even to the increasing number of patients who undergo an ad hoc procedure, consisting of angioplasty with or without stent placement, simultaneously with diagnostic catheterization. Therefore, a key secondary objective of CART-2 is to determine whether pre-treatment with AGI-1067 for a shorter duration, combined with prolonged treatment after PCI, will prevent post-PCI restenosis. Thus far, 12-month follow-up angiography has been performed in the 425 patients and QCA analysis of the results should be available soon.

Effects of synthetic antioxidants

Probucol

Cholesterol-lowering and antioxidant properties
    Probucol is a potent synthetic antioxidant, which was developed in the 1960s by Dow Chemicals Co.[54]. Probucol has a structural formula, which bears little resemblance to any other lipid-lowering agent. It is a highly lipophilic cholesterol-lowering molecule with strong antioxidant properties. Probucol is structurally related to butylated hydroxytoluene (BHT), an antioxidant widely used as a food additive. Probucol absorption is generally limited to 7% of the initial dose. It circulates in plasma in association with lipoproteins (primarily in LDL), apparently dissolved in the lipid core. The major route of elimination is via the bile and feces, and lipid clearance is negligible. Probucol is a lipophilic chain-breaking antioxidant that allows LDL to resist oxidative modification[55-57]. This property is probably responsible for the reduction of macrophage accumulation in the arterial wall observed in treated animals[58]. Probucol has been shown to inhibit atherosclerosis in WHHL rabbits, independent of its cholesterol-lowering effect[59]. It also inhibits macrophage secretion of interleukin-1, a proinflammatory cytokine, which has SMC proliferating, and metalloproteinase activating effects[60]. Endothelial function is improved by probucol when it is administered in patients with proven coronary artery

disease[61]. This beneficial effect is correlated with the protection against oxidation offered by probucol.

Minor and major side effects

Most minor adverse reactions associated with probucol are generally mild to moderate and of short duration. The most frequent symptom associated with its use is diarrhea, which occurs in approximately 10% of patients. Other adverse gastro-intestinal reactions include flatulence, abdominal pain, nausea and vomiting. These symptoms are usually transient and seldom require stopping the medication. During clinical studies, probucol was discontinued in about 2% of patients because of adverse gastro-intestinal side effects.

Two serious adverse effects associated with the use of probucol have been prolongation of the QT interval and reduction of HDL cholesterol. Prolongation of the QT interval has been documented with the use of probucol since its introduction. A prolonged QT interval (>450 msec.) has been reported in 22% of women and in 7% of men in a review of several studies[62]. Despite this prolongation of the QT interval, there was no increase in the incidence of ventricular arrhythmias or deaths in patients treated with probucol in the MVP trial. Although probucol was prescribed more than three million times from 1979 to 1994, only 16 tachyarrythmic events have been reported[62-65]. Potentially predisposing factors (e.g. hypokaliemia, use of type 1a antiarrythmic agents) were identified in 14 of the 16 patients with tachyarrythmias. Of the 11 patients (included in the initial 16) who had torsades de pointe, only two did not have any identifiable risk factor. There was a clear gender difference in the susceptibility to tachyarrythmias. Female patients accounted for 15 of the 16 patients with events, and all 11 patients with torsades de pointe were women.

Probucol lowers LDL cholesterol by approximately 10% in patients[54] via modifications of LDL characteristics resulting in an increase in their catabolism[62]. However, HDL level is also lowered by up to 40%, possibly due to enhancement of reverse cholesterol transport from peripheral tissues to the liver[67]. It has been hypothesized that the lack of beneficial effects of probucol on progression of femoral atherosclerosis in the Probucol Quantitative Regression Swedish Trial (PQRST) was due to this prolonged reduction in HDL levels[68,69]. Nevertheless, the risk associated with lowering of HDL levels for only a period of six months is probably low.

AGI-1067

Cholesterol-lowering and antioxidant properties

AGI-1067, the mono-succinic acid ester of probucol, is a phenolic antioxidant member of a novel class of agents termed "vascular protectants"[70]. It has strong antioxidant properties equipotent to those of probucol and anti-inflammatory properties[71-73]. AGI-1067 also exhibits greater water solubility and cell permeability than probucol. AGI-1067 has the ability to selectively block the expression of oxidation-sensitive inflammatory genes that code for VCAM-1 and MCP-1 through the NF-kappa B independent mechanism (*Table 1*).

Table 1. AGI-1067 and Probucol Pre-Clinical Comparison

Activities	AGI-1067	Probucol
♦ Phenolic antioxidant	+++	+++
♦ VCAM-1 expression inhibitor	+++	-
♦ MCP-1 expression inhibitor	+++	-
♦ E-selectin expression inhibitor	+++	-
♦ SMC proliferation inhibitor	+++	-
♦ LDL-lowering	+++	+/-
♦ HDL-lowering	+/-	+++
♦ Cellular permeability	++	-
♦ Potential to prolong QTc interval	-	++
♦ Stability	++	+
♦ Anti-atherosclerotic models		
- Monkeys	+++	+
- Rabbits	+++	+
- LDLr-KO mice	+++	+
- ApoE-KO mice	+++	-
♦ Inhibition of LPS-induced TNF-α and IL-1β release from HAECs and hPBMCs	+++	-

Although AGI-1067 and probucol are equipotent antioxidants, they produce different effects on VCAM-1 expression in human aortic endothelial cells. AGI-1067 produces a concentration-related decrease in TNF-alpha stimulated VCAM-1 expression in the concentration range of 2.5 to 10 μmol/L while probucol was shown to have no effect at concentration as high as 100 μmol/L[72]. It is notable that ICAM-1 expression is not inhibited by AGI-1067, which demonstrates that this agent is not a global inhibitor of inflammatory response genes. Because ICAM-1 is the counter ligand to neutrophils, immune surveillance by these cells should not be affected by inhibiting only VCAM-1. AGI-1067 is also a powerful inhibitor of SMC proliferation in experimental studies (*Table 1*).

In CART-1, over a six-month period, AGI-1067 did not decrease LDL-cholesterol levels as compared to placebo. However, this was also the case for probucol over this short time period. As stated earlier, AGI-1067 did not prolong QT interval in CART-1[48]. However, AGI-1067 resulted in dose-related decreases in HDL-cholesterol in that study, although to a lesser extent than probucol[48]. The decrease was maximum at two weeks and, in contrast to probucol, did not progress further. Overall, HDL lowering was < 20% after six weeks of therapy with AGI-1067. The clinical significance of this modest reduction is unclear. High HDL-cholesterol values are generally thought to protect against atherosclerosis, and reduced levels have been associated with a higher risk of cardiovascular events[74]. However, this relationship is not uniformly supported by transgenic animal models[75,76]. In addition, patients with genetic abnormalities resulting in very high or low levels of HDL-cholesterol are not necessarily at reduced or elevated cardiovascular risk, respectively[77]. It has been suggested that the serum level of HDL-cholesterol does not necessarily reflect the efficacy of reverse cholesterol transport[78,79]. The reduction in HDL associated with the higher AGI-1067 dosages may in fact reflect enhanced reverse cholesterol transport and may prove to be atheroprotective or neutral.

Prevention of restenosis using synthetic antioxidants

Probucol

Possible mechanisms

The powerful antioxidant effects of probucol may prevent endothelial dysfunction, LDL oxidation and macrophage and metalloproteinase activation[37,53,80-82]. These actions could limit SMC activation, migration, proliferation and contraction; matrix degradation and deposition; and cross-linking of new collagen fibers. By ultimately limiting SMC contraction, collagen formation and cross-linking, and endothelial dysfunction, probucol may modify vascular remodeling and allow greater vessel enlargement after balloon angioplasty. Other mechanisms of action have to be considered, however, in view of the disappointing results with multivitamins in the MVP study. The hypocholesterolemic effect of probucol is weak and unlikely by itself to be responsible for the positive MVP results, considering that high-dose lovastatin started seven to ten days before angioplasty failed to prevent restenosis in a recent trial[83]. The role of probucol in reverse cholesterol transport and interleukin-1 secretion, however, may have contributed to the beneficial effects of the drug. In particular, inhibition by probucol of the secretion of interleukin-1 by macrophages[60] may have decreased secretion of metalloproteinases[84] and modified remodeling of the extracellular matrix.

IVUS data

Whether probucol acts through prevention of neointimal formation, improvement in arterial remodeling, or both, cannot be adequately addressed by angiography. We have, therefore, obtained IVUS data in MVP patients after angioplasty and at follow-up, with operators blinded to the results[19]. By providing topographic views of coronary arteries with high resolution, IVUS allows quantitative assessment of changes in lumen and wall dimensions[85]. Before determining how probucol acted in the MVP study, it is important to clarify the mechanisms of lumen loss and restenosis after balloon angioplasty. Indeed, conflicting animal and human data exist concerning the relative role of neointima formation and vascular remodeling in lumen loss after angioplasty[19]. In control patients from the MVP study, the increase in wall area (mean: 1.50 mm2) was greater than the decrease in lumen area (-1.21 mm2) with a slight increase in external elastic membrane area (0.29 mm2). However, the change in lumen area correlated better with the change in external elastic membrane area (r =0.53, p=0.002) than it did with the change in wall area (r=-0.13, p=0.49). These results indicate that the direction (enlargement or constriction) and extent (inadequate or adequate compensatory enlargement) of vascular remodeling in response to neointima formation after balloon angioplasty determine the magnitude of lumen loss at follow-up. In other words, data from MVP[19] and from other studies[20] suggest that lumen loss after balloon angioplasty is caused by the combination of inadequate or deleterious vessel remodeling and neointima formation.

Probucol in the MVP study significantly reduced lumen loss chiefly by improving vascular remodeling[19]. Compared to the placebo group, there was a reduction in lumen loss of 88% or 1.06 mm2 when probucol was administered alone. A striking improvement of compensatory vessel enlargement after coronary angioplasty was mainly responsible for the favourable effect of probucol on lumen loss. There was a mean enlargement in external elastic membrane area of 1.74 mm2 from early post-angioplasty to follow-up in patients treated with probucol alone compared to 0.29 mm2 in patients given placebo (*Figure 6*).

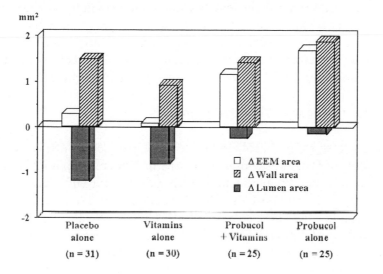

Figure 6. **Changes in lumen, wall and external elastic membrane (EEM) areas as assessed by IVUS in the MVP trial.** Probucol allowed for an almost perfect match between neointima formation (increase in wall area) and vascular remodeling (increase in EEM area) resulting in minimal lumen loss. In contrast, groups not treated with probucol had an important mismatch between neointimal formation and compensatory vascular remodeling[29]

AGI-1067

Animal studies have demonstrated dual pharmacological activities of AGI-1067: 1) the ability to block the expression of oxidation-sensitive inflammatory genes, including genes that code for VCAM-1 and MCP-1[72], and 2) the ability to lower total plasma LDL cholesterol levels. The LDL cholesterol lowering effect of AGI-1067 is due to enhanced clearance of plasma VLDL and LDL. AGI-1067 exhibits strong antioxidant activity equipotent to probucol.

Results from CART-1 have shown that, like probucol, AGI-1067 improves lumen size at the site of stent placement six months after PCI. Moreover, as a result of the two-week pre-treatment period, this benefit is present immediately after PCI. Thus, countering oxidative stress may promptly improve endothelial function and reduce vasomotor tone. Balloon injury induces an immediate release of reactive oxygen species and this release may be inhibited by powerful antioxidants. Lumen enlargement early after PCI in CART-1 was also present after stent deployment. Furthermore, these early effects on lumen volume persisted at follow-up, despite the fact that study medication had been stopped for five months.

These results demonstrate that both probucol and AGI-1067 effectively prevent restenosis not only in vessels without but also in those with coronary stenting. Sirolimus- and paclitaxel-eluting stents strongly suppress neointimal hyperplasia after PCI with presumably little effect on vascular remodeling. Therefore, it seems reasonable to postulate that, by its effect on vascular remodeling, AGI-1067 can act synergistically with DES.

Reason for inefficacy of multivitamins

In contrast to probucol, multivitamins had no significant effect on angiographic or IVUS restenosis and on major clinical endpoints in the MVP trial. Vitamin E is a lipophilic antioxidant present in LDL[86] and in cellular membranes[87]. A daily dose of 1400 IU was chosen based on data showing higher serum levels at doses over 1000 IU daily[88]. We also administered an additional dose of 2000 IU of vitamin E 12 hours before angioplasty because stability in plasma levels of hydrogen peroxide was observed with such a regimen during bypass surgery[89]. We opted for a multivitamin complex because of the capacity of vitamin C to regenerate the antioxidant activity of vitamin E[90] and because beta-carotene can modulate endothelial function and possibly interact directly with nuclear receptors[91]. Considering that probucol and multivitamins both are antioxidants, it is not clear why multivitamins did not prevent restenosis whereas probucol did. Moderately intense dietary intervention was done in all patients in the MVP trial and included limitation of vitamin intake, instruction to avoid vitamin and mineral supplements, and teaching the American Heart Association step 1 diet. Smoking habits, which may modify antioxidant requirements, were similar in all groups. Probucol may simply be a more powerful antioxidant at LDL and cellular levels than multivitamins. Alternatively, other properties may have contributed to this result. Indeed, the effects of probucol, vitamin E and beta-carotene on atherosclerosis[91] and vascular reactivity[92] are not clearly related to their antioxidant properties in animal studies. The improvement in vascular remodeling after angioplasty observed with the combination of vitamin C and E in one animal study[93] contrasts with the lack of effect of multivitamins on remodeling in the MVP trial. The possible prooxidant effects of the higher doses of vitamin C and E[47,94] and the addition of beta-carotene to the combination may explain the discrepant results.

Conclusions

The synthetic antioxidants probucol and AGI-1067 are effective in reducing the rate of restenosis after PCI. Probucol is no longer available in most countries. However, AGI-1067 is currently being rigorously evaluated as a clinically relevant antioxidant agent in the prevention of restenosis after PCI in the Canadian Atherosclerosis and Restenosis Trial (CART-2). If the CART-2 results confirm and extend the findings of CART-1, AGI-1067 will not only contribute to firmly establish the oxidative stress/inflammatory hypothesis, but this novel antioxidant agent will also presumably find major clinical applications.

DES have shown marked antiproliferative effects and strong effectiveness in the prevention of restenosis after PCI in mild to moderate coronary lesions. In addition to their current high cost, their usefulness in complex and multiple coronary lesions remains to be established. If, in CART-2, the strong antioxidant AGI-1067 proves to be as effective in the prevention of restenosis after PCI as suggested in CART-1, it may find some interesting applications. In addition, its potential synergetic action with DES will require further assessment.

References

1. Smith SC, Jr., Dove JT, Jacobs, AK, et al. ACC/AHA guidelines for percutaneous coronary intervention (revision of the 1993 PTCA guidelines)-executive summary: a report of the American College of Cardiology/American Heart Association task force on practice guidelines (Committee to revise the 1993 guidelines for percutaneous transluminal coronary angioplasty) endorsed by the Society for Cardiac Angiography and Interventions. Circulation 2001;103:3019-41.

2. Landau C, Lange RA, Hillis, LD. Percutaneous transluminal coronary angioplasty. N Engl J Med 1994;330:981-93.

3. The Bypass Angioplasty Revascularization Investigation (BARI) Investigators. Comparison of coronary bypass surgery with angioplasty in patients with multivessel disease. N Engl J Med 1996;335:217-25.

4. Nobuyoshi M, Kimura T, Nosaka H, et al. Restenosis after successful percutaneous transluminal coronary angioplasty: Serial angiographic follow-up of 299 patients. J Am Coll Cardiol 1988;12:616-23.

5. Bourassa MG, Lespérance J, Eastwood C, et al. Physiologic, anatomic and procedural factors predictive of restenosis after percutaneous transluminal coronary angioplasty. J Am Coll Cardiol 1991;18:368-76.

6. Mercado N, Boersma E, Wijns W, et al. Clinical and quantitative coronary angiographic predictors of coronary restenosis: a comparative analysis from the balloon-to-stent era. J Am Coll Cardiol 2001;38:645-52.

7. Brophy JM, Belisle P, Joseph L. Evidence for use of coronary stents. A hierarchical Bayesian meta-analysis. Ann Intern Med 2003;138:777-86.

8. Morice M, Serruys PW, Sousa JE, et al. A randomized comparison of a sirolimus-eluting stent with a standard stent for coronary revascularization. N Engl J Med 2002;346:1773-80.

9. Moses JW, Leon MB, Popma JJ, et al. Sirolimus-eluting stent versus standard stents in patients with stenosis in a native coronary artery. N Engl J Med 2003;349:1315-23.

10. Grube E, Silber S, Hauptmann KE, et al. TAXUS-1: six- and twelve-month results from a randomized, double-blind trial on a slow-release paclitaxel-eluting stent for de novo coronary lesions. Circulation 2003;107:38-42.

11. Stone GW, Ellis SG, Cox DA, et al. A polymer-based, paclitaxel-eluting stent in patients with coronary artery disease. N Engl J Med 2004;350:221-31.

12. Hernandez RA, Macaya C, Iniguez A, et al. Midterm outcome of patients with asymptomatic restenosis after coronary balloon angioplasty. J Am Coll Cardiol 1992;19:1402-9.

13. Bourassa MG. Silent myocardial ischemia after coronary angioplasty: distinguishing the shadow from the substance. J Am Coll Cardiol 1992;19:1410-1.

14. Sheppard R, Schechter D, Azoulay A, Witt H, Garzon P, Eisenberg MJ. Results of a routine exercise treadmill testing strategy early after percutaneous transluminal coronary angioplasty. Can J Cardiol 2001;17:407-14.

15. Lespérance J, Bourassa MG, Schwartz L, et al. Definition and measurement of restenosis after successful coronary angioplasty: implications for clinical trials. Am Heart J 1993;125:1394-1408.

16. Lespérance J, Bilodeau L, Reiber JHC, Koning G, Hudon G, Bourassa MG. Issues in the performance of quantitative coronary angiography in clinical research trials. *In:* What is New in Cardiovascular Imaging? J.H.C. Reiber and E.E. van der Wall (eds.): Kluwer Academic Publishers, The Netherlands 1998:31-46.

17. Currier JW, Faxon DP. Restenosis after percutaneous transluminal coronary angioplasty: have we been aiming at the wrong target? J Am Coll Cardiol 1995;25:516-20.

18. Strauss BH, Chisholm RJ, Keely FW, Gotlieb AI, Logan RA, Armstrong PW. Extracellular matrix remodeling after balloon angioplasty injury in a rabbit model of restenosis. Circ Res 1994;75:650-8.

19. Coté G, Tardif JC, Lespérance J, et al. Effects of probucol on vascular remodeling after coronary angioplasty. Circulation 1999;99:30-5.

20. Mintz GS, Popma JJ, Pichard AD, et al. Arterial remodeling after coronary angioplasty: a serial intravascular ultrasound study. Circulation 1996;94:35-43.

21. Langille BL, O'Donnell F. Reductions in arterial diameter produced by chronic decreases in blood flow are endothelium-dependent. Science 1986;231:405-7.

22. Serruys PW, de Jaegere P, Kiemeneij F, et al. for the Benestent Study Group. A comparison of balloon-expandable stent implantation with balloon angioplasty in patients with coronary artery disease. N Engl J Med 1994;331:489-95.

23. Hoffman R, Mintz GS, Dusaillant GR, et al. Patterns and mechanisms of in-stent restenosis. Circulation 1996;94:1247-54.

24. Kornowski R, Mintz GS, Kent KM, et al. Increased restenosis in diabetes mellitus after coronary interventions is due to exaggerated intimal hyperplasia. A serial intravascular ultrasound study. Circulation 1997;95:1366-9.

25. Rodès J, Tardif JC, Lespérance J, et al. Prevention of restenosis after angioplasty in small coronary arteries with probucol. Circulation 1998;97:429-36.

26. Bertrand O, Mongrain R, Tardif JC, Bourassa MG. Prevention of restenosis using ionizing radiation. Rev Med Liege 1998;53:419-24.

27. Teirstein P, Massulo V, Jani S, et al. Catheter-based radiotherapy to inhibit restenosis after coronary stenting. N Engl J Med 1997;336;1697-703.

28. Meerkin D, Tardif JC, Crocker IR, et al. Effects of intracoronary beta-radiation therapy after coronary angioplasty: an intravascular ultrasound study. Circulation 1999;99:1660-5.

29. Tardif JC, Coté G, Lespérance J, et al. Probucol and multivitamins in the prevention of restenosis after coronary angioplasty. N Engl J Med 1997;337:365-72.

30. Tardif JC, Coté G, Lespérance J, et al. Impact of residual plaque burden after balloon angioplasty in the multivitamins and probucol (MVP) trial. Circulation 1998;98:I-89 (abstract).

31. Lee YJ, Yamaguchi H, Daida H, et al. Pharmacological interventions to modify restenosis. Circulation 1991;84:II-299 (abstract).

32. Setsuda M, Inden M, Hiraoka N, et al. Probucol therapy in the prevention of restenosis after successful percutaneous transluminal coronary angioplasty. Clinical Therapeutics 1993;15:374-81.

33. Watanabe K, Sekyia M, Ikeda S, Miyagawa M, Hashida K. Preventive effects of probucol on restenosis after percutaneous transluminal coronary angioplasty. Am Heart J 1996;13:23-9.

34. Lee YJ, Daida H, Yokoi H, et al. Effectiveness of probucol in preventing restenosis after percutaneous transluminal coronary angioplasty. Jpn Heart J. 1996;37:327-32.

35. Yokoi H, Daida H, Kuwabara Y, et al. Effectiveness of an antioxidant in preventing restenosis after percutaneous transluminal coronary angioplasty. The Probucol Angioplasty Restenosis Trial. J Am Coll Cardiol 1997;30:855-62.

36. Yokoi H, Daida H, Yamaguchi H, Kuwabara Y, for the PART Group. Effectiveness of probucol in preventing restenosis after percutaneous transluminal coronary angioplasty in small coronary arteries: a subgroup analysis of the Probucol Angioplasty Restenosis Trial (PART). J Am Coll Cardiol 1997;29:418A (abstract).

37. Roberts MJD, Young IS, Trouton TG, et al. Transient release of lipid peroxides after coronary artery balloon angioplasty. Lancet 1990;336:143-5.

38. Iuliano L, Pratico D, Greco C, et al. Angioplasty increases coronary sinus F2-isoprostane formation: evidence for an in vivo oxidative stress during PTCA. J Am Coll Cardiol 2001;37:76-80.

39. Kugiyama K, Kerns SA, Morissett JD, Roberts R, Henry PD. Impairment of endothelium-dependent arterial relaxation by lysolecithin in modified low-density lipoproteins. Nature 1990;344:160-2.

40. Steinberg D, Parthasarathy S, Carew TE, Khoo JC, Witzum JL. Beyond cholesterol: modifications of low-density lipoprotein that increase its atherogenicity. N Engl J Med 1989;320:915-24.

41. Rajapopalan S, Meng XP, Ramasamy S, Harrison DG, Galis ZS. Reactive oxygen species produced by macrophage-derived foam cells regulate the activity of matrix metalloproteinases in vitro. J Clin Invest 1996;98:2572-9.

42. Bendeck MP, Zempo N, Clowes AW, Galardy RE, Reidy MA. Smooth muscle cell migration and matrix metalloproteinase expression after arterial injury in the rat. Circ Res 1994;75:539-45.

43. Reiser K, McCormick RJ, Rucker RB. Enzymatic and non-enzymatic cross-linking of collagen and elastin. FASEB J 1992;6:2439-49.

44. O'Keefe JH, Jr., Stone GW, McCallister BD, et al. Lovastatin plus probucol for prevention of restenosis after percutaneous transluminal coronary angioplasty. Am J Cardiol 1996;77:649-52.

45. Reaven PD, Parthasarathy S, Beltz WF, Witzum JL. Effect of probucol dosage on plasma lipid and lipoprotein levels and on protection of low density lipoprotein against in vitro oxidation in humans. Arterioscler Thromb 1992;12:318-24.

46. Edelman ER. Vessel size, antioxidants, and restenosis. Never too small, not too little, but often too late. Circulation 1998;97:416-20.

47. Bowry VW, Ingold KU, Stocker R. Vitamin E in human low-density lipoprotein: when and how this antioxidant becomes a pro-oxidant. Biochem J 1992;288:341-4.

48. Tardif JC, Grégoire J, Schwartz L, et al. Effects of AGI-1067 and probucol after percutaneous coronary interventions. Circulation 2003;107:552-8.

49. Anderson TJ, Meredith IT, Yeung AC, Frei B, Selwyn AP, Ganz P. The effect of cholesterol-lowering and antioxidant therapy on endothelium-dependent coronary vasomotion. N Engl J Med 1995;332:488-93.

50. McLean LR, Thomas CE, Weintraub B, et al. Modulation of the physical state of cellular cholesteryl esters by probucol. J Biol Chem 1992;267:12291-8.

51. Tardif JC. The future of intravascular ultrasound in the detection and management of coronary artery disease. Can J Cardiol 2000;16 (Suppl.D): 12D-15D.

52. Nunes GL, Robinson K, Kalynych A, et al. Vitamins C and E inhibit O_2-production in the pig coronary artery. Circulation 1997;96:3593-601.

53. Tardif JC, Grégoire J, L'Allier PL. Prevention of restenosis with antioxidants. Mechanisms and implications. Am J Cardiovasc Drugs 2002;2:323-34.

54. Buckley MMT, Goa KL, Price AH, et al. Probucol, a reappraisal of the pharmacological properties and therapeutic use in hypercholesterolemia. Drugs 1989;37:761-800

55. Parthasarathy S, Young SG, Witzum JL, Pittman RC, Steinberg D. Probucol inhibits oxidative modification of low density lipoprotein. J Clin Invest 1986;77:641-4.

56. Chisholm GM III, Morel DW. Lipoprotein oxidation and cytotoxicity effect of probucol on streptomycin-treated rats. Am J Cardiol 1988;62:20B-26B.

57. Sasahara M, Raines EW, Chait A, et al. Inhibition of hypercholesterolemia-induced atherosclerosis in the non-human primate by probucol. Is the extent of atherosclerosis related to the resistance of LDL to oxidation? J Clin Invest 1994;94:155-64.

58. Steinberg D, Parthasarathy S, Carew TE. In vivo inhibition of foam cell development by probucol in Watanabe rabbits. Am J Cardiol 1988;62:6B-12B.

59. Carew TE, Schwenke DC, Steinberg D. Antiatherogenic effect of probucol unrelated to its hypocholesterolemic effect: evidence that antioxidants in vivo can selectively inhibit low density lipoprotein degradation in macrophage-rich fatty streaks and slow the progression of atherosclerosis in Watanabe heritable hyperlipidemic rabbit. Proc Natl Acad Sci USA 1987;84:7725-9.

60. Ku G, Doherty NS, Wolos JA, Jackson RL. Inhibition by probucol of interleukin-1 secretion and its implication in atherosclerosis. Am J Cardiol 1988;62:77B-81B.

61. Anderson TJ, Meredith IT, Charbonneau F, et al. Endothelium-dependent coronary vasomotion relates to the susceptibility of LDL to oxidation in humans. Circulation 1996;93:1647-50.

62. Reinoehl J, Frankovich D, Machado C, et al. Probucol-associated tachyarrythmic events and QT prolongation: importance of gender. Am Heart J 1996;131:1184-91.

63. Gohn DC, Simmons TW. Polymorphic ventricular tachycardia (torsades de pointe) associated with the use of probucol. N Engl J Med 1992;326:1435-6.

64. Kajinami K, Takeoshi N, Mabuchi H. Propranolol for probucol-induced QT prolongation with polymorphic ventricular tachycardia. Lancet 1993;341:124-5.

65. Matsuhashi H, Onodera S, Kawamura Y, et al. Probucol-induced QT prolongation and torsades de pointe. Jpn J Med 1989;28:612-5.

66. Naruszewicz M, Carew TE, Pittman RC, et al. A novel mechanism by which probucol lowers LDL levels demonstrated in the LDL-receptor deficient rabbit. J Lipid Res 1984;25:1206-13.

67. Schwartz CJ. The probucol experience: a review of the past and a look at the future. Am J Cardiol 1988;62:1B-5B.

68. Walldius G, Erikson U, Olsson AG, et al. The effect of probucol on femoral atherosclerosis: the Probucol Quantitative Regression Swedish Trial (PQRST). Am J Cardiol 1994;74:875-83.

69. Johansson J, Olsson AG, Bergstrand L, et al. Lowering of HDL2b by probucol partly explains the failure of the drug to affect femoral atherosclerosis in subjects with hypercholesterolemia. A Probucol Quantitative Regression Swedish Trial (PQRST) report. Arterioscler Thromb Vasc Biol 1995;15:1049-56.

70. Meng CQ, Somers PK, Rachita CL, et al. Novel phenolic antioxidants as multifunctional inhibitors of inducible VCAM-1 expression for use in atherosclerosis. Bioorg Med Chem Lett 2003;12:2545-8.

71. Kunsch C, Medford RM. Oxidative stress as a regulator of gene expression in the vasculature. Circ Res 1999;85:753-66.

72. Marui N, Offerman MK, Swerlick R, et al. Vascular cell adhesion molecule-1 (VCAM-1) gene transcription and expression are regulated through an antioxidant-sensitive mechanism in human vascular endothelial cells. J Clin Invest 1993;92:1866-74.

73. Wasserman MA, Sundell CL, Kunsch C, et al. Chemestry and pharmacology of vascular protectants: a novel approach to the treatment of atherosclerosis and coronary artery disease. Am J Cardiol 2003;91 (suppl.):34A-40A.

74. Gordon DG, Rifkind BM. High-density lipoprotein - the clinical implications of recent studies. N Engl J Med 1989;321:1311-6.

75. Hayek T, Masucci-Magoulas L, Jiang X, et al. Decreased early atherosclerotic lesions in hypertriglyceridemic mice expressing cholesteryl ester transfer protein transgene. J Clin Invest 1995;96:2071-4.

76. Busch SJ, Barnhart RL, Martin GA, et al. Human hepatic triglyceride lipase expression reduces high density lipoprotein and aortic cholesterol in cholesterol-fed transgenic mice. J Biol Chem 1994;269:16376-82.

77. de Backer G, de Backer D, Kornitzer M. Epidemiological aspects of high density lipoprotein cholesterol. Atherosclerosis 1998;137 (Suppl.):S1-S6.

78. von Eckardstein A, Nofer JR, Assmann G. High density lipoproteins and arteriosclerosis. Role of cholesterol efflux and reverse cholesterol transport. Arterioscler Thromb Vasc Biol 2001;21:13-27.

79. von Eckardstein A, Nofer JR, Assmann G. Acceleration of reverse cholesterol transport. Curr Opin Cardiol 2000;15:348-54.

80. Kuzuya M, Naito M, Funaki C, Hayashi T, Asai K, Kuzuya F. Probucol prevents oxidative injury in endothelial cells. J Lipid Res 1991;32:197-204.

81. Yamamoto A, Hara H, Takaichi S, et al. Effect of probucol on macrophages, leading to regression of xanthomas and atheromatous vascular lesions. Am J Cardiol 1988;62:31B-36B.

82. Chang MY, Sasahara M, Chait A, et al. Inhibition of hypercholesterolemia-induced atherosclerosis in the non-human primate by probucol. Cellular composition and proliferation. Arterioscler Thromb Vasc Biol 1995;15:1631-40.

83. Weintraub Ws, Boccuzzi SJ, Klein JL, et al. Lack of effect of lovastatin on restenosis after coronary angioplasty. N Engl J Med 1994;331:1331-7.

84. Galis ZS, Muszynski M, Sukhova GK, et al. Cytokine-stimulated human vascular smooth muscle cells synthetize a complement of enzymes required for extracellular matrix digestion. Circ Res 1994;75:181-9.

85. Tardif JC, Pandian NG. Intravascular ultrasound imaging in peripheral arterial and coronary artery disease. Curr Opin Cardiol 1994;9:627-33.

86. Jialal I, Grundy SM. Effect of dietary supplementation with alpha-tocopherol on the oxidative modification of low density lipoprotein. J Lipid Res 1992;33:899-906.

87. Burton GW, Ingold KU. Vitamin E as an in vitro and in vivo antioxidant. Ann N Y Acad Soi 1989,570:7-22.

88. Brin MF, Fahn S, Loftus S, McMahon D, Flaster, E. Relationship between dose of vitamin E administered and blood level. Ann N Y Acad Sci 1989;570:421-4.

89. Cavarocchi NC, England MD, O'Brien JF, et al. Superoxide generation during cardiopulmonary bypass: is there a role for vitamin E? J Surg Res 1986;40:519-27.

90. Kagan VE, Serbinova EA, Forte T, Scita G, Packer L. Recycling of vitamin E in human low density lipoproteins. J Lipid Res 1992;33:385-97.

91. Shaish A, Daugherty A, O'Sullivan F, Schonfeld G, Heinecke JW. Beta-carotene inhibits atherosclerosis in hypercholesterolemic rabbits. J Clin Invest 1995;96:2075-82.

92. Keaney JF Jr., Gaziano JM, Xu A, et al. Dietary antioxidants preserve endothelium-dependent vessel relaxation in cholesterol-fed rabbits. Proc Natl Acad Sci USA 1993;90:11880-4.

93. Nunes GI, Sgoutas DS, Redden RA, et al. Combination of vitamin C and E alters the response to coronary balloon injury in the pig. Arterioscler Thromb Vasc Biol 1995;15:156-65.

94. Keaney JF Jr., Gaziano JM, Xu A, et al. Low-dose alpha-tocopherol improves and high-dose alpha-tocopherol worsens endothelial vasodilator function in cholesterol-fed rabbits. J Clin Invest 1994;93:844-51.

Chapter 15

OXIDATIVE STRESS IN HYPERTENSION

Ernesto L. Schiffrin and Rhian M. Touyz
Clinical Research Institute of Montreal, University of Montreal, Quebec, Canada

Introduction

Reactive oxygen species (ROS) participate in normal cell signaling as mediators that regulate vascular function[1]. ROS are produced by all layers of the vascular wall: endothelium, smooth muscle and adventitia[2]. The major ROS are superoxide anion, hydrogen peroxide (H_2O_2), hydroxyl radical ($\bullet OH$), nitric oxide (NO) and peroxynitrite ($ONOO^-$). Under physiological conditions, ROS are produced in low concentrations and act as signaling molecules that regulate vascular smooth muscle cell (VSMC) contraction and relaxation, and participate in VSMC growth[3-5]. Under pathophysiological conditions, these free radicals play roles in various conditions such as hypertension, diabetes, atherosclerosis, ischemia-reperfusion injury, ischemic heart disease and congestive cardiac failure)[4-9]. Oxidant excess associated with increased production of ROS or decreased antioxidant capacity results in scavenging of NO, lipid peroxidation, upregulation of adhesion molecules, leading to the different manifestations of endothelial dysfunction, as well as increased contractility and growth of VSMC, apoptosis, macrophage infiltration and migration in the vascular wall with inflammation and increased deposition of extracellular matrix proteins, contributing to vascular injury associated with cardiovascular disease[10].

In experimental hypertension and in hypertension in humans increased generation of ROS has been demonstrated by many studies[8,9,11,12]. Antioxidants may reduce blood pressure in animal models of hypertension, prevent target organ damage and improve vascular structure and function[12]. Inactivation of the genes for the enzymes that form ROS in mice results in lowering of their blood pressure. The blood pressure elevation that follows angiotensin II infusion does not occur in these mice[13,14]. Antioxidants have also demonstrated some beneficial effects in some studies in essential hypertension in humans[15-18]. Cultured VSMCs and isolated arteries from hypertensive rats and humans exhibit increased ROS production, whereas antioxidant capacity is reduced[11,12,19]. All these data support the hypothesis that oxidant excess plays a role in the development and progression of hypertension, and in the target organ damage associated with elevated blood pressure.

ROS and oxidative stress in the vasculature

Production of ROS in blood vessels

In the vasculature, superoxide, H_2O_2 NO, OONO- and •OH are all produced to varying degrees. Their concentration in tissues is regulated by superoxide dismutase (SOD), of which there are three isoforms, CuZnSOD, MnSOD and extracellular SOD (EC-SOD)[20], by catalase, thioredoxin, glutathione, anti-oxidant vitamins and other small molecules[21-23]. An imbalance in ROS generation and antioxidant capacity will induce ROS excess and oxidative stress. The resulting oxidative damage is an important mechanism participating in vascular injury in hypertension[5-7,10,12].

The most important source of ROS in blood vessels appears to be NAD(P)H oxidase[1,8]. This is a multi-subunit enzyme[2,24] with NAD(P)H as the electron donor. The best characterized NAD(P)H oxidase is found in phagocytes, in neutrophils, monocytes and macrophages[25]. This phagocytic NAD(P)H oxidase has several subunits: p47phox (phox for PHagocyte OXidase), p67phox, p40phox, p22phox and gp91phox[43,44]. Small G proteins Rac 2 (Rac 1 in some cells) and Rap1A also participate in the generation of the active enzyme. p40phox, p47phox and p67phox are cytosolic, p22phox and gp91phox are in the cell membrane present as a heterodimeric flavoprotein, cytochrome b558. Phosphorylation of p47phox upon stimulation results in the formation of a complex with the other cytosolic subunits and translocation to the membrane. Association with cytochrome b558 (containing p22phox and gp91phox) results in the assembly of the active oxidase. Phosphorylation of p47phox and p67phox are critical for activation of NAD(P)H oxidase[26] whereas phosphorylated p40phox has recently been reported to negatively regulate NAD(P)H oxidase[27].

Non-phagocytic NAD(P)H oxidase is the main source of ROS in blood vessels[2,28,29], present and active in the endothelium[30], the VSMCs in the media[28,29,31], and in the adventitia[32]. In contrast to the phagocytic NAD(P)H oxidase that is activated upon stimulation and generates superoxide anion in bursts into the extracellular milieu[25,33], vascular

NAD(P)H oxidase is constitutively active, and slowly produces superoxide inside the cell that then acts as an intracellular messenger molecule[2,33-35]. Whereas all subunits of NAD(P)H are found in the endothelium and the adventitia, only p47phox and p22phox appear to be expressed consistently in VSMCs of the media of blood vessels[2]. gp91phox is not present in rat aortic VSMCs while p22phox and p47phox are present. In human resistance arteries, all of the major subunits, including gp91phox, are expressed[29]. The newly discovered homologues of gp91phox (nox2, nox for NAD(P)H Oxidase), nox1, nox4 and nox5 are found in the vasculature[36,37]. Nox1 may be a substitute for gp91phox in rat aortic VSMCs[24,29]. Nox1 is regulated by NoxO1 (Nox organizer 1) and NoxA1 (Nox activator 1)[38], although precise roles for these in vascular cells are unclear. Nox1 is upregulated in vascular injury[2]. Nox4, on the other hand, may be involved in constitutive production of superoxide in non-proliferating cells, and indeed is expressed in all vascular cell types[39], and may be the major catalytic component of NAD(P)H oxidase in the endothelium[37].

The activity of vascular NAD(P)H oxidase is modulated by many different factors that include cytokines, growth factors and vasoactive peptides[2]. Stretch, pulsatile strain and shear stress may activate NAD(P)H oxidase[2,40]. Angiotensin II not only stimulates NAD(P)H oxidase but also enhances the expression of the subunits of NAD(P)H oxidase. Angiotensin II induces ROS generation by endothelial cells, VSMCs and adventitial fibroblasts[2,29,31] via stimulation of AT_1 receptors[41]. In fact, ROS may downregulate AT_1 receptors[42]. Angiotensin II was first shown to stimulate NAD(P)H oxidase *in vivo* after infusion into rats to mediate angiotensin II-induced hypertension[43]. The activation of NAD(P)H oxidase is both acute and chronic following the increased expression of its different subunits[2,24,29]. Mechanisms linking AT_1 receptors to NAD(P)H oxidase activation in vascular cells include stimulation of phospholipase D, phospholipase A, protein kinase C, c-Src, phosphoinositide 3kinase, and a role of the small G proteins RhoA and Rac[26,33].

Platelet-derived growth factor (PDGF), transforming growth factor-β (TGF-β), tumor necrosis factor (TNF)-α and thrombin also activate NAD(P)H oxidase in VSMCs[44-46]. Endothelin-1 via ET_A receptors increases NAD(P)H oxidase activity in human endothelial cells[47]. Peroxisome proliferator-activated receptor (PPAR) activators (thiazolidinediones or glitazones, antidiabetic insulinomimetic agents), statins and antihypertensive drugs such as β-blockers, calcium channel blockers, angiotensin converting enzyme inhibitors and angiotensin receptor blockers decrease the expression of NAD(P)H oxidase subunits and its activity[48-52], which may have therapeutic consequences in hypertension and other forms of cardiovascular disease.

Nitric oxide synthase (NOS) is present in the endothelium as a dimer that functions as an oxygenase and generates NO when tetrahydrobiopterin (BH_4), which comes from folic acid, is present in high concentrations. It functions as a reductase that generates superoxide when the enzyme is present as a monomer ("NOS uncoupling") because BH_4 is not present in high concentrations[53]. Endothelial NOS (eNOS) uncoupling occurs in atherosclerosis[54], diabetes[55], hyperhomocysteinemia[56] and hypertension[57]. In hypertension, increased NAD(P)H oxidase-derived ROS oxidizes BH_4 resulting in uncoupling of eNOS, thus further enhancing free radical generation[57]. GTP cyclohydrolase (GTPCH) I is the enzyme responsible for regenerating BH_4, and gene transfer of this enzyme will restore BH_4 levels, reduce superoxide and result in correction of impaired endothelium-dependent relaxation in DOCA-salt hypertensive rats[58]. In vessels from diabetic and hypertensive patients sepiapterin, a precursor of BH_4, reduces superoxide anion generation, underlining the role played by uncoupled eNOS in ROS generation[59]. NOS may become an important source of superoxide when there is moderate to severe endothelial dysfunction and BH_4 deficiency (due to folic acid deficiency).

ROS may also be produced in blood vessels by xanthine oxidase, cytochrome P450, mitochondrial respiratory chain enzymes and phagocyte-derived myeloperoxidase[60]. However, their participation in ROS generation in blood vessels except for xanthine oxidase, appears minor. Indeed, there is increasing evidence that the latter may be an important contributor to ROS production, including mediating NAD(P)H oxidase-initiated generation of superoxide in the longterm[61].

Vascular actions of ROS

The best-established direct targets of ROS signaling are protein tyrosine phosphatases[62,63] and transcription factors[64]. ROS-induced inhibition of tyrosine phosphatases results in increased tyrosine phosphorylation, modulating receptor protein tyrosine kinases such as the EGFR, IGF-1R and PDGFR and non-receptor tyrosine kinases, such as Src, FAK, PI3K, JAK2[62,65].

Nuclear factor κB (NFκB) and activator protein 1 (AP-1) modulate expression of inflammatory genes such as monocyte chemotactic protein-1 (MCP-1), adhesion molecules like vascular cell adhesion molecule-1 (VCAM-1) and intracellular adhesion molecule-1 (ICAM-1), and interleukins[66], all associated with vascular responses and remodeling in hypertension and atherosclerosis. Increased activation of vascular NFκB and AP-1 and associated inflammatory responses occur in hypertensive rats, attributed, in part, to oxidative stress[67]. Other molecules that are redox-sensitive include protooncogenes and transcription factors including c-Myb, early growth response-1 (egr-1), p53, Sp-1, and hypoxia-inducible factor (HIF-1)[64]. Most redox-sensitive molecules possess conserved cysteines, which are susceptible to oxidative modification[68]. Redox-sensitivity of protein degradation is another mode of regulation by ROS.

ROS activate many other signaling pathways including mitogen-activated protein (MAP) kinases, including ERK1/2, p38MAP kinase, JNK and ERK5, that are involved in cell growth, inflammation, apoptosis and cell differentiation respectively[69]. In cultured VSMCs, angiotensin II-induced stimulation of ROS does not however activate ERK1/2[69-72]. MAP kinases may not be direct substrates of ROS, but may be activated by upstream modulators such as MEKs, tyrosine kinases and phosphatases that are redox-sensitive. PDGFR and EGFR are stimulated by ROS-mediated inhibition of protein tyrosine phosphatases that result in reduced dephosphorylation of these receptors[73]. ROS participate in the transactivation of PDGFR and EGFR by angiotensin II. Non-receptor tyrosine kinases (Src, JAK2, Pyk2 and Akt) that are involved in cardiovascular remodeling and injury are also redox-dependent[1,62,65,73].

ROS also modulate intracellular free Ca^{2+} concentration ($[Ca^{2+}]_i$). Superoxide and H_2O_2 increase $[Ca^{2+}]_i$ in VSMCs and endothelial cells, in part via inositol-trisphosphate-induced Ca^{2+} mobilization, increased Ca^{2+} influx and decreased Ca^{2+}-ATPase activation[74]. Plasma membrane K^+ channels in VSMCs that relate to hyperpolarization-induced relaxation are opened by redox-dependent mechanisms[62,65,73]. Contractile responses to H_2O_2 are enhanced in arteries from spontaneously hypertensive rats (SHR) compared with normotensive counterparts[75], suggesting that in hypertension oxidant excess, in addition to impaired endothelium-dependent vasodilation (due to increased quenching of NO by superoxide⁻), contributes to altered contractility.

Oxidative excess leads to cell proliferation and hypertrophy, vascular injury and remodeling[1,4,10]. ROS induce apoptosis and differentiation depending on the specific ROS generated, their concentration and subcellular distribution. At high concentrations (>100 µmol/L) H_2O_2 and peroxynitrite stimulate apoptosis and anoikis (cell detachment and shedding), whereas at low concentrations they induce growth and cell differentiation[76,77]. ROS modulate vascular structure in hypertension via increased extracellular matrix deposition. By influencing vascular MMP2 and MMP9, they may promote matrix degradation, including that of the basement membrane and elastin respectively[78]. Redox-sensitive activation of inflammation through expression of MCP-1, osteopontin and interleukin-6, adhesion molecules (VCAM-1 and ICAM-1), lipid peroxidation and cell migration, participates in vascular remodeling in hypertension[79,80].

Decreased NO bioavailability due to oxidant excess plays an important role in the impaired endothelium-mediated vasodilation found often in hypertension and usually in hypercholesterolemia[12,81]. Peroxynitrite generated by ROS acting on NO has pro-inflammatory properties. Endothelial function may be improved by anti-oxidant vitamins, probucol, SOD or sepiapterin (precursor of BH_4) in experimental models of hypertension, hypercholesterolemia and diabetes, and in hypertensive patients[56].

Hydrogen peroxide dilates pulmonary, coronary and mesenteric arteries and has been considered an endothelium-derived relaxing factor[82]. In rat aorta, angiotensin II stimulates vasoconstriction via H_2O_2[83], whereas in human and porcine vessels, ROS do not mediate angiotensin II action[84]. ROS-mediated contractile effects are enhanced in aortic and mesenteric arteries from SHR[75]. At present the exact role of superoxide anion and H_2O_2 respect to vascular contraction/dilation under physiological and pathophysiological conditions remains unclear.

ROS in hypertension

Genetic hypertension

Genetic models of hypertension, such as SHR and stroke-prone SHR (SHRSP)[15] exhibit enhanced NAD(P)H oxidase-mediated superoxide generation in conduit (aorta) and resistance arteries (mesenteric), and in the kidney[12,85]. This is associated with increased expression of its subunits (p22phox and p47phox)[2]. Enhanced oxidative stress occurs as well in the heart in SHR and SHRSP compared with normotensive Wistar Kyoto rats (WKY), and the expression of the redox-regulating protein thioredoxin is inhibited[86]. Polymorphisms have been identified in the promoter region of the $p22^{phox}$ gene in SHR, which could contribute to increase NAD(P)H oxidase activity[87]. Increased expression of p47phox has been demonstrated in the renal vasculature, macula densa, and distal nephron from young SHR, suggesting that increased NAD(P)H oxidase-mediated oxidative stress may precede the development of hypertension[88]. Indeed, mice in which the p47phox gene has been inactivated do not develop hypertension in response to Ang II infusion[89]. Treatment with antioxidant vitamins, NAD(P)H oxidase inhibitors, SOD mimetics, folic acid and AT_1 receptor blockers decrease vascular superoxide production and may blunt development of blood pressure elevation in genetic hypertension[11,12,18, 90,91].

Experimentally-induced hypertension

Oxidative excess has been demonstrated in experimental hypertension, such as that which is induced by angiotensin II infusion[67,92], in Dahl-salt-sensitive rats[93], in obesity-associated hypertension[94], in mineralocorticoid hypertension[95,96], in 2-kidney, 1-clip Goldblatt hypertensive rats[97] and in models of postmenopausal hypertension[98]. Increased activation of vascular NAD(P)H oxidase[2] and xanthine oxidase[98] and uncoupling of eNOS[53-55] seem to be the main mechanisms involved in increased superoxide production. Inhibitors of NAD(P)H oxidase and xanthine oxidase (apocynin that may inhibit both enzymes or allopurinol that inhibits xanthine oxidase), and antioxidants or SOD mimetics prevent development of most models of experimental hypertension[12,15,86,99] except for norepinephrine-induced hypertension[92]. These treatments are followed by improved endothelial function, regression of vascular remodeling and reduced vascular inflammation. The findings in norepinephrine-induced hypertension suggest that blood pressure does not directly induce oxidative stress in hypertension.

Human hypertension

In humans most of the findings regarding ROS are based on increased levels of plasma and urine thiobarbituric acid reducing substances (TBARS) and 8-epi-isoprostanes, considered to be systemic markers of lipid peroxidation and oxidative stress. Essential hypertensive patients have been shown to produce excessive amounts of ROS[100,101] and exhibit decreases in their antioxidant capacity[102]. In never-treated mild-to-moderate hypertension, however, lipid peroxidation is not increased[103], which suggests that oxidative stress is not important in early uncomplicated human hypertension. Oxidative stress has been demonstrated on the other hand in patients with renovascular hypertension[104], malignant hypertension[105] and in pre-eclampsia[106].

Activation of the renin-angiotensin system is a major mediator of NAD(P)H oxidase activation and ROS production in human hypertension[107]. Antihypertensive action of angiotensin receptor blockers and angiotensin converting enzyme inhibitors may in large measure be the result of inhibition of NAD(P)H oxidase activity and decreased ROS production[108]. p22*phox* gene polymorphisms may play a role in altered NAD(P)H oxidase-generation of superoxide in humans, particularly the -930(A/G) polymorphism[87]. In contrast, homozygous individuals with the T allele of the C242T CYBA polymorphism may have reduced vascular oxidative stress[109].

Although the hypothesis of oxidative excess in hypertension appears well supported by evidence, clinical trials with antioxidants have not been confirmatory except for some small studies[16-18,110-113]. Currently, there is no support for administration of antioxidants in the prevention and management of hypertension except for the use of blockers of the renin-angiotensin-aldosterone system[114]. The Cambridge Heart Antioxidant Study (CHAOS)

(2002 patients), Alpha Tocopherol, Beta-Carotene Cancer Prevention Study (ATBC) (27,271 males), GISSI-Prevenzione trial (3,658 patients), Heart Outcomes Prevention Evaluation (HOPE) study (2,545 subjects), MRC/BHF Heart Protection Study (20,536 adults), Primary Prevention Project (PPP) (4,495 patients) and Antioxidant Supplementation in Atherosclerosis Prevention (ASAP) study (520 subjects) were trials in cardiovascular disease with negative results except for CHAOS[115]. Supplementation with daily vitamin E and slow-release vitamin C for six years in ASAP reduced progression of carotid atherosclerosis. However, none of the large multicenter studies was associated with reduction in blood pressure or other cardiovascular end points. Thus, clinical trials have been disappointing despite promising findings from experimental and epidemiological studies. Patients may have had disease that was too advanced for prevention with antioxidants. The antioxidants used may be ineffective, or doses and duration of treatment may have been insufficient. Antioxidants have pro-oxidant properties, which may result in opposite effects from those desired, or they may not reach adequate concentrations in the intracellular compartments and organelles where ROS are generated. Also, they may not scavenge the specific species involved in hypertensive vascular damage. Reduction of ROS generation by inhibition of NAD(P)H oxidase by, for example, blockade of the renin-angiotensin-aldosterone system may be more effective, and indeed has been shown to induce lowering of blood pressure, regression of vascular remodeling and improved endothelial function[96,109,116]. Homologues of NAD(P)H oxidase subunits may be novel therapeutic agents for vascular disease and hypertension[117]. The beneficial effects of other agents such as some β-adrenergic blockers (carvedilol) and some Ca^{2+} channel blockers may be mediated, in part, by decreasing vascular oxidative stress[50,118].

Conclusions

ROS such as superoxide and H_2O_2 are produced in the vessel wall and have important signaling properties through oxidative modification of proteins and activation of transcription factors that affect vascular structure and function. Alterations in the activity of NAD(P)H oxidase, xanthine oxidase, NOS, mitochondrial enzymes or SOD, in thioredoxin or the glutathione systems, or reduced scavenging by anti-oxidants, will result in oxidative excess, which contributes to vascular injury. Oxidative stress is increased in experimental and clinical hypertension, especially those with severe, salt-sensitive and renovascular hypertension. Treatments that alter ROS by decreasing production and/or enhancing antioxidant defence mechanisms may regress vascular remodeling, prevent further vascular injury and reduce blood pressure and associated target organ damage in hypertensive patients, although currently available antioxidants have so far failed to achieve this. Accordingly, it is recommended that the general population consume a balanced diet rich in vegetables and fruits which contain antioxidants, and whole grains. Antioxidant supplementation is not recommended for the prevention or treatment of hypertension, consistent with guidelines of the American Heart Association[119] and the Canadian Hypertension Society[120]. These recommendations are supported by the Dietary Approaches to Stop Hypertension (DASH) trial and a recent study from the UK, which demonstrated that subjects consuming high fruit and vegetable diets had significantly reduced blood pressure[121].

Acknowledgements

The work of the authors was supported by grants 13570, 37917, 44018 and a Group grant to the Multidisciplinary Research Group on Hypertension, all from the Canadian Institutes of Health Research (previously called the Medical Research Council of Canada). RMT received a scholarship from the Fonds de la recherche en santé du Québec.

References

1. Griendling KK, Sorescu D, Lassegue B, Ushio-Fukai M. Modulation of protein kinase activity and gene expression by reactive oxygen species and their role in vascular physiology and pathophysiology. Arterioscler Thromb Vasc Biol 2000;20:2175-83.

2. Lassegue B, Clempus RE. Vascular NAD(P)H oxidases: specific features, expression, and regulation. Am J Physiol Regul Integr Comp Physiol 2003;285:R277-97.

3. Touyz RM, Schiffrin EL. Ang II-stimulated superoxide production is mediated via phospholipase D in human vascular smooth muscle cells. Hypertension 1999;34:976-82.

4. Rao GN, Berk BC. Active oxygen species stimulate vascular smooth muscle cell growth and proto-oncogene expression. Circ Res 1992;70:593-9.

5. Zafari AM, Ushio-Fukai M, Akers M, Griendling K. Role of NADH/NADPH oxidase-derived H_2O_2 in angiotensin II-induced vascular hypertrophy. Hypertension 1998;32:488-95.

6. Cosentino F, Sill JC, Katusic ZS. Role of superoxide anions in the mediation of endothelium-dependent contractions. Hypertension 1994;23:229-35.

7. Harrison DG. Cellular and molecular mechanisms of endothelial cell dysfunction. J Clin Invest 1997;108:2153-7.

8. Kerr S, Brosnan J, McIntyre M, Reid JL, Dominiczak AF, Hamilton CA. Superoxide anion production is increased in a model of genetic hypertension. Role of endothelium. Hypertension 1999;33:1353-8.

9. Zalba G, San Jose G, Moreno MU, et al. Oxidative stress in arterial hypertension: role of NAD(P)H oxidase. Hypertension 2001;38:1395-9.

10. Landmesser U, Harrison DG. Oxidative stress and vascular damage in hypertension. Coron Artery Dis 2001;12:455-61.

11. Schnackenberg CG, Welch W, Wilcox CS. Normalization of blood pressure and renal vascular resistance in SHR with a membrane-permeable superoxide dismutase mimetic. Role of nitric oxide. Hypertension 1999;32:59-64.

12. Chen X, Touyz RM, Park JB, Schiffrin EL. Antioxidant effects of vitamins C and E are associated with altered activation of vascular NAD(P)H oxidase and superoxide dismutase in stroke-prone SHR. Hypertension 2001;38, 606-11.

13. Bendall JK, Cave AC, Heymes C, Gall N, Shah AM. Pivotal role of a gp91(phox)-containing NADPH oxidase in angiotensin II-induced cardiac hypertrophy in mice. Circulation 2002;105:293-6.

14. Li JM, Shah AM. Mechanism of endothelial cell NADPH oxidase activation by angiotensin II. Role of the p47phox subunit. J Biol Chem 2003;278:12094-100.

15. Sharma RC, Hodis HN, Mack WJ. Probucol suppresses oxidant stress in hypertensive arteries. Immunohistochemical evidence. Am J Hypertens 1996;9:577-90.

16. Duffy SJ, Gokce N, Holbrook M, et al. Treatment of hypertension with ascorbic acid. Lancet 1999;354:2048-9.

17. Fotheby MD, Williams JC, Forster LA, Craner P, Ferns GA. Effect of vitamin C on ambulatory blood pressure and plasma lipids in older patients. J Hypertens 2000;18:411-5.

18. Mullan B, Young IS, Fee H, McCance DR. Ascorbic acid reduces blood pressure and arterial stiffness in type 2 diabetes. Hypertension 2002;40:804-9.

19. Touyz RM, Schiffrin EL. Increased generation of superoxide by angiotensin II in smooth muscle cells from resistance arteries of hypertensive patients: role of phospholipase D-dependent NAD(P)H oxidase-sensitive pathways. J Hypertens 2001;19:1245-54.

20. Fridovich I. Superoxide anion radical, superoxide dismutases, and related matters. J Biol Chem 1997;272:18515-7.

21. Halliwell B. Antioxidant defence mechanisms: from the beginning to the end (of the beginning). Free Radic Res 1999;31:261-72.

22. Yamawaki H, Haendeler J, Berk BC. Thioredoxin: a key regulator of cardiovascular homeostasis. Circ Res 2003;93:1029-33.

23. Schafer FQ, Buettner GR. Redox environment of the cell as viewed through the redox state of the glutathione disulfide/glutathione couple. Free Radic Biol Med 2001;30:1191-212.

24. Griendling KK, Sorescu D, Ushio-Fukai M. NAD(P)H oxidase: role in cardiovascular biology and disease. Circ Res 2000;86:494-501.

25. Babior BM, Lambeth JD, Nauseef W. The neutrophil NADPH oxidase. Arch Biochem Biophys. 2002;397:342-4.

26. Touyz RM, Yao G, Schiffrin EL. c-Src Induces phosphorylation and translocation of p47phox: role in superoxide generation by angiotensin II in human vascular smooth muscle cells. Arterioscler Thromb Vasc Biol 2003;23:981-7.

27. Lopes LR, Dagher MC, Gutierrez A, et al. Phosphorylated p40phox as a negative regulator of NADPH oxidase. Biochemistry 2004;43:3723-30.

28. Berry C, Hamilton CA, Brosnan MJ, et al. Investigation into the sources of superoxide in human blood vessels: angiotensin II increases superoxide production in human internal mammary arteries. Circulation 2000;101:2206-12.

29. Touyz RM, Chen X, He G, Quinn MT, Schiffrin EL. Expression of a gp91phox-containing leukocyte-type NADPH oxidase in human vascular smooth muscle cells – modulation by Ang II. Circ Res.2002;90:1205-13.

30. Muzaffar S, Jeremy JY, Angelini GD, Stuart-Smith K, Shukla N. Role of the endothelium and nitric oxide synthases in modulating superoxide formation induced by endotoxin and cytokines in porcine pulmonary arteries. Thorax 2003;58:598-604.

31. Griendling KK, Minieri CA, Ollerenshaw JD, Alexander RW. Angiotensin II stimulates NADH and NADPH oxidase activity in cultured vascular smooth muscle cells. Circ Res 1994;74:1141-8.

32. Rey FE, Pagano PJ. The reactive adventitia: fibroblast oxidase in vascular function. Arterioscler Thromb Vasc Biol 2002;22:1962-71.

33. Seshiah PN, Weber DS, Rocic P, Valppu L, Taniyama Y, Griendling KK. Angiotensin II stimulation of NAD(P)H oxidase activity. Upstream mediators. Circ Res 2002;91:406-13.

34. De Leo FR, Ulman KV, Davis AR,Jutila KL, Quinn MT. Assembly of the human neutrophil NADPH oxidase involves binding of p67phox and flavocytochrome b to a common functional domain in p47phox. J Biol Chem 1996;271:17013-20.

35. Li JM, Shah AM. Intracellular localization and preassembly of the NADPH oxidase complex in cultured endothelial cells. J Biol Chem 2002;277:19952-60

36. Hilenski LL, Clempus RE, Quinn MT, Lambeth JD, Griendling KK. Distinct subcellular localizations of Nox1 and Nox4 in vascular smooth muscle cells. Arterioscler Thromb Vasc Biol 2004;24:1-8.

37. Ago T, Kitazono T, Ooboshi H, et al. Nox4 as the major catalytic component of an endothelial NAD(P)H oxidase. Circulation 2004;109:227-33.

38. Banfi B, Clark RA, Steger K, Krause K-H. Two novel proteins activate superoxide generation by the NADPH oxidase Nox1. J Biol Chem 2003;278:3510-3.

39. Lassegue B, Sorescu D, Szocs K, et al. Novel gp91(phox) homologues in vascular smooth muscle cells: nox1 mediates angiotensin II-induced superoxide formation and redox-sensitive signaling pathways. Circ Res 2001;88:888-94.

40. Grote K, Flach I, Luchtefeld M, et al. Mechanical stretch enhances mRNA expression and proenzyme release of matrix metalloproteinase-2 (MMP-2) via NAD(P)H oxidase-derived reactive oxygen species. Circ Res 2003;92:80-6.

41. Privratsky JR, Wold LE, Sowers JR, Quinn MT, Ren J. AT$_1$ blockade prevents glucose-induced cardiac dysfunction in ventricular myocytes: role of the AT$_1$ receptor and NADPH oxidase. Hypertension 2003;42:206-12.

42. Nickenig G, Strehlow K, Baumer AT, et al. Negative feedback regulation of reactive oxygen species on AT1 receptor gene expression. Br J Pharmacol 2000;131:795-803.

43. Rajagopalan S, Kurz S, Munzel T. Angiotensin II mediated hypertension in the rat increases vascular superoxide production via membrane NADH/NADPH oxidase activation: contribution to alterations of vasomotor tone. J Clin Invest 1996;97:1916-23.

44. Marumo T, Schini-Kerth VB, Fisslthaler B, Busse R. Platelet-derived growth factor-stimulated superoxide anion production modulates activation of transcription factor NF-kappaB and expression of monocyte chemoattractant protein 1 in human aortic smooth muscle cells. Circulation 1997;96:2361-7.

45. De Keulenaer GW, Alexander RW, Ushio-Fukai M, Ishizaka N, Griendling KK. Tumour necrosis factor alpha activates a p22phox-based NADH oxidase in vascular smooth muscle. Biochem J 1998;329:653-7.

46. Gorlach A, Diebold I, Schini-Kerth VB, et al. Thrombin activates the hypoxia-inducible factor-1 signaling pathway in vascular smooth muscle cells: Role of the p22(phox)-containing NADPH oxidase. Circ Res 2001;89:47-54.

47. Duerrschmidt N, Wippich N, Goettsch W, Broemme HJ, Morawietz H. Endothelin-1 induces NAD(P)H oxidase in human endothelial cells. Biochem Biophys Res Commun 2000;269:713-7.

48. Diep QN, Amiri F, Touyz RM, et al. PPARalpha activator effects on Ang II-induced vascular oxidative stress and inflammation. Hypertension 2002;40:866-71.

49. Wassmann S, Laufs U, Muller K, et al. Cellular antioxidant effects of atorvastatin in vitro and in vivo. Arterioscler Thromb Vasc Biol 2002;22:300-5.

50. Dandona P, Karne R, Ghanim H, Hamouda W, Aljada A, Magsino CH. Carvedilol inhibits reactive oxygen species generation by leukocytes and oxidative damage to amino acids. Circulation 2000;101:122-4.

51. Ohtahara A, Hisatome I, Yamamoto Y, Furuse M, Sonoyama K, Furuse Y. The release of the substrate for xanthine oxidase in hypertensive patients was suppressed by angiotensin converting enzyme inhibitors and α1-blockers. J Hypertens 2001;19:575-82.

52. Taddei S, Virdis A, Ghiadoni L, et al. Effect of calcium antagonist or beta blockade treatment on nitric oxide-dependent vasodilation and oxidative stress in essential hypertensive patients. J Hypertens 2001;19:1379-86.

53. Cosentino F, Barker JE, Brand MP, et al. Reactive oxygen species mediate endothelium-dependent relaxations in tetrahydrobiopterin-deficient mice. Arterioscler Thromb Vasc Biol 2001;21:496-502.

54. Vasquez-Vivar J, Duquaine D, Whitsett J, Kalyanaraman B, Rajagopalan S. Altered tetrahydrobiopterin metabolism in atherosclerosis: implications for use of oxidized tetrahydrobiopterin analogues and thiol antioxidants. Arterioscler Thromb Vasc Biol 2002;22:1655-61.

55. Bagi Z, Koller A. Lack of nitric oxide mediation of flow-dependent arteriolar dilation in type I diabetes is restored by sepiapterin. J Vasc Res 2003;40:47-57

56. Virdis A, Iglarz M, Neves MF, et al. Effect of hyperhomocystinemia and hypertension on endothelial function in methylenetetrahydrofolate reductase-deficient mice. Arterioscler Thromb Vasc Biol 2003;23:1352-7.

57. Landmesser U, Dikalov S, Price SR, et al. Oxidation of tetrahydrobiopterin leads to uncoupling of endothelial cell nitric oxide synthase in hypertension. J Clin Invest 2003;111:1201-9.

58. Zheng JS, Yang XQ, Lookingland KJ et al. Gene transfer of human guanosine 5'-triphosphate cyclohydrolase I restores vascular tetrahydrobiopterin level and endothelial function in low renin hypertension. Circulation 2003;108:1238-45.

59. Guzik TJ, Mussa S, Gastaldi D, et al. Mechanisms of increased vascular superoxide production in human diabetes mellitus: role of NAD(P)H oxidase and endothelial nitric oxide synthase. Circulation 2002;105:1656-62.

60. Taniyama Y, Griendling KK. Reactive oxygen species in the vasculature: molecular and cellular mechanisms. Hypertension 2003;42:1075-81.

61. Spiekermann S, Landmesser U, Dikalov S et al. Electron spin resonance characterization of vascular xanthine and NAD(P)H oxidase activity in patients with coronary artery disease: Relation to endothelium-dependent vasodilation. Circulation 2003;107:1383-9.

62. Touyz RM, Schiffrin EL. Signal transduction mechanisms mediating the physiological and pathophysiological actions of angiotensin II in vascular smooth muscle cells. Pharmacol Rev 2000;52: 639-72.

63. Lee SR, Kwon KS, Kim SR, Rhee SG. Reversible inactivation of protein-tyrosine phosphatase 1B in A431 cells stimulated with epidermal growth factor. J Biol Chem 1998;273:15366-72.

64. Turpaev KT. Reactive oxygen species and regulation of gene expression. Biochemistry 2002;67:281-92.

65. Touyz RM, Wu XH, He G, Salomon S, Schiffrin EL. Increased angiotensin II-mediated Src signaling via epidermal growth factor receptor transactivation is associated with decreased C-terminal Src kinase activity in vascular smooth muscle cells from spontaneously hypertensive rats. Hypertension 2002;39:479-85.

66. Brigelius-Flohe R, Banning A, Kny M, Bol GF. Redox events in interleukin-1 signaling. Arch Biochem Biophys 2004;423:66-73.

67. Virdis A, Neves MF, Amiri F, Touyz RM, Schiffrin EL. Role of NAD(P)H oxidase on vascular alterations in angiotensin II-infused mice. J Hypertension 2004;22:535-42.

68. Haddad JJ. Antioxidant and prooxidant mechanisms in the regulation of redox(y)-sensitive transcription factors. Cell Signal 2002;14:879-97.

69. Touyz RM, Yao G, Viel E, Amiri F, Schiffrin EL. Angiotensin II and endothelin-1 regulate MAP kinases through different redox-dependent mechanisms in human vascular smooth muscle cells. J Hypertens 2004;22:1141-9.

70. Viedt C, Soto U, Krieger-Brauer HI, et al. Differential activation of mitogen-activated protein kinases in smooth muscle cells by angiotensin II: involvement of p22phox and reactive oxygen species. Arterioscler Thromb Vasc Biol 2000;20:940-8.

71. Ushio-Fukai M, Alexander RW, Akers M, Griendling KK. p38 Mitogen-activated protein kinase is a critical component of the redox-sensitive signaling pathways activated by angiotensin II. Role in vascular smooth muscle cell hypertrophy. J Biol Chem 1998;273:15022-9.

72. Touyz RM, Cruzado M, Tabet F, Yao G, Salomon S, Schiffrin EL. Redox-dependent MAP kinase signaling by Ang II in vascular smooth muscle cells – role of receptor tyrosine kinase transactivation. Can J Physiol Pharmacol 2003;81:159-67.

73. Droge, W. Free radicals in the physiological control of cell function. Physiol Rev 2001;82:47-95.

74. Lounsbury KM, Hu Q, Ziegelstein RC. Calcium signaling and oxidant stress in the vasculature. Free Radic Biol Med 2000;28: 1362-9.

75. Gao YJ, Lee RM. Hydrogen peroxide induces a greater contraction in mesenteric arteries of spontaneously hypertensive rats through thromboxane A(2) production. Br J Pharmacol 2001;134: 1639-46.

76. Deshpande NN, Sorescu D, Seshiah P, et al. Mechanism of hydrogen peroxide-induced cell cycle arrest in vascular smooth muscle. Antioxid Redox Signal 2002;4:845-54.

77. Li AE, Ito H, Rovira II, et al. A role for reactive oxygen species in endothelial cell anoikis. Circ Res 1999;85:304-10.

78. Rajagopalan S, Meng XP, Ramasamy S, Harrison DG, Galis ZS. Reactive oxygen species produced by macrophage-derived foam cells regulate the activity of vascular matrix metalloproteinases in vitro. J Clin Invest 1996;98:2572-9.

79. Muller DN, Dechend R, Mervaala EMA, et al. NFκB inhibition ameliorates angiotensin II-induced inflammatory damage in rats. Hypertension 2000;35:193-201.

80. Luft FC. Mechanisms and cardiovascular damage in hypertension. Hypertension 2001;37:594-8.

81. Alexander RW. Hypertension and the pathogenesis of atherosclerosis. Oxidative stress and the mediation of arterial inflammatory response: a new perspective. Hypertension 1995;25:155-61.

82. Yada T, Shimokawa H, Hiramatsu O, et al. Hydrogen peroxide, an endogenous endothelium-derived hyperpolarizing factor, plays an important role in coronary autoregulation in vivo. Circulation 2003;107:1040-5.

83. Torrecillas G, Boyano-Adanez MC, Medina J, et al. The role of hydrogen peroxide in the contractile response to angiotensin II. Mol Pharmacol 2001;59:104-12.

84. Schuijt MP, Tom B, De Vries R, et al. Superoxide does not mediate the acute vasoconstrictor effects of angiotensin II: a study in human and porcine arteries. J Hypertens 2003;21:2335-44.

85. Zalba G, Beaumont FJ, San Jose G, et al. Vascular NADH/NADPH oxidase is involved in enhanced superoxide production in spontaneously hypertensive rats. Hypertension 2000;35:1055-61.

86. Tanito M, Nakamura H, Kwon YW, et al. Enhanced oxidative stress and impaired thioredoxin expression in spontaneously hypertensive rats. Antioxid Redox Signal 2004;6:89-97.

87. Zalba G, San Jose G, Beaumont FJ, Fortuno MA, Fortuno A, Diez J. Polymorphisms and promoter overactivity of the p22(phox) gene in vascular smooth muscle cells from spontaneously hypertensive rats. Circ Res 2001;88:217-22.

88. Chabrashvili T, Tojo A, Onozato ML, et al. Expression and cellular localization of classic NADPH oxidase subunits in the spontaneously hypertensive rat kidney. Hypertension 2002;39:269-74.

89. Landmesser U, Cai H, Dikalov S, et al. Role of p47(phox) in vascular oxidative stress and hypertension caused by angiotensin II. Hypertension 2002;40:511-5.

90. Hong HJ, Hsiao G, Cheng TH, Yen MH. Supplemention with tetrahydrobiopterin suppresses the development of hypertension in spontaneously hypertensive rats. Hypertension 2001;38:1044-8.

91. Zhan CD, Sindhu RK, Vaziri ND. Up-regulation of kidney NAD(P)H oxidase and calcineurin in SHR: reversal by lifelong antioxidant supplementation. Kidney Int 2004;65:219-27.

92. Laursen JB, Rajagopalan S, Galis Z, Tarpey M, Freeman BA, Harrison DG. Role of superoxide in angiotensin II-induced but not catecholamine-induced hypertension. Circulation 1997;95:588-93.

93. Tojo A, Onozato ML, Kobayashi N, Goto A, Matsuoka H, Fujita T. Angiotensin II and oxidative stress in Dahl Salt-sensitive rat with heart failure. Hypertension 2002;40: 834-9.

94. Dobrian AD, Davies MJ, Schriver SD, Lauterio TJ, Prewitt RL. Oxidative stress in a rat model of obesity-induced hypertension. Hypertension 2001;37:554-60.

95. Li L, Fink GD, Watts SW, et al. Endothelin-1 increases vascular superoxide via endothelin(A)-NADPH oxidase pathway in low-renin hypertension. Circulation 2003;107:1053-8.

96. Virdis A, Fritsch Neves M, Amiri F, et al. Spironolactone improves angiotensin-induced vascular changes and oxidative stress. Hypertension 2002;40:504-10.

97. Welch WJ, Mendonca M, Aslam S, Wilcox CS. Roles of oxidative stress and AT_1 receptors in renal hemodynamics and oxygenation in the postclipped 2K,1C kidney. Hypertension 2003;41:692-6.

98. Fortepiani LA, Zhang H, Racusen L, Roberts LJ 2nd, Reckelhoff JF. Characterization of an animal model of postmenopausal hypertension in spontaneously hypertensive rats. Hypertension 2003;41:640-5.

99. Park JB, Touyz RM, Chen X, Schiffrin EL. Chronic treatment with a superoxide dismutase mimetic prevents vascular remodeling and progression of hypertension in salt-loaded stroke-prone spontaneously hypertensive rats. Am J Hypertens 2002;15:78-84.

100. Minuz P, Patrignani P, Gaino S, Degan M, Menapace L, Tommasoli R. Increased oxidative stress and platelet activation in patients with hypertension and renovascular disease. Circulation 2002;106:2800-5.

101. Lacy F, Kailasam MT, O'Connor DT, Schmid-Schonbein GW, Parmer RJ. Plasma hydrogen peroxide production in human essential hypertension: role of heredity, gender, and ethnicity. Hypertension 2000;36:878-84.

102. Russo C, Olivieri O, Girelli D, et al. Anti-oxidant status and lipid peroxidation in patients with essential hypertension. J Hypertens 1998;16:1267-71.

103. Cracowski JL, Baguet JP, Ormezzano O, et al. Lipid peroxidation is not increased in patients with untreated mild-to-moderate hypertension. Hypertension 2003;41:286-8.

104. Higashi Y, Sasaki S, Nakagawa K et al. Endothelial function and oxidative stress in renovascular hypertension. N Engl J Med 2002;346:1954-62.

105. Lip GY, Edmunds E, Nuttall SL, Landray MJ, Blann AD, Beevers DG. Oxidative stress in malignant and non-malignant phase hypertension. J Hum Hypertens 2002;16: 333-6.

106. Lee VM, Quinn PA, Jennings SC, Ng LL. Neutrophil activation and production of reactive oxygen species in pre-eclampsia. J Hypertens 2003;21:395-402.

107. Schiffrin EL, Touyz RM. Inflammation and vascular hypertrophy induced by angiotensin II: role of NADPH oxidase-derived reactive oxygen species independently of blood pressure elevation? Arterioscler Thromb Vasc Biol 2003;23: 707-9.

108. Schiffrin EL, Touyz RM. Multiple actions of angiotensin II in hypertension: Benefits of AT_1 receptor blockade. J Am Coll Cardiol 2003;42:911-3.

109. Wyche KE, Wang SS, Griendling KK, et al. C242T CYBA polymorphism of the NADPH oxidase is associated with reduced respiratory burst in human neutrophils. Hypertension 2004;43:1246-51.

110. Mullan B, Young IS, Fee H, McCance DR. Ascorbic acid reduces blood pressure and arterial stiffness in type 2 diabetes. Hypertension 2002;40:804-9.

111. Galley HF, Thornton J, Howdle PD, Walker BE, Webster NR. Combination oral antioxidant supplementation reduces blood pressure. Clin Sci 1997;92: 361-5.

112. Kim MY, Sasaki S, Sasazuki S, Okubo S, Hayashi M, Tsugane S. Lack of long-term effect of vitamin C supplementation on blood pressure. Hypertension 2002;40:797-803.

113. Chen J, He J, Hamm L, Batuman V, Whelton PK. Serum antioxidant vitamins and blood pressure in the United States population. Hypertension 2002;40:810-6.

114. Hamilton CA, Miller WH, Al-Benna S, et al. Strategies to reduce oxidative stress in cardiovascular disease. Clin Sci 2004;106:219-34.

115. Vivekananthan DP, Penn MS, Sapp SK, Hsu A, Topol EJ. Use of antioxidant vitamins for the prevention of cardiovascular disease: meta-analysis of randomised trials. Lancet 2003;361:2017-23.

116. Schiffrin EL, Park J-B, Intengan HD, Touyz RM. Correction of arterial structure and endothelial dysfunction in human essential hypertension by the angiotensin receptor antagonist losartan. Circulation 2000;101:1653-9.

117. Rey FE, Cifuentes ME, Kiarash A, et al. Novel competitive inhibitor of NAD(P)H oxidase assembly attenuates vascular O2- and systolic blood pressure in mice. Circ Res 2001;89:408-14.

118. Ghiadoni L, Magagna A, Versari D, et al. Different effect of antihypertensive drugs on conduit artery endothelial function. Hypertension 2003;41:1281-6.

119. Tribble DL. Antioxidant consumption and risk of coronary heart disease: emphasis on vitamin C, vitamin E and β-carotene. A statement for the healthcare professionals from the American Heart Association. Circulation 1999;99:591-5.

120. Touyz RM, Campbell N, Logan A, Gledhill N, Petrella R, Padwal R, Canadian Hypertension Education Program. The 2004 Canadian recommendations for the management of hypertension: Part III-Lifestyle modifications to prevent and control hypertension. Can J Cardiol 2004;20:55-83.

121. John JH, Ziebland S, Yudkin P, Roe LS, Neil HAW. Effects of fruit and vegetable consumption on plasma antioxidant concentrations and blood pressure: a randomized controlled trial. Lancet 2002;359:1969-73.

Chapter 16

OXIDATIVE STRESS IN THE DEVELOPMENT OF DIABETES AND ITS COMPLICATIONS

Jean-Louis Chiasson, Rémi Rabasa-Lhoret and Ashok K. Srivastava
Research Centre, Centre hospitalier de l'Université de Montréal and Departments of Nutrition and Medicine, Université de Montréal, Montréal, Canada

Introduction

The prevalence of diabetes is increasing to epidemic proportions worldwide. It has been estimated that the overall diabetic population will grow from 150 to 300 million by the year 2025[1]. Furthermore, the long-term complications associated with diabetes mellitus are major causes of blindness, end-stage renal disease, non-traumatic amputations[2,3], and cardiovascular disease[4]. Diabetes is the seventh leading cause of death in the United States[5]. This excess morbidity and mortality translates into increased healthcare expenditures that are 2.5- to 6.5-fold higher than for non-diabetic subjects[6].

It is generally accepted that hyperglycemia is the major factor responsible for diabetes-related complications. Epidemiological studies have shown a strong relationship between glycemic control and the development of microvascular complications, and this has been confirmed in prospective intervention trials for both type 1 and type 2 diabetes[7,8]. The relationship between hyperglycemia and cardiovascular disease has been more difficult to establish. However, a number of epidemiological investigations have demonstrated the association between dysglycemia and cardiovascular disease[9]. The Diabetes Epidemiology Collaborative analysis Of Diagnostic criteria in Europe (DECODE) study[10] has shown that post-prandial hyperglycemia is the strongest predictor of cardiovascular disease. Most prospective intervention trials, including the United Kingdom Prospective Diabetes Study (UKPDS), have all fallen short of achieving a significant reduction in cardiovascular disease[8]. Only the Diabetes mellitus, Insulin Glucose infusion in Acute Myocardial Infarction (DIGAMI) study[11] post-acute myocardial infarction in patients with diabetes was able to establish that intensive insulin treatment was associated with absolute risk reduction of 11% ($p = 0.01$). It should be mentioned that in the latter study, post-prandial as well as fasting hyperglycemia was treated aggressively.

There is now accumulating evidence that oxidative stress resulting from hyperglycemia could be involved in the development of diabetes as well as in the micro- and macrovascular complications of the disease. However, the cause and effect relationship between oxidative stress and the development of diabetes and its complications remains to be established.

Hyperglycemia and oxidative stress

Existent *in vitro* and *in vivo* data indicate that reactive oxygen species (ROS) formation can be a direct consequence of hyperglycemia. Michael Brownlee[12] recently reviewed the biochemistry and molecular cell biology of diabetic complications, and provided evidence that the different mechanisms involved in the pathogenesis of diabetes-related complications result from a single hyperglycemia-induced process: the overproduction of superoxide by the mitochondrial electron transport chain[13,14]. It has been found that the inhibition of hyperglycemia-induced overproduction of superoxide by manganese superoxide dismutase completely prevents increases in the polyol pathway, advanced glycation end-product (AGE) formation, protein kinasae C activation (PKC) and the hexosamine pathway in endothelial cells[12].

Supportive data in humans suggest that hyperglycemia is associated with heightened oxidative stress. Ceriello *et al.*[15] were among the first to report augmented superoxide anion generation in diabetic serum which correlated with plasma glucose. Furthermore, Berg *et al.*[16] discovered that intensive insulin therapy in type 1 diabetic subjects through continuous subcutaneous insulin infusion resulted in a 31% reduction of plasma lipid hydroperoxides compared to the control group ($p < 0.001$). A significant correlation between glycated hemoglobin and hydroperoxide levels ($p < 0.04$) was apparent in these studies. They were the first to report that improved glycemic control reduced oxidative stress, as assessed by plasma hydroperoxide levels in type 1 diabetes patients. Marfella *et al.*[17] demonstrated in healthy subjects submitted to two-hour hyperglycemic clamp (15 mmol/L) that nitrotyrosine levels, a marker of oxidative stress, rose 2.5-fold over baseline. The same group also looked at the effect of a mixed meal on nitrotyrosine in insulin-treated type 2 diabetic patients compared to healthy controls. The diabetic subjects were studied twice, once with the short-acting insulin Actrapid® before meal and once with the rapid-acting insulin NovoRapid® in randomized order. While baseline glycemia was similar for both tests, two-hour plasma glucose was significantly lower after NovoRapid® insulin ($p < 0.04$); similarly, nitrotyrosine elevation after meals was significantly reduced with lower post-prandial plasma glucose ($p < 0.03$). This was the first demonstration that post-prandial hyperglycemia is associated with a significant increase in oxidative stress.

It was, therefore, suggested that spiking hyperglycemia was more potent in inducing oxidative stress than continuous hyperglycemia. This was confirmed in endothelial cells by Quagliaro *et al.*[18]. In their study, human umbilical vein endothelial cells were cultured for 14 days in medium containing either 5 mM glucose, 20 mM glucose or 5 mM glucose alternating every 24 hours with 20 mM glucose. Exposure of the endothelial cells to continuous high glucose (25 mM glucose) was associated with a two-fold increment of the oxidative stress markers nitrotyrosine and 8-hydroxydeoxyguanosine as well as PKC activity and apoptosis. However, intermittent hyperglycemia was even more potent in inducing oxidative stress, PKC activation and apoptosis; these phenomena were totally inhibited by Mn (III) tetrakis (4-henzoic acid) porphyrine chloride, a superoxide inhibitor. These observations strongly suggest that spiking hyperglycemia is worse than continuous hyperglycemia.

More recently, Ceriello *et al.*[19] have shown in non-diabetic and type 2 diabetic subjects that not only glucose, but also a high fat meal could induce oxidative stress, as measured by nitrotyrosine (*Figure 1*). After a high carbohydrate meal, the rise in nitrotyrosine peaked at one and two hours in the non-diabetic and diabetic subjects respectively and returned to baseline by two and four hours. After the high-fat meal, the rise in nitrotyrosine was much slower but also more prolonged, reaching a peak at two and four hours, respectively. A combined high-carbohydrate, high-fat meal produced a cumulative effect on the rise in post-prandial nitrotyrosine. This indicates that a mixed meal containing both carbohydrates and fat is a strong inducer of oxidative stress.

All these studies in non-diabetic and diabetic subjects suggest that hyperglycemia, particularly spiking post-prandial hyperglycemia, is linked with an elevation of oxidative stress. Furthermore, post-prandial hyperlipidemia is also associated with heightened oxidative stress. Accumulating evidence is now showing that free fatty acids (FFA) are involved in the pathogenesis of insulin resistance[20] and impaired insulin secretion[21], and could be major determinants of type 2 diabetes. Could oxidative stress be the pathogenic mediator involved in the development of diabetes?

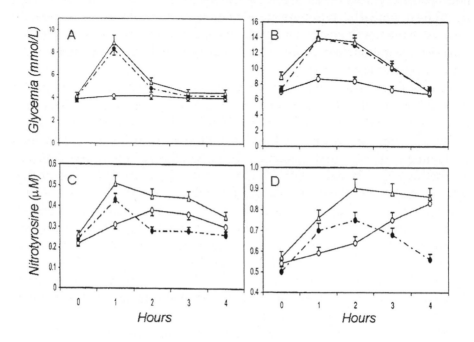

Figure 1. **Effects of high-fat load (O), 75 g glucose (l) and high-fat load plus 75 g glucose (D) on plasma glucose (A + B) and nitrotyrosine in healthy normal subjects (A + C) and in type 2 diabetic patients (B + D).** Data are expressed as means ± SE. Reproduced with permission from reference[19].

Oxidative stress and the development of diabetes

Obesity and decreased physical activity are products of Western industrialized societies[22]. Most obese subjects have elevated FFA[23,24], primarily because of an increased lipolysis rate from the expanded fat cell mass[25,26]. Elevated FFA have been disclosed to mediate, at least in part, impairment of insulin secretion[21,27,28] and insulin action[20,29] in non-diabetic subjects, major defects leading to the development of diabetes.

We would like to present the following evidence in support of chronic oxidative stress as the major mechanism involved in the pathogenesis of type 2 diabetes mellitus (*Figure 2*). A large volume of data indicate that hyperlipidemia is associated with increased oxidative stress[19,30,31]; since obesity is often accompanied by elevated FFA levels, ROS production is very likely to be a common occurrence in obese subjects. The ROS produced by hyperlipidemia will activate PKC and a number of stress enzymes (ERK 1/2, JNK/SAPK, p38^{mapk} and ERK5)[32]. These will induce serine/threonine phosphorylation of the insulin receptor and IRS 1-2, leading to insulin resistance due to attenuation of the insulin signaling cascade[33]. Furthermore, islet cells are low in antioxidant enzyme content and activities, and are thus vulnerable to rising ROS[34]; these include superoxide, hydrogen peroxide, nitric oxide and hydroxyl radicals. Among them, hydroxyl radicals are the most toxic, because they pass freely through membrane barriers to the cell nucleus where they react strongly with DNA[35]. Hydroxyl radicals inhibit PDX-1 transcription, which is necessary for insulin synthesis[35].

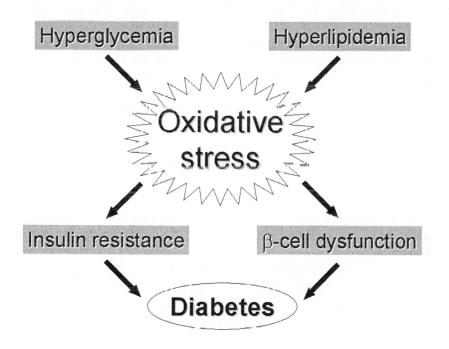

Figure 2. **Schematic representation of the involvement of oxidative stress induced by hyperglycemia and hyperlipidemia in the development of diabetes through an effect on insulin sensitivity and insulin secretion.**

Furthermore, Sakuraba *et al.*[36] have shown that decreased beta cell mass in type 2 diabetic patients correlates with increased oxidative stress-related tissue damage. It is, therefore, possible that in genetically susceptible individuals, the oxidative stress induced by hyperlipidemia could lead to decreased insulin secretion and action, resulting in the development of glucose intolerance characterized by post-prandial hyperglycemia. This moderate post-prandial hyperglycemia will exacerbate the resulting oxidative stress[37,38], and further contribute to the deterioration of insulin action and secretion, thus accelerating the progression to diabetes. Such a view is compatible with the observations that type 2 diabetes is associated with elevated markers of oxidative stress[39-44]. Finally, there is abundant literature suggesting that increased oxidative stress in poorly-controlled diabetics could be responsible for diabetes-related complications[12,43,45].

Oxidative stress and diabetes-related complications

Much data has accumulated supporting the involvement of oxidative stress in the development of both microvascular and macrovascular complications. In 2001, Michael Brownlee[12] described the molecular mechanism leading to diabetic complications. He detailed the four main hypotheses on how hyperglycemia can induce diabetes complications: 1) augmented polyol pathway flux; 2) increased AGE formation; 3) PKC isoform activation; and 4) enhanced hexosamine pathway flux. He provided evidence that these four different pathogenic mechanisms result from a single hyperglycemia-induced process; ROS overproduction[13,14]. The molecular events involved in hyperglycemia-induced ROS production have been demonstrated in endothelial cell cultures.

Intracellular glucose oxidation starts in the glycolytic pathway in the cytoplasm, generating NADH and pyruvate. Cytoplasmic NADH can donate reducing equivalents to the mitochondrial electron transport chain or reduce pyruvate to lactate. Pyruvate can also be transported into the mitochondria where it is oxidized in the TCA cycle to CO_2 and H_2O with the production of NADH and $FADH_2$. The latter reducing equivalents provide energy for ATP production through oxidative phosphorylation by the electron transport chain. Electron flow through the system produces superoxide which is normally neutralized by antioxidant enzymes. During hyperglycemia, however, the electrochemical potential difference generated by the proton gradient across the inner mitochondrial membranes is high, and the half-life of the superoxide generating system is prolonged, resulting in increased superoxide production. Heightened ROS production is now known to be involved in increases of polyol pathway flux, AGE formation, PKC activation and hexosamine pathway flux. These mechanisms have been shown to be involved in the microvascular complications of diabetes.

As discussed above, spiking post-prandial hyperglycemia is probably more deleterious than chronic hyperglycemia. The acute rise in plasma glucose produces an increment of the glomerular filtration rate in diabetic patients[46]. This effect is even greater in patients who already have albuminuria[47]. The intermittent exposure of mesangial cells to high glucose concentrations stimulates collagen overproduction, a crucial event in the pathogenesis of diabetic nephropathy[48,49]. These observations are consistent with clinical data showing a definite relationship between post-prandial plasma glucose and the development of nephropathy[50,51]. Even in the case of retinopathy, acute post-prandial hyperglycemia has been found to augment retinal perfusion[52] and the development of eye complications[50]. Similar observations have been made between acute hyperglycemia and the occurrence of diabetic neuropathy. Hyperglycemia acutely induced in type 1 diabetes causes impairment of motor and sensory nerve conduction velocity[53,54]. It has now been shown that tight glycemic control is associated with decreased oxidative stress[16], and delays the appearance and the progression of specific complications in both type 1[7] and type 2 diabetes[8]. This would be consistent with the oxidative stress hypothesis in the pathogenesis of diabetes-specific microvascular complications.

There is also strong evidence that post-prandial hyperglycemia and hyperlipidemia are important contributing factors in the development of atherosclerosis in both diabetic and non-diabetic subjects[55]. Numerous epidemiological studies have confirmed the relationship between post-prandial hyperglycemia and cardiovascular disease (CVD)[56]. It has also been shown that post-prandial hypertriglyceridemia is an independent risk factor for CVD[57,58]. These are associated with small-dense LDL cholesterol that is prone to oxidation[59]. LDL oxidation increases after meals[41] and is directly related to the degree of hyperglycemia[42]. This post-prandial state is also linked with augmented coagulation activity[60,61] as well as with the heightened expression of adhesion molecules on the endothelial surface[19,62], resulting in enhanced adhesion of mononuclear cells and endothelial dysfunction, a first step in the formation of atherosclerosis[62]. In summary, it is proposed that post-prandial hyperglycemia and hyperlipidemia culminate in increased ROS production and the development of microvascular and macrovascular complications in diabetes mellitus (*Figure 3*).

Antioxidants in the prevention of diabetes and its complications

A number of studies have shown that in high-risk populations, type 2 diabetes mellitus can be prevented or at least delayed (*Table 1*). The Da Qing study was the first to reveal in impaired glucose tolerance (IGT) subjects that lifestyle modification, diet and exercise could decrease the development of diabetes by 39%[63]. This observation was confirmed by the Finnish Diabetes Prevention Study (DPS) and the Diabetes Prevention Program (DPP) demonstrating that diet and exercise could lower the conversion rate of IGT to diabetes by 58%[64,65]. The DPP also showed that metformin treatment in IGT was associated with a 30% risk reduction of diabetes[65].

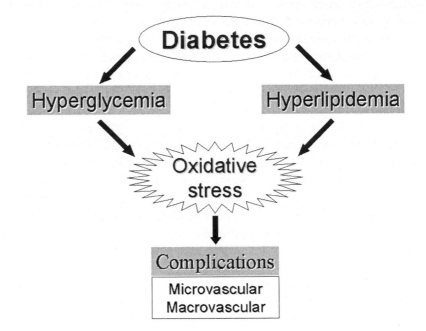

Figure 3. **Schematic representation of the involvement of oxidative stress induced by hyperglycemia and hyperlipidemia in the development of diabetes-related complications.**

The Study to Prevent Non-Insulin-Dependent Diabetes Mellitus Trial (STOP-NIDDM) reported that the α-glucosidase inhibitor, acarbose, by lowering post-prandial plasma glucose, could decrease the risk of conversion of IGT to diabetes by 36%[66]. The Troglitazone in Prevention of Diabetes (TRIPOD) study also demonstrated the efficacy of troglitazone, a thiazolidinedione, in reducing by 50% the incidence of diabetes in Hispanic women with a history of gestational diabetes[67]. More recently, it was shown that decreasing post-prandial lipidemia with orlistat could lower the risk of diabetes by 37.3%[68]. It has also been noted in subgroup analysis, that angiotensin-converting enzyme (ACE) inhibitors, statins and angiotensin II receptor antagonists (ARA) were associated with a reduced incidence of diabetes[69-71]. All these interventions have one thing in common: they all possess antioxidant activity. Both specific diet and regular exercise have been suggested to be accompanied by an increase in antioxidant capacity[72-74]. Acarbose and orlistat reduce post-prandial hyperglycemia and hyperlipidemia, respectively and thus should theoretically be associated with decreased oxidative stress production[16,19,38]. A number of studies have now established that statins have antioxidant properties[19,75,76]. This is also the case for ACE inhibitors[77], and would be expected to be true for ARA as well.

Table 1: Intervention studies on the prevention of type 2 diabetes

Studies	No. of subjects	Interventions	Follow-up (yr)	Relative risk reduction (%)
Lifestyle modifications				
Da Qing (1997)	577	Diet and/or exercise	6.0	39
DPS (2001)	522	Diet and exercise	3.2	58
DPP (2002)	2,161	Diet and exercise	2.8	58
Drug Interventions				
DPP (2002)	2,151	Metformin	2.8	31
STOP-NIDDM (2002)	1,429	Acarbose	3.3	36
TRIPOD (2002)	236	Troglitazone	2.5	50

Intensive treatment of diabetes, both type 1 and type 2 reduces the development of microvascular complications[7,8]. Since intensive treatment of hyperglycemia is associated with decreased ROS production[78], this would be compatible with an antioxidant effect.

The past 25 years have witnessed the establishment of Aspirin®, ACE inhibitors and lipid-lowering drugs in lowering the risk of cardiovascular events[79] (*Table 2*). Again, this would be compatible with an antioxidant effect. It has been shown that Aspirin® inhibits glucose-induced superoxide production in Sprague-Dawley rats[80]. Ceriello et al.[19] have recently demonstrated that simvastatin treatment for three months totally normalizes the post-prandial rise in nitrotyrosine and adhesion molecules. Furthermore, decreasing post-prandial hyperglycemia with acarbose in subjects with IGT and type 2 diabetes is associated with significant risk reduction of cardiovascular disease[81,82] (*Figure 4*). Hanefeld et al.[83] have reported that acarbose slows the progression of intima-media thickness in IGT subjects, an accepted surrogate for atherosclerosis.

Table 2: Prevention of cardiovascular disease*

	Relative risk reduction	2-year event rate
None	---	8%
Aspirin®	25%	6%
β-blockers	25%	4-5%
Lipid-lowering drugs (by 1-5 mmol)	30%	3-0%
ACE inhibitors	25%	2-3%

*Adapted from: reference 79.

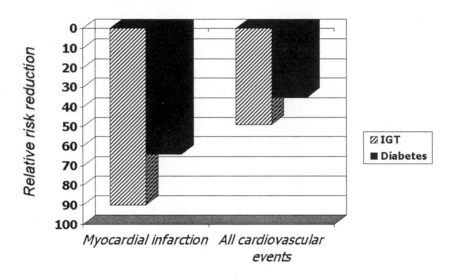

Figure 4

Figure 4. **The effects of lowering post-prandial hyperglycemia with acarbose on the incidence of myocardial infarction and overall cardiovascular events in subjects with IGT (hatched bars) and type 2 diabetes (black bars).** Adapted from references[81,82].

Proving the oxidative stress hypothesis in intervention studies with specific antioxidant therapy has proven to be difficult. The HOPE study with vitamin E was totally negative[84]. Whether this is due to the potential pro-oxidant effects of vitamin E or whether the results are confounded by other nutritional pharmacological factors remains to be established[85]. It has, however, been shown in a small number of patients with coronary artery disease that acute and chronic treatment with ascorbic acid reverses endothelial vasomotor dysfunction[86,87].

Overall, these observations could be compatible with a beneficial effect of antioxidant therapy in the prevention of diabetes and its complications.

Conclusion

It is now well-established that hyperglycemia and hyperlipidemia are associated with increased oxidative stress. The resulting oxidative stress can augment insulin resistance and decrease beta-cell function, major factors involved in the development of type 2 diabetes. Oxidative stress is also believed to be involved in the development of microvascular and macrovascular complications associated with diabetes. Though it is suggested that antioxidant therapy can prevent diabetes and its complications, this still needs to be confirmed by well-designed, randomized trials with specific antioxidant drugs.

References

1. King H, Aubert RE, Herman WH. Global burden of diabetes, 1995-2025. Prevalence, numerical estimates, and projections. Diabetes Care 1998;21:1414-31.
2. Eastman RC, Javitt JC, Herman WH et al. Model of complications of NIDDM. I. Model construction and assumptions. Diabetes Care 1997;20:725-34.
3. Caputo GM, Cavanagh PR, Ulbrecht JS, Gibbons GW, Karchmer AW. Assessment and management of foot disease in patients with diabetes. N Engl J Med 1994;331:854-60.
4. Haffner SM, Lehto S, Rönnemaa T, Pyörälä K, Laakso M. Mortality from coronary heart disease in subjects with type 2 diabetes and in nondiabetic subjects with and without prior myocardial infarction. N Engl J Med 1998;339:229-34.
5. Geiss LS, Herman WH, Smith PJ. Mortality in non-insulin-dependent diabetes. Diabetes in America. National Institutes of Health, 1995:233-55.
6. American Diabetes Association. Economic consequences of diabetes mellitus in the U.S. in 1997. Diabetes Care 1998;21:296-309.
7. DCCT Research Group. The effect of intensive treatment of diabetes on the development and progression of long-term complications in insulin-dependent diabetes mellitus. N Engl J Med 1993;329:977-86.
8. UK Prospective Diabetes Study Group. Intensive blood-glucose control with sulphonylureas or insulin compared with conventional treatment and risk of complications in patients with type 2 diabetes (UKPDS 33). Lancet 1998;352:837-53.
9. Coutinho M, Gerstein HC, Wang Y, Yusuf S. The relationship between glucose and incident cardiovascular events. A metaregression analysis of published data from 20 studies of 95,783 individuals followed for 12.4 years. Diabetes Care 1999;22:233-40.
10. The DECODE Study Group EDEG. Glucose tolerance and mortality: comparison of WHO and American Diabetes Association diagnostic criteria. Diabetes Epidemiology: Collaborative analysis of diagnostic criteria in Europe. Lancet 1999;354:617-21.
11. Malmberg K. Prospective randomised study of intensive insulin treatment on long term survival after acute myocardial infarction in patients with diabetes mellitus. DIGAMI (Diabetes Mellitus, Insulin Glucose Infusion in Acute Myocardial Infarction) Study Group (see comments). BMJ 1997;314:1512-5.
12. Brownlee M. Biochemistry and molecular cell biology of diabetic complications. Nature 2001;414:813-20.
13. Du XL, Edelstein D, Rossetti L et al. Hyperglycemia-induced mitochondrial superoxide overproduction activates the hexosamine pathway and induces plasminogen activator inhibitor-1 expression by increasing Sp1 glycosylation. Proc Natl Acad Sci U S A 2000;97:12222-6.
14. Nishikawa T, Edelstein D, Du XL et al. Normalizing mitochondrial superoxide production blocks three pathways of hyperglycaemic damage. Nature 2000;404:787-90.
15. Ceriello A, Giugliano D, Quatraro A, Dello RP, Lefebvre PJ. Metabolic control may influence the increased superoxide generation in diabetic serum. Diabet Med 1991;8:540-2.

16. Berg TJ, Nourooz-Zadeh J, Wolff SP et al. Hydroperoxides in plasma are reduced by intensified insulin treatment. A randomized controlled study of IDDM patients with microalbuminuria. Diabetes Care 1998;21:1295-300.

17. Marfella R, Quagliaro L, Nappo F, Ceriello A, Giugliano D. Acute hyperglycemia induces an oxidative stress in healthy subjects. J Clin Invest 2001;108:635-6.

18. Quagliaro L, Piconi L, Assaloni R et al. Intermittent high glucose enhances apoptosis related to oxidative stress in human umbilical vein endothelial cells: the role of protein kinase C and NAD(P)H-oxidase activation. Diabetes 2003;52:2795-804.

19. Ceriello A, Quagliaro L, Piconi L et al. Effect of postprandial hypertriglyceridemia and hyperglycemia on circulating adhesion molecules and oxidative stress generation and the possible role of simvastatin treatment. Diabetes 2004;53:701-10.

20. Boden G. Role of fatty acids in the pathogenesis of insulin resistance and NIDDM. Diabetes 1997;46:3-10.

21. Carpentier A, Zinman B, Leung N et al. Free fatty acid-mediated impairment of glucose-stimulated insulin secretion in nondiabetic Oji-Cree individuals from the Sandy Lake community of Ontario, Canada: a population at very high risk for developing type 2 diabetes. Diabetes 2003;52:1485-95.

22. Zimmet P. Globalization, coca-colonization and the chronic disease epidemic: can the Doomsday scenario be averted? J Intern Med 2000;247:301-10.

23. Gorden ES. Non-esterified fatty acids in blood of obese and lean subjects. Am J Clin Nutr 1960;8:740-7.

24. Reaven GM, Hollenbeck C, Jeng C-Y, Wu MS, Chen Y-D. Measurement of plasma glucose, free fatty acid, lactate and insulin for 24 hour in patients with NIDDM. Diabetes 1988;37:1020-4.

25. Bjorntorp P, Bergman H, Varnauskas E. Plasma free fatty acid turnover rate in obesity. Acta Med Scand 1969;185:351-6.

26. Jensen MD, Haymond MW, Rizza RA, Cryer PE, Miles JM. Influence of body fat distribution on free fatty acid metabolism in obesity. J Clin Invest 1989;83:1168-73.

27. Paolisso G, Tagliamonte MR, Rizzo MR et al. Lowering fatty acids potentiates acute insulin response in first degree relatives of people with type II diabetes. Diabetologia 1998;41:1127-32.

28. Carpentier A, Mittelman SD, Bergman RN, Giacca A, Lewis GF. Prolonged elevation of plasma free fatty acids impairs pancreatic beta-cell function in obese nondiabetic humans but not in individuals with type 2 diabetes. Diabetes 2000;49:399-408.

29. McGarry JD. Banting Lecture 2001: Dysregulation of fatty acid metabolism in the etiology of type 2 diabetes. Diabetes 2002;51:7-18.

30. Wojtczak L, Schonfeld P. Effect of fatty acids on energy coupling processes in mitochondria. Biochim Biophys Acta 1993;1183:41-57.

31. Bakker SJ, IJzerman RG, Teerlink T et al. Cytosolic triglycerides and oxidative stress in central obesity: the missing link between excessive atherosclerosis, endothelial dysfunction, and beta-cell failure? Atherosclerosis 2000;148:17-21.

32. Srivastava AK. High glucose-induced activation of protein kinase signaling pathways in vascular smooth muscle cells: A potential role in the pathogenesis of vascular dysfunction in diabetes (review). Intern J Mol Med 2001;9:85-9.

33. Evans JL, Goldfine ID, Maddux BA, Grodsky GM. Are oxidative stress-activated signaling pathways mediators of insulin resistance and beta-cell dysfunction? Diabetes 2003;52:1-8.

34. Grankvist K, Marklund SL, Taljedal IB. CuZn-superoxide dismutase, Mn-superoxide dismutase, catalase and glutathione peroxidase in pancreatic islets and other tissues in the mouse. Biochem J 1981;199:393-8.

35. Robertson RP, Harmon J, Tran PO, Tanaka Y, Takahashi H. Glucose toxicity in beta-cells: type 2 diabetes, good radicals gone bad, and the glutathione connection. Diabetes 2003;52:581-7.

36. Sakuraba H, Mizukami H, Yagihashi N et al. Reduced beta-cell mass and expression of oxidative stress-related DNA damage in the islet of Japanese Type II diabetic patients. Diabetologia 2002;45:85-96.

37. Brown JP, Josse RG. 2002 clinical practice guidelines for the diagnosis and management of osteoporosis in Canada. CMAJ 2002;167(Suppl):S1-34.

38. Ceriello A, Quagliaro L, Catone B et al. Role of hyperglycemia in nitrotyrosine postprandial generation. Diabetes Care 2002;25:1439-43.

39. Ceriello A, Mercuri F, Quagliaro L et al. Detection of nitrotyrosine in the diabetic plasma: evidence of oxidative stress. Diabetologia 2001;44:834-8.

40. Ceriello A. The possible role of postprandial hyperglycaemia in the pathogenesis of diabetic complications. Diabetologia 2003;46 Suppl 1:M9-16.

41. Diwadkar VA, Anderson JW, Bridges SR, Gowri MS, Oelgten PR. Postprandial low-density lipoproteins in type 2 diabetes are oxidized more extensively than fasting diabetes and control samples. Proc Soc Exp Biol Med 1999;222:178-84.

42. Ceriello A, Bortolotti N, Motz E et al. Meal-generated oxidative stress in diabetes. The protective effect of red wine. Diabetes Care 1999;22:2084-5.

43. Giugliano D, Ceriello A, Paolisso G. Oxidative stress and diabetic vascular complications. Diabetes Care 1996;19:257-67.

44. Ceriello A, Bortolotti N, Crescentini A et al. Antioxidant defences are reduced during the oral glucose tolerance test in normal and non-insulin-dependent diabetic subjects. Eur J Clin Invest 1998;28:329-33.

45. Mullarkey CJ, Edelstein D, Brownlee M. Free radical generation by early glycation products: a mechanism for accelerated atherogenesis in diabetes. Biochem Biophys Res Commun 1990;173:932-9.

46. Skott P, Vaag A, Hother-Nielsen O et al. Effects of hyperglycaemia on kidney function, atrial natriuretic factor and plasma renin in patients with insulin-dependent diabetes mellitus. Scand J Clin Lab Invest 1991;51:715-27.

47. Remuzzi A, Viberti G, Ruggenenti P et al. Glomerular response to hyperglycemia in human diabetic nephropathy. Am J Physiol 1990;259:F545-52.

48. Takeuchi A, Throckmorton DC, Brogden AP et al. Periodic high extracellular glucose enhances production of collagens III and IV by mesangial cells. Am J Physiol 1995;268:F13-9.

49. Steffes MW, Bilous RW, Sutherland DE, Mauer SM. Cell and matrix components of the glomerular mesangium in type I diabetes. Diabetes 1992;41:679-84.

50. Shichiri M, Kishikawa H, Ohkubo Y, Wake N. Long-term results of the Kumamoto Study on optimal diabetes control in type 2 diabetic patients. Diabetes Care 2000;23 Suppl 2:B21-9.

51. Hasslacher C, Ritz E. Effect of control of diabetes mellitus on progression of renal failure. Kidney Int Suppl 1987;22:S53-6.

52. Grunwald JE, Brucker AJ, Schwartz SS et al. Diabetic glycemic control and retinal blood flow. Diabetes 1990;39:602-7.

53. Ward JD, Barnes CG, Fisher DJ, Jessop JD, Baker RW. Improvement in nerve conduction following treatment in newly diagnosed diabetics. Lancet 1971;1:428-30.

54. Gregersen G. Variations in motor conduction velocity produced by acute changes of the metabolic state in diabetic patients. Diabetologia 1968;4:273-7.

55. Ceriello A. The post-prandial state and cardiovascular disease: relevance to diabetes mellitus. Diabetes Metab Res Rev 2000;16:125-32.

56. Bonora E. Postprandial peaks as a risk factor for cardiovascular disease: epidemiological perspectives. Int J Clin Pract Suppl 2002:5-11.

57. Groot PH, van Stiphout WA, Krauss XH et al. Postprandial lipoprotein metabolism in normolipidemic men with and without coronary artery disease. Arterioscler Thromb 1991;11:653-62.

58. Patsch JR, Miesenbock G, Hopferwieser T et al. Relation of triglyceride metabolism and coronary artery disease. Studies in the postprandial state. Arterioscler Thromb 1992;12:1336-45.

59. McKeone BJ, Patsch JR, Pownall HJ. Plasma triglycerides determine low density lipoprotein composition, physical properties, and cell-specific binding in cultured cells. J Clin Invest 1993;91:1926-33.

(60) Ceriello A, Taboga C, Tonutti L et al. Post-meal coagulation activation in diabetes mellitus: the effect of acarbose. Diabetologia 1996;39:469-73.

60. Ceriello A. Fibrinogen and diabetes mellitus: is it time for intervention trials? Diabetologia 1997;40:731-4.

61. Ceriello A, Falleti E, Bortolotti N et al. Increased circulating intercellular adhesion molecule-1 levels in type II diabetic patients: the possible role of metabolic control and oxidative stress. Metabolism 1996;45:498-501.

62. Giugliano D, Marfella R, Coppola L et al. Vascular effects of acute hyperglycemia in humans are reversed by L-arginine. Evidence for reduced availability of nitric oxide during hyperglycemia. Circulation 1997;95:1783-90.

63. Pan XR, Li G-W, Hu Y-H et al. The Da Qing IGT and Diabetes Study. Effects of diet and exercise in preventing NIDDM in people with impaired glucose tolerance. Diabetes Care 1997;20:537-44.

64. Tuomilehto J, Lindstrom J, Eriksson JG et al. Prevention of type 2 diabetes mellitus by changes in lifestyle among subjects with impaired glucose tolerance. N Engl J Med 2001;344:1343-50.

65. Knowler WC, Barrett-Connor E, Fowler SE et al. Reduction in the incidence of type 2 diabetes with lifestyle intervention or metformin. N Engl J Med 2002;346:393-403.

66. Chiasson JL, Josse RG, Gomis R et al. Acarbose for prevention of type 2 diabetes mellitus: the STOP-NIDDM randomised trial. Lancet 2002;359:2072-7.

67. Buchanan TA, Xiang AH, Peters RK et al. Response of pancreatic beta-cells to improved insulin sensitivity in women at high risk for type 2 diabetes. Diabetes 2000;49:782-8.

68. Torgerson JS, Hauptman J, Boldrin MN, Sjostrom L. XENical in the prevention of diabetes in obese subjects (XENDOS) study: a randomized study of orlistat as an adjunct to lifestyle changes for the prevention of type 2 diabetes in obese patients. Diabetes Care 2004;27:155-61.

69. Vermes E, Ducharme A, Bourassa MG et al. Enalapril reduces the incidence of diabetes in patients with chronic heart failure: insight from the Studies Of Left Ventricular Dysfunction (SOLVD). Circulation 2003;107:1291-6.

70. Freeman DJ, Norrie J, Sattar N et al. Pravastatin and the development of diabetes mellitus: evidence for a protective treatment effect in the West of Scotland Coronary Prevention Study. Circulation 2001;103:357-62.

71. Dahlof B, Devereux RB, Kjeldsen SE et al. Cardiovascular morbidity and mortality in the Losartan Intervention For Endpoint reduction in hypertension study (LIFE): a randomised trial against atenolol. Lancet 2002;359:995-1003.

72. Reaven P. Dietary and pharmacologic regimens to reduce lipid peroxidation in non-insulin-dependent diabetes mellitus. Am J Clin Nutr 1995;62(Suppl):1483S-9.

73. de Lorgeril M, Renaud S, Mamelle N et al. Mediterranean alpha-linolenic acid-rich diet in secondary prevention of coronary heart disease. Lancet 1994;343:1454-9.

74. Lawson DL, Chen L, Mehta JL. Effects of exercise-induced oxidative stress on nitric oxide release and antioxidant activity. Am J Cardiol 1997;80:1640-2.

75. Takemoto M, Node K, Nakagami H et al. Statins as antioxidant therapy for preventing cardiac myocyte hypertrophy. J Clin Invest 2001;108:1429-37.

76. Shishehbor MH, Aviles RJ, Brennan ML et al. Association of nitrotyrosine levels with cardiovascular disease and modulation by statin therapy. JAMA 2003;289:1675-80.

77. Dzau VJ. Theodore Cooper Lecture: Tissue angiotensin and pathobiology of vascular disease: a unifying hypothesis. Hypertension 2001;37:1047-52.

78. Dornhorst A, Powell SH, Pensky J. Aggravation by propranolol of hyperglycaemic effect of hydrochlorothiazide in type II diabetics without alteration of insulin secretion. Lancet 1985;1:123-6.

79. Yusuf S. Two decades of progress in preventing vascular disease. Lancet 2002;360:2-3.

80. El Midaoui A, Wu R, De Champlain J. Prevention of hypertension, hyperglycemia and vascular oxidative stress by aspirin treatment in chronically glucose-fed rats. J Hypertens 2002;20:1407-12.

81. Chiasson JL, Josse RG, Gomis R et al. Acarbose treatment and the risk of cardiovascular disease and hypertension in patients with impaired glucose tolerance. The STOP-NIDDM Trial. JAMA 2003;290:486-94.

82. Hanefeld M, Cagatay M, Petrowitsch T et al. Acarbose reduces the risk for myocardial infarction in type 2 diabetic patients: meta-analysis of seven long-term studies. Eur Heart J 2004;25:10-6.

83. Hanefeld M, Chiasson JL, Koehler C et al. Acarbose slows progression of intima-media thickness of the carotid arteries in subjects with impaired glucose tolerance. Stroke 2004;35:1073-8.

84. Heart Outcomes Prevention Evaluation Study Investigators. Vitamin E supplementation and cardiovascular events in high-risk patients. N Engl J Med 2000;42:154-60.

85. Bowry VW, Ingold KU, Stocker R. Vitamin E in human low-density lipoprotein. When and how this antioxidant becomes a pro-oxidant. Biochem J 1992;288:341-4.

86. Levine GN, Frei B, Koulouris SN et al. Ascorbic acid reverses endothelial vasomotor dysfunction in patients with coronary artery disease. Circulation 1996;93:1107-13.

87. Gokce N, Keaney JF, Jr., Frei B et al. Long-term ascorbic acid administration reverses endothelial vasomotor dysfunction in patients with coronary artery disease. Circulation 1999;99:3234-40.

Chapter 17

ANTI-INFLAMMATORY AND ANTIOXIDANT FUNCTIONS OF HIGH DENSITY LIPOPROTEINS

Ryan E. Moore and Daniel J. Rader
The Institute for Translational Medicine and Experimental Therapeutics and the Cardiovascular Institute, University of Pennsylvania School of Medicine

Initiation and progression of atherosclerosis

Most hypotheses proposed to explain the development of atherosclerosis include low-density lipoproteins (LDL) (and other atherogenic lipoproteins) entering the sub-intimal space, macrophage uptake of LDL leading to the formation of foam cells, and an important role for oxidation of LDL and inflammation. There is agreement that a certain level of serum LDL (or other atherogenic lipoproteins) is an absolute requirement for the development of atherosclerosis. There is also agreement that LDL and macrophages must enter the sub-intimal space as an early step in the development of atherosclerosis. There is agreement that inflammation, entry of LDL to within the subendothelial space, retention of LDL within the subendothelial space, and oxidation of LDL all occur early in the development of a lesion, though uncertainty remains regarding the exact sequence of these events. There is also agreement that macrophages within the subendothelial space must ingest LDL that has in some way been modified, whether by oxidation, aggregation or other processes, leading to the generation of cholesterol overloaded foam cells as the principle cell type present in an early lesion. At this point, a chronic inflammatory process may be initiated that further promotes LDL entry, retention, and oxidation within the subendothelial space, as well as monocyte/macrophage, T-cell, and vascular smooth muscle cell (SMC) entry to within the subendothelial space. Interaction of these cells with each other, with endothelial cells, and with LDL begets further inflammation and a vicious cycle resulting in sustained expansion of the developing lesion.

The oxidation hypothesis of atherosclerosis

By the 1970s, the fact that LDL is atherogenic was well established, as was the fact that macrophages are the cell type that gives rise to foam cells. However, investigators struggled to demonstrate that LDL was atherogenic *in vitro,* namely it did not support foam cell formation when incubated with macrophages[1,2]. In the search for a mechanistic link between LDL and foam cell formation, Brown, Goldstein and colleagues observed that acetylation of LDL leads to extensive macrophage cholesterol uptake and foam cell formation[3]. This process of oxidized LDL uptake was later shown to be mediated by scavenger receptors present on macrophages[4]. Brown and Goldstein acknowledged that there was no known means by which LDL was acetylated *in vivo* and went on to speculate that other, yet unknown, modifications of LDL could facilitate its recognition by the same receptor responsible for the uptake of acetyl-LDL[2]. It was later demonstrated that incubation of LDL with endothelial cells resulted in its conversion to a form that could be taken up by macrophages[5].

Offering an explanation for the observation that LDL incubated with cells resulted in its conversion to a form that could be taken up by macrophages to support foam cell formation, Steinberg, Witztum and colleagues proposed the oxidative modification hypothesis of atherosclerosis which stated that oxidation represents a biological modification of LDL analogous to the chemical modifications described by Brown and Goldstein[6]. The hypothesis holds that LDL in its native state is not atherogenic, and that it becomes atherogenic only after oxidative modification. It is believed that as LDL transverses the subendothelial space of lesion-prone arterial sites, LDL lipids are subject to oxidation, and as a consequence, apolipoprotein B (apoB) lysine residues are modified so that the net negative charge of the particle increases[7]. This modification of apoB renders LDL susceptible to macrophage uptake via scavenger pathways allowing for the formation of cholesterol ester-laden foam cells[8].

Vascular reactive oxygen species (ROS) and generation of Ox-LDL

Cells within the vessel wall, including endothelial cells, SMCs, and fibroblasts are capable of producing ROS that are capable of directly or indirectly participating in nonenzymatic oxidation reactions with LDL. Superoxide ($O_2^-\cdot$) is believed to be a key molecule because many other ROS are formed as a consequence of reactions involving superoxide[9]. NADPH oxidase exhibits low basal activity for superoxide ($O_2^-\cdot$) generation in vascular cells[10] that can be induced by various inflammatory stimuli as well as mechanical forces such as sheer stress[11]. Lesion monocytes and macrophages can also be activated to generate high levels of superoxide via the NADPH oxidase system[12]. Endothelial cell xanthine oxidase produces superoxide and can be induced by oscillatory sheer stress[13]. Superoxide is also produced in cells as a consequence of mitochondrial respiration[14]. Nitric oxide synthase (NOS) produces nitric oxide (NO·) which has a number of anti-atherogenic effects including the inhibition of platelet adherence and aggregation, leukocyte adhesion and infiltration, vascular SMC proliferation, and oxidative modification of LDL[15]. However, NOS can become uncoupled resulting in production of superoxide[16]. In addition, NO· reacts readily with superoxide, leading to the formation of the potent oxidant, peroxynitrite (ONOO⁻)[2,9,17-19]. Transition metals are also known to be strong catalysts of oxidation reactions[2]. The heme-containing enzyme myeloperoxidase is capable of generating the potent oxidant, hypochlorous acid (HOCL), as well as other secondary oxidation products that are capable of oxidizing LDL[20]. Lipoxygenases are non-heme iron-containing dioxygenases that catalyze the insertion of molecular oxygen into free and esterified polyunsaturated fatty acids resulting in their oxidation to fatty acid hydroperoxides[2,21]. Lipoxygenases are therefore able to directly oxidize LDL phospholipids that contain an unsaturated fatty acid in the sn2 position. In addition, lipoxygenases can generate oxidants including lipid peroxyl radical (LOO·)[22] that may participate in nonenzymatic lipid peroxidation of LDL phospholipids[23-25].

Fatty acid hydroperoxides have been proposed to play an important role in the formation of oxidized phospholipids in LDL[26]. In a model proposed by Navab and colleagues (*figure 1*)[27,28], the first step in the oxidation of LDL is that LDL is "seeded" with ROS before it can be oxidized. These reactive species are believed to include fatty acid hydroperoxides that are formed through the lipoxygenase pathway, and other lipid hydroperoxides, including fatty acid hydroperoxides, that are formed through nonenzymatic reactions with other vascular ROS. Once LDL becomes trapped within the subendothelial space, it receives additional reactive seeding molecules formed through both lipoxygenase and nonenzymatic pathways. Finally, once LDL acquires a threshold amount of lipid hydroperoxides, 1-palmitoyl-2-arachidonoyl-sn-glycero-3-phosphorylcholine (PAPC) can become oxidized leading to the formation ox-PAPC and a form of LDL that is known as "minimally modified LDL" (mmLDL; *figure 2*)[26]. Minimally modified LDL is characterized by the presence of biologically active PAPC-derived oxidized phospholipids such as 1-palmitoyl-2-oxovaleryl-sn-glycero-3-phosphorylcholine (POVPC), 1-palmitoyl-2-gluraryl-sn-glycero-3-phosphorylcholine (PGPC), and 1-palmitoyl-2-(5,6 epoxyisoprostane E2)-sn-glycero-3-phosphorylcholine (PEIPC)[29-36] in the absence of significant modification of apoB. Unlike the more extensively oxidized LDL initially described by Steinberg and Witztum, minimally modified LDL retains its ability to be taken up by the LDL receptor and is not taken up by scavenger receptors.

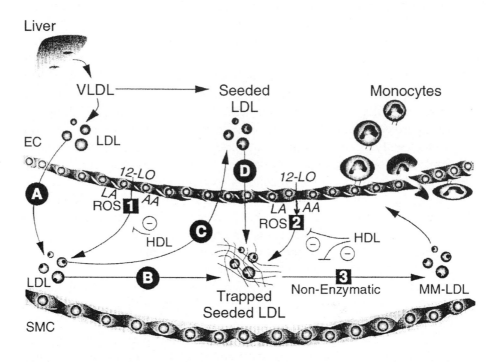

Figure 1. **A three-step model for LDL oxidation by artery wall cells:** Step 1: LDL is seeded. Step 2: LDL is trapped in the artery wall and receives further seeding molecules. Step 3: When a critical level of seeding molecules relative to phospholipids is reached in the LDL, a nonenzymatic oxidation process generates POVPC, PGPC, and PEIPC. LDL that is formed from the hydrolysis of VLDL in the circulation may contain seeding molecules. Alternatively, LDL may enter the subendothelial space (A), where it is seeded with ROS delivered from the artery wall cells (likely by the action of 12-lipoxygenase (12-LO) on linoleic (LA) and arachidonic (AA) acids (step 1). While the diagram depicts this as occurring in the subendothelial space, step one might actually occur in the microcirculation. If the LDL is seeded in the subendothelial space it might remain there, becoming trapped in the extracellular matrix (B), or the seeded LDL could exit into the circulation (C) and reenter the subendothelial space at another site, where it would become trapped in the extracellular matrix (D). In step 2, the artery wall cells generate and transfer additional or different ROS to the trapped seeded LDL. This transfer could occur within the cell, at the cell surface, or in an adjacent protected microdomain. After this transfer of ROS to the seeded and trapped LDL, a nonenzymatic propagation of lipid oxidation occurs (step 3). This results in the formation of specific oxidized phospholipids that induce NF-kB activation, monocyte binding, MCP-1 production, and M-CSF production and that are present in mildly oxidized LDL (minimally modified LDL; MM-LDL). As indicated, normal high-density lipoproteins (HDL) is capable of blocking each and every step in the formation of MM-LDL. From reference[27].

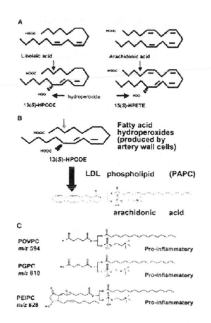

Figure 2. A: The formation of the fatty acid hydroperoxides 13-hydroperoxyoctadecadienoic acid (HPODE) and 15-hydroperoxyeicosatetraenoic acid (HPETE). B: The action of HPODE on an LDL-derived phospholipid, 1-palmitoyl-2-arachidonoyl-sn-glycero-3-phosphorylcholine (PAPC). C: Three of the proinflammatory oxidized phospholipids in minimally modified LDL. POVPC, 1-palmitoyl-2-oxovaleryl-sn-glycero-3-phosphorylcholine; PGPC, 1-palmitoyl-2-glutaryl-sn-glycero-3-phosphorylcholine; PEIPC, 1-palmitoyl-2-(5,6-epoxyisoprostane E2)-sn-glycero-3-phosphorylcholine. From reference[26].

Atherogenic properties of mmLDL and oxLDL

Minimally modified LDL has been demonstrated to exhibit a number of properties that promote the development of atherosclerosis. Minimally modified LDL induces aortic endothelial cells to produce monocyte chemoattractant protein-1 (MCP-1), macrophage colony-stimulating factor (M-CSF), and interleukin-8 (Il-8) which are pro-inflammatory, pro-atherogenic mediators, and also stimulate aortic endothelial cells to bind monocytes[37-43]. A recent study has demonstrated that administration of LDL that contains ox-PAPC to mice induces MCP-1, keratinocyte-derived chemokine (KC), tissue factor (TF), interleukin-6 (IL-6), heme oxygenase 1 (HO-1), and early growth response 1 (EGR-1) *in vivo*[44]. The same study demonstrated that oxidized phospholipids triggered rolling and firm adhesion of monocytes in a P-selectin and KC-dependent manner[44].

Specific molecular species present in minimally modified LDL such as POVPC, PGPC, and PEIPC have been shown to be responsible for some of the biological activity of minimally modified LDL. Direct measurement of these specific oxidized phospholipids has suggested that they exist at concentrations that would be biologically active *in vivo*[31].

In addition to the effects of minimally modified LDL that contains only oxidized phospholipids, LDL that has been further oxidized leading to modification of apoB, (and which still also contains oxidized phospholipids), has been demonstrated to induce expression of cell adhesion molecules such as vascular cell adhesion molecule-1 (VCAM-1) and intercellular adhesion molecule-1 (ICAM-1)[45,46], to be directly chemotactic for monocytes, macrophages and T-cells[47,48], and to upregulate the expression of scavenger receptors on macrophages[49]. Oxidative modification of LDL has also been shown to increase the ability of LDL to bind to the extracellular matrix[50]. Therefore, oxidation of LDL plays an important role not only in allowing LDL to be taken up by macrophages leading to the formation of foam cells, but also in promoting entry of monocytes/macrophages to the sub-intimal space where the process of LDL uptake occurs. Additional pro-atherogenic effects of oxidized LDL are summarized in *table 1*.

Table 1. **Potential proatherogenic activities of oxidized LDL**

Supports macrophage foam cell formation.

Chemotactic for monocytes and T cells and chemostatic for tissue macrophages.

Cytotoxic and can induce apoptosis.

Mitogenic for smooth muscle cells and macrophages.

Alters inflammatory gene expression in vascular cells.

Increases expression of macrophage scavenger receptors.

Is immunogenic and elicits autoantibody formation and activated T cells.

Undergoes aggregation, which independently leads to enhanced uptake.

A substrate for sphingomyelinase.

Induces tissue factor expression and platelet aggregation.

Impairs NO bioavailability and bioactivity.

Binds C-reactive protein activating the complement pathway.

From reference[2].

Plasma high-density lipoprotein (HDL) and apoA-I levels are inversely associated with atherosclerosis

Much of the early epidemiological research conducted in support of the lipid hypothesis of atherosclerosis sought to establish a link between total serum cholesterol levels, and/or LDL cholesterol levels and coronary disease (CAD). The fact that increased levels of LDL result in increased risk of CAD was conclusively established. Yet in addition to demonstrating the positive relationship between LDL cholesterol and CAD, investigators came also to appreciate that there may be an inverse relationship between HDL cholesterol levels and CAD. Starting in the 1970s and 1980s, a number of case-control and prospective epidemiological studies have shown that there is an independent and inverse relationship between circulating HDL cholesterol levels and CAD[51-60]. It has been calculated that for every one mg/dL increase in the amount of circulating HDL cholesterol there is a 2-3% decrease in the risk of CAD[61,62]. A similar inverse relationship has been demonstrated between the plasma level of apolipoprotein A-I (apoA-I), the primary protein component of HDL, and CAD[63-70]. ApoA-I has been identified as a risk factor for CAD, independent of HDL cholesterol[71]. A number of studies have identified apoA-I to be as good as or better than HDL cholesterol as a predictor of CAD[70-74].

With the establishment of animal models, investigators have been able to investigate the roles of HDL and apoA-I in atherosclerosis in ways not possible in humans. A number of studies have employed strategies to increase the levels of HDL and apoA-I. Studies in cholesterol-fed rabbits involving repeated injections of either HDL[75] or apoA-I[76] have demonstrated inhibition of progression or even regression of atherosclerotic lesions. Several studies of hepatic overexpression of apoA-I in mice have also demonstrated inhibition of progression or regression of atherosclerotic lesions. Human apoA-I transgenic mice have reduced lesion progression compared to non-transgenic mice: fed a high-fat, high-cholesterol diet on a wild-type background[77], on an apoE knockout background[78,79], and in mice that overexpress human apo(a), a pro-atherogenic apolipoprotein distinct from apoA-I[80]. In addition, somatic adenovirus-mediated hepatic gene transfer of human apoA-I resulted in inhibition of atherosclerosis progression in apoE knockout mice[81], and regression of preexisting lesions in LDL receptor knockout mice[82]. Expression of apoA-I in macrophages has also been demonstrated to inhibit atherosclerosis progression[83-85]. Conversely, apoA-I deficiency has been shown to result in markedly increased atherosclerosis and increased oxidized phospholipids in the plasma of LDL-receptor deficient mice fed a chow diet[86]. ApoA-I has also been demonstrated to result in increased atherosclerosis in human apoB transgenic mice fed a high-fat, high-cholesterol diet[87,88].

HDL structure and metabolism

HDL are heterogeneous, differing in size, density, and protein composition. It has been suggested that different HDL sub-populations may have important differences in function. Like all lipoproteins, mature HDL has a hydrophobic core of cholesteryl ester and triglyceride surrounded by polar phospholipids and apolipoproteins[89,90]. Unesterified cholesterol distributes between the surface of the particle and the particle core[89]. ApoA-I is the most abundant apolipoprotein on HDL, followed by apoA-II, with apoA-IV, apoC's, apoE and apoJ being found in low amounts[89,90]. Additional proteins that have enzyme activity can also be found associated with HDL, including lecithin-cholesterol aclytransferase (LCAT), cholesterol ester transfer protein (CETP), phospholipid transfer protein (PLTP), paraoxonase-1 (PON-1), platelet-activating factor acetylhydrolase (PAF-AH), and possibly others[89,90]. Factors that affect the lipid composition of the HDL particle determine both the size and density[89,90]. Using ultracentrifugation, human HDL can be isolated and separated into a large, more buoyant HDL_2 fraction (d=1.063-1.0125 g/ml), and smaller, more dense HDL_3 fraction (d=1.0125-1.250 g/ml). When subjected to electrophoresis, both HDL_2 and HDL_3 exhibit α-electrophoretic mobility[89,90]. Less well characterized by ultracentrifugation, but representing the apoA-I found at a density greater than 1.250 g/ml is a smaller particle that is referred to as lipid-poor apoA-I, nascent HDL, or preβ–HDL. As the name implies, these apoA-I containing particles exhibit preβ-electrophoretic mobility[89,90]. Preβ–HDL usually contain apoA-I in association with a few phospholipid molecules; however in some cases, preβ–HDL may contain only apoA-I[89,90]. Apolipoprotein A-I is synthesized and secreted by both the liver and intestine[90]. The current paradigm (*figure 3*) is that nascent apoA-I interacts with peripheral cells to acquire phospholipids and cholesterol through an active transport process that is mediated by the cellular protein ATP-binding cassette transporter A1 (ABCA1)[90]. Within the HDL particle, unesterified cholesterol can be esterified to cholesteryl ester through the addition of a fatty acid to the cholesterol molecule through the action of the HDL associated enzyme LCAT, leading to the formation of a mature HDL_3 particle[90]. Further acquisition of cholesterol and its esterification results in the formation of the larger HDL_2 particle. HDL cholesteryl ester can be taken up selectively by scavenger receptor class B type I (SR-BI) in the liver or can be transferred to apoB containing lipoproteins in exchange for triglyceride through the action of CETP. Conversely, PLTP can transfer phospholipids from apoB containing lipoproteins to HDL[90].

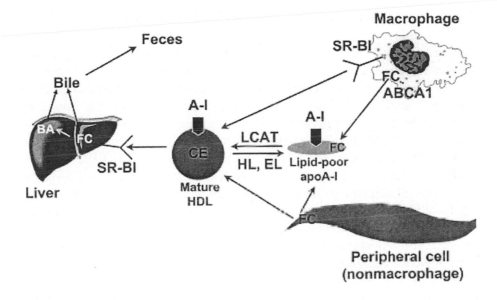

Figure 3. **High-density lipoprotein (HDL) and reverse cholesterol transport.** Peripheral cells, both macrophages and non-macrophages, must efflux excess free cholesterol (FC) to acceptors in the extracellular environment. Lipid-poor apolipoprotein A-I (A-1) interacts with peripheral cells and acquires FC and phospholipid (PC) through a transport process facilitated by the cellular protein adenosine triphosphate–binding cassette protein A1 (ABCA1). Mature HDL can also acquire cholesterol from macrophages via the scavenger receptor class BI (SR-BI). Unesterified cholesterol in HDL is converted to cholesteryl ester (CE) within the HDL particle by the enzyme lecithin cholesterol acyltransferase (LCAT). HDL cholesterol can be taken up selectively by the liver through the action of SR-BI. The liver secretes free cholesterol directly into the bile or converts it into bile acids (BA), which are then secreted into the bile. Ultimately, biliary sterols are excreted in the feces. HDL CE can also be selectively transferred to apolipoprotein B–containing lipoproteins in exchange for triglyceride through the action of CE transfer protein (CETP) (not shown). Hepatic lipase (HL) and endothelial lipase (EL) hydrolyze HDL lipids, generating smaller HDL particles and promoting their catabolism. From reference[90].

In addition to the lipid transfer proteins described above, HDL is also remodeled by lipases such as hepatic lipase (HL), endothelial lipase (EL), and others[90]. Hepatic lipase converts larger HDL$_2$ particles to smaller HDL$_3$ particles through hydrolysis of triglyceride and phospholipid[91]. Overexpression of hepatic lipase results in reduced levels of HDL cholesterol in the plasma whereas hepatic lipase deficiency results in increased HDL[90]. Endothelial lipase also has the ability to hydrolyze triglycerides[92] and is particularly efficient in hydrolyzing phospholipids[93]. Overexpression of endothelial lipase results in reduction of HDL particle size and/or formation of delipidated HDL, as well as a drastic reduction of plasma HDL cholesterol levels[94].

HDL and apoA-I participate in reverse cholesterol transport

One of the primary mechanisms by which HDL and apoA-I are believed to inhibit atherosclerosis is through their participation in a process known as reverse cholesterol transport, whereby excess cholesterol is transported from peripheral cells, including lesion macrophages, back to the liver for excretion in the bile (*figure 3*)[95-98]. A key feature of the atherosclerotic lesion is the presence of cholesterol overloaded macrophages. As the macrophage continues to ingest oxidized or modified LDL through scavenger receptors, it eventually becomes cholesterol overloaded resulting in the pro-inflammatory, pro-atherogenic foam cell phenotype. The crucial nature of macrophage cholesterol overloading is highlighted by the fact that macrophages from mice lacking scavenger receptors are protected from cholesterol overloading, which results in the mice being protected from the development of atherosclerosis[99-101]. Therefore, removal of excess cholesterol from lesion macrophages by apoA-I and HDL has the potential to reverse the process of foam cell formation and is considered to be anti-atherogenic.

Antioxidant mechanisms of atheroprotection by HDL and apoA-I

In addition to participating in reverse cholesterol transport, HDL and apoA-I are believed to inhibit atherosclerosis through inhibition of oxidation and/or removal and destruction of pro-inflammatory/pro-atherogenic products of oxidation. A number of studies have demonstrated a variety of mechanisms whereby HDL and apoA-I counteract the effects of oxidation. HDL has been shown to inhibit the oxidation of LDL by transition metals in cell free systems[102-105]. ApoA-I has also been demonstrated to reduce peroxides of phospholipids and cholesterol to the corresponding hydroxide through the oxidation of its own methionine residues at positions 112 and 148[106]. The fact that oxidized methionine (Met(O)) formed in proteins can be reduced by peptide Met(O) reductase[107-109] raises the possibility that apoA-I could act as a redox-cycling "active site" in a pseudo-enzymatic way, providing a peroxidase-like activity[106]. The implied reduction of HDL lipid hydroperoxides to lipid hydroxides by the proposed 2-electron reaction (*figure 4*) would represent an antioxidant defense, as it prevents the participation of lipid hydroperoxides (LOOH) in secondary radical or other potentially damaging reactions[106].

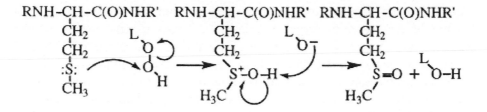

Figure 4. Proposed mechanism for the reduction of HDL-associated LOOH by human apoAI and apoAII. HDL's LOOH are reduced to the corresponding lipid hydroxides (LOH) via direct 2-electron transfer from the sulfide of thioethers of the oxidation-prone Met112 and Met148 residues of human apoAI and Met26 of apoAII, resulting in formation of their respective Met(O). From reference[106].

In an attempt to establish a physiologic assay to assess the roles of HDL and apoA-I in oxidation of LDL, Navab and colleagues developed a system in which LDL is incubated with co-cultures of freshly isolated human aortic endothelial cells and human aortic SMCs resulting in oxidization of LDL. Following incubation with the cells, LDL is removed and lipid hydroperoxides in the LDL are measured. Fresh media that does not contain lipoproteins is then added to the cells, which continue to produce MCP-1 in response to their prior exposure to oxidized LDL, resulting in the appearance of monocyte chemotactic activity in the media[27,28]. Therefore, monocyte chemotactic activity in the media can be used as an index of LDL oxidation by artery wall cells.

Using this system, HDL and apoA-I were shown to inhibit 12-lipoxygenase mediated formation of lipid hydroperoxides ("seeding molecules") in LDL, which are capable of carrying out non-enzymatic oxidation of lipoprotein phospholipids[27,28]. In addition, incubation of freshly isolated LDL with apoA-I was shown to result in transference of lipid hydroperoxides from the LDL to apoA-I, rendering the LDL resistant to oxidation by the artery wall cells[27,28]. However, if the lipids that were transferred from LDL to apoA-I during the pre-incubation were isolated from apoA-I via a lipid extraction and added back to the LDL, the LDL again became susceptible to oxidation by the artery wall cells[27,28]. Similar results were obtained when LDL was isolated from mice or humans six hours after intravenous administration of apoA-I. Whereas LDL from saline or apoA-II treated mice or saline treated humans was oxidized by the artery wall cells resulting in significant monocyte migration, LDL from apoA-I treated mice or humans was significantly less susceptible to oxidation by the cells and induced significantly less monocyte migration[27,28]. Interestingly, pre-incubation of the artery wall cells with either HDL or apoA-I also rendered the cells unable to oxidize freshly isolated LDL, implying that HDL and apoA-I have the ability to remove reactive seeding molecules from both LDL, the target of oxidation, as well as from the artery wall cells, a source of the reactive oxygen species[27,28]. Taken together, these results suggest that a significant component of the antioxidant effects of HDL and apoA-I may be rooted in their ability to transport reactive lipids.

It has been suggested that other HDL associated proteins besides apoA-I, such as PON-1, PAF-AH, LCAT, and possibly others mediate antioxidant effects[26,89,110]. Rather than the prevention of oxidation, the antioxidant effects of PON-1, PAF-AH and LCAT are believed to be related to the ability of these enzymes to hydrolyze oxidized phospholipids thereby leading to their destruction[111]. All three enzymes are almost completely HDL-associated in mice. In humans, PON-1 and LCAT are also HDL-associated, while the majority of PAF-AH present in humans is associated with LDL[111,112].

PAF-AH is a serine esterase that was initially characterized in its role to hydrolyze the pro-inflammatory phospholipid, platelet activating factor (PAF)[113-115]. PAF-AH has also been demonstrated to hydrolyze oxidized phospholipids with short acyl groups (less than six carbons) at the sn2 position without affecting the non-oxidized parent compounds[111,115-119]. HPLC analysis was able to demonstrate that active oxidized phospholipid species present in minimally modified LDL were destroyed after PAF-AH treatment, which also eliminated the ability of minimally modified LDL to induce endothelial cells to bind monocytes[120]. In addition, the ability of HDL to prevent the formation of minimally modified LDL was lost when the HDL was pre-incubated with a serine esterase inhibitor that effectively inhibits PAF-AH function[120].

Like PAF-AH, PON-1 can hydrolyze a variety of oxidized phospholipids, including phosphatidylcholine isoprostane and phosphatidylcholines that contain C9 and C5 core aldehydes or acids in the sn2 position[121], yet it does not hydrolyze the non-oxidized parent compounds. ApoA-I is not required for association of PON-1 with HDL, yet the stability of PON-1 activity is increased in the presence of apoA-I[122]. Similar to studies in which a serine esterase inhibitor was added to HDL to inhibit PAF-AH activity, HDL from PON-1 knockout mice is unable to inhibit the formation of minimally oxidized LDL by artery wall cells[123]. Both HDL and LDL isolated from PON-1 knockout mice are more susceptible to oxidation by artery wall cells[123]. In addition, PON-1 knockout mice have increased levels of IDL and LDL-associated oxidized phospholipids (POVPC, PGPC, and PEIPC) *in vivo*[124]. Lipid peroxides in serum, LDL, and macrophages are also elevated in PON-1 knockout mice[125]. Supporting the concept that PON-1 antioxidant function plays a physiological role in inhibiting atherosclerosis, PON-1 deficiency results in increased atherosclerosis in the absence of any effects on plasma lipids[123,124]. Conversely, overexpression of PON-1 results in increased ability of HDL to prevent LDL from being oxidized by artery wall cells, and also results in reduced atherosclerosis[126].

Although the major function of LCAT is esterification of cholesterol within HDL, studies have suggested that LCAT may also have antioxidant and anti-inflammatory functions[127-131]. LCAT has been shown to hydrolyze PAF to lyso-PAF and acetate[127]. Oxidized phospholipids that have a short-chain at the sn2 position are structurally similar to PAF, and purified LCAT has been shown to hydrolyze oxidized phospholipids isolated from oxidized plasma[129] as well as oxidized phospholipids that were derived from oxidation of synthetic phosphatidylcholine[129]. Incubation of purified human LCAT with either LDL or palmitoyl-linoleoyl phosphatidylcholine (PLPC) was also shown to inhibit the oxidation-dependant accumulation of conjugated dienes and lipid hydroperoxides[130]. LCAT has also been shown to prevent spontaneous oxidation, copper-mediated oxidation, and lipoxygenase-catalyzed oxidation of lipids and was also shown to inhibit the increased in net negative charge that occurs during oxidation of LDL[130].

An interesting model of apoA-I/HDL antioxidant function is that apoA-I and HDL may acquire oxidized phospholipids and reactive lipid hydroperoxides from LDL and peripheral cells, thereby removing them from an area where they have pro-inflammatory effects. Then once the oxidized lipids are HDL-associated, HDL enzymes effectively hydrolyze them, leading to their destruction. Alternatively, another possibility is that HDL may bring antioxidant enzyme activity to LDL and cells, resulting in hydrolysis of oxidized phospholipids that are still associated with LDL or the cells.

Anti-inflammatory mechanisms of atheroprotection by HDL and apoA-I

ApoA-I and HDL have also been described to have a number of anti-inflammatory effects. Atherosclerosis has been described as a chronic inflammatory disorder characterized by accumulation of macrophages and T-cells within the subendothelial space associated with increased levels of inflammatory markers in the plasma[132]. The macrophages that accumulate within the lesion are derived from blood monocytes that first adhere to the endothelium before migrating to within the subendothelial space. This monocyte-endothelium interaction is mediated by cell adhesion molecules including VCAM-1, ICAM-1, E-selectin and P-selectin[133-137] that are upregulated by pro-inflammatory cytokines and oxidized LDL at the sites of developing atherosclerotic lesions[132,138]. Following adherence to the endothelium, monocyte migration into the artery wall is promoted by chemotactic factors such as oxidized LDL, as well as chemokines such as

MCP-1 that are produced by endothelial cells in response to oxidized LDL, shear stress, and vascular injury[132,139].

Oxidation of LDL converts it to a pro-atherogenic particle, which can in part be attributed to the inflammatory effects of oxidized LDL. Therefore, the antioxidant effects of HDL and apoA-I described above can also be considered to be anti-inflammatory. Interestingly, the ability of HDL and apoA-I to transport lipid hydroperoxides and possibly oxidized phospholipids away from LDL and cells, resulting in effects that are antioxidant and anti-inflammatory, may represent one common mechanism by which the lipid transport, antioxidant and anti-inflammatory properties of HDL and apoA-I are linked. Consistent with this concept are studies by Navab and colleagues demonstrating that HDL and apoA-I inhibit monocyte transmigration in response to oxidized LDL[27,28,140]. Furthermore the inhibition of monocyte migration has been shown to be promoted by the HDL associated antioxidant enzymes, PON-1 and PAF-AH[141], providing another link between HDL antioxidant and anti-inflammatory function. The ability of HDL and apoA-I to participate in macrophage reverse cholesterol transport may also have anti-inflammatory effects by reversing the pro-inflammatory foam cell phenotype.

In addition to antioxidant and reverse cholesterol transport functions of HDL and apoA-I that have indirect anti-inflammatory effects, studies have demonstrated that native HDL, apoA-I, and recombinant HDL (rHDL) can directly inhibit other aspects of the process whereby leukocytes enter the subendothelial space[132]. Both native HDL and rHDL have been shown to inhibit the cytokine-induced expression of VCAM-1, ICAM-1, and E-selectin by human umbilical vein endothelial cells in a concentration-dependent manner within the range of physiological HDL levels[132,142-145]. The inhibition of adhesion molecule expression was associated with a reduction in mRNA levels[132,142,145]. The inhibition of VCAM-1 was dependent on the duration of pre-treatment of the cells with HDL up to 16 hours prior to the addition of tumor necrosis factor alpha (TNF-α). It was not required that HDL be present at the time that the TNF-α was added to the cells for the inhibitory effect to occur, indicating that HDL was not physically blocking TNF-α from binding its receptor[146]. The inhibitory effect of pre-incubation of HDL with the cells persisted from several hours after the HDL was removed, suggesting that exposure of the cells to the HDL modifies the cells in some way to make them resistant to TNF-α - induced expression of VCAM-1[132,146]. It has been suggested that the inhibitory effect of HDL may be derived from inhibition of endothelial cell sphingosine kinase which catalyzes phosphoralyzation of sphingosine to form sphingosine-1-phosphate, which is part of the pathway by which TNF-α stimulates nuclear translocation of NF-κB to upregulate transcription of message for cell adhesion molecules[132,145].

The ability of HDL to inhibit endothelial cell adhesion protein expression has also been demonstrated *in vivo*[132]. Alternative daily infusion of rHDL containing apoA-I and phosphatidylcholine to apoE knockout mice with carotid peri-arterial collars resulted in 40% reductions in VCAM-1 expression and monocyte infiltration within one week as well as reduction in the development of neointima after three weeks[147]. In another study, a single infusion of rHDL inhibited E-selectin expression in the microvasculature after subcutaneous administration of interleukin IL-1 in pigs[148]. A recent study in normocholesterolemia, nonatherosclerotic rabbits demonstrated that intravenous administration of rHDL inhibited peri-arterial collar mediated generation of superoxide in vascular tissue. The same study also demonstrated that administration of either rHDL or lipid-free apoA-I inhibited vascular VCAM-1, ICAM-1 and MCP-1 expression in vivo[149]. However, another study in which the human apoA-I transgene was overexpressed in apoE knockout mice showed apoA-I overexpression to have no effect on endothelial VCAM-1 expression or monocyte adherence at an early lesion stage despite[150].

Other anti-inflammatory effects that have been reported for HDL and apoA-I include binding and neutralization of lipopolysaccharide (LPS), a pro-inflammatory bacterial cell wall component[151] that is an important mediator of septic shock. Infection has been linked to atherosclerosis; therefore neutralization of LPS may contribute to HDL anti-atherogenic function. ApoA-I has been shown to inhibit the T-cell contact mediated activation of monocytes to produce interleukin 1 beta (IL-1β) and TNF-α[152], which would also be predicted to be an anti-atherogenic effect. HDL has been shown to increase synthesis of prostacyclin, a vasoactive prostanoid that has vasodilatory effects and also functions to inhibits leukocyte-endothelial interactions[153]. In addition, apoA-I has been shown to increase the half life of prostacyclin[154]. Thromboxane A_2 has effects that oppose those of prostacyclin, and HDL_2 has been shown to inhibit its formation from endothelial cells in a dose dependent manner[155]. HDL has also been reported to activate endothelial nitric oxide synthase (eNOS) to promote the production of NO which, like prostacyclin, has vasodilatory effects, as well as inhibitory effects on leukocyte-endothelial interactions[156]. Anticoagulant and antiplatelet effect of HDL have also been described[89,157,158].

Increasing HDL levels and function in the treatment of atherosclerosis

There is abundant evidence both *in vitro* and in animals that supports a central role for oxidation of LDL in the pathogenesis of atherosclerosis, yet the results of trials in which humans have been administered exogenous antioxidants such as vitamin E have demonstrated either little beneficial effect[159-161] or less benefit than was hoped[162-166]. In 2004, the American Heart Association Council on Nutrition concluded that "Collectively, for the most part, clinical trials have failed to demonstrate a beneficial effect of antioxidant supplements on cardiovascular disease (CVD) morbidity and mortality"[167]. It has been argued that the apparent lack of protection afforded by antioxidant therapy may be due in part to lack of efficacy of the antioxidants used in preventing oxidation of LDL within the vessel wall[166]. In fact, most antioxidant trials to date have not made any attempt to assess the efficacy of their antioxidant regimen, making it impossible to know whether the oxidation hypothesis of atherosclerosis is irrelevant to humans, or if the antioxidants used in the human trials simply did not work[168]. By analogy, it is unimaginable that a trial for a new lipid lowering drug that is intended to reduce the risk of cardiovascular disease would be conducted without measuring plasma lipids[168]. Clearly there is a need for better understanding of oxidative mechanisms *in vivo*, better biochemical markers by which to evaluate candidate antioxidant compounds, and novel, more effective antioxidant compounds and strategies to fully test the oxidation hypothesis of atherosclerosis.

Increasing the levels and/or improving the function of HDL and apoA-I represent a promising strategy for the treatment of CVD. Increasing reverse cholesterol transport is certainly an important goal of HDL-based therapies. However, increasing the antioxidant and anti-inflammatory properties of HDL may be particularly important goals, especially considering that some HDL raising strategies may potentially inhibit reverse cholesterol transport. It has been suggested that endogenous antioxidant defense mechanisms may have greater capacity to inhibit the oxidation of LDL than exogenous antioxidant supplements[166]. It has also been suggested that exogenous antioxidants may not reach high enough concentrations in vascular tissue to be effective[166]. Another potential advantage of endogenous antioxidants is that they may have better access to vascular tissues than exogenous antioxidants. There are a number of existing drugs, as well as new strategies at the forefront of development that are targeted at increasing the level of HDL and/or improving HDL function. Increasing the level of HDL or improving its antioxidant and anti-inflammatory function may therefore be a viable approach in the effort to reduce CVD.

HDL-raising strategies: current and future

Lifestyle

The current first line therapy for increasing HDL-cholesterol (HDL-C) levels is lifestyle modification. There is a clear inverse correlation between obesity and visceral adiposity with HDL-C levels[169]. Sustained weight loss is associated with an increase in HDL-C, and exercise can raise HDL-C, especially intense regular exercise and long distance running[169]. Cigarette smoking is correlated with significantly lower serum HDL-C levels[169], and smoking cessation is strongly advised for the HDL-raising effect as well as for overall cardiovascular benefit. Consumption of ethanol has also been shown to increase HDL-C levels[170-172]. In addition, a variety of other antioxidant properties have been attributed to alcohol, particularly red wine which also contains a variety of polyphenols[170]. These effects include scavenging ROS, inhibiting peroxidation of LDL, and others[170]. The apparent health benefits of alcohol consumption are maximal when consumption is moderate, one to two drinks per day[173]. With higher levels of alcohol consumption in the range of three to five drinks per day, the health benefits are lost or potentially counteracted by other adverse health effects[173]. Higher alcohol consumption clearly has negative health effects that outweigh any potential benefits[173].

Fibrates

Fibrates, which are agonists of peroxisome proliferator-activated receptor-α (PPAR-α), can raise HDL-C by 10-20%[174]. The HDL effect is dependent in part on triglyceride levels. In the Helsinki Heart Study, a primary prevention trial of gemfibrozil in dyslipidemic middle-aged men, there was an 11% increase in HDL-C levels and significant reduction in major CAD events, especially in the subgroup of patients with elevated triglycerides[175]. An 18% increase in HDL-C levels was also observed in the Bezafibrate Infarction Prevention Study[176]. In the Veterans Affairs HDL Intervention Trial there was a modest 6% increase in HDL-C that was associated with a significant 22% reduction in events[177]. The effects of fibrate-mediated PPAR-α activation that may be responsible for increasing HDL levels include increased hepatic synthesis of apoA-I[178,179], hepatic down regulation of SR-BI expression[180], and increased lipoprotein lipase expression.

Niacin

The effect of niacin is slightly greater than fibrates or statins and has been shown to result in about a 15-30% increase in HDL-C levels[174]. The exact HDL-raising mechanism of niacin has not yet been fully elucidated[181]. However, it is currently the most potent HDL-raising therapy available, and its use is rising, especially the combination of an extended-release preparation with statins. In the HDL Atherosclerosis Treatment Study (HATS), this combination proved to be safe as well as effective in increasing HDL by 26% and reducing both clinical events and in slowing angiographic progression of CAD[182,183]. Niacin in combination with fibrates has been proven to reduce cardiovascular mortality and is generally considered safe[184]. In a recently published randomized controlled trial of the sequential addition of gemfibrozil plus short acting niacin plus cholestyramine compared with placebo, there was a 36% increase in HDL-C, significant decrease in coronary stenosis, and a nonsignificant decrease cardiovascular outcomes[185]. In addition to its lipid effects, *in vitro* studies have suggested that niacin may have other anti-atherogenic effects[181,186]. It has been suggested that niacin may exhibit antioxidant and anti-inflammatory effects by preventing copper-induced and endothelial cell-mediated oxidation of LDL, and may also prevent the TNF-α- induced transcription of VCAM-1 and MCP-1[181].

Specific PPAR- alpha, delta, and gamma agonists

In addition to fibrates, a number of selective, potent PPAR-α agonists have recently been reported, some of which are in clinical trails[187-191]. Agonists of PPAR-γ, the thiazolidinediones, have primarily been used to improve insulin sensitivity in type II diabetes. In this patient population, they have been shown to exhibit a modest effect on HDL-C, with an average HDL-C elevation around 10%[192]. Studies have not yet been conducted to investigate if the HDL-C raising effect of PPAR-γ agonists will translate into improved clinical cardiovascular outcomes. There are also several dual PPAR-α/ PPAR-γ agonists in clinical trials, including muraglitazar, tesaglitazar, and naveglitazar. Other similar compounds have showed promising results, however, trials have been discontinued because of adverse preclinical findings in rodents[191]. Ragaglitazar, demonstrated beneficial effects on both insulin sensitivity and lipids and was well-tolerated by patients[193,194]. Therapy with dual PPAR agonists is currently intended for type 2 diabetics with atherogenic dyslipidemia.

In addition to their effects on HDL, it has been suggested that both PPAR-α and PPAR-γ agonists may exert anti-inflammatory effects[195,196], including inhibition of NF-κB signaling and suppression of the secretion of pro-inflammatory cytokines. In addition PPAR-γ activators have been shown to inhibit expression of VCAM-1 and ICAM-1 in activated endothelial cells and significantly reduce monocyte/macrophage homing to atherosclerotic plaques[197]. PPAR-γ agonists have also been shown to inhibit MCP-1 stimulated migration of monocytes[198], likely through down regulation of CCR2, the receptor for MCP-1[199].

Cholesteryl ester transfer protein (CETP) inhibitors

Observational studies have demonstrated that certain lifestyle factors are associated with plasma CETP levels. For example, alcohol and physical exercise, which are known to increase HDL-C, are associated with decreased CETP concentration; in contrast, smoking, which decreases HDL-C, is associated with elevated CETP activity[200]. In a recent nested case-control study among participants of the prospective European Prospective Investigation into Cancer and Nutrition-Norfolk (EPIC-Norfolk) cohort study, healthy individuals were followed for an average of six years for the development of CAD in relation to CETP levels[201]. Overall, the risk of CAD increased with increasing CETP quintiles, reaching statistical significance for the highest quintile[201]. CETP levels were also significantly correlated with lower levels of HDL-C and increased levels of total cholesterol and LDL-C[201]. The findings support the concept that CETP inhibition could reduce CAD risk[202].

Two small molecule-inhibitors of CETP have been studied in humans to date, JTT-705 and torcetrapib. In a randomized, double-blind, placebo-controlled trial of the efficacy and safety of JTT-705 in healthy subjects, treatment with 900mg of JTT-705 for four weeks led to a 37% decrease in CETP activity, a 34% increase in HDL-C, and increased levels of apoA-I[200]. In a phase I multidose study of torcetrapib, increases in HDL-C were seen, with up to 91% increase in HDL-C at the maximal dose of 120 mg twice daily[203]. A four week, single-blind, placebo-controlled crossover study of torcetrapib in a small group of patients with HDL-C levels <40 mg/dL, in which a subset were also treated with atorvastatin, showed increases in HDL concentrations by 46% with torcetrapib 120 mg daily and by 61% in the combination treatment group[204]. Treatment with torcetrapib 120mg twice daily increased HDL-C by 106%[204]. ApoA-I levels were increased by 13% in the twice daily treatment group[204]. A shift in distribution of particle size was also seen, with a shift towards increased mean HDL and LDL particle sizes[204]. There is still uncertainty as to the effect of CETP inhibition will have on atherosclerotic disease, and it may be particularly dependent on the balance between HDL reverse cholesterol transport, antioxidant and anti-inflammatory effects. The effects of CETP inhibition on inflammation, thrombosis, endothelial function, and oxidation also warrant intensive study[205].

Infusion of apoA-I Milano

In humans, a single amino acid substitution in apoA-I causes a variant of apolipoprotein A-I known as apoA-I Milano that was discovered in Northern Italy[206]. Individuals with this mutation are characterized by very low HDL-C but do not have increased risk of atherosclerosis[206,207]. ApoA-I Milano has faster catabolism than normal apoA-I, explaining the accompanying low HDL[206]. In addition, it may have properties that are more atheroprotective than wild-type apoA-I, although the two have not been extensively directly compared[206].

In a human trial, a recombinant apoA-I Milano/phospholipid complex infusion was studied in patients with acute coronary syndrome for effect on coronary atherosclerosis as measured by intravascular ultrasound[208]. In this small double-blind placebo-controlled trial, patients who received the five weekly infusions of ApoA-I Milano/phospholipids complex had a significant regression in total atheroma volume of 4.2% from baseline[208]. There was a non significant increase in the mean percent atheroma volume in the placebo group[208]. This study is the best example to date that directly targeting HDL-C may have an impact on atherosclerosis in humans and a relatively rapid effect at that, despite limitations of the study[206].

ApoA-I mimetic peptides

Other apoA-I based therapeutics are in clinical development, including synthetic peptides that can mimic apoA-I in promoting cholesterol efflux from macrophages as well as other antioxidant and anti-inflammatory effects[209]. Most such peptides must be administered intravenously. However, D-4F is an apoA-I mimetic peptide that is synthesized from amino acids with d-sterochemistry (as opposed to endogenous amino acids with l-sterochemistry) resulting in resistance to proteolysis in the gastro-intestinal (GI) tract and oral bioavailability[209]. D-4F is based on the apoA-I mimetic peptide 4F that contains 18 amino acids and was designed to contain a class A amphipathic helix, with a polar and a nonpolar face, and positively charged residues at the polar-nonpolar interface and negatively charged residues at the center of the polar face, providing a structure that allows it to bind lipids similar to apoA-I[209]. Oral administration of D-4F does not result in increased levels of HDL-C, yet D-4F has been shown in mice to promote the formation of preß-HDL with increased paraoxonase activity. Treatment with D-4F also increases the ability of HDL to inhibit oxidation of LDL by artery wall cells. Treatment of mice and monkeys with D-4F reduces VLDL, LDL and HDL associated lipid hydroperoxides *in vivo*, rendering LDL less susceptible to oxidation by artery wall cells and converting HDL from a form that is pro-inflammatory form to a form that is anti-inflammatory[209]. D-4F has been shown to dramatically reduce atherosclerosis in mice[209]. D-

4F also promotes macrophage cholesterol efflux and reverse cholesterol transport *in vivo*[209]. D-4F is an excellent example of a HDL based therapy that has the potential to improve HDL antioxidant, anti-inflammatory, as well as reverse cholesterol transport function.

Statins: cholesterol reduction accompanied by possible antioxidant and anti-inflammatory effects

Statins represent the first line in primary and secondary prevention of CAD. The effectiveness of statins in preventing vascular disease is attributed primarily to their significant LDL-lowering effects and modest HDL-raising effects. On average, statins can raise HDL-C by 5-10%[174]. The mechanism for statin-induced increases in HDL-C is probably in part due to reduction in CETP[210]. In addition, it has been proposed that statins inhibit the Rho-signaling pathway, which in turn activates PPAR-α, thereby inducing the transcription of the apoA-I gene[61].

However it has been suggested that statins may also have other potentially atheroprotective effects beyond lowering the level of LDL and raising the level of HDL[211-213]. In the West of Scotland Coronary Prevention Study (WOSCOPS), the Scandinavian Simvastatin Survival Study (4S), and the Heart Protection Study (HPS), it was noted that clinical benefit associated with statin therapy was independent of LDL cholesterol levels[214-216]. In the secondary prevention Cholesterol and Recurrent Events (CARE) study, pravastatin significantly reduced the serum levels of c-reactive protein (CRP); however, change in LDL-cholesterol was not a significant predictor of this effect. In addition, pravastatin treatment resulted in a greater reduction of risk in subjects with higher baseline inflammatory markers than in subjects with lower baseline inflammatory markers, despite similar levels of plasma lipids in both groups[217,218]. Hypercholesterolemia results in impaired endothelial function as assessed by endothelium-dependent vasodilation[219,220] which can be reversed by LDL apheresis[221]. Studies with statins have also demonstrated restoration of endothelial function, which, in some cases, occured prior to significant reduction in serum cholesterol[222-224], suggesting that there are additional effects of statins on endothelial function beyond the effects associated with reducing serum cholesterol[225].

A number of cholesterol-independent effects of statins may potentially contribute to their ability to reduce CVD. Cholesterol-independent reduction of superoxide formation in hypercholesterolemic human subjects in response to statins has been observed[226]. Studies have demonstrated that statins have inhibitory actions on superoxide production from NAD(P)H oxidase that are independent of LDL lowering. The effect on NAD(P)H oxidase has been attributed to reduced synthesis of mevalonic acid, resulting in the prevention of isoprenylation of p21 Rac, which is critical for the assembly of NADPH oxidase after activation of protein kinase C[227,228]. It has also been suggested that statins may increase the levels of tetrahydrobiopterin that is a cofactor for eNOS, thereby preventing uncoupling of eNOS and shifting the balance toward production of NO rather than superoxide[229]. Statins have also been shown to promote eNOS function by inhibiting expression of caveolin, an inhibitor of eNOS[230,231]. Statins have been shown to increase eNOS activity via posttranslational activation of the phosphatidylinositol 3-kinase/protein kinase Akt pathway[232]. Statins have also been shown to attenuate P-selectin expression and leukocyte adhesion in normocholesterolemic animals by increasing NO in an eNOS dependent manner[233]. In cholesterol-fed rabbits, a dose of fluvastatin that was insufficient to have any effect on plasma lipids resulted in reduced susceptibility of LDL to ex vivo copper-induced oxidation, reduced vascular superoxide generation, and reduced atheromatous plaque formation, independent of any cholesterol-lowering effect[234]. Statins have also been demonstrated to increase the serum activity of paraoxonase-1[235]. Atorvastatin has been shown to reduce the formation of atherogenic[236] myeloperoxidase-derived and nitric-oxide-derived oxidants in human subjects independent of effects on plasma lipids[237]. Metabolites of atorvastatin that are formed *in vivo* have been shown to possess antioxidative potential and the ability to protect LDL, VLDL, and HDL from oxidation[238]. Fluvastatin has also been shown to directly scavenge ROS[239] and also inhibit peroxynitrite-mediated oxidation of LDL lipids and nitration of apoB[240]. Therefore, although the lipid effects of statins most likely represent the primary mechanism by which they inhibit atherosclerosis, there is significant evidence that the non lipid effects may also play an anti-atherogenic role.

References

1. Goldstein JL, Brown MS. The low-density lipoprotein pathway and its relation to atherosclerosis. Ann Rev Biochem 1977;46:897-930.

2. Stocker R, Keaney JF, Jr. Role of oxidative modifications in atherosclerosis. Physiol Rev 2004;84:1381-478.

3. Goldstein JL, Ho YK, Basu SK, Brown MS. Binding site on macrophages that mediates uptake and degradation of acetylated low density lipoprotein, producing massive cholesterol deposition. Proc Natl Acad Sci U S A 1979;76:333-7.

4. Krieger M, Acton S, Ashkenas J, Pearson A, Penman M, Resnick D. Molecular flypaper, host defense, and atherosclerosis. Structure, binding properties, and functions of macrophage scavenger receptors. J Biol Chem 1993;268:4569-72.

5. Henriksen T, Mahoney EM, Steinberg D. Enhanced macrophage degradation of low density lipoprotein previously incubated with cultured endothelial cells: recognition by receptors for acetylated low density lipoproteins. Proc Natl Acad Sci U S A 1981;78:6499-503.

6. Steinberg D, Parthasarathy S, Carew TE, Khoo JC, Witztum JL. Beyond cholesterol. Modifications of low-density lipoprotein that increase its atherogenicity. N Engl J Med 1989;320:915-24.

7. Haberland ME, Fogelman AM, Edwards PA. Specificity of receptor-mediated recognition of malondialdehyde-modified low density lipoproteins. Proc Natl Acad Sci U S A 1982;79:1712-6.

8. Haberland ME, Olch CL, Folgelman AM. Role of lysines in mediating interaction of modified low density lipoproteins with the scavenger receptor of human monocyte macrophages. J Biol Chem 1984;259:11305-11.

9. Hamilton CA, Miller WH, Al-Benna S, et al. Strategies to reduce oxidative stress in cardiovascular disease. Clin Sci (Lond) 2004;106:219-34.

10. Pagano PJ, Clark JK, Cifuentes-Pagano ME, Clark SM, Callis GM, Quinn MT. Localization of a constitutively active, phagocyte-like NADPH oxidase in rabbit aortic adventitia: enhancement by angiotensin II. Proc Natl Acad Sci U S A 1997;94:14483-8.

11. Ushio-Fukai M, Tang Y, Fukai T, et al. Novel role of gp91(phox)-containing NAD(P)H oxidase in vascular endothelial growth factor-induced signaling and angiogenesis. Circ Res 2002;91:1160-7.

12. Badwey JA, Karnovsky ML. Active oxygen species and the functions of phagocytic leukocytes. Ann Rev Biochem 1980;49:695-726.

13. McNally JS, Davis ME, Giddens DP, et al. Role of xanthine oxidoreductase and NAD(P)H oxidase in endothelial superoxide production in response to oscillatory shear stress. Am J Physiol Heart Circ Physiol 2003;285:H2290-7.

14. Chance B, Sies H, Boveris A. Hydroperoxide metabolism in mammalian organs. Physiol Rev. 1979;59:527-605.

15. Davignon J, Ganz P. Role of endothelial dysfunction in atherosclerosis. Circulation. 2004;109:III27-32.

16.   Vasquez-Vivar J, Kalyanaraman B, Martasek P, et al Superoxide generation by endothelial nitric oxide synthase: the influence of cofactors. Proc Natl Acad Sci U S A 1998;95:9220-5.

17.   Darley-Usmar VM, Hogg N, O'Leary VJ, Wilson MT, Moncada S. The simultaneous generation of superoxide and nitric oxide can initiate lipid peroxidation in human low density lipoprotein. Free Radic Res Commun 1992;17:9-20.

18.   Graham A, Hogg N, Kalyanaraman B, O'Leary V, Darley-Usmar V, Moncada S. Peroxynitrite modification of low-density lipoprotein leads to recognition by the macrophage scavenger receptor. FEBS Lett 1993;330:181-5.

19.   Hogg N, Kalyanaraman B, Joseph J, Struck A, Parthasarathy S. Inhibition of low-density lipoprotein oxidation by nitric oxide. Potential role in atherogenesis. FEBS Lett 1993;334:170-4.

20.   Kawamura M, Heinecke JW, Chait A. Increased uptake of alpha-hydroxy aldehyde-modified low density lipoprotein by macrophage scavenger receptors. J Lipid Res 2000;41:1054-9.

21.   Funk CD, Cyrus T. 12/15-lipoxygenase, oxidative modification of LDL and atherogenesis. Trends Cardiovasc Med 2001;11:116-24.

22.   Chamulitrat W, Mason RP. Lipid peroxyl radical intermediates in the peroxidation of polyunsaturated fatty acids by lipoxygenase. Direct electron spin resonance investigations. J Biol Chem 1989;264:20968-73.

23.   Neuzil J, Upston JM, Witting PK, Scott KF, Stocker R. Secretory phospholipase A2 and lipoprotein lipase enhance 15-lipoxygenase-induced enzymic and nonenzymic lipid peroxidation in low-density lipoproteins. Biochemistry 1998;37:9203-10.

24.   Upston JM, Neuzil J, Stocker R. Oxidation of LDL by recombinant human 15-lipoxygenase: evidence for alpha-tocopherol-dependent oxidation of esterified core and surface lipids. J Lipid Res 1996;37:2650-61.

25.   Upston JM, Neuzil J, Witting PK, Alleva R, Stocker R. Oxidation of free fatty acids in low density lipoprotein by 15-lipoxygenase stimulates nonenzymic, alpha-tocopherol-mediated peroxidation of cholesteryl esters. J Biol Chem 1997;272:30067-74.

26.   Navab M, Ananthramaiah GM, Reddy ST, et al. The oxidation hypothesis of atherogenesis: the role of oxidized phospholipids and HDL. J Lipid Res 2004;45:993-1007.

27.   Navab M, Hama SY, Anantharamaiah GM, et al. Normal high density lipoprotein inhibits three steps in the formation of mildly oxidized low density lipoprotein: steps 2 and 3. J Lipid Res 2000;41:1495-508.

28.   Navab M, Hama SY, Cooke CJ, et al. Normal high density lipoprotein inhibits three steps in the formation of mildly oxidized low density lipoprotein: step 1. J Lipid Res 2000;41:1481-94.

29.   Watson AD, Leitinger N, Navab M, et al. Structural identification by mass spectrometry of oxidized phospholipids in minimally oxidized low density lipoprotein that induce monocyte/endothelial interactions and evidence for their presence in vivo. J Biol Chem 1997;272:13597-607.

30. Watson AD, Subbanagounder G, Welsbie DS, et al. Structural identification of a novel pro-inflammatory epoxyisoprostane phospholipid in mildly oxidized low density lipoprotein. J Biol Chem 1999;274:24787-98.

31. Subbanagounder G, Leitinger N, Schwenke DC, et al. Determinants of bioactivity of oxidized phospholipids. Specific oxidized fatty acyl groups at the sn-2 position. Arterioscler Thromb Vasc Biol 2000;20:2248-54.

32. Subbanagounder G, Deng Y, Borromeo C, Dooley AN, Berliner JA, Salomon RG. Hydroxy alkenal phospholipids regulate inflammatory functions of endothelial cells. Vascul Pharmacol 2002;38:201-9.

33. Subbanagounder G, Wong JW, Lee H, et al. Epoxyisoprostane and epoxycyclopentenone phospholipids regulate monocyte chemotactic protein-1 and interleukin-8 synthesis. Formation of these oxidized phospholipids in response to interleukin-1beta. J Biol Chem 2002;277:7271-81.

34. Poliakov E, Brennan ML, Macpherson J, et al. Isolevuglandins, a novel class of isoprostenoid derivatives, function as integrated sensors of oxidant stress and are generated by myeloperoxidase in vivo. Faseb J 2003;17:2209-20.

35. Marathe GK, Prescott SM, Zimmerman GA, McIntyre TM. Oxidized LDL contains inflammatory PAF-like phospholipids. Trends Cardiovasc Med 2001;11:139-42.

36. Marathe GK, Zimmerman GA, Prescott SM, McIntyre TM. Activation of vascular cells by PAF-like lipids in oxidized LDL. Vascul Pharmacol 2002;38:193-200.

37. Berliner JA, Territo MC, Sevanian A, et al. Minimally modified low density lipoprotein stimulates monocyte endothelial interactions. J Clin Invest 1990;85:1260-6.

38. Cushing SD, Berliner JA, Valente AJ, et al. Minimally modified low density lipoprotein induces monocyte chemotactic protein 1 in human endothelial cells and smooth muscle cells. Proc Natl Acad Sci U S A 1990;87:5134-8.

39. Rajavashisth TB, Andalibi A, Territo MC, et al. Induction of endothelial cell expression of granulocyte and macrophage colony-stimulating factors by modified low-density lipoproteins. Nature 1990;344:254-7.

40. Schwartz D, Andalibi A, Chaverri-Almada L, et al. Role of the GRO family of chemokines in monocyte adhesion to MM-LDL-stimulated endothelium. J Clin Invest 1994;94:1968-73.

41. Liao F, Berliner JA, Mehrabian M, et al. Minimally modified low density lipoprotein is biologically active in vivo in mice. J Clin Invest 1991;87:2253-7.

42. Vora DK, Fang ZT, Liva SM, et al. Induction of P-selectin by oxidized lipoproteins. Separate effects on synthesis and surface expression. Circ Res 1997;80:810-8.

43. Cushing SD, Fogelman AM. Monocytes may amplify their recruitment into inflammatory lesions by inducing monocyte chemotactic protein. Arterioscler Thromb 1992;12:78-82.

44. Furnkranz A, Schober A, Bochkov VN, et al. Oxidized phospholipids trigger atherogenic inflammation in murine arteries. Arterioscler Thromb Vasc Biol 2005;25:633-8.

45. Khan BV, Parthasarathy SS, Alexander RW, Medford RM. Modified low density lipoprotein and its constituents augment cytokine-activated vascular cell adhesion molecule-1 gene expression in human vascular endothelial cells. J Clin Invest 1995;95:1262-70.

46. Cominacini L, Garbin U, Pasini AF, et al. Antioxidants inhibit the expression of intercellular cell adhesion molecule-1 and vascular cell adhesion molecule-1 induced by oxidized LDL on human umbilical vein endothelial cells. Free Radic Biol Med 1997;22:117-27.

47. Quinn MT, Parthasarathy S, Fong LG, Steinberg D. Oxidatively modified low density lipoproteins: a potential role in recruitment and retention of monocyte/macrophages during atherogenesis. Proc Natl Acad Sci U S A 1987;84:2995-8.

48. McMurray HF, Parthasarathy S, Steinberg D. Oxidatively modified low density lipoprotein is a chemoattractant for human T lymphocytes. J Clin Invest 1993;92:1004-8.

49. Mietus-Snyder M, Friera A, Glass CK, Pitas RE. Regulation of scavenger receptor expression in smooth muscle cells by protein kinase C: a role for oxidative stress. Arterioscler Thromb Vasc Biol 1997;17:969-78.

50. Wang X, Greilberger J, Ratschek M, Jurgens G. Oxidative modifications of LDL increase its binding to extracellular matrix from human aortic intima: influence of lesion development, lipoprotein lipase and calcium. J Pathol 2001;195:244-50.

51. Miller GJ. High density lipoproteins and atherosclerosis. Ann Rev Med 1980;31:97-108.

52. Miller GJ, Miller NE. Plasma-high-density-lipoprotein concentration and development of ischaemic heart-disease. Lancet 1975;1:16-9.

53. Miller NE. Associations of high-density lipoprotein subclasses and apolipoproteins with ischemic heart disease and coronary atherosclerosis. Am Heart J 1987;113:589-97.

54. Miller NE, Thelle DS, Forde OH, Mjos OD. The Tromso heart-study. High-density lipoprotein and coronary heart-disease: a prospective case-control study. Lancet 1977;1:965-8.

55. Abbott RD, Wilson PW, Kannel WB, Castelli WP. High density lipoprotein cholesterol, total cholesterol screening, and myocardial infarction. The Framingham Study. Arteriosclerosis 1988;8:207-11.

56. Castelli WP, Garrison RJ, Wilson PW, Abbott RD, Kalousdian S, Kannel WB. Incidence of coronary heart disease and lipoprotein cholesterol levels. The Framingham Study. JAMA 1986;256:2835-8.

57. Gordon T, Castelli WP, Hjortland MC, Kannel WB, Dawber TR. High density lipoprotein as a protective factor against coronary heart disease. The Framingham Study. Am J Med 1977;62:707-14.

58. Gordon T, Kannel WB, Castelli WP, Dawber TR. Lipoproteins, cardiovascular disease, and death. The Framingham study. Arch Intern Med 1981;141:1128-31.

59. Gordon DJ, Probstfield JL, Garrison RJ, et al. High-density lipoprotein cholesterol and cardiovascular disease. Four prospective American studies. Circulation 1989;79:8-15.

60. Gordon DJ, Rifkind BM. High-density lipoprotein--the clinical implications of recent studies. N Engl J Med 1989;321:1311-6.

61. Shah PK, Kaul S, Nilsson J, Cercek B. Exploiting the vascular protective effects of high-density lipoprotein and its apolipoproteins: an idea whose time for testing is coming, part I. Circulation 2001;104:2376-83.

62. Ng DS. Treating low HDL--from bench to bedside. Clin Biochem 2004;37:649-59.

63. Genest J Jr., Marcil M, Denis M, Yu L. High density lipoproteins in health and in disease. J Invest Med 1999;47:31-42.

64. Fager G, Wiklund O, Olofsson SO, Wilhelmsson C, Bondjers G. Serum apolipoprotein levels in relation to acute myocardial infarction and its risk factors. Apolipoprotein A-I levels in male survivors of myocardial infarction. Atherosclerosis 1980;36:67-74.

65. Puchois P, Kandoussi A, Fievet P, et al. Apolipoprotein A-I containing lipoproteins in coronary artery disease. Atherosclerosis 1987;68:35-40.

66. Bigot-Corbel E, Amory-Touz MC, Mainard F. [HDL-cholesterol or apolipoprotein AI: which parameter to choose?]. Ann Biol Clin (Paris) 1996;54:349-52.

67. Forte TM, McCall MR. The role of apolipoprotein A-I-containing lipoproteins in atherosclerosis. Curr Opin Lipidol 1994,5:354-64.

68. Fruchart JC, Castro G, Duriez P. Apolipoprotein-AI-containing particles and atherosclerosis. Isr J Med Sci 1996;32:498-502.

69. Rader DJ, Hoeg JM, Brewer HB Jr. Quantitation of plasma apolipoproteins in the primary and secondary prevention of coronary artery disease. Ann Intern Med 1994;120:1012-25.

70. Lamarche B, Moorjani S, Lupien PJ, et al. Apolipoprotein A-I and B levels and the risk of ischemic heart disease during a five-year follow-up of men in the Quebec cardiovascular study. Circulation 1996;94:273-8.

71. Francis MC, Frohlich JJ. Coronary artery disease in patients at low risk-apolipoprotein AI as an independent risk factor. Atherosclerosis 2001;155:165-70.

72. Maciejko JJ, Holmes DR, Kottke BA, Zinsmeister AR, Dinh DM, Mao SJ. Apolipoprotein A-I as a marker of angiographically assessed coronary-artery disease. N Engl J Med 1983;309:385-9.

73. Franzen J, Fex G. Low serum apolipoprotein A-I in acute myocardial infarction survivors with normal HDL cholesterol. Atherosclerosis 1986;59:37-42.

74. Kwiterovich PO Jr., Coresh J, Smith HH, Bachorik PS, Derby CA, Pearson TA. Comparison of the plasma levels of apolipoproteins B and A-1, and other risk factors in men and women with premature coronary artery disease. Am J Cardiol 1992;69:1015-21.

75. Badimon JJ, Badimon L, Fuster V. Regression of atherosclerotic lesions by high density lipoprotein plasma fraction in the cholesterol-fed rabbit. J Clin Invest 1990;85:1234-41.

76. Miyazaki A, Sakuma S, Morikawa W, et al. Intravenous injection of rabbit apolipoprotein A-I inhibits the progression of atherosclerosis in cholesterol-fed rabbits. Arterioscler Thromb Vasc Biol 1995;15:1882-8.

77. Rubin EM, Krauss RM, Spangler EA, Verstuyft JG, Clift SM. Inhibition of early atherogenesis in transgenic mice by human apolipoprotein AI. Nature 1991;353:265-7.

78. Plump AS, Scott CJ, Breslow JL. Human apolipoprotein A-I gene expression increases high density lipoprotein and suppresses atherosclerosis in the apolipoprotein E-deficient mouse. Proc Natl Acad Sci U S A 1994;91:9607-11.

79. Paszty C, Maeda N, Verstuyft J, Rubin EM. Apolipoprotein AI transgene corrects apolipoprotein E deficiency-induced atherosclerosis in mice. J Clin Invest 1994;94:899-903.

80. Liu AC, Lawn RM, Verstuyft JG, Rubin EM. Human apolipoprotein A-I prevents atherosclerosis associated with apolipoprotein[a] in transgenic mice. J Lipid Res 1994;35:2263-7.

81. Benoit P, Emmanuel F, Caillaud JM, et al. Somatic gene transfer of human ApoA-I inhibits atherosclerosis progression in mouse models. Circulation 1999;99:105-10.

82. Tangirala RK, Tsukamoto K, Chun SH, Usher D, Pure E, Rader DJ. Regression of atherosclerosis induced by liver-directed gene transfer of apolipoprotein A-I in mice. Circulation 1999;100:1816-22.

83. Ishiguro H, Yoshida H, Major AS, et al. Retrovirus-mediated expression of apolipoprotein A-I in the macrophage protects against atherosclerosis in vivo. J Biol Chem 2001;276:36742-8.

84. Major AS, Dove DE, Ishiguro H, et al. Increased cholesterol efflux in apolipoprotein AI (ApoAI)-producing macrophages as a mechanism for reduced atherosclerosis in ApoAI((-/-)) mice. Arterioscler Thromb Vasc Biol 2001;21:1790-5.

85. Su YR, Ishiguro H, Major AS, et al. Macrophage apolipoprotein A-I expression protects against atherosclerosis in ApoE-deficient mice and up-regulates ABC transporters. Mol Ther 2003;8:576-83.

86. Moore RE, Kawashiri MA, Kitajima K, et al. Apolipoprotein A-I deficiency results in markedly increased atherosclerosis in mice lacking the LDL receptor. Arterioscler Thromb Vasc Biol 2003;23:1914-20.

87. Voyiaziakis E, Goldberg IJ, Plump AS, Rubin EM, Breslow JL, Huang LS. ApoA-I deficiency causes both hypertriglyceridemia and increased atherosclerosis in human apoB transgenic mice. J Lipid Res 1998;39:313-21.

88. Hughes SD, Verstuyft J, Rubin EM. HDL deficiency in genetically engineered mice requires elevated LDL to accelerate atherogenesis. Arterioscler Thromb Vasc Biol 1997;17:1725-9.

89. Nofer JR, Kehrel B, Fobker M, Levkau B, Assmann G, von Eckardstein A. HDL and arteriosclerosis: beyond reverse cholesterol transport. Atherosclerosis 2002;161:1-16.

90. Rader DJ. High-density lipoproteins and atherosclerosis. Am J Cardiol 2002;90:62i-70i.

91. Connelly PW. The role of hepatic lipase in lipoprotein metabolism. Clin Chim Acta 1999;286:243-55.

92. McCoy MG, Sun GS, Marchadier D, Maugeais C, Glick JM, Rader DJ. Characterization of the lipolytic activity of endothelial lipase. J Lipid Res 2002;43:921-9.

93. Rader DJ, Jaye M. Endothelial lipase: a new member of the triglyceride lipase gene family. Curr Opin Lipidol 2000;11:141-7.

94. Jaye M, Lynch KJ, Krawiec J, et al. A novel endothelial-derived lipase that modulates HDL metabolism. Nat Genet 1999;21:424-8.

95. Glomset JA. The plasma lecithins: cholesterol acyltransferase reaction. J Lipid Res 1968;9:155-67.

96. Rader DJ. Regulation of reverse cholesterol transport and clinical implications. Am J Cardiol 2003;92:42J-49J.

97. Reichl D, Miller NE. Pathophysiology of reverse cholesterol transport. Insights from inherited disorders of lipoprotein metabolism. Arteriosclerosis 1989;9:785-97.

98. Barter PJ, Rye KA. Molecular mechanisms of reverse cholesterol transport. Curr Opin Lipidol 1996;7:82-7.

99. Suzuki H, Kurihara Y, Takeya M, et al. A role for macrophage scavenger receptors in atherosclerosis and susceptibility to infection. Nature 1997;386:292-6.

100. Nozaki S, Kashiwagi H, Yamashita S, et al. Reduced uptake of oxidized low density lipoproteins in monocyte-derived macrophages from CD36-deficient subjects. J Clin Invest 1995;96:1859-65.

101. Febbraio M, Podrez EA, Smith JD, et al. Targeted disruption of the class B scavenger receptor CD36 protects against atherosclerotic lesion development in mice. J Clin Invest 2000;105:1049-56.

102. Hessler JR, Robertson AL, J., Chisolm GM, 3rd. LDL-induced cytotoxicity and its inhibition by HDL in human vascular smooth muscle and endothelial cells in culture. Atherosclerosis 1979;32:213-29.

103. Parthasarathy S, Barnett J, Fong LG. High-density lipoprotein inhibits the oxidative modification of low-density lipoprotein. Biochim Biophys Acta 1990;1044:275-83.

104. Berliner JA, Navab M, Fogelman AM, et al. Atherosclerosis: basic mechanisms. Oxidation, inflammation, and genetics. Circulation 1995;91:2488-96.

105. Sanguinetti SM, Brites FD, Fasulo V, et al. HDL oxidability and its protective effect against LDL oxidation in Type 2 diabetic patients. Diabetes Nutr Metab 2001;14:27-36.

106. Garner B, Waldeck AR, Witting PK, Rye KA, Stocker R. Oxidation of high density lipoproteins. II. Evidence for direct reduction of lipid hydroperoxides by methionine residues of apolipoproteins AI and AII. J Biol Chem 1998;273:6088-95.

107. Shechter Y, Burstein Y, Patchornik A. Selective oxidation of methionine residues in proteins. Biochemistry 1975;14:4497-503.

108. Brot N, Weissbach H. Biochemistry and physiological role of methionine sulfoxide residues in proteins. Arch Biochem Biophys 1983;223:271-81.

109. Glaser CB, Karic L, Parmelee S, Premachandra BR, Hinkston D, Abrams WR. Studies on the turnover of methionine oxidized alpha-1-protease inhibitor in rats. Am Rev Respir Dis 1987;136:857-61.

110. Assmann G, Gotto AM, Jr. HDL cholesterol and protective factors in atherosclerosis. Circulation 2004;109:III8-14.

111. Tselepis AD, John Chapman M. Inflammation, bioactive lipids and atherosclerosis: potential roles of a lipoprotein-associated phospholipase A2, platelet activating factor-acetylhydrolase. Atheroscler Suppl 2002;3:57-68.

112. Tsaoussis V, Vakirtzi-Lemonias C. The mouse plasma PAF acetylhydrolase: I. Characterization and properties. J Lipid Mediat Cell Signal 1994;9:301-15.

113. Farr RS, Cox CP, Wardlow ML, Jorgensen R. Preliminary studies of an acid-labile factor (ALF) in human sera that inactivates platelet-activating factor (PAF). Clin Immunol Immunopathol 1980;15:318-30.

114. Farr RS, Wardlow ML, Cox CP, Meng KE, Greene DE. Human serum acid-labile factor is an acylhydrolase that inactivates platelet-activating factor. Fed Proc 1983;42:3120-2.

115. Wardlow ML, Cox CP, Meng KE, Greene DE, Farr RS. Substrate specificity and partial characterization of the PAF-acylhydrolase in human serum that rapidly inactivates platelet-activating factor. J Immunol 1986;136:3441-6.

116. Stafforini DM, Prescott SM, McIntyre TM. Human plasma platelet-activating factor acetylhydrolase. Purification and properties. J Biol Chem 1987;262:4223-30.

117. Steinbrecher UP, Pritchard PH. Hydrolysis of phosphatidylcholine during LDL oxidation is mediated by platelet-activating factor acetylhydrolase. J Lipid Res 1989;30:305-15.

118. Stremler KE, Stafforini DM, Prescott SM, Zimmerman GA, McIntyre TM. An oxidized derivative of phosphatidylcholine is a substrate for the platelet-activating factor acetylhydrolase from human plasma. J Biol Chem 1989;264:5331-4.

119. Smiley PL, Stremler KE, Prescott SM, Zimmerman GA, McIntyre TM. Oxidatively fragmented phosphatidylcholines activate human neutrophils through the receptor for platelet-activating factor. J Biol Chem 1991;266:11104-10.

120. Watson AD, Navab M, Hama SY, et al. Effect of platelet activating factor-acetylhydrolase on the formation and action of minimally oxidized low density lipoprotein. J Clin Invest 1995;95:774-82.

121. Ahmed Z, Ravandi A, Maguire GF, et al. Multiple substrates for paraoxonase-1 during oxidation of phosphatidylcholine by peroxynitrite. Biochem Biophys Res Commun 2002;290:391-6.

122. Sorenson RC, Bisgaier CL, Aviram M, Hsu C, Billecke S, La Du BN. Human serum Paraoxonase/Arylesterase's retained hydrophobic N-terminal leader sequence associates with HDLs by binding phospholipids: apolipoprotein A-I stabilizes activity. Arterioscler Thromb Vasc Biol 1999;19:2214-25.

123. Shih DM, Gu L, Xia YR, et al. Mice lacking serum paraoxonase are susceptible to organophosphate toxicity and atherosclerosis. Nature 1998;394:284-7.

124. Shih DM, Xia YR, Wang XP, et al. Combined serum paraoxonase knockout/apolipoprotein E knockout mice exhibit increased lipoprotein oxidation and atherosclerosis. J Biol Chem 2000;275:17527-35.

125. Rozenberg O, Rosenblat M, Coleman R, Shih DM, Aviram M. Paraoxonase (PON1) deficiency is associated with increased macrophage oxidative stress: studies in PON1-knockout mice. Free Radic Biol Med 2003;34:774-84.

126. Tward A, Xia YR, Wang XP, et al. Decreased atherosclerotic lesion formation in human serum paraoxonase transgenic mice. Circulation 2002;106:484-90.

127. Liu M, Subbaiah PV. Hydrolysis and transesterification of platelet-activating factor by lecithin-cholesterol acyltransferase. Proc Natl Acad Sci U S A 1994;91:6035-9.

128. Aron L, Jones S, Fielding CJ. Human plasma lecithin-cholesterol acyltransferase. Characterization of cofactor-dependent phospholipase activity. J Biol Chem 1978;253:7220-6.

129. Goyal J, Wang K, Liu M, Subbaiah PV. Novel function of lecithin-cholesterol acyltransferase. Hydrolysis of oxidized polar phospholipids generated during lipoprotein oxidation. J Biol Chem 1997;272:16231-9.

130. Vohl MC, Neville TA, Kumarathasan R, Braschi S, Sparks DL. A novel lecithin-cholesterol acyltransferase antioxidant activity prevents the formation of oxidized lipids during lipoprotein oxidation. Biochemistry 1999;38:5976-81.

131. Itabe H, Hosoya R, Karasawa K, et al. Metabolism of oxidized phosphatidylcholines formed in oxidized low density lipoprotein by lecithin-cholesterol acyltransferase. J Biochem (Tokyo) 1999;126:153-61.

132. Barter PJ, Nicholls S, Rye KA, Anantharamaiah GM, Navab M, Fogelman AM. Antiinflammatory properties of HDL. Circ Res 2004;95:764-72.

133. Carlos TM, Schwartz BR, Kovach NL, et al. Vascular cell adhesion molecule-1 mediates lymphocyte adherence to cytokine-activated cultured human endothelial cells. Blood 1990;76:965-70.

134. Blankenberg S, Barbaux S, Tiret L. Adhesion molecules and atherosclerosis. Atherosclerosis 2003;170:191-203.

135. Lawrence MB, Springer TA. Leukocytes roll on a selectin at physiologic flow rates: distinction from and prerequisite for adhesion through integrins. Cell 1991;65:859-73.

136. Davies MJ, Gordon JL, Gearing AJ, et al. The expression of the adhesion molecules ICAM-1, VCAM-1, PECAM, and E-selectin in human atherosclerosis. J Pathol 1993;171:223-9.

137. Springer TA. Adhesion receptors of the immune system. Nature 1990;346:425-34.

138. O'Brien KD, McDonald TO, Chait A, Allen MD, Alpers CE. Neovascular expression of E-selectin, intercellular adhesion molecule-1, and vascular cell adhesion molecule-1 in human atherosclerosis and their relation to intimal leukocyte content. Circulation 1996;93:672-82.

139. Reape TJ, Groot PH. Chemokines and atherosclerosis. Atherosclerosis 1999;147:213-25.

140. Navab M, Imes SS, Hama SY, et al. Monocyte transmigration induced by modification of low density lipoprotein in cocultures of human aortic wall cells is due to induction of monocyte chemotactic protein 1 synthesis and is abolished by high density lipoprotein. J Clin Invest 1991;88:2039-46.

141. Van Lenten BJ, Hama SY, de Beer FC, et al. Anti-inflammatory HDL becomes pro-inflammatory during the acute phase response. Loss of protective effect of HDL against LDL oxidation in aortic wall cell cocultures. J Clin Invest 1995;96:2758-67.

142. Cockerill GW, Rye KA, Gamble JR, Vadas MA, Barter PJ. High-density lipoproteins inhibit cytokine-induced expression of endothelial cell adhesion molecules. Arterioscler Thromb Vasc Biol 1995;15:1987-94.

143. Calabresi L, Franceschini G, Sirtori CR, et al. Inhibition of VCAM-1 expression in endothelial cells by reconstituted high density lipoproteins. Biochem Biophys Res Commun 1997;238:61-5.

144. Park SH, Park JH, Kang JS, Kang YH. Involvement of transcription factors in plasma HDL protection against TNF-alpha-induced vascular cell adhesion molecule-1 expression. Int J Biochem Cell Biol 2003;35:168-82.

145. Xia P, Vadas MA, Rye KA, Barter PJ, Gamble JR. High density lipoproteins (HDL) interrupt the sphingosine kinase signaling pathway. A possible mechanism for protection against atherosclerosis by HDL. J Biol Chem 1999;274:33143-7.

146. Clay MA, Pyle DH, Rye KA, Vadas MA, Gamble JR, Barter PJ. Time sequence of the inhibition of endothelial adhesion molecule expression by reconstituted high density lipoproteins. Atherosclerosis 2001;157:23-9.

147. Dimayuga P, Zhu J, Oguchi S, et al. Reconstituted HDL containing human apolipoprotein A-1 reduces VCAM-1 expression and neointima formation following periadventitial cuff-induced carotid injury in apoE null mice. Biochem Biophys Res Commun 1999;264:465-8.

148. Cockerill GW, Huehns TY, Weerasinghe A, et al. Elevation of plasma high-density lipoprotein concentration reduces interleukin-1-induced expression of E-selectin in an in vivo model of acute inflammation. Circulation 2001;103:108-12.

149. Nicholls SJ, Dusting GJ, Cutri B, et al. Reconstituted high-density lipoproteins inhibit the acute pro-oxidant and proinflammatory vascular changes induced by a periarterial collar in normocholesterolemic rabbits. Circulation 2005;111:1543-50.

150. Dansky HM, Charlton SA, Barlow CB, et al. Apo A-I inhibits foam cell formation in Apo E-deficient mice after monocyte adherence to endothelium. J Clin Invest 1999;104:31-9.

151. Levine DM, Parker TS, Donnelly TM, Walsh A, Rubin AL. In vivo protection against endotoxin by plasma high density lipoprotein. Proc Natl Acad Sci U S A 1993;90:12040-4.

152. Hyka N, Dayer JM, Modoux C, et al. Apolipoprotein A-I inhibits the production of interleukin-1beta and tumor necrosis factor-alpha by blocking contact-mediated activation of monocytes by T lymphocytes. Blood 2001;97:2381-9.

153. Vinals M, Martinez-Gonzalez J, Badimon JJ, Badimon L. HDL-induced prostacyclin release in smooth muscle cells is dependent on cyclooxygenase-2 (Cox-2). Arterioscler Thromb Vasc Biol 1997;17:3481-8.

154. Yui Y, Aoyama T, Morishita H, Takahashi M, Takatsu Y, Kawai C. Serum prostacyclin stabilizing factor is identical to apolipoprotein A-I (Apo A-I). A novel function of Apo A-I. J Clin Invest 1988;82:803-7.

155. Oravec S, Demuth K, Myara I, Hornych A. The effect of high density lipoprotein subfractions on endothelial eicosanoid secretion. Thromb Res 1998;92:65-71.

156. Yuhanna IS, Zhu Y, Cox BE, et al. High-density lipoprotein binding to scavenger receptor-BI activates endothelial nitric oxide synthase. Nat Med 2001;7:853-7.

157. Griffin JH, Kojima K, Banka CL, Curtiss LK, Fernandez JA. High-density lipoprotein enhancement of anticoagulant activities of plasma protein S and activated protein C. J Clin Invest 1999;103:219-27.

158. Griffin JH, Fernandez JA, Deguchi H. Plasma lipoproteins, hemostasis and thrombosis. Thromb Haemost 2001;86:386-94.

159. Hennekens CH, Buring JE, Manson JE, et al. Lack of effect of long-term supplementation with beta carotene on the incidence of malignant neoplasms and cardiovascular disease. N Engl J Med 1996;334:1145-9.

160. Yusuf S, Dagenais G, Pogue J, Bosch J, Sleight P. Vitamin E supplementation and cardiovascular events in high-risk patients. The Heart Outcomes Prevention Evaluation Study Investigators. N Engl J Med 2000;342:154-60.

161. Waters DD, Alderman EL, Hsia J, et al. Effects of hormone replacement therapy and antioxidant vitamin supplements on coronary atherosclerosis in postmenopausal women: a randomized controlled trial. JAMA 2002;288:2432-40.

162. Stephens NG, Parsons A, Schofield PM, Kelly F, Cheeseman K, Mitchinson MJ. Randomised controlled trial of vitamin E in patients with coronary disease: Cambridge Heart Antioxidant Study (CHAOS). Lancet 1996;347:781-6.

163. Boaz M, Smetana S, Weinstein T, et al. Secondary prevention with antioxidants of cardiovascular disease in endstage renal disease (SPACE): randomised placebo-controlled trial. Lancet 2000;356:1213-8.

164. Salonen RM, Nyyssonen K, Kaikkonen J, et al. Six-year effect of combined vitamin C and E supplementation on atherosclerotic progression: the Antioxidant Supplementation in Atherosclerosis Prevention (ASAP) Study. Circulation 2003;107:947-53.

165. Tepel M, van der Giet M, Statz M, Jankowski J, Zidek W. The antioxidant acetylcysteine reduces cardiovascular events in patients with end-stage renal failure: a randomized, controlled trial. Circulation 2003;107:992-5.

166. Griendling KK, FitzGerald GA. Oxidative stress and cardiovascular injury: Part II: animal and human studies. Circulation 2003;108:2034-40.

167. Kris-Etherton PM, Lichtenstein AH, Howard BV, Steinberg D, Witztum JL. Antioxidant vitamin supplements and cardiovascular disease. Circulation 2004;110:637-41.

168. Steinberg D, Witztum JL. Is the oxidative modification hypothesis relevant to human atherosclerosis? Do the antioxidant trials conducted to date refute the hypothesis? Circulation 2002;105:2107-11.

169. Ginsberg HN. Nonpharmacologic management of low levels of high-density lipoprotein cholesterol. Am J Cardiol 2000;86:41L-45L.

170. Cordova AC, Jackson LS, Berke-Schlessel DW, Sumpio BE. The cardiovascular protective effect of red wine. J Am Coll Surg 2005;200:428-39.

171. Perret B, Ruidavets JB, Vieu C, et al. Alcohol consumption is associated with enrichment of high-density lipoprotein particles in polyunsaturated lipids and increased cholesterol esterification rate. Alcohol Clin Exp Res 2002;26:1134-40.

172. Araya J, Rodrigo R, Orellana M, Rivera G. Red wine raises plasma HDL and preserves long-chain polyunsaturated fatty acids in rat kidney and erythrocytes. Br J Nutr 2001;86:189-95.

173. Klatsky AL, Friedman GD, Armstrong MA, Kipp H. Wine, liquor, beer, and mortality. Am J Epidemiol 2003;158:585-95.

174. Executive Summary of The Third Report of The National Cholesterol Education Program (NCEP) Expert Panel on Detection, Evaluation, And Treatment of High Blood Cholesterol In Adults (Adult Treatment Panel III). JAMA 2001;285:2486-97.

175. Manninen V, Elo MO, Frick MH, et al. Lipid alterations and decline in the incidence of coronary heart disease in the Helsinki Heart Study JAMA 1988;260:641-51.

176. Secondary prevention by raising HDL cholesterol and reducing triglycerides in patients with coronary artery disease: the Bezafibrate Infarction Prevention (BIP) study. Circulation 2000;102:21-7.

177. Rubins HB, Robins SJ, Collins D, et al. Gemfibrozil for the secondary prevention of coronary heart disease in men with low levels of high-density lipoprotein cholesterol. Veterans Affairs High-Density Lipoprotein Cholesterol Intervention Trial Study Group. N Engl J Med 1999;341:410-8.

178. Kockx M, Princen HM, Kooistra T. Fibrate-modulated expression of fibrinogen, plasminogen activator inhibitor-1 and apolipoprotein A-I in cultured cynomolgus monkey hepatocytes -- role of the peroxisome proliferator-activated receptor-alpha. Thromb Haemost 1998;80:942-8.

179. Neele DM, Kaptein A, Huisman H, de Wit EC, Princen HM. No effect of fibrates on synthesis of apolipoprotein(a) in primary cultures of cynomolgus monkey and human hepatocytes: apolipoprotein A-I synthesis increased. Biochem Biophys Res Commun 1998;244:374-8.

180. Mardones P, Pilon A, Bouly M, et al. Fibrates down-regulate hepatic scavenger receptor class B type I protein expression in mice. J Biol Chem 2003;278:7884-90.

181. Meyers CD, Kamanna VS, Kashyap ML. Niacin therapy in atherosclerosis. Curr Opin Lipidol 2004;15:659-65.

182. Brown BG, Zhao XQ, Chait A, et al. Simvastatin and niacin, antioxidant vitamins, or the combination for the prevention of coronary disease. N Engl J Med 2001;345:1583-92.

183. Zhao XQ, Morse JS, Dowdy AA, et al. Safety and tolerability of simvastatin plus niacin in patients with coronary artery disease and low high-density lipoprotein cholesterol (The HDL Atherosclerosis Treatment Study). Am J Cardiol 2004;93:307-12.

184. Carlson LA, Rosenhamer G. Reduction of mortality in the Stockholm Ischaemic Heart Disease Secondary Prevention Study by combined treatment with clofibrate and nicotinic acid. Acta Med Scand 1988;223:405-18.

185. Whitney EJ, Krasuski RA, Personius BE, et al. A randomized trial of a strategy for increasing high-density lipoprotein cholesterol levels: effects on progression of coronary heart disease and clinical events. Ann Intern Med 2005;142:95-104.

186. Rosenson RS. Antiatherothrombotic effects of nicotinic acid. Atherosclerosis 2003;171:87-96.

187. Brown PJ, Stuart LW, Hurley KP, et al. Identification of a subtype selective human PPARalpha agonist through parallel-array synthesis. Bioorg Med Chem Lett 2001;11:1225-7.

188. Miyachi H, Nomura M, Tanase T, et al. Design, synthesis and evaluation of substituted phenylpropanoic acid derivatives as peroxisome proliferator-activated receptor (PPAR) activators: novel human PPARalpha-selective activators. Bioorg Med Chem Lett 2002;12:77-80.

189. Xu Y, Mayhugh D, Saeed A, et al. Design and synthesis of a potent and selective triazolone-based peroxisome proliferator-activated receptor alpha agonist. J Med Chem 2003;46:5121-4.

190. Kuwabara K, Murakami K, Todo M, et al. A novel selective peroxisome proliferator-activated receptor alpha agonist, 2-methyl-c-5-[4-[5-methyl-2-(4-methylphenyl)-4-oxazolyl]butyl]-1,3-dioxane -r-2-carboxylic acid (NS-220), potently decreases plasma triglyceride and glucose levels and modifies lipoprotein profiles in KK-Ay mice. J Pharmacol Exp Ther 2004;309:970-7.

191. Melnikova I. Raising HDL cholesterol. Nat Rev Drug Discov 2005;4:185-6.

192. Yki-Jarvinen H. Thiazolidinediones. N Engl J Med 2004;351:1106-18.

193. Skrumsager BK, Nielsen KK, Muller M, Pabst G, Drake PG, Edsberg B. Ragaglitazar: the pharmacokinetics, pharmacodynamics, and tolerability of a novel dual PPAR alpha and gamma agonist in healthy subjects and patients with type 2 diabetes. J Clin Pharmacol 2003;43:1244-56.

194. Saad MF, Greco S, Osei K, et al. Ragaglitazar improves glycemic control and lipid profile in type 2 diabetic subjects: a 12-week, double-blind, placebo-controlled dose-ranging study with an open pioglitazone arm. Diabetes Care 2004;27:1324-9.

195. Moore KJ, Fitzgerald ML, Freeman MW. Peroxisome proliferator-activated receptors in macrophage biology: friend or foe? Curr Opin Lipidol 2001;12:519-27.

196. Linsel-Nitschke P, Tall AR. HDL as a target in the treatment of atherosclerotic cardiovascular disease. Nat Rev Drug Discov 2005;4:193-205.

197. Pasceri V, Wu HD, Willerson JT, Yeh ET. Modulation of vascular inflammation in vitro and in vivo by peroxisome proliferator-activated receptor-gamma activators. Circulation 2000;101:235-8.

198. Kintscher U, Goetze S, Wakino S, et al. Peroxisome proliferator-activated receptor and retinoid X receptor ligands inhibit monocyte chemotactic protein-1-directed migration of monocytes. Eur J Pharmacol 2000;401:259-70.

199. Han KH, Chang MK, Boullier A, et al. Oxidized LDL reduces monocyte CCR2 expression through pathways involving peroxisome proliferator-activated receptor gamma. J Clin Invest 2000;106:793-802.

200. de Grooth GJ, Klerkx AH, Stroes ES, Stalenhoef AF, Kastelein JJ, Kuivenhoven JA. A review of CETP and its relation to atherosclerosis. J Lipid Res 2004;45:1967-74.

201. Boekholdt SM, Kuivenhoven JA, Wareham NJ, et al. Plasma levels of cholesteryl ester transfer protein and the risk of future coronary artery disease in apparently healthy men and women: the prospective EPIC (European Prospective Investigation into Cancer and nutrition)-Norfolk population study. Circulation 2004;110:1418-23.

202. Wolfe ML, Rader DJ. Cholesteryl ester transfer protein and coronary artery disease: an observation with therapeutic implications. Circulation 2004;110:1338-40.

203. Clark RW, Sutfin TA, Ruggeri RB, et al. Raising high-density lipoprotein in humans through inhibition of cholesteryl ester transfer protein: an initial multidose study of torcetrapib. Arterioscler Thromb Vasc Biol 2004;24:490-7.

204. Brousseau ME, Schaefer EJ, Wolfe ML, et al. Effects of an inhibitor of cholesteryl ester transfer protein on HDL cholesterol. N Engl J Med 2004;350:1505-15.

205. van der Steeg WA, Kuivenhoven JA, Klerkx AH, Boekholdt SM, Hovingh GK, Kastelein JJ. Role of CETP inhibitors in the treatment of dyslipidemia. Curr Opin Lipidol 2004;15:631-6.

206. Rader DJ. High-density lipoproteins as an emerging therapeutic target for atherosclerosis. JAMA 2003;290:2322-4.

207. Sirtori CR, Calabresi L, Franceschini G, et al. Cardiovascular status of carriers of the apolipoprotein A-I(Milano) mutant: the Limone sul Garda study. Circulation 2001;103:1949-54.

208. Nissen SE, Tsunoda T, Tuzcu EM, et al. Effect of recombinant ApoA-I Milano on coronary atherosclerosis in patients with acute coronary syndromes: a randomized controlled trial. JAMA 2003;290:2292-300.

209. Navab M, Anantharamaiah GM, Reddy ST, et al. Human apolipoprotein A-I and A-I mimetic peptides: potential for atherosclerosis reversal. Curr Opin Lipidol 2004;15:645-9.

210. Klerkx AH, de Grooth GJ, Zwinderman AH, Jukema JW, Kuivenhoven JA, Kastelein JJ. Cholesteryl ester transfer protein concentration is associated with progression of atherosclerosis and response to pravastatin in men with coronary artery disease (REGRESS). Eur J Clin Invest 2004;34:21-8.

211. Laufs U. Beyond lipid-lowering: effects of statins on endothelial nitric oxide. Eur J Clin Pharmacol 2003;58:719-31.

212. Mason RP, Walter MF, Jacob RF. Effects of HMG-CoA reductase inhibitors on endothelial function: role of microdomains and oxidative stress. Circulation 2004;109:II34-41.

213. Rosenson RS. Statins in atherosclerosis: lipid-lowering agents with antioxidant capabilities. Atherosclerosis 2004;173:1-12.

214. MRC/BHF Heart Protection Study of cholesterol lowering with simvastatin in 20,536 high-risk individuals: a randomised placebo-controlled trial. Lancet 2002;360:7-22.

215. Influence of pravastatin and plasma lipids on clinical events in the West of Scotland Coronary Prevention Study (WOSCOPS). Circulation 1998;97:1440-5.

216. Baseline serum cholesterol and treatment effect in the Scandinavian Simvastatin Survival Study (4S). Lancet 1995;345:1274-5.

217. Ridker PM, Rifai N, Pfeffer MA, et al. Inflammation, pravastatin, and the risk of coronary events after myocardial infarction in patients with average cholesterol levels. Cholesterol and Recurrent Events (CARE) Investigators. Circulation 1998;98:839-44.

218. Ridker PM, Rifai N, Pfeffer MA, Sacks F, Braunwald E. Long-term effects of pravastatin on plasma concentration of C-reactive protein. The Cholesterol and Recurrent Events (CARE) Investigators. Circulation 1999;100:230-5.

219. Liao JK, Bettmann MA, Sandor T, Tucker JI, Coleman SM, Creager MA. Differential impairment of vasodilator responsiveness of peripheral resistance and conduit vessels in humans with atherosclerosis. Circ Res 1991;68.1027-34.

220. Libby P. Molecular bases of the acute coronary syndromes. Circulation 1995;91:2844-50.

221. Tamai O, Matsuoka H, Itabe H, Wada Y, Kohno K, Imaizumi T. Single LDL apheresis improves endothelium-dependent vasodilatation in hypercholesterolemic humans. Circulation 1997;95:76-82.

222. Anderson TJ, Meredith IT, Yeung AC, Frei B, Selwyn AP, Ganz P. The effect of cholesterol-lowering and antioxidant therapy on endothelium-dependent coronary vasomotion. N Engl J Med 1995;332:488-93.

223. Treasure CB, Klein JL, Weintraub WS, et al. Beneficial effects of cholesterol-lowering therapy on the coronary endothelium in patients with coronary artery disease. N Engl J Med 1995;332:481-7.

224. O'Driscoll G, Green D, Taylor RR. Simvastatin, an HMG-coenzyme A reductase inhibitor, improves endothelial function within 1 month. Circulation 1997;95:1126-31.

225. Liao JK, Laufs U. Pleiotropic effects of statins. Ann Rev Pharmacol Toxicol 2005;45:89-118.

226. Sanguigni V, Pignatelli P, Caccese D, et al. Increased superoxide anion production by platelets in hypercholesterolemic patients. Thromb Haemost 2002;87:796-801.

227. Wagner AH, Kohler T, Ruckschloss U, Just I, Hecker M. Improvement of nitric oxide-dependent vasodilatation by HMG-CoA reductase inhibitors through attenuation of endothelial superoxide anion formation. Arterioscler Thromb Vasc Biol 2000;20:61-9.

228. Yasunari K, Maeda K, Minami M, Yoshikawa J. HMG-CoA reductase inhibitors prevent migration of human coronary smooth muscle cells through suppression of increase in oxidative stress. Arterioscler Thromb Vasc Biol 2001;21:937-42.

229. Hattori Y, Nakanishi N, Kasai K. Statin enhances cytokine-mediated induction of nitric oxide synthesis in vascular smooth muscle cells. Cardiovasc Res 2002;54:649-58.

230. Plenz GA, Hofnagel O, Robenek H. Differential modulation of caveolin-1 expression in cells of the vasculature by statins. Circulation 2004;109:e7-8; author reply e7-8.

231. Pelat M, Dessy C, Massion P, Desager JP, Feron O, Balligand JL. Rosuvastatin decreases caveolin-1 and improves nitric oxide-dependent heart rate and blood pressure variability in apolipoprotein E-/- mice in vivo. Circulation 2003;107:2480-6.

232. Brouet A, Sonveaux P, Dessy C, Moniotte S, Balligand JL, Feron O. Hsp90 and caveolin are key targets for the proangiogenic nitric oxide-mediated effects of statins. Circ Res 2001;89:866-73.

233. Lefer AM, Campbell B, Shin YK, Scalia R, Hayward R, Lefer DJ. Simvastatin preserves the ischemic-reperfused myocardium in normocholesterolemic rat hearts. Circulation 1999;100:178-84.

234. Rikitake Y, Kawashima S, Takeshita S, et al. Anti-oxidative properties of fluvastatin, an HMG-CoA reductase inhibitor, contribute to prevention of atherosclerosis in cholesterol-fed rabbits. Atherosclerosis 2001;154:87-96.

235. Fuhrman B, Koren L, Volkova N, Keidar S, Hayek T, Aviram M. Atorvastatin therapy in hypercholesterolemic patients suppresses cellular uptake of oxidized-LDL by differentiating monocytes. Atherosclerosis 2002;164:179-85.

236. Shishehbor MH, Aviles RJ, Brennan ML, et al. Association of nitrotyrosine levels with cardiovascular disease and modulation by statin therapy. JAMA 2003;289:1675-80.

237. Shishehbor MH, Brennan ML, Aviles RJ, et al. Statins promote potent systemic antioxidant effects through specific inflammatory pathways. Circulation 2003;108:426-31.

238. Aviram M, Rosenblat M, Bisgaier CL, Newton RS. Atorvastatin and gemfibrozil metabolites, but not the parent drugs, are potent antioxidants against lipoprotein oxidation. Atherosclerosis 1998;138:271-80.

239. Yamamoto A, Hoshi K, Ichihara K. Fluvastatin, an inhibitor of 3-hydroxy-3-methylglutaryl-CoA reductase, scavenges free radicals and inhibits lipid peroxidation in rat liver microsomes. Eur J Pharmacol 1998;361:143-9.

240. Yamaguchi Y, Matsuno S, Kagota S, Haginaka J, Kunitomo M. Peroxynitrite-mediated oxidative modification of low-density lipoprotein by aqueous extracts of cigarette smoke and the preventive effect of fluvastatin. Atherosclerosis 2004;172:259-65.

Chapter 18

OXIDATIVE STRESS IN HEART FAILURE

Douglas B. Sawyer[1] and Wilson S. Colucci[2]
*Cardiovascular Medicine Section, Department of Medicine[1] and Myocardial Biology Unit[2],
Boston University School of Medicine, Boston, MA*

Introduction

Oxidative stress is increased in heart failure and may contribute to many of the structural and functional changes that characterize disease progression. Oxidative stress exists when there is a net increase in reactive oxygen species (ROS). ROS are the byproduct of aerobic metabolism. Since the myocardium is metabolically very active, it is a rich source of ROS. The production of ROS is balanced by an efficient antioxidant system. When the production of ROS exceeds the capacity of these antioxidant systems, oxidative stress occurs. The generation of ROS begins with the formation of superoxide anion (O_2^-) as the result of the one electron reduction of molecular oxygen (*Figure 1*). The unpaired electron in O_2^- is an unstable free radical that is highly reactive and may react with other oxygen containing species and organic molecules.

Increased oxidative stress in heart failure

There is both indirect and direct evidence of increased oxidative stress in humans with heart failure. Oxidation products of several organic molecules including lipids, proteins and nucleic acids can be measured, and if increased, provide indirect evidence of oxidative stress in heart failure. In patients with heart failure the level of the lipid peroxidation product malonyldialdehyde (MDA) is increased in the plasma, the level of pentane (a volatile lipid peroxidation product) is increased in exhaled air, and the level of total thiols is decreased in the plasma[1-3]. More direct evidence of increased myocardial oxidative stress comes from demonstration that the level of 8-iso-prostaglandin $F_{2\alpha}$ (8-isoprostane) is increased in the pericardial fluid obtained from patients with heart failure[4].

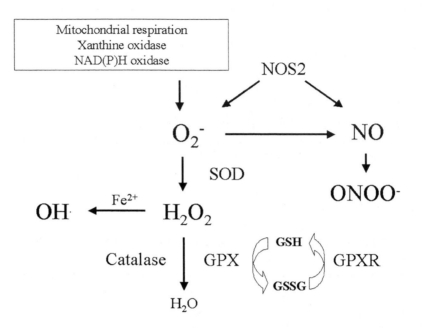

***Figure 1.* Reactive oxygen species (ROS) and antioxidant enzyme systems.** The enzymatic or non-enzymatic formation of superoxide anion leads to the formation of other ROS. ROS are removed by the enzymes superoxide dismutase (SOD), glutathione peroxidase (GPx) and catalase. The presence of Fe+2 or nitric oxide (NO) can allow the formation of hydroxyl radical (OH·) and peroxynitrite (ONOO-), respectively. These latter reactions are favored when the activity of SOD is decreased. O2- can increase the formation of OH· by reducing Fe3+ to Fe2+. Glutathione (GSH) plays a central role in cellular antioxidant defenses not only as a reducing agent for the action of GPx, but also through direct reactions with ROS. Glutathione is recycled by the enzyme glutathione reductase, which requires NADPH.

8-Isoprostanes are formed by the peroxidation of arachidonic acid through a noncyclooxygenase-mediated reaction catalyzed by free radicals[5]. As with circulating oxidation products, the level of 8-isoprostanes correlates with NYHA functional class in patients with heart failure.

Antioxidant systems in the heart

A major component of the antioxidant system consists of antioxidant enzymes including superoxide dismutases (SOD), catalase and peroxidases (*Figure 1*). In cardiac myocytes, the mitochondrial enzyme manganese superoxide dismutase (MnSOD; SOD2) predominates, accounting for approximately 70% of the SOD activity in the heart and 90% of that in the cardiac myocyte[6]. The remainder consists of cytosolic Cu/ZnSOD (SOD1), with less than 1% contributed by extracellular-SOD (ECSOD; SOD3)[7]. MnSOD thus plays a major role in controlling mitochondrial ROS generated during normal oxidative phosphorylation. Glutathione peroxidase (GPx) and to a lesser extent, catalase, also play a critical role in regulating ROS in the myocardium by handling H_2O_2, the product of SOD. GPx catalyzes the removal of H_2O_2 via the oxidation of reduced glutathione (GSH) that is recycled from oxidized glutathione (GSSG) by the NADPH-dependent glutathione reductase (GRed). GPx activity thus requires GSH. Glutathione reductase (Gred) generates GSH by the NADPH-dependent recycling of GSSG. Like MnSOD, GPx localizes to the mitochondria.

Glutathione is an important soluble antioxidant that acts both to replenish GPx and as a direct scavenger of ROS and reactive nitrogen species. As noted above, GSH is replenished the action of GRed on GSSG, and by *de novo* synthesis of GSH. The ratio of GSH/GSSG thus serves as a measure of net myocardial oxidative stress within the cell. Certain vitamins contribute to the cell's antioxidant defense system. However, vitamins do not reduce the levels of ROS, but rather, act to protect target molecules. For example, α-tocopherol and ascorbic acid act together to prevent lipid peroxidation and membrane breakdown.

Sources of ROS in the failing heart

There are a number of potential sources of ROS in the myocardium. Several enzyme systems are present that generate O_2^-. Among these, the mitochondria appear to be an important source of myocardial ROS in the failing heart. A small fraction of the electrons that pass through the mitochondrial electron transport chain may 'leak', thereby reacting with molecular oxygen to form O_2^-. Using electroparamagnetic resonance (EPR) with an O_2^- spin-trap it was shown that ROS are increased 2.8-fold in mitochondria from failing hearts in association with a decrease in the activity of electron transport complex I, thereby leading to the suggestion that in heart failure there is a functional uncoupling of the mitochondria that contributes to increased ROS formation.

There is also evidence that oxidases may contribute to ROS generation in the myocardium. Xanthine oxidase activity is increased in the failing heart, and xanthine oxidase inhibitors improve myocardial energetics in a dog model of heart failure and in humans with heart failure[8]. Another oxidase implicated in myocardial failure is NADPH oxidase, a plasmalemmal enzyme[9] that generates O_2^- in the cytosol. NADPH oxidase was first described in the neutrophil, where it is responsible for cytotoxic levels of

$ROS^{(10)}$. In other cells types, NADPH oxidases produce much lower levels of ROS that act as signaling molecules[11]. Finally, the non-enzymatic autooxidation reaction of organic molecules such as catecholamines and thiol-containing compounds (e.g., cysteine and GSH) can form O_2^-, and has been implicated in heart failure.

Role of ROS in myocardial remodeling failure

Myocardial remodeling is a term that describes changes in the structure and function of the heart. When caused by pathologic stimuli such as chronic hypertension or loss of functional muscle due to infarction, the remodeling process often leads to dysfunction and failure. At the cellular level, mechanisms that contribute to remodeling include myocyte hypertrophy, myocyte slippage, myocyte apoptosis and/or alterations in the turnover and properties of the extracellular matrix[12]. *In vitro* and *in vivo* studies have suggested that the stimuli for ventricular remodeling may include increased wall stress, inflammatory cytokines and neurohormones including catecholamines and peptide hormones such as angiotensin. A growing body of evidence suggests that ROS may mediate the effects of these and other remodeling stimuli (*Figure 2*).

Regulation of myocyte growth by ROS

It is now appreciated that ROS can regulate growth pathways in many cell types. Among the first demonstrations of the role of ROS in growth was obtained in vascular smooth muscle cells, where it was shown that angiotensin mediates hypertrophy via the production of O_2^- by NADPH oxidase[13]. We and others have demonstrated that ROS can mediate growth responses in cardiac myocytes. An early proof of principle was obtained by inhibiting the activity of SOD in cultured cardiac myocytes, leading to an increase in cellular O_2^- levels[14]. Partial inhibition for 24 hours caused myocyte growth associated and induction of a fetal gene pattern with increased expression of fetal genes (e.g., ANF) and decreased expression of adult genes (e.g., SERCA2). These effects of were inhibited by antioxidants, thus suggesting that a small increase in intracellular oxidative stress due to inhibition of an endogenous antioxidant can cause hypertrophy.

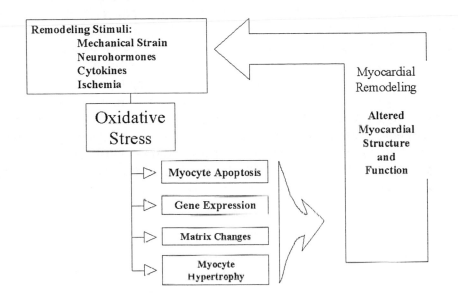

Figure 2. **The potential role of oxidative stress in the pathogenesis of myocardial remodeling.** Oxidative stress may be a central mediator of changes in cellular structure and function that are stimulated by inflammatory cytokines, neurohormones or mechanical strain. (MMP, metalloproteinase; TIMP, tissue inhibitor of metalloproteinases)

To examine whether ROS may be involved in mediating the growth effects of hypertrophic stimuli, we subjected cardiac myocytes in culture to mechanical strain, a well known stimulus for myocyte hypertrophy[15]. A low level of mechanical strain applied for 24 hours caused an amplitude-dependent increase in ROS formation that was associated with myocyte hypertrophy that could be prevented by the use of antioxidants such as SOD. Another frequently used model for myocyte hypertrophy is α-adrenergic receptor (α-AR) stimulation[16]. We and others have shown that α-AR stimulation also induces ROS formation in cultured myocytes, and that the ROS play a critical role in mediating the hypertrophic response[17]. Likewise, it has been shown in cultured myocytes that hypertrophy in response to angiotensin or TNF-α is mediated by ROS[18].

The source of ROS for these and other hypertrophic stimuli is not fully understood, and likely varies with the stimulus. However, we have provided indirect evidence that an NADPH oxidase is involved in mediating the effect of hypertrophic response to α-AR stimulation in cultured myocytes[19]. The neutrophil NADPH oxidase is a complex consisting of at least four major sub-units, including two membrane-spanning components (p22phox and gp91phox), and two cytosolic components (p67phox and p47phox)[11]. A similar oxidase system has been identified in many cell types in the cardiovascular system. The NADPH oxidases typically consist of four or more sub-units, although it now appears that some isoforms may function with fewer subunits. We and others have demonstrated that at least four of the major sub-units of NADPH oxidase (p22phox, gp91phox, p67phox and p47phox) are expressed in rat ventricular myocytes[19]. In wild type mice the chronic administration of a sub-pressor dose of angiotensin caused cardiac hypertrophy, whereas in mice deficient in gp91phox hypertrophy was inhibited[20]. In contrast, pressure overload-induced hypertrophy was not attenuated in these mice[21,22], suggesting that NADPH oxidase, or at least the gp91phox-dependent isoform, is not involved in mediating this hypertrophic stimulus.

Role of ROS in regulating myocyte calcium

A characteristic of myocardial failure is abnormal calcium homeostasis due to alterations in the expression and/or activity of Ca^{+2} handling proteins. It appears that these changes may be due in part to oxidative stress. For example, the decreased expression and activity of sarcoplasmic reticulum Ca^{+2} ATPase (SERCA2) in the failing heart may to contribute to contractile dysfunction in heart failure[23]. As noted above, ROS can decrease SERCA2 expression in cultured cardiac myocytes[14], thus suggesting that oxidative stress may contribute to dysregulation of calcium homeostasis by altering the expression of SERCA2 and/or other calcium handling proteins. ROS may also directly affect the function of calcium handling proteins. For example, studies in isolated cardiac myocytes suggest that ROS and reactive nitrogen species can directly affect the function of both the voltage-dependent Ca^{2+} channel and the calcium release channel[24-25]. More recently, Adachi et al. have shown that ROS can regulate the function of SERCA2 via a variety of post-translational oxidative modifications of reactive thiol and tyrosine groups[26,27].

Role of ROS in myocyte apoptosis

ROS also appear to play a central role in mediating apoptosis in cardiac myocytes. There is evidence that ROS mediate hypertrophy in cardiac myocytes and that the quantity and/or quality of the ROS differs from the ROS involved in mediating hypertrophy. Some evidence suggests that apoptosis is caused by levels of ROS that are higher than those associated with hypertrophy. For example, we found that the addition of low levels of exogenous H_2O_2, on the order of 10 μM, caused hypertrophy; whereas higher concentrations, on the order of 100 – 300 μM, caused apoptosis[28].

Likewise, we found that, in contrast to low amplitude mechanical strain, which causes hypertrophy, high amplitude strain results in a larger increase in ROS resulting in apoptosis[15].

Distal effector mechanisms for ROS

ROS may mediate their actions either indirectly via the regulation of distal signaling pathways (e.g., mitogen-activated protein kinases) or directly via their actions on target proteins (e.g., SERCA2). ROS are well known to activate[29] stress-responsive protein kinases of the mitogen-activated protein kinase (MAPK) superfamily which includes the extracellularly-responsive kinases (ERK) and two stress-responsive MAPK subfamilies, the p38-kinases and the c-Jun N-terminal kinases (JNK)[30].

In adult rat ventricular myocytes in culture, we found that incubation with graded concentrations of exogenous H_2O_2 leads to the sequential activation of ERK at low concentrations on the order of 10 µM that cause hypertrophy, and activation of JNK at higher concentrations on the order of 200 µM that cause apoptosis[28]. Likewise, the hypertrophic effect of the low H_2O_2 concentration was inhibited by the MEK inhibitor U0126, whereas the apoptotic effect of the higher concentration of H_2O_2 was opposed by a dominant-negative JNK adenovirus, and was potentiated by U0126. These observations suggest that the concentration-dependent effects of ROS on myocyte hypertrophy and survival are due, at least in part, to the differential activation of specific kinase signaling pathways.

Mitochondria are involved in the regulation of apoptosis in many cell types. In cardiac myocytes, ROS appear to act via JNK to cause the release of cytochrome c from the intermembrane space. Stimulation of β-adrenergic receptors (βAR) causes apoptosis in adult rat ventricular myocytes[31]. We found that βAR stimulation for 24 hours caused apoptosis that is inhibited by an SOD/catalase-mimetic or infection with an adenovirus expressing catalase[32]. Inhibition of the mitochondrial permeability transition pore with bongkrekic acid also decreased βAR-stimulated apoptosis, as did the caspase inhibitor zVAD. βAR-stimulation caused JNK activation which was abolished by an SOD/catalase-mimetic; and an adenovirus expressing dominant-negative JNK or a JNK inhibitor (SP600125) prevented βAR-stimulated apoptosis and cytochrome c release. Taken together, these observations suggest that βAR-stimulated apoptosis involves ROS-dependent activation of JNK and the mitochondrial death pathway.

While relatively little is known about the immediate targets of ROS, it appears that activation of the ERK pathway is mediated by an oxidative post-translational modification of Ras, which is known to have redox-sensitive cysteine residues. We found that αAR stimulation caused a decrease in on the number of free thiols on Ras as measured using biotinylated iodoacetamide[33]. The decrease in free (i.e., reduced) thiols was reversed by exposure to the reducing agent dithiothreitol (DTT) indicating that it was due to an oxidative post-translational modification (*Figure 3*). This effect was also abolished by adenoviral overexpression of thioredoxin-1, an enzyme that reduces thiol groups, and potentiated by the TRX system inhibitor azaleic acid. Likewise, αAR-stimulated Ras activation was abolished by TRX1 overexpression and potentiated by azaleic acid. TRX1 overexpression inhibited the αAR-stimulated phosphorylation of ERK; and prevented cellular hypertrophy, sarcomere reorganization and protein synthesis; whereas azaleic acid potentiated αAR-stimulated protein synthesis. Taken together, these observations demonstrate that αAR-stimulated hypertrophic signaling in cardiac myocytes is mediated via a TRX1-sensitive post-translational oxidative modification of thiols on Ras.

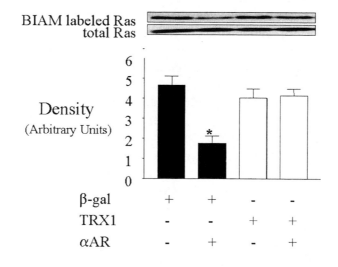

Figure 3. Effects of αAR stimulation and the overexpression of thioredoxin-1 (TRX1) on the abundance of free thiols on Ras. Free (i.e., reduced) thiols were measured by labeling with biotinylated iodoacetamide (BIAM). αAR stimulation (5 min) decreased the abundance of free thiols on Ras, and this decrease was completely reversed by the addition of DTT to the lysate buffer, suggesting that the aAR-stimulated thiol modification is oxidative in nature. Adenoviral overexpression of TRX1 had no effect on basal free thiols, but prevented the αAR-stimulated decrease. Overexpression of β-galactosidase (b-gal) had no effect on the abundance of basal or αAR-stimulated free thiols on Ras. Reproduced from[33]

ROS regulation of interstitial matrix turnover by cardiac fibroblasts.

An important mechanism in myocardial remodeling involves alterations in the interstitial matrix. The interstitial matrix proteins connect to the sarcomere via integrins and intermediate filaments, and thereby provide mechanical coupling between individual cardiac myocytes. The turnover of interstitial matrix proteins, of which collagen is the most important, is regulated by the balance between synthesis and degradation, the latter primarily due to the action of matrix metalloproteinases (MMPs)[34]. In cardiac fibroblasts in culture, we have found that both collagen synthesis and MMP activity are regulated in part by ROS[35]. ROS caused a decrease in procollagen mRNA expression and collagen synthesis. Conversely, ROS increased fibroblast MMP activity as measured by in-gel zymography. The combined effects of decreased synthesis and increased degradation may lead to abnormalities in interstitial collagen that would promote myocyte slippage and chamber dilation. The functional importance of ROS-mediated changes in interstitial matrix is suggested by the demonstration in the mouse heart that treatment with an antioxidant reduced the extent of ventricular dilation and suppressed MMP activity early after a myocardial infarction[36].

Reactive nitrogen species

Nitric oxide (NO) is a free radical that can modify the myocardial response to ROS both directly and indirectly. NO is a free radical gas that is buffered in the cell by reactions with glutathione and, like ROS, can react reversibly with sulfhydryl groups of proteins forming S-nitrosothiols that lead to alterations in protein function[37]. NO can react chemically with ROS to either decrease or increase the net oxidative stress in the cell. In the normal myocardium, NO is produced at low levels by NOS3, and perhaps NOS1. By contrast, the inducible isoform of nitric oxide synthase (NOS2) is capable of producing high levels of cellular NO. While NOS2 is not expressed in the normal myocardium, its induction by exposure to cytokines or other stimuli leads to a marked increase in the production of NO. Of note, there is evidence for increased expression and activity of the NOS2 in the myocardium of patients with both idiopathic and ischemic dilated cardiomyopathies[38-40].

At low levels, NO formed by NOS3 may reduce net oxidative stress by decreasing the production of O_2^- through inhibition of oxidative enzymes[41]. NO can also oppose hypertrophic stimuli through the activation of guanylate cyclase[42] and may promote cell survival by inactivating apoptotic proteases. The functional importance of NOS3 is suggested by the demonstration that mice deficient in NOS3 exhibit worse ventricular remodeling and function late after myocardial infarction[43]. At higher levels, NO may increase oxidative stress by directly reacting with O_2^- to generate peroxynitrite $(ONOO^-)$[45]. $ONOO^-$ is a toxic free radical that can react with many cell constituents. The formation of $ONOO^-$ is favored when the levels of O_2^- or NO are high, and/or the level of SOD is low.

High concentrations of NO can have direct toxic effects on cardiac myocytes. The cytotoxic effect of cytokines are mediated in part by NO[45]. Cytokine-induced apoptosis is prevented by interventions that reduce either NO or O_2^-, further suggesting a role for $ONOO^-$[46]. In contrast to the detrimental affect of NOS3 deficiency, mice deficient in NOS2 have improved myocardial remodeling and function late post-myocardial infarction[47].

Summary

Oxidative stress is elevated systemically and in the myocardium of patients with chronic myocardial failure. While the cause of increased ROS in this setting is not known, it may relate to a) increased production via mitochondria or the activation of oxidases including NADPH oxidase and xanthine oxidase, and/or b) decreased antioxidant activity. *In vitro* in cardiac myocytes, ROS can exert important effects on myocyte growth and survival. At low concentrations ROS can stimulate growth and appear to mediate the hypertrophic effects of several growth stimuli including mechanical strain, α-adrenergic receptor stimulation and various peptides. These effects are mediated, at least part, via the activation of the ERK signaling pathway. At higher concentrations ROS lead to apoptosis of cardiac myocytes that is mediated in part via the activation of the JNK signaling pathway and activation of the mitochondrial death pathway, with the release of cytochrome c. ROS act in part by causing the oxidative post-translational modifications of target proteins such as Ras and SERCA2, in which reversible modifications of reactive thiol and tyrosine groups lead to changes in protein function. Advances in our understanding of the sources of ROS and the mechanisms by which they regulate myocardial structure and function should provide new insight into the treatment and prevention of myocardial dysfunction.

References

1. McMurray J, Chopra M, Abdullah I, Smith WE, Dargie HJ. Evidence of oxidative stress in chronic heart failure in humans. Eur Heart J 1993;14:1493-8.

2. Diaz-Velez CR, Garcia-Castineiras S, Mendoza-Ramos E, Hernandez-Lopez E. Increased malondialdehyde in peripheral blood of patients with congestive heart failure. Am Heart J 1996;131:146-52.

3. Sobotka PA, Brottman MD, Weitz Z, Birnbaum AJ, Skosey JL, Zarling EJ. Elevated breath pentane in heart failure reduced by free radical scavenger. Free Radic Biol Med 1993;14:643-7.

4. Mallat Z, Philip I, Lebret M, Chatel D, Maclouf J, Tedgui A. Elevated levels of 8-iso-prostaglandin F2alpha in pericardial fluid of patients with heart failure: a potential role for in vivo oxidant stress in ventricular dilatation and progression to heart failure. Circulation 1998;97:1536-9.

5. Liu TZ, Stern A, Morrow JD. The isoprostanes: unique bioactive products of lipid peroxidation. An overview [In Process Citation]. J Biomed Sci 1998;5:415-20.

6. Assem M, Teyssier JR, Benderitter M et al. Pattern of supcroxide dismutase enzymatic activity and RNA changes in rat heart ventricles after myocardial infarction. Am J Pathol 1997;151:549-55.

7. Carlsson LM, Jonsson J, Edlund T, Marklund SL. Mice lacking extracellular superoxide dismutase are more sensitive to hyperoxia. Proc Natl Acad Sci U S A 1995;92:6264-8.

8. Saavedra WF, Paolocci N, St John ME et al. Imbalance between xanthine oxidase and nitric oxide synthase signaling pathways underlies mechanoenergetic uncoupling in the failing heart. Circ Res 2002;90:297-304.

9. Griendling KK, Minieri CA, Ollerenshaw JD, Alexander RW. Angiotensin II stimulates NADH and NADPH oxidase activity in cultured vascular smooth muscle cells. Circ Res 1994;74:1141-8.

10. Babior BM. NADPH oxidase: an update. Blood 1999;93:1464-76.

11. Griendling KK, Sorescu D, Ushio-Fukai M. NAD(P)H oxidase: role in cardiovascular biology and disease. Circ Res 2000;86:494-501.

12. Maytin M, Colucci WS. Molecular and cellular mechanisms of myocardial remodeling. J Nucl Cardiol 2002;9:319-27.

13. Ushio-Fukai M, Zafari AM, Fukui T, Ishizaka N, Griendling KK. p22phox is a critical component of the superoxide-generating NADH/NADPH oxidase system and regulates angiotensin II-induced hypertrophy in vascular smooth muscle cells. J Biol Chem 1996;271:23317-21.

14. Siwik DA, Tzortzis JD, Pimental DR et al. Inhibition of copper-zinc superoxide dismutase induces cell growth, hypertrophic phenotype, and apoptosis in neonatal rat cardiac myocytes in vitro. Circ Res 1999;85:147-53.

15. Pimentel DR, Amin JK, Xiao L et al. Reactive oxygen species mediate amplitude-dependent hypertrophic and apoptotic responses to mechanical stretch in cardiac myocytes. Circ Res 2001;89:453-60.

16. Simpson P. Stimulation of hypertrophy of cultured neonatal rat heart cells through an alpha 1-adrenergic receptor and induction of beating through an alpha 1- and beta 1-adrenergic receptor interaction. Evidence for independent regulation of growth and beating. Circ Res 1985;56:884-94.

17. Amin JK, Xiao L, Pimental DR et al. Reactive oxygen species mediate alpha-adrenergic receptor-stimulated hypertrophy in adult rat ventricular myocytes. J Mol Cell Cardiol 2001;33:131-9.

18. Nakamura K, Fushimi K, Kouchi H et al. Inhibitory effects of antioxidants on neonatal rat cardiac myocyte hypertrophy induced by tumor necrosis factor-alpha and angiotensin II. Circulation 1998;98:794-9.

19. Xiao L, Pimentel DR, Wang J, Singh K, Colucci WS, Sawyer DB. Role of reactive oxygen species and NAD(P)H oxidase in alpha(1)- adrenoceptor signaling in adult rat cardiac myocytes. Am J Physiol Cell Physiol 2002;282:C926-34.

20. Bendall JK, Cave AC, Heymes C, Gall N, Shah AM. Pivotal role of a gp91(phox)-containing NADPH oxidase in angiotensin II-induced cardiac hypertrophy in mice. Circulation 2002;105:293-6.

21. Maytin M, Siwik DA, Ito M et al. Pressure overload-induced myocardial hypertrophy in mice does not require gp91phox. Circulation 2004;109:1168-71.

22. Byrne JA, Grieve DJ, Bendall JK et al. Contrasting roles of NADPH oxidase isoforms in pressure-overload versus angiotensin II-induced cardiac hypertrophy. Circ Res 2003;93:802-5.

23. Monte FD, Hajjar RJ. Targeting calcium cycling proteins in heart failure through gene transfer. J Physiol 2003;546:49-61.

24. Campbell DL, Stamler JS, Strauss HC. Redox modulation of L-type calcium channels in ferret ventricular myocytes. Dual mechanism regulation by nitric oxide and S-nitrosothiols. J Gen Physiol 1996;108:277-93.

25. Xu L, Eu JP, Meissner G, Stamler JS. Activation of the cardiac calcium release channel (ryanodine receptor) by poly-S-nitrosylation. Science 1998;279:234-7.

26. Adachi T, Matsui R, Xu S et al. Antioxidant improves smooth muscle sarco/endoplasmic reticulum Ca(2+)-ATPase function and lowers tyrosine nitration in hypercholesterolemia and improves nitric oxide-induced relaxation. Circ Res 2002;90:1114-21.

27. Adachi T, Pimentel DR, Heibeck T et al. S-glutathiolation of Ras mediates redox-sensitive signaling by angiotensin II in vascular smooth muscle cells. J Biol Chem 2004;279:29857-62.

28. Kwon SH, Pimentel DR, Remondino A, Sawyer DB, Colucci WS. H(2)O(2) regulates cardiac myocyte phenotype via concentration-dependent activation of distinct kinase pathways. J Mol Cell Cardiol 2003;35:615-21.

29. Sugden PH, Clerk A. "Stress-responsive" mitogen-activated protein kinases (c-Jun N-terminal kinases and p38 mitogen-activated protein kinases) in the myocardium. Circ Res 1998;83:345-52.

30. Jiang Y, Gram H, Zhao M et al. Characterization of the structure and function of the fourth member of p38 group mitogen-activated protein kinases, p28d. J Biol Chem 1997;272:30122-8.

31. Communal C, Singh K, Pimentel DR, Colucci WS. Norepinephrine stimulates apoptosis in adult rat ventricular myocytes by activation of the b-adrenergic pathway. Circulation 1998;98:1329-34.

32. Remondino A, Kwon SH, Communal C et al. Beta-adrenergic receptor-stimulated apoptosis in cardiac myocytes is mediated by reactive oxygen species/c-Jun NH2-terminal kinase-dependent activation of the mitochondrial pathway. Circ Res 2003;92:136-8.

33. Kuster GM, Pimentel DR, Adachi T et al. Alpha adrenergic receptor-stimulated hypertrophy in adult rat ventricular myocytes is mediated via thioredoxin-1-sensitive oxidative modification of thiols on Ras. Circulation 2005;111:1192-8.

34. Spinale FG, Coker ML, Bond BR, Zellner JL. Myocardial matrix degradation and metalloproteinase activation in the failing heart: a potential therapeutic target. Cardiovasc Res 2000;46:225-38.

35. Siwik DA, Pagano PJ, Colucci WS. Oxidative stress regulates collagen synthesis and matrix metalloproteinase activity in cardiac fibroblasts. Am J Physiol Cell Physiol 2001;280:C53-C60.

36. Kinugawa S, Tsutsui H, Hayashidani S et al. Treatment with dimethylthiourea prevents left ventricular remodeling and failure after experimental myocardial infarction in mice: role of oxidative stress. Circ Res 2000;87:392-8.

37. Stamler JS, Simon DI, Osborne JA et al. S-nitrosylation of proteins with nitric oxide: synthesis and characterization of biologically active compounds. Proc Natl Acad Sci U S A 1992;89:444-8.

38. Haywood GA, Sneddon JF, Bashir Y, Jennison SH, Gray HH, McKenna WJ. Adenosine infusion for the reversal of pulmonary vasoconstriction in biventricular failure. A good test but a poor therapy. Circulation 1992;86:896-902.

39. Habib F, Dutka D, Crossman D, Oakley CM, Cleland JG. Enhanced basal nitric oxide production in heart failure: another failed counter-regulatory vasodilator mechanism? [see comments]. Lancet 1994;344:371-3.

40. Habib FM, Springall DR, Davies GJ, Oakley CM, Yacoub MH, Polak JM. Tumour necrosis factor and inducible nitric oxide synthase in dilated cardiomyopathy [see comments]. Lancet 1996;347:1151-5.

41. Xie YW, Wolin MS. Role of nitric oxide and its interaction with superoxide in the suppression of cardiac muscle mitochondrial respiration. Involvement in response to hypoxia/reoxygenation. Circulation 1996;94:2580-6.

42. Calderone A, Thaik CM, Takahashi N, Chang DL, Colucci WS. Nitric oxide, atrial natriuretic peptide, and cyclic GMP inhibit the growth-promoting effects of norepinephrine in cardiac myocytes and fibroblasts. J Clin Invest 1998;101:812-8.

43. Scherrer-Crosbie M, Ullrich R, Bloch KD et al. Endothelial nitric oxide synthase limits left ventricular remodeling after myocardial infarction in mice. Circulation 2001;104:1286-91.

44. Beckman JS, Koppenol WH. Nitric oxide, superoxide, and peroxynitrite: the good, the bad, and ugly. Am J Physiol 1996;271:C1424-37.

45. Pinsky DJ, Cai B, Yang X, Rodriguez C, Sciacca RR, Cannon PJ. The lethal effects of cytokine-induced nitric oxide on cardiac myocytes are blocked by nitric oxide synthase antagonism or transforming growth factor beta. J Clin Invest 1995;95:677-85.

46. Arstall MA, Sawyer DB, Fukazawa R, Kelly RA. Cytokine-mediated apoptosis in cardiac myocytes: the role of inducible nitric oxide synthase induction and peroxynitrite generation [see comments]. Circ Res 1999;85:829-40.

47. Sam F, Sawyer DB, Xie Z et al. Mice lacking inducible nitric oxide synthase have improved left ventricular contractile function and reduced apoptotic cell death late after myocardial infarction. Circ Res 2001;89:351-6.

Chapter 19

USE OF ANTIOXIDANTS IN PATIENTS WITH CONGESTIVE HEART FAILURE

Anique Ducharme, Jean Lucien Rouleau, Michel White
Montreal Heart Institute, Montreal, Quebec, Canada

Introduction

Dramatic improvement in the knowledge of the pathophysiology and management of congestive heart failure (CHF) has occurred in the last decade. Pharmacological developments, including the use of angiotensin converting enzyme (ACE) inhibitors[1,2] have substantially reduced morbidity and mortality in CHF patients with depressed systolic function. Unfortunately, the beneficial effect of these agents reaches a peak within a few months after initiation of therapy, with angiotensin II blood levels returning towards baseline, an escape phenomenon of angiotensin II inhibition by ACE-I. More recently, beta-adrenergic blockade[3-6], angiotensin receptor blockers[7] and the aldosterone blockers, spironolactone[8] and epleronone[9] have been shown to improve survival when given to CHF patients on background ACE-inhibitors therapy.

In parallel with drug development, electrophysiological devices such as implantable defibrillators have been shown to substantially decrease sudden death[10] and, when combined with resynchronization therapy, hospitalization for heart failure[11]. Nevertheless, despite the use of such therapies, mortality from progressive heart failure remains unacceptably high. Thus it appears that attenuation of neurohumoral pathways may not be sufficient to allow adequate control of the progressive left ventricular (LV) remodeling process occurring in these patients.

This chapter reviews the pathophysiology of CHF, including mechanisms involving neurohumoral activation and those potentially related to inflammation, apoptosis and oxidative stress. The second part focuses on antioxidant interventions that may attenuate oxidative damage, including water-soluble antioxidants (such as vitamin C), lipid-soluble antioxidant (mitochondrial coenzyme Q10), factors that inhibit free radical formation (such as allopurinol), as well as cardiovascular drugs used clinically in patients with CHF, which have potent antioxidant properties.

Neurohumoral activation in CHF

Heart failure has evolved from a pure hemodynamic, to a neurohumoral and more recently an inflammatory condition. Although neurohumoral activation is necessary to maintain vital status after an acute event such as a myocardial infarction, there is growing evidence suggesting that increased levels of circulating vasoconstrictive hormones such as norepinephrine, endothelin-I, angiotensin-II and vasopressin contribute to heart failure progression in humans[12-15]. Data obtained using radio-tracer techniques or selective sampling of vascular beds have shown that a specific increase in neurohumoral activation such as increased cerebral, cardiac and renal norepinephrine spillover occurs in CHF, leading to increased plasma levels of neurohormones[16]. Changes in cardiac adrenergic activity may occur early in the disease process and has been closely linked to clinical outcomes and, in some cases, to mortality. As a response to chronic tissue-specific neurohumoral activation, there is significant downregulation in ß-adrenergic and parallel changes in the angiotensin signal transduction pathways[17]. To counterbalance these vasoconstrictive agents, vasodilatory hormones such as adrenomedullin, atrial and brain natriuretic peptides and prostaglandins are secreted[18-20]. Furthermore, abnormalities in nitric oxide (NO) formation and/or resistance to the effect of NO is present both experimentally and in patients with CHF[21-23].

Evidence that inflammation occurs in CHF

In addition to neurohormonal activation, several markers of chronic inflammation are increased in CHF. Circulatory levels of tumor necrosis factor alpha (TNFα) and other cytokines such as interleukin (IL)-1, -2, -6 - 12 and -18 are elevated in patients with CHF, especially with advanced disease[24-26]. Some of these cytokine soluble receptors such as TNF receptors (R) I and II are also increased and their elevation correlates with disease severity and changes in functional clinical status[27,28]. The mechanisms for the increase in immune activation in heart failure are largely unknown. One hypothesis is that cytokines are released from the bowel in patients with severe cardiac cachexia[29]. In addition, high circulating levels of angiotensin-II, norepinephrine and possibly other hormones appear to promote inflammation both experimentally and in patients with CHF[27,30,31]. Beyond neurohumoral activation and cachexia, hypoperfusion and/or hypoxemia to the peripheral organs including the gut may contribute to the release of endotoxins and, thus to the release of cytokines and an increase in oxidative stress. The high prevalence of depression in these patients may also contribute to increase the levels of proinflammatory cytokines such as IL-6. In addition proinflammatory risk factors exist in patients with CHF because of the high prevalence of coronary artery disease and the importance of hypertension as a significant risk factor for the development of this condition in North America.

The limited data on this issue suggest a rather non-specific increase in the level of proinflammatory markers in heart failure. The increase in proinflammatory cytokines such as IL-18 results in the production of other cardiotoxic cytokines such as IL-6 and C-reactive protein (CRP). These primary proinflammatory cytokines also activate the endothelium and the expression of adhesion molecules and the selectins needed to recruit inflammatory cells to the vascular wall. Plasma levels IL-1, IL-6, TNF plasma and CRP, and also in some adhesion molecules have been reported to be increased in CHF. Moreover, some of these markers appear to correlate with NYHA class and the severity of disease.

As reported for neurohormones, changes in tissue-specific cytokines have been observed both in animal models and in humans[25,31]. Intramyocardial content in TNFα is increased in explanted hearts from patients with ischemic heart failure or dilated cardiomyopathy (CMP). In addition, TNF R-I and R-II are downregulated in explanted failing human hearts to a similar degree as reported for beta-I and angiotensin-II type I receptor density, suggesting that the neurohumoral system may be linked to inflammatory pathways in CHF patients[25,31].

Oxidative stress and CHF

Oxidative stress occurs when an imbalance exists between free radicals production and endogenous antioxidant defenses, provoking tissue damage through oxidative modification of essential cellular biomolecules[32]. In the failing heart, various mechanisms of free radical production have been proposed; the most important sources include the mitochondrial respiratory chain enzymes, xanthine oxidase, non-phagocytic NADPH oxidase, neutrophil NADPH oxidase, and autooxidation of catecholamines[33-35]. Neurohumoral activation and increased markers of inflammation systemically and at the tissue level promote tissue damage and oxidative stress. Recent clinical evidence suggests a relationship between markers of oxidative stress, catecholamines levels and impairment in cardiac chronotopic response, implying a relationship between the regulation of the ß-adrenergic signal transduction pathway and oxidative stress in heart failure. Angiotensin-II induces cell damage and the formation of peroxynitrite, an oxidized and toxic metabolite of NO[36,37]. The failing human myocardium appears especially vulnerable to the effect of angiotensin-II, and exposure of the nonfailing heart to angiotensin- II produces little change in the expression of the mitogen pathway (MAP kinase) as opposed to a 100% increase in the expression of MAP kinase in explanted failing human hearts[38]. Similarly, catecholamines promote direct tissue injury through oxygen-derived free radical formation[16,17].

There is evidence suggesting that oxidative stress is increased in CHF. Experimentally, increased oxidative stress becomes apparent during transition from hypertrophy to heart failure, suggesting that oxidation may represent a triggering mechanism for heart failure development[39]. Patients with CHF of ischemic and non-ischemic etiology have increased oxygen-derived free radical production[40,41] and increased malondialdehyde levels compatible with increased lipid peroxidation by reactive oxygen species (ROS)[42]; these products of lipid peroxidation detected in plasma represent indirect evidences of increased oxidative stress. On the other hand, decreased antioxidant defenses seem to be also present in CHF patients and may contribute to further increase in oxidative stress. Despite some controversy about antioxidant enzymes activity in CHF[43,44], dietary intake and blood levels of some antioxidant vitamins and micronutrients (mainly vitamin C and selenium) seem to be decreased in CHF patients[45]. This can be secondary to increased metabolic requirements and/or malabsorption due to gut edema. This leads to impaired nutritional status and vitamin and micronutrient depletion[46].

Despite some controversial observations[47], there are evidences suggesting a significant association between oxidative stress and the severity of HF[42,48,49]. A good correlation is found between markers of oxidative stress such as pericardial levels of 8-iso-PGF2α[50], plasma levels of lipid peroxides and malondialdehyde levels[42], and indexes of functional capacity, such as NYHA class and peak exercise oxygen consumption[50-54]. Recently, we have shown that the intermediate oxidized metabolites of catecholamines called plasma adrenolutin are increased in patients with heart failure and correlate with a poor prognosis independently of other important predictors of survival[55]. The mechanism for an increase in oxidative stress remains largely unknown. However, an increase in oxidative stress is likely to play an important role in disease progression. In fact, the increase in oxidative stress could thus contribute to endothelial dysfunction, myocyte apoptosis and necrosis, fibroblast proliferation, deposition of extracellular matrix proteins, cardiac remodeling, and impairment in cardiac contractile reserve and consequently progressive deterioration of the failing heart.

Oxidative stress in cardiac tissues

Regardless of the exact sources, increased free radical activity seems to be implicated in several pathophysiological mechanisms of CHF and its progression. Twenty years ago, Singal *et al.* suggested that oxidation at the tissue level was increased in experimental models of CHF[56]. Although systemic markers of oxidative stress are increased in human CHF, there are limited data about actual changes in these markers and in antioxidant enzymes content in the non-failing and failing human heart. Prasad *et al.* have found that polymorphonuclear leucocyte-mediated production of oxygen-derived free radicals is increased four-fold in patients with heart failure as compared to controls[57]. They reported that superoxide production in cardiac tissues increases as a result of reduced antioxidant reserves in heart failure in the transition from LV hypertrophy to overt LV dysfunction[57]. Data from Baumer *et al.* have demonstrated a significant decrease in cardiac antioxidant enzymes (30% reduction in catalase activity) in the failing compared to non-failing explanted human heart[43].

Oxidative stress in the vascular wall

The important role of the endothelium in the regulation of tissue perfusion in CHF is being increasingly recognized, the presence of endothelial dysfunction being implicated in the systemic vasoconstriction and reduced peripheral perfusion found in these patients[58]. This reduction of vasodilatory capacity affects both myocardial and skeletal muscle vascular beds, and may result in myocardial ischemia, LV dysfunction, arrhythmias, systemic hypoperfusion, and poor exercise tolerance[59]. The underlying mechanisms are unclear but likely involve many distinct mechanisms. Endothelial regulation of vascular tone is mediated predominantly by endothelium-derived NO, which promotes vasorelaxation. The presence of endothelial dysfunction in patients with heart failure may be related to a decrease in NO production and/or a resistance to its effect[60-62]. The low output state of CHF patients leads to a reduction in blood flow, and thus to a decreased in shear stress, resulting in diminished production of endothelial NO at rest and with stress[62]. This is associated with decline in expression of endothelial NO synthase (eNOS) and cyclooxygenase-1, the enzyme responsible for production of prostacyclin[23]. In addition, neurohumoral stimulation, with endothelin-I, norepinephrine, angiotensin-II and vasopressin all contribute to increased arterial vascular resistance and thus afterload in patients with CHF. These may be related to the endothelial dysfunction caused by either a direct effect or by increase in oxidative stress[36]. In addition to the detrimental effects of neurohumoral activation, levels of many cytokines such as TNFα, IL-1, 2, 6 and their soluble receptors such as TNF-RI and TNF-RII are increased in animal models and in patients with CHF. Increased circulating levels of the cytokine TNFα has been associated with the degradation of eNOS mRNA[24].

In contrast, other studies have reported an enhanced basal production of NO in heart failure[60-62], suggesting that an actual resistance to the effect of NO may be causing the endothelial dysfunction. Recent evidence showed that endothelial dysfunction may occur despite an increase in vascular eNOS and sGC expression as a result of increased NADH-dependent vascular production of superoxide anion which rapidly scavenges NO in the vascular wall in the setting of CHF[61]. Thus, a net reduction in the bioavailability of NO occurs despite an increase in NO generation. The source of the superoxide anion appears to be the vascular smooth muscle cells, since removal of the endothelium does not significantly attenuate ROS production. Both NO and superoxide are radicals. When exposed to each other, they undergo a radical-radical reaction to form peroxinitrite anion, a highly reactive-toxic molecule[62]. Recently it has been recognized that ROS, and especially peroxynitrite, can oxidize tetrahydrobiopterin, a critical co-factor of NO synthase.

Finally, Landmesser *et al.* have demonstrated that the activity of extracellular superoxide dismutase (a major endothelium-bound antioxidant enzyme) is markedly reduced in CHF patients, while xanthine oxidase is significantly increased[63]. These alterations are closely related to an impairment of endothelium-dependent vasodilation, and suggest an association between oxidative stress and endothelial dysfunction.

Link between oxygen-derived free radical formation and apoptosis

There is growing evidence suggesting that programmed cell death, or apoptosis, is increased in heart failure, and may contribute to ventricular remodeling both after myocardial infarction[64,65] and in CHF[65,66]. The cause for accelerated apoptosis remains largely unknown but many mechanisms described above may play an important role, particularly increased oxidative stress. Experimentally, at the myocyte level, oxidative stress has been shown to induce apoptosis, leading to myocyte loss[41,67]. Oxygen containing free radicals may induce DNA damage and subsequent apoptosis. In addition, inflammatory cytokines such as TNFα appear to induce apoptosis as well. Fas, a transmembrane protein belonging to the TNF receptor family, regulates T-cell apoptosis and is expressed in cardiac myocytes. Thus, the Fas/Fas-ligand system as well as TNFα may be involved in the development or progression of cardiac or vascular lesions by mediating apoptosis. In addition, apoptosis can also be modulated by growth factors and other cytokines[68-70]. Interestingly, these apoptotic changes seem to precede the development of LV dysfunction, suggesting that apoptosis contributes to LV remodeling[71,72]. In addition, processes such as fibrosis, collagen deposition, and metalloproteinase activation[73], which all participate in the remodeling of the failing myocardium, can be induced by free radicals derived from myofibroblasts during experimental CHF[35,74]. Better knowledge of how apoptosis can be regulated will undoubtedly provide new therapeutic modalities including gene therapy to influence cardiac and vascular remodeling.

Use of antioxidants in heart failure

The accumulation of knowledge on the interrelationship between CHF and oxidative stress has prompted researchers to evaluate the effect of antioxidants on various pathophysiological parameters of CHF. Although a direct correlation between markers of oxidative stress and ventricular performance has not been clearly established, there appears to be a strong association between oxidative stress and several underlying pathological processes, such as apoptosis, remodeling, mechanoenergetic uncoupling, and endothelial dysfunction. Thus antioxidant interventions that exert favorable effects on these processes may also have potential clinical benefits in this setting.

Exercise

In patients with CHF, regular exercise improves endothelium-dependent vasodilation and reduces systemic levels of hypoxanthine, a marker of oxidative stress[75,76]. The mechanisms for such observations are not well known. Exercise-induced increase in cardiac output and peripheral blood flow are associated with increased shear stress which is known to stimulate eNOS expression and to increase Cu/Zn SOD expression and free radical scavengers in aortic endothelial cells[77].

Natural (endogenous) antioxidants (table 1)

Several experimental studies have demonstrated the beneficial effects of antioxidant vitamins in CHF animals[39,78-80]. Antioxidant vitamins can inhibit cardiac myocyte hypertrophy, apoptosis, and the transition of hypertrophy to heart failure. Additionally, a combination of beta-carotene, vitamin C, and vitamin E reduces myocardial oxidative stress, attenuates cardiac dysfunction and prevents myocardial beta-receptor down-regulation and sympathetic nerve terminal dysfunction in a rabbit model of tachycardia-induced cardiomyopathy[80].

Table 1. Use of antioxidants in heart failure

	Author	Model	End-point	Results
Antioxidants vitamins				
Vitamin E	AK. Dhalla [39]	Coarctation-Induced Hypertension	Oxidative stress markers	Improved
	A. Ghatak [81]	CHF patients	Oxidative stress markers	Improved
	ME. Keith [82]	CHF patients (NYHA II-IV)	Oxidative stress Quality of Life	No change
	S. Yusuf [83]	High risk patients	Clinical	No change
Vitamin C	B. Hornig [86]	CHF patients	Endothelial function O.S. Markers	Improved
	L. Rossia [87]	CHF patients	Endothelial function O.S. Markers	Improved
	K. Ito [88]	Non ischemic CHF patients	Endothelium function	No change
	BM. Richartz[89]	Non ischemic CHF patients	Endothelium function	No change
Ubiquinone (coenzyme Q-10)	PH. Langsjoen [150]	Idiopathic CMP (n=19) NYHA III - IV	LVEF and NYHA class	Improved
	C. Hofman-Bang [151]	CHF patients (n=79)	LVEF Exercise capacity Quality of Life	Improved Improved Improved
	PS. Watson [92]	CHF patients (n=30)	LVEF Hemodynamics Quality of Life	No change
	M. Khatta [93]	CHF patients (n=55) NYHA III - IV	Oxygen consumption Exercise duration, LVEF	No change No change
Allopurinol	N. Doehner [129]	CHF hyperuricemic patients	Endothelial function	
	CA. Farguharson[130]	CHF patients	Endothelial function	Improved
	TP. Cappola[132]	Dilated CMP (9)	O_2 consumption, dp/dt Stroke volume	Improved Improved
Lipid lowering agents				
Probucol	YT. Sia [147]	MI rats	LV Remodeling Cardiac Fibrosis Apoptosis	Improved Improved Improved
	N. Siveski-Iliskovic [152]	Adriamycin rat model	LV remodeling	Complete protection
	R. Nakamuna [149]	Rapid-pacing dogs	LV Remodeling MCP-1 MPPs Activity	Improved Improved Improved
	L. Tavazzi [153]	CHF patients NYHA II – IV (n=7000)	All-cause mortality	Ongoing
	J. Kjekshus [154]	CAD patients (n=7027)	Hospitalizations for Heart Failure	Reduce

CHF: congestive heart failure; NYHA: New-York Heart Association; CAD: coronary artery disease; CMP cardiomypoathy

Experimentally, the transition from hypertrophy to heart failure in coarctation-induced hypertension is associated with increased oxidative stress and can be prevented by treatment with the antioxidant **vitamin E**[39]. However, few data on the effectiveness of natural antioxidants in clinical studies of patients with CHF are presently available. Vitamin E, a major lipid-soluble antioxidant, has been tested in a few human trials[81,82]. Although vitamin E supplementation improved markers of oxidative stress in one study[81], in another, 12 weeks of vitamin E supplementation failed to demonstrate any significant improvement in markers of oxidative stress (malondialdehyde, isoprostanes and breath pentane and ethane), neurohumoral markers of prognosis (TNFα, epinephrine, ANP) or quality of life[82]. Negative results regarding cardiovascular events after vitamin E supplementation have also been reported in coronary artery disease (CAD) patients[83]. Interestingly, some investigators argue that antioxidants such as vitamin E may be an ineffective anti-oxidant, and under certain circumstances may even enhance oxidative stress[63,84].

Data are also conflicting concerning the use of **vitamin C** in patients with CHF, a water-soluble antioxidant. In several cardiovascular diseases, vitamin C has been shown to increases the bioavailability of NO and to attenuate endothelial dysfunction. It has a favorable effect on endothelial NO synthase activity by increasing tetrahydrobiopterin availability[85]. In patients with CHF, beneficial effects of pharmacological doses of vitamin C on endothelial dysfunction have also been demonstrated[85,86], possibly through suppression of endothelial cell apoptosis and decrease neutrophil superoxide generation[85]. Amelioration of oxidative stress derived from TNFα and angiotensin II stimulation seem to have a role in this antiapoptotic effect[87]. In one study, vitamin C failed to improve endothelium-dependent vasodilation in patients with idiopathic dilated CMP, and the authors suggested that comorbidities such as CAD more than CHF per se might be responsible for endothelial dysfunction[88]. Subsequently, Richartz *et al.* have shown that vitamin C acutely improves endothelial dysfunction in patients with idiopathic dilated CMP[89]. In a different setting, Mak and Newton have suggested a role for ROS on adrenergic-mediated myocardial contractility. They have shown that vitamin C administration amplified the inotropic response to dobutamine in patients with normal LV function[90]. Whether vitamin C has beneficial effects on the inotropic state of patients with CHF remains unanswered, but one may hypothesize that ROS contributes to the loss of β-adrenergic responsiveness after prolonged β-adrenergic stimulation[91].

The lipid-soluble antioxidant mitochondrial **coenzyme Q10** (ubiquinone) has also been evaluated in patients with CHF. Coenzyme Q10 has a role in mitochondrial oxidative phosphorylation and may act as a free radical scavenger, by preventing lipid peroxydation. Moreover, the extent of deficiency of this coenzyme correlates with clinical severity of CHF. Few studies have been published, and their results are conflicting, most of them failing to prove any clinical benefit in CHF[47,92,93]. In one of these, Khatta *et al.* evaluated the effects of coenzyme Q10 in a small, randomized and controlled study of 55 patients with NYHA class III and IV CHF. No change could be demonstrated on VO2 max and echocardiographic parameters[93].

Drugs with antioxidant properties

At the present time, the interest in targeting oxidative stress in CHF has shifted from the use of antioxidant vitamins to drugs specifically designed to inhibit the relevant radical-producing enzymes and to cardiovascular drugs with free radical scavenging properties. In fact, several cardiovascular drugs commonly used have demonstrated intrinsic antioxidant properties. These include propranolol[94], captopril[95], losartan[96], calcium channel blockers[97], statins[98,99], trimetazidine[100], aspirin[101], amiodarone[102], and others. In addition, it has been suggested that the anti-inflammatory action of some of these drugs correlates with their antioxidant capacity. The impact of these drugs on CHF-induced oxidative stress has not yet been clarified. The independent study of a potential antioxidant effect of these agents is difficult, since many interfere with neurohormonal processes that are also able to induce in vivo oxidative stress by themselves. Despite this difficulty, the potential impact of redox manipulations on ventricular and endothelial function represents a promising area that should be investigated in CHF patients[103] A variety of conventional cardiovascular drugs (already used in the treatment of CHF) as well as new antioxidant agents have been studied for this purpose.

Angiotensin inhibitors and other vasodilators

Recent experimental studies have shown that treatment with either ACE inhibitors or angiotensin receptor antagonists decreases vascular superoxide production in models of angiotensin II-driven hypertension[104] and in apolipoprotein E deficient mice[95]. Using a rat myocardial infarction model, Khaper *et al.* have demonstrated that losartan, in addition to improving cardiac remodeling, reduces oxidative stress and increases myocardial antioxidant enzymes[96]. Interestingly, the direct vasodilator hydralazine, which has been used for many years as a treatment for heart failure, also possesses antioxidant properties[62,105]. Hydralazine inhibits NADH oxidase, a major source of ROS in heart failure, both in the endothelium and in vascular smooth muscle cells[62,105]. Furthermore, previous animal studies have shown that angiotensin II and cytokines such as TNFα can stimulate the activity and/or expression of this oxidase. Thus one could speculate that the well-established long term benefit of vasodilators in heart failure may be due in part to suppression of NADH oxidase activity and to a concomitant decrease in vascular oxidative stress[62].

Beta-adrenergic blockers

Beta-adrenergic blockers had been traditionally contraindicated in CHF patients because of their known negative inotropic effects. However, following the recognition of the important role of activation of the sympathetic nervous system in heart failure, the potential benefit of beta-blockade in these patients has been demonstrated since 1975, with beneficial effects on symptoms, exercise tolerance and LV function in patients with dilated CMP[106]. This report was followed by several small clinical trials involving the use of different beta-blockers in patients with idiopathic dilated or ischemic CMP. Although the results of these early trials were not always consistent, large-scale randomized clinical trials have shown significant mortality reduction in patients on ACE inhibitors background therapy[4-6,107]. Three agents had been used: metoprolol, bisoprolol, two selective beta 1 receptor blockers, and carvedilol, a non-selective beta-blocker with antioxidant properties. Beta-blockers counteract the direct cardiotoxic effect of high catecholamines levels, released either locally in the myocardium or systemically in patients with CHF. This decrease in sympathetic drive likely contributes to decreased local tissue levels of oxidized catecholamine metabolites such as adrenochromes and adrenolutins.

Anti-inflammatory effect of carvedilol

Being an antagonist of beta- and alpha-adrenergic receptors, carvedilol exerts potent antiischemic and cardioprotective effects on the myocardium. In animal models of myocardial infarction, carvedilol significantly reduces the inflammatory response to ischemic injury and significantly reduces infarct size[108]. Yue *et al.* have shown that carvedilol suppresses the expression of intercellular adhesion molecules (ICAM-1) in a manner that parallels its ability to inhibit neutrophil adhesion to endothelial cells [109].

Antoxidant and anti-apoptotic effects of carvedilol

Carvedilol, also possesses a carbazol functional group, which is responsible for its in vitro antioxidant activity. Carvedilol substantially decreases oxidative stress in the failing human heart, by suppression of lipid peroxidation in myocardial cell membranes, inhibition of superoxide ion release from activated neutrophils, inhibition of endothelial cell apoptosis[110], protection of endothelial and vascular smooth muscle cells from oxygen radical-mediated injury[109,111], and inhibition of the formation of oxidized LDL[111,112]. Furthermore, carvedilol seems to preserve the endogenous antioxidant systems (vitamin E and glutathione) that are normally consumed when tissues or organs are exposed to oxidative stress[112]. Several metabolites of carvedilol are extremely potent antioxidants, being 50- to 100-fold more potent than carvedilol and 1000- to 10,000-fold more potent than vitamin E[113], and may contribute significantly to the overall antioxidant activity of the drug. In addition to its potent anti-ischemic effect, carvedilol may attenuate oxygen free radical driven transcriptional events leading to apoptosis and cardiac remodeling[114]. However, it is unclear if these beneficial effects are unique to carvedilol or apply to other beta-blockers. Propranolol has also been demonstrated to have antioxidant properties[94]. Moreover, in a recent randomized clinical trial, Kukin et al. have shown that metoprolol and carvedilol exert a similar beneficial effect on an index of oxidative stress. In fact changes in TBARS level were similar in both group after six months of therapy[115].

As stated previously, both metoprolol and bisoprolol, which are selective beta-1 receptor blockers without direct antioxidant activity, have been shown to significantly decrease total and cardiovascular mortality in patients with CHF[5,6]. Thus blockade of increased systemic and cardiac adrenergic activity in these patients provides clinical benefits, which are independent of a direct antioxidant effect. One could however postulate that these drugs decrease cardiac injury at least in part by preventing the generation of oxidized metabolites of catecholamines such as adenochromes and adrenolutins. Di Lenarda et al. have shown that carvedilol improves LV ejection fraction and cardiac remodeling and decreases ventricular arrhythmias in patients with idiopathic dilated CMP who fail to improve on chronic metoprolol therapy[116]. The recently published COMET trial in patients with symptomatic CHF has shown a mortality benefit of carvedilol over metoprolol[117] in CHF patients. Although the dose of metoprolol used might have been sub-optimal, this additional benefit of carvedilol may be dependent on its antioxidant properties.

Calcium channel blockade in CHF

Despite the efficacy of calcium channel blockers in reducing systemic vascular resistance, they are not recommended routinely for the treatment of CHF. Some agents have deleterious effects on symptoms and survival of these patients[118,119], presumably due to depression of cardiac contractility, bradycardia and activation of the neurohormonal systems. However, data from the first Prospective Randomized Amlodipine Survival Evaluation (PRAISE)-1 trial[120] were provocative by demonstrating that amlodipine, a newer long-acting 1,4- dihydropyridine, did not have any deleterious cardiovascular effects in patients with CHF, and increased survival in the subset of patients with non-ischemic dilated CMPs. Although the exact mechanisms responsible for these possible benefits are still poorly understood, the significant antioxidant properties of amlodipine and its ability to promote NO production in the coronary circulation have been proposed[121]. Unfortunately, PRAISE II, specifically designed to evaluate the effect of amlodipine on all-cause mortality in patients with severe heart failure due to a nonischemic CMP, failed to demonstrate a mortality benefit over placebo.

Several studies have reported that calcium channel blockers exhibit antioxidant properties in various cell membranes and may thereby possess cytoprotective effects[121-123]. Oxygen free radical damage to membranes and lipoproteins is believed to constitute an early step in the development of atherosclerosis and inhibition of lipid peroxidation by calcium channel blockers, together with protection against irreversible cell injury and LV dysfunction following myocardial ischemic insult, may be one of the protective mechanisms of calcium-channel blockers[124,125]. In addition, amlodipine has been shown to release NO from coronary microvessels of animals[126] and human with end-stage heart failure in a dose-dependent manner[127]. Since NO plays a major role in the regulation of many biologic functions including vasodilation and mitochondrial respiration[128], this finding can be important and at least partly explain the difference between amlodipine and other calcium channel blockers in the treatment of heart failure.

Allopurinol

Allopurinol is a potent inhibitor of xanthine oxidase and has been shown to improve the endothelial function of patients with CHF. There appears to be two mechanism responsible for this beneficial effect. First, allopurinol presumably blocks the production of free radicals mediated by this enzyme and second by its direct hydroxyl radical-scavenging action[129-131]. Moreover, Cappola *et al.* have demonstrated that short-term administration of allopurinol improves cardiac efficiency in patients with idiopathic dilated CMP by decreasing myocardial oxygen consumption[132]. Thus allopurinol seems to favorably alter the mechanoenergetic uncoupling present in patients with CHF, possibly via its antioxidant properties. Whether these favorable effects can be translated into clinical benefits warrants further investigation with a large scale randomized trial.

Lipid lowering agents

In addition to the beneficial effects of statins on coronary events, recent evidence suggests other potential beneficial effects of these agents on progression of CHF, mainly through anti-inflammatory and antioxidant actions. Data on established CHF are scarce. Experimentally, administration of statins markedly attenuates ischemia-reperfusion injury in the brain and heart[133,134], a process characterized by a polymorphonuclear leukocyte (PMN)-mediated inflammatory response[135,136]. On reperfusion, activated PMNs can stimulate tissue injury by producing a variety of cytotoxic substances, including oxygen-derived free radicals, inflammatory cytokines and proteases[137]. Many of these substances also mediate vascular endothelial dysfunction as well as myocardial cell injury[138]. Statin therapy leads to a significant reduction in PMN infiltration and adherence (P-selectin levels), an effect apparently mediated by enhanced endothelial release of NO, upregulation of endothelial NO synthesis[139] as well as by inhibition of hypoxia-mediated inhibition of NOS activity[140]. Moreover, statins have been shown to reduce monocyte CD11b expression, which participates in promoting leucocyte and monocyte adhesion to the endothelium[141], and inhibits neutrophil and monocyte chemotaxis in human blood cells[142]. In CHF patients, treatment with statins improves endothelial function[143], and interferes with the systemic inflammatory response[144]. Node *et al.* performed a small randomized clinical trial of 63 non-ischemic CHF patients using short-term (14 weeks) low-dose simvastatin (5-10 mg/d) or placebo[145]. Despite only a modest reduction in serum cholesterol, statin-treated patients had a lower NYHA functional class, associated with improved LV ejection fraction and decreased plasma concentrations of tumor necrosis factor-alpha, interleukin-6 and brain natriuretic peptide, but not of aldosterone or norepinephrine. This was associated with improved flow-mediated vasodilatation, a marker of endothelial function. These findings suggest that statins may have therapeutic benefits in patients with heart failure that result from both their lipid lowering effects and from effect that occurs irrespective of serum cholesterol levels. Thus, statins are potent and effective cardioprotective agents that seem to have important biological effects independent of their cholesterol-lowering effects, and may act at least partly through reduction of oxidative stress.

Probucol is a weak lipid-lowering agent, which possesses antioxidant properties. Clinically, it has been shown to decreases restenosis after angioplasty[146]. In CHF, using different experimental models, probucol has been shown to have a beneficial effect on mortality, LV remodeling, pulmonary congestion and neurohormonal activation, and to improve hemodynamics and renal function. The authors conclude that theses beneficial effects may be related mainly to the antioxidant properties of the drug[147], and secondly to its anti-inflammatory effect[147,148,148,149].

Future directions

Experimental data suggest that oxidative stress may play a significant role in heart failure progression. Many of the agents commonly used to treat CHF patients may exert their beneficial effects in part by reducing oxidative stress in patients with CHF. Likewise, the clinical benefits observed with carvedilol over metoprolol in these patients may be related at least in part to its antioxidant properties[117]. Finally, in view of the importance of endothelial dysfunction, inflammation and apoptosis in heart failure, new agents with primary antioxidant properties may become an important component of the treatment of patients with CHF. Accordingly and despite encouraging animal studies and theoretical principles (ex. statins), all anti-oxidants were not created equal and clinical studies showing a benefit are required, preferably using a powerful antioxidant.

Conclusions

A review of the recent literature provides substantial evidence that oxidative stress contributes to myocardial dysfunction, ventricular remodeling, cardiomyocyte apoptosis, and endothelial dysfunction in CHF. These pathophysiological alterations are believed to have a major impact on the pathogenesis and progression of CHF, and possibly exert a detrimental influence on the prognostic of these patients. Several experimental studies have shown that a decrease in oxidative stress may favorably impact on pathophysiological pathways involved in the progression of CHF. New approaches focused on the inhibition of the sources of oxidative stress (xanthine oxidase, catecholamines, angiotensin II, TNFα) are currently being evaluated. Several cardiovascular drugs acting on components of neurohormonal activation, or having metabolic and anti-inflammatory action, seem to possess intrinsic antioxidant properties. These drugs may substantially expand and simplify antioxidant interventions and provide new directions for future research. Despite encouraging preliminary results, well-designed clinical trials are needed to further clarify the exact role of oxidative stress in CHF. Targeting oxidative stress is a promising and exciting new avenue in the treatment of heart failure. Whether this will translate in clinical benefit for the patients with CHF remains to be determined.

References

1. Effect of enalapril on survival in patients with reduced left ventricular ejection fractions and congestive heart failure. The SOLVD Investigators. N Engl J Med 1991;325:293-302.

2. Effect of enalapril on mortality and the development of heart failure in asymptomatic patients with reduced left ventricular ejection fractions. The SOLVD Investigators. N Engl J Med 1992;327:685-91.

3. Packer M, Bristow MR, Cohn JN, et al. The effect of carvedilol on morbidity and mortality in patients with chronic heart failure. U.S. Carvedilol Heart Failure Study Group. N Engl J Med 1996;334:1349-55.

4. Packer M, Coats AJ, Fowler MB, et al. Effect of carvedilol on survival in severe chronic heart failure. N Engl J Med 2001;344:1651-8.

5. Effect of metoprolol CR/XL in chronic heart failure: Metoprolol CR/XL Randomised Intervention Trial in Congestive Heart Failure (MERIT-HF). Lancet 1999;353:2001-7.

6. The Cardiac Insufficiency Bisoprolol Study II (CIBIS-II): a randomised trial. Lancet 1999;353:9-13.

7. Pfeffer MA, Swedberg K, Granger CB, et al. Effects of candesartan on mortality and morbidity in patients with chronic heart failure: the CHARM-Overall programme. Lancet 2003;362:759-66.

8. Pitt B, Zannad F, Remme WJ, et al. The effect of spironolactone on morbidity and mortality in patients with severe heart failure. Randomized Aldactone Evaluation Study Investigators. N Engl J Med 1999;341:709-17.

9. Pitt B, Williams G, Remme W, et al. The EPHESUS trial: eplerenone in patients with heart failure due to systolic dysfunction complicating acute myocardial infarction. Eplerenone Post-AMI Heart Failure Efficacy and Survival Study. Cardiovasc Drugs Ther 2001;15:79-87.

10. Moss AJ, Zareba W, Hall WJ, et al. Prophylactic implantation of a defibrillator in patients with myocardial infarction and reduced ejection fraction. N Engl J Med 2002;346:877-83.

11. Bristow MR, Saxon LA, Boehmer J, et al. Cardiac-resynchronization therapy with or without an implantable defibrillator in advanced chronic heart failure. N Engl J Med 2004;350:2140-50.

12. Rouleau JL, Kortas C, Bichet D, de Champlain J. Neurohumoral and hemodynamic changes in congestive heart failure: lack of correlation and evidence of compensatory mechanisms. Am Heart J 1988;116:746-57.

13. Stewart DJ, Cernacek P, Costello KB, Rouleau JL. Elevated endothelin-1 in heart failure and loss of normal response to postural change. Circulation 1992;85:510-7.

14. Cohn JN, Levine TB, Olivari MT, et al. Plasma norepinephrine as a guide to prognosis in patients with chronic congestive heart failure. N Engl J Med 1984;311:819-23.

15. Dzau VJ, Colucci WS, Hollenberg NK, Williams GH. Relation of the renin-angiotensin-aldosterone system to clinical state in congestive heart failure. Circulation 1981;63:645-51.

16. Kaye DM, Lefkovits J, Jennings GL, Bergin P, Broughton A, Esler MD. Adverse consequences of high sympathetic nervous activity in the failing human heart. J Am Coll Cardiol 1995;26:1257-63.

17. Lefkowitz RJ, Caron MG, Stiles GL. Mechanisms of membrane-receptor regulation. Biochemical, physiological, and clinical insights derived from studies of the adrenergic receptors. N Engl J Med 1984;310:1570-9.

18. Hall C, Rouleau JL, Moye L, et al. N-terminal proatrial natriuretic factor. An independent predictor of long-term prognosis after myocardial infarction. Circulation 1994;89:1934-42.

19. Nishikimi T, Saito Y, Kitamura K, et al. Increased plasma levels of adrenomedullin in patients with heart failure. J Am Coll Cardiol 1995;26:1424-31.

20. Packer M. Interaction of prostaglandins and angiotensin II in the modulation of renal function in congestive heart failure. Circulation 1988;77:164-173.

21. Kubo SH, Rector TS, Bank AJ, Williams RE, Heifetz SM. Endothelium-dependent vasodilation is attenuated in patients with heart failure. Circulation 1991;84:1589-96.

22. Drexler H, Hayoz D, Munzel T, et al. Endothelial function in chronic congestive heart failure. Am J Cardiol 1992;69:1596-601.

23. Smith CJ, Sun D, Hoegler C, et al. Reduced gene expression of vascular endothelial NO synthase and cyclooxygenase-1 in heart failure. Circ Res 1996;78:58-64.

24. Levine B, Kalman J, Mayer L, Fillit HM, Packer M. Elevated circulating levels of tumor necrosis factor in severe chronic heart failure. N Engl J Med 1990;323:236-41.

25. Shan K, Kurrelmeyer K, Seta Y, et al. The role of cytokines in disease progression in heart failure. Curr Opin Cardiol 1997;12:218-23.

26. Yndestad A, Damas JK, Geir EH, et al. Increased gene expression of tumor necrosis factor superfamily ligands in peripheral blood mononuclear cells during chronic heart failure. Cardiovasc Res 2002;54:175-82.

27. Ferrari R, Bachetti T, Confortini R, et al. Tumor necrosis factor soluble receptors in patients with various degrees of congestive heart failure. Circulation 1995;92:1479-86.

28. Parissis JT, Venetsanou KF, Mentzikof DG, Ziras NG, Kefalas CG, Karas SM. Tumor necrosis factor-alpha serum activity during treatment of acute decompensation of cachectic and non-cachectic patients with advanced congestive heart failure. Scand Cardiovasc J 1999;33:344-50.

29. Anker SD, Egerer KR, Volk HD, Kox WJ, Poole-Wilson PA, Coats AJ. Elevated soluble CD14 receptors and altered cytokines in chronic heart failure. Am J Cardiol 1997;79:1426-30.

30. Samsonov M, Lopatin J, Tilz GP, et al. The activated immune system and the renin-angiotensin-aldosterone system in congestive heart failure. J Intern Med 1998;243:93-8.

31. Werdan K. The activated immune system in congestive heart failure--from dropsy to the cytokine paradigm. J Intern Med 1998;243:87-92.

32. Korantzopoulos P, Papaioannides D, Galaris D, Kokkoris S. On the role of oxidative stress in accelerated atherosclerosis observed in rheumatic diseases. Joint Bone Spine 2003;70:311-2.

33. Dhalla NS, Temsah RM, Netticadan T. Role of oxidative stress in cardiovascular diseases. J Hypertens 2000;18:655-73.

34. Ide T, Tsutsui H, Kinugawa S, et al. Mitochondrial electron transport complex I is a potential source of oxygen free radicals in the failing myocardium. Circ Res 1999;85:357-63.

35. Sorescu D, Griendling KK. Reactive oxygen species, mitochondria, and NAD(P)H oxidases in the development and progression of heart failure. Congest Heart Fail 2002;8:132-40.

36. Tan LB, Jalil JE, Pick R, Janicki JS, Weber KT. Cardiac myocyte necrosis induced by angiotensin II. Circ Res 1991;69:1185-95.

37. Lefkowitz RJ, Caron MG, Stiles GL. Mechanisms of membrane-receptor regulation. Biochemical, physiological, and clinical insights derived from studies of the adrenergic receptors. N Engl J Med 1984;310:1570-9.

38. Sharov VG, Todor A, Suzuki G, Morita H, Tanhehco EJ, Sabbah HN. Hypoxia, angiotensin-II, and norepinephrine mediated apoptosis is stimulus specific in canine failed cardiomyocytes: a role for p38 MAPK, Fas-L and cyclin D1. Eur J Heart Fail 2003;5:121-9.

39. Dhalla AK, Hill MF, Singal PK. Role of oxidative stress in transition of hypertrophy to heart failure. J Am Coll Cardiol 1996;28:506-14.

40. Belch JJ, Bridges AB, Scott N, Chopra M. Oxygen free radicals and congestive heart failure. Br Heart J 1991;65:245-8.

41. Hare JM. Oxidative stress and apoptosis in heart failure progression. Circ Res 2001;89:198-200.

42. Diaz-Velez CR, Garcia-Castineiras S, Mendoza-Ramos E, Hernandez-Lopez E. Increased malondialdehyde in peripheral blood of patients with congestive heart failure. Am Heart J 1996;131:146-52.

43. Baumer AT, Flesch M, Wang X, Shen Q, Feuerstein GZ, Bohm M. Antioxidative enzymes in human hearts with idiopathic dilated cardiomyopathy. J Mol Cell Cardiol 2000;32:121-30.

44. Dieterich S, Bieligk U, Beulich K, Hasenfuss G, Prestle J. Gene expression of antioxidative enzymes in the human heart: increased expression of catalase in the end-stage failing heart. Circulation 2000;101:33-9.

45. De Lorgeril M, Salen P, Accominotti M, et al. Dietary and blood antioxidants in patients with chronic heart failure. Insights into the potential importance of selenium in heart failure. Eur J Heart Fail 2001;3:661-9.

46. Witte KK, Clark AL, Cleland JG. Chronic heart failure and micronutrients. J Am Coll Cardiol 2001;37:1765-74.

47. Mak S, Newton GE. The oxidative stress hypothesis of congestive heart failure: radical thoughts. Chest 2001;120:2035-46.

48. Ferrari R, Guardigli G, Mele D, Percoco GF, Ceconi C, Curello S. Oxidative stress during myocardial ischaemia and heart failure. Curr Pharm Des 2004;10:1699-711.

49. Sawyer DB, Colucci WS. Mitochondrial oxidative stress in heart failure: "oxygen wastage" revisited. Circ Res 2000;86:119-20.

50. Mallat Z, Philip I, Lebret M, Chatel D, Maclouf J, Tedgui A. Elevated levels of 8-iso-prostaglandin F2alpha in pericardial fluid of patients with heart failure: a potential role for in vivo oxidant stress in ventricular dilatation and progression to heart failure. Circulation 1998;97:1536-9.

51. Nishiyama Y, Ikeda H, Haramaki N, Yoshida N, Imaizumi T. Oxidative stress is related to exercise intolerance in patients with heart failure. Am Heart J 1998;135:115-20.

52. Keith M, Geranmayegan A, Sole MJ, et al. Increased oxidative stress in patients with congestive heart failure. J Am Coll Cardiol 1998;31:1352-6.

53. Mak S, Lehotay DC, Yazdanpanah M, Azevedo ER, Liu PP, Newton GE. Unsaturated aldehydes including 4-OH-nonenal are elevated in patients with congestive heart failure. J Card Fail 2000;6:108-14.

54. Polidori MC, Savino K, Alunni G, et al. Plasma lipophilic antioxidants and malondialdehyde in congestive heart failure patients: relationship to disease severity. Free Radic Biol Med 2002;32:148-52.

55. Roulcau JL, Pitt B, Dhalla NS, ct al. Prognostic importance of the oxidized product of catecholamines, adrenolutin, in patients with severe heart failure. Am Heart J 2003;145:926-32.

56. Singal PK, Beamish RE, Dhalla NS. Potential oxidative pathways of catecholamines in the formation of lipid peroxides and genesis of heart disease. Adv Exp Med Biol 1983;161:391-401

57. Prasad K, Gupta JB, Kalra J, Bharadwaj B. Oxygen free radicals in volume overload heart failure. Mol Cell Biochem 1992;111:55-9.

58. Adamopoulos S, Parissis JT, Kremastinos DT. Endothelial dysfunction in chronic heart failure: clinical and therapeutic implications. Eur J Intern Med 2002;13:233-9.

59. Belardinelli R. Endothelial dysfunction in chronic heart failure: clinical implications and therapeutic options. Int J Cardiol 2001;81:1-8.

60. Habib F, Dutka D, Crossman D, Oakley CM, Cleland JG. Enhanced basal nitric oxide production in heart failure: another failed counter-regulatory vasodilator mechanism? Lancet 1994;344:371-3.

61. Bauersachs J, Bouloumie A, Fraccarollo D, Hu K, Busse R, Ertl G. Endothelial dysfunction in chronic myocardial infarction despite increased vascular endothelial nitric oxide synthase and soluble guanylate cyclase expression: role of enhanced vascular superoxide production. Circulation 1999;100:292-8.

62. Munzel T, Harrison DG. Increased superoxide in heart failure: a biochemical baroreflex gone awry. Circulation 1999;100:216-8.

63. Landmesser U, Spiekermann S, Dikalov S, et al. Vascular oxidative stress and endothelial dysfunction in patients with chronic heart failure: role of xanthine-oxidase and extracellular superoxide dismutase. Circulation 2002;106:3073-8.

64. Olivetti G, Quaini F, Sala R, et al. Acute myocardial infarction in humans is associated with activation of programmed myocyte cell death in the surviving portion of the heart. J Mol Cell Cardiol 1996;28:2005-16.

65. Hill MF, Singal PK. Right and left myocardial antioxidant responses during heart failure subsequent to myocardial infarction. Circulation 1997;96:2414-20.

66. Olivetti G, Abbi R, Quaini F, et al. Apoptosis in the failing human heart. N Engl J Med 1997;336:1131-41.

67. Buttke TM, Sandstrom PA. Oxidative stress as a mediator of apoptosis. Immunol Today 1994;15:7-10.

68. Yonish-Rouach E, Resnitzky D, Lotem J, Sachs L, Kimchi A, Oren M. Wild-type p53 induces apoptosis of myeloid leukaemic cells that is inhibited by interleukin-6. Nature 1991;352:345-7.

69. Williams GT, Smith CA, Spooncer E, Dexter TM, Taylor DR. Haemopoietic colony stimulating factors promote cell survival by suppressing apoptosis. Nature 1990;343:76-9.

70. Evan GI, Wyllie AH, Gilbert CS, et al. Induction of apoptosis in fibroblasts by c-myc protein. Cell 1992;69:119-28.

71. Singal PK, Khaper N, Palace V, Kumar D. The role of oxidative stress in the genesis of heart disease. Cardiovasc Res 1998;40:426-32.

72. Cesselli D, Jakoniuk I, Barlucchi L, et al. Oxidative stress-mediated cardiac cell death is a major determinant of ventricular dysfunction and failure in dog dilated cardiomyopathy. Circ Res 2001;89:279-86.

73. Ducharme A, Frantz S, Aikawa M, et al. Targeted deletion of matrix metalloproteinase-9 attenuates left ventricular enlargement and collagen accumulation after experimental myocardial infarction. J Clin Invest 2000;106:55-62.

74. Hunt MJ, Aru GM, Hayden MR, Moore CK, Hoit BD, Tyagi SC. Induction of oxidative stress and disintegrin metalloproteinase in human heart end-stage failure. Am J Physiol Lung Cell Mol Physiol 2002;283:L239-45.

75. Katz SD, Yuen J, Bijou R, LeJemtel TH. Training improves endothelium-dependent vasodilation in resistance vessels of patients with heart failure. J Appl Physiol 1997;82:1488-92.

76. Hambrecht R, Fiehn E, Weigl C, et al. Regular physical exercise corrects endothelial dysfunction and improves exercise capacity in patients with chronic heart failure. Circulation 1998;98:2709-15.

77. Inoue N, Ramasamy S, Fukai T, Nerem RM, Harrison DG. Shear stress modulates expression of Cu/Zn superoxide dismutase in human aortic endothelial cells. Circ Res 1996;79:32-7.

78. Qin F, Rounds NK, Mao W, Kawai K, Liang CS. Antioxidant vitamins prevent cardiomyocyte apoptosis produced by norepinephrine infusion in ferrets. Cardiovasc Res 2001;51:736-48.

79. Nakamura K, Fushimi K, Kouchi H, et al. Inhibitory effects of antioxidants on neonatal rat cardiac myocyte hypertrophy induced by tumor necrosis factor-alpha and angiotensin II. Circulation 1998;98:794-9.

80. Shite J, Qin F, Mao W, Kawai H, Stevens SY, Liang C. Antioxidant vitamins attenuate oxidative stress and cardiac dysfunction in tachycardia-induced cardiomyopathy. J Am Coll Cardiol 2001;38:1734-40.

81. Ghatak A, Brar MJ, Agarwal A, et al. Oxy free radical system in heart failure and therapeutic role of oral vitamin E. Int J Cardiol 1996;57:119-27.

82. Keith ME, Jeejeebhoy KN, Langer A, et al. A controlled clinical trial of vitamin E supplementation in patients with congestive heart failure. Am J Clin Nutr 2001;73:219-24.

83. Yusuf S, Sleight P, Pogue J, Bosch J, Davies R, Dagenais G. Effects of an angiotensin-converting-enzyme inhibitor, ramipril, on cardiovascular events in high-risk patients. The Heart Outcomes Prevention Evaluation Study Investigators. N Engl J Med 2000;342:145-53.

84. Griendling KK, Harrison DG. Out, damned dot: studies of the NADPH oxidase in atherosclerosis. J Clin Invest 2001;108:1423-4.

85. Ellis GR, Anderson RA, Lang D, et al. Neutrophil superoxide anion--generating capacity, endothelial function and oxidative stress in chronic heart failure: effects of short- and long-term vitamin C therapy. J Am Coll Cardiol 2000;36:1474-82.

86. Hornig B, Arakawa N, Kohler C, Drexler H. Vitamin C improves endothelial function of conduit arteries in patients with chronic heart failure. Circulation 1998;97:363-8.

87. Rossig L, Hoffmann J, Hugel B, et al. Vitamin C inhibits endothelial cell apoptosis in congestive heart failure. Circulation 2001;104:2182-7.

88. Ito K, Akita H, Kanazawa K, et al. Comparison of effects of ascorbic acid on endothelium-dependent vasodilation in patients with chronic congestive heart failure secondary to idiopathic dilated cardiomyopathy versus patients with effort angina pectoris secondary to coronary artery disease. Am J Cardiol 1998;82:762-7.

89. Richartz BM, Werner GS, Ferrari M, Figulla HR. Reversibility of coronary endothelial vasomotor dysfunction in idiopathic dilated cardiomyopathy: acute effects of vitamin C. Am J Cardiol 2001;88:1001-5.

90. Mak S, Newton GE. Vitamin C augments the inotropic response to dobutamine in humans with normal left ventricular function. Circulation 2001;103:826-30.

91. Givertz MM, Sawyer DB, Colucci WS. Antioxidants and myocardial contractility: illuminating the "Dark Side" of beta-adrenergic receptor activation? Circulation 2001;103:782-3.

92. Watson PS, Scalia GM, Galbraith A, Burstow DJ, Bett N, Aroney CN. Lack of effect of coenzyme Q on left ventricular function in patients with congestive heart failure. J Am Coll Cardiol 1999;33:1549-52.

93. Khatta M, Alexander BS, Krichten CM, et al. The effect of coenzyme Q10 in patients with congestive heart failure. Ann Intern Med 2000;132:636-40.

94. Khaper N, Rigatto C, Seneviratne C, Li T, Singal PK. Chronic treatment with propranolol induces antioxidant changes and protects against ischemia-reperfusion injury. J Mol Cell Cardiol 1997;29:3335-44.

95. Hayek T, Attias J, Smith J, Breslow JL, Keidar S. Antiatherosclerotic and antioxidative effects of captopril in apolipoprotein E-deficient mice. J Cardiovasc Pharmacol 1998;31:540-4.

96. Khaper N, Singal PK. Modulation of oxidative stress by a selective inhibition of angiotensin II type 1 receptors in MI rats. J Am Coll Cardiol 2001;37:1461-6.

97. Sevanian A, Shen L, Ursini F. Inhibition of LDL oxidation and oxidized LDL-induced cytotoxicity by dihydropyridine calcium antagonists. Pharm Res 2000;17:999-1006.

98. Delbosc S, Morena M, Djouad F, Ledoucen C, Descomps B, Cristol JP. Statins, 3-hydroxy-3-methylglutaryl coenzyme A reductase inhibitors, are able to reduce superoxide anion production by NADPH oxidase in THP-1-derived monocytes. J Cardiovasc Pharmacol 2002;40:611-7.

99. Delbosc S, Cristol JP, Descomps B, Mimran A, Jover B. Simvastatin prevents angiotensin II-induced cardiac alteration and oxidative stress. Hypertension 2002;40:142-7.

100. Tselepis A, Doulias P, Lourida E, Glantzounis G, Tsimoyiannis E, Galaris D. Trimetazidine protects low-density lipoproteins from oxidation and cultured cells exposed to $H(2)O(2)$ from DNA damage. Free Radic Biol Med 2001;30:1357-64.

101. Lopez-Farre A, Riesco A, Digiuni E, et al. Aspirin-stimulated nitric oxide production by neutrophils after acute myocardial ischemia in rabbits. Circulation 1996;94:83-7.

102. Ide T, Tsutsui H, Kinugawa S, Utsumi H, Takeshita A. Amiodarone protects cardiac myocytes against oxidative injury by its free radical scavenging action. Circulation 1999;100:690-2.

103. Zafari AM, Harrison DG. Free radicals in heart failure: therapeutic targets for old and new drugs. Congest Heart Fail 2002;8:129-30.

104. Rajagopalan S, Meng XP, Ramasamy S, Harrison DG, Galis ZS. Reactive oxygen species produced by macrophage-derived foam cells regulate the activity of vascular matrix metalloproteinases in vitro. Implications for atherosclerotic plaque stability. J Clin Invest 1996;98:2572-9.

105. Munzel T, Kurz S, Rajagopalan S, et al. Hydralazine prevents nitroglycerin tolerance by inhibiting activation of a membrane-bound NADH oxidase. A new action for an old drug. J Clin Invest 1996;98:1465-70.

106. Waagstein F, Hjalmarson A, Varnauskas E, Wallentin I. Effect of chronic beta-adrenergic receptor blockade in congestive cardiomyopathy. Br Heart J 1975;37:1022-36.

107. Packer M, Bristow MR, Cohn JN, et al. The effect of carvedilol on morbidity and mortality in patients with chronic heart failure. U.S. Carvedilol Heart Failure Study Group. N Engl J Med 1996;334:1349-55.

108. Bril A, Slivjak M, DiMartino MJ, et al. Cardioprotective effects of carvedilol, a novel beta adrenoceptor antagonist with vasodilating properties, in anaesthetised minipigs: comparison with propranolol. Cardiovasc Res 1992;26:518-25.

109. Yue TL, Wang X, Gu JL, Ruffolo RR, Jr., Feuerstein GZ. Carvedilol, a new vasodilating beta-adrenoceptor blocker, inhibits oxidation of low-density lipoproteins by vascular smooth muscle cells and prevents leukocyte adhesion to smooth muscle cells. J Pharmacol Exp Ther 1995;273:1442-9.

110. Rossig L, Haendeler J, Mallat Z, et al. Congestive heart failure induces endothelial cell apoptosis: protective role of carvedilol. J Am Coll Cardiol 2000;36:2081-9.

111. Yue TL, Cheng HY, Lysko PG, et al. Carvedilol, a new vasodilator and beta adrenoceptor antagonist, is an antioxidant and free radical scavenger. J Pharmacol Exp Ther 1992;263:92-8.

112. Yue TL, McKenna PJ, Gu JL, Cheng HY, Ruffolo RR, Jr., Feuerstein GZ. Carvedilol, a new antihypertensive agent, prevents lipid peroxidation and oxidative injury to endothelial cells. Hypertension 1993;22:922-8.

113. Feuerstein R, Yue TL. A potent antioxidant, SB209995, inhibits oxygen-radical-mediated lipid peroxidation and cytotoxicity. Pharmacology 1994;48:385-91.

114. Gottlieb RA, Burleson KO, Kloner RA, Babior BM, Engler RL. Reperfusion injury induces apoptosis in rabbit cardiomyocytes. J Clin Invest 1994;94:1621-8.

115. Kukin ML, Kalman J, Charney RH, et al. Prospective, randomized comparison of effect of long-term treatment with metoprolol or carvedilol on symptoms, exercise, ejection fraction, and oxidative stress in heart failure. Circulation 1999;99:2645-51.

116. Di Lenarda A, Sabbadini G, Salvatore L, et al. Long-term effects of carvedilol in idiopathic dilated cardiomyopathy with persistent left ventricular dysfunction despite chronic metoprolol. The Heart-Muscle Disease Study Group. J Am Coll Cardiol 1999;33:1926-34.

117. Poole-Wilson PA, Swedberg K, Cleland JG, et al. Comparison of carvedilol and metoprolol on clinical outcomes in patients with chronic heart failure in the Carvedilol Or Metoprolol European Trial (COMET): randomised controlled trial. Lancet 2003;362:7-13.

118. Elkayam U, Amin J, Mehra A, Vasquez J, Weber L, Rahimtoola SH. A prospective, randomized, double-blind, crossover study to compare the efficacy and safety of chronic nifedipine therapy with that of isosorbide dinitrate and their combination in the treatment of chronic congestive heart failure. Circulation 1990;82:1954-61.

119. Goldstein RE, Boccuzzi SJ, Cruess D, Nattel S. Diltiazem increases late-onset congestive heart failure in postinfarction patients with early reduction in ejection fraction. The Adverse Experience Committee; and the Multicenter Diltiazem Postinfarction Research Group. Circulation 1991;83:52-60.

120. Packer M, O'Connor CM, Ghali JK, et al. Effect of amlodipine on morbidity and mortality in severe chronic heart failure. Prospective Randomized Amlodipine Survival Evaluation Study Group. N Engl J Med 1996;335:1107-14.

121. Mason RP, Mak IT, Trumbore MW, Mason PE. Antioxidant properties of calcium antagonists related to membrane biophysical interactions. Am J Cardiol 1999;84:16L-22L.

122. Janero DR, Burghardt B, Lopez R. Protection of cardiac membrane phospholipid against oxidative injury by calcium antagonists. Biochem Pharmacol 1988;37:4197-203.

123. Mak IT, Weglicki WB. Comparative antioxidant activities of propranolol, nifedipine, verapamil, and diltiazem against sarcolemmal membrane lipid peroxidation. Circ Res 1990;66:1449-52.

124. Ross R. The pathogenesis of atherosclerosis: a perspective for the 1990s. Nature 1993;362:801-9.

125. Steinberg D. Antioxidants and atherosclerosis. A current assessment. Circulation 1991;84:1420-5.

126. Zhang X, Hintze TH. Amlodipine Releases Nitric Oxide From Canine Coronary Microvessels: An Unexpected Mechanism of Action of a Calcium Channel Blocking Agent. Circulation 1998;97:576-80.

127. Zhang X, Kichuk MR, Mital S, et al. Amlodipine promotes kinin-mediated nitric oxide production in coronary microvessels of failing human hearts. Am J Cardiol 1999;84:27L-33L.

128. Moncada S, Palmer RM, Higgs EA. Nitric oxide: physiology, pathophysiology, and pharmacology. Pharmacol Rev 1991;43:109-42.

129. Doehner W, Schoene N, Rauchhaus M, et al. Effects of xanthine oxidase inhibition with allopurinol on endothelial function and peripheral blood flow in hyperuricemic patients with chronic heart failure: results from 2 placebo-controlled studies. Circulation 2002;105:2619-24.

130. Farquharson CA, Butler R, Hill A, Belch JJ, Struthers AD. Allopurinol improves endothelial dysfunction in chronic heart failure. Circulation 2002;106:221-6.

131. Landmesser U, Drexler H. Allopurinol and endothelial function in heart failure: future or fantasy? Circulation 2002;106:173-5.

132. Cappola TP, Kass DA, Nelson GS, et al. Allopurinol improves myocardial efficiency in patients with idiopathic dilated cardiomyopathy. Circulation 2001;104:2407-11.

133. Lefer AM, Campbell B, Shin YK, Scalia R, Hayward R, Lefer DJ. Simvastatin preserves the ischemic-reperfused myocardium in normocholesterolemic rat hearts. Circulation 1999;100:178-84.

134. Endres M, Laufs U, Huang Z, et al. Stroke protection by 3-hydroxy-3-methylglutaryl (HMG)-CoA reductase inhibitors mediated by endothelial nitric oxide synthase. Proc Natl Acad Sci U S A 1998;95:8880-5.

135. Tsao PS, Aoki N, Lefer DJ, Johnson G, III, Lefer AM. Time course of endothelial dysfunction and myocardial injury during myocardial ischemia and reperfusion in the cat. Circulation 1990;82:1402-12.

136. Entman ML, Michael L, Rossen RD, et al. Inflammation in the course of early myocardial ischemia. FASEB J 1991;5:2529-37.

137. Weiss SJ. Tissue destruction by neutrophils. N Engl J Med 1989;320:365-76.

138. Buerke M, Weyrich AS, Lefer AM. Isolated cardiac myocytes are sensitized by hypoxia-reoxygenation to neutrophil-released mediators. Am J Physiol 1994;266:H128-36.

139. Laufs U, La F, V, Plutzky J, Liao JK. Upregulation of endothelial nitric oxide synthase by HMG CoA reductase inhibitors. Circulation 1998;97:1129-35.

140. Laufs U, Fata VL, Liao JK. Inhibition of 3-hydroxy-3-methylglutaryl (HMG)-CoA reductase blocks hypoxia-mediated down-regulation of endothelial nitric oxide synthase. J Biol Chem 1997;272:31725-9.

141. Weber C, Erl W, Weber KS, Weber PC. HMG-CoA reductase inhibitors decrease CD11b expression and CD11b-dependent adhesion of monocytes to endothelium and reduce increased adhesiveness of monocytes isolated from patients with hypercholesterolemia. J Am Coll Cardiol 1997;30:1212-7.

142. Dunzendorfer S, Rothbucher D, Schratzberger P, Reinisch N, Kahler CM, Wiedermann CJ. Mevalonate-dependent inhibition of transendothelial migration and chemotaxis of human peripheral blood neutrophils by pravastatin. Circ Res 1997;81:963-9.

143. Koh KK. Effects of statins on vascular wall: vasomotor function, inflammation, and plaque stability. Cardiovasc Res 2000;47:648-57.

144. Albert MA, Danielson E, Rifai N, Ridker PM. Effect of statin therapy on C-reactive protein levels: the pravastatin inflammation/CRP evaluation (PRINCE): a randomized trial and cohort study. JAMA 2001;286:64-70.

145. Node K, Fujita M, Kitakaze M, Hori M, Liao JK. Short-term statin therapy improves cardiac function and symptoms in patients with idiopathic dilated cardiomyopathy. Circulation 2003;108:839-43.

146. Tardif JC, Cote G, Lesperance J, et al. Probucol and multivitamins in the prevention of restenosis after coronary angioplasty. Multivitamins and Probucol Study Group. N Engl J Med 1997;337:365-72.

147. Sia YT, Lapointe N, Parker TG, et al. Beneficial effects of long-term use of the antioxidant probucol in heart failure in the rat. Circulation 2002;105:2549-55.

148. Siveski-Iliskovic N, Hill M, Chow DA, Singal PK. Probucol protects against adriamycin cardiomyopathy without interfering with its antitumor effect. Circulation 1995;91:10-5.

149. Nakamura R, Egashira K, Machida Y, et al. Probucol attenuates left ventricular dysfunction and remodeling in tachycardia-induced heart failure: roles of oxidative stress and inflammation. Circulation 2002;106:362-7.

150. Langsjoen PH, Folkers K. Long-term efficacy and safety of coenzyme Q10 therapy for idiopathic dilated cardiomyopathy. Am J Cardiol 1990;65:521-3.

151. Hofman-Bang C, Rehnquist N, Swedberg K, Wiklond I, Astrom H. Coenzyme Q10 as an adjunctive in the treatment of chronic congestive heart failure. The Q10 Study Group. J Card Failure 1995;1:101-7.

152. Siveski-Iliskovic N, Hill M, Singal PK. Probucol protects against adriamycin cardiomyopathy without interfering with its antitumor effect. Circulation 1995;9:10-5.

153. Tavazzi L, Tognoni G, Frazosi MG, Latini R, Maggioni AP, Marchioli R, Nicolosi GL, Porcu M. Rationale and design of the GISSI heart failure trial: a large trial to assess the effects of n-3 polyunsaturated fatty acids and rosuvastatin in symptomatic congestive heart failure. Eur J Heart Fail 2004;6:635-41.

154. Kjekshus J, Pedersen TR, Olsson AG, Faergeman O, Pyörälä K. The effects of simvastatin or the incidence of heart failure in patients with coronary heart disease. J Card Failure 1997;3:259-51.

Index